INTRODUCTION TO ORGANIC AND NEUROGENIC DISORDERS OF COMMUNICATION

CURRENT SCOPE OF PRACTICE

CAROLE T. FERRAND

RONALD L. BLOOM
Hofstra University

ALLYN AND BACON
Boston • London • Toronto • Sydney • Tokyo • Singapore

Executive Editor: Stephen D. Dragin
Editorial Assistant: Christine Svitila
Marketing Manager: Kathy Hunter
Editorial Production Service: Chestnut Hill Enterprises, Inc.
Manufacturing Buyer: Megan Cochran
Cover Administrator: Suzanne Harbison

Copyright © 1997 by Allyn & Bacon
A Viacom Company
Needham Heights, MA 02194

Internet: www.abacon.com
America Online: keyword: College Online

Library of Congress Cataloging-in-Publication Data
Ferrand, Carole T.
    Introduction to organic and neurogenic disorders of communication
  : current scope of practice / Carole T. Ferrand and Ronald L. Bloom.
        p.   cm.
    Includes bibliographical references and index.
    ISBN 0-205-16867-1 (case)
    1. Communicative disorders.   I. Bloom, Ronald L.   II. Title.
RC423.F47 1997
616.85'5–dc20   96-41887
                                                          CIP

Printed in the United States of America
10   9   8   7   6   5   4   01

CTF—To the memory of my father, Issy Friedman,
whose love of teaching inspired my own

RLB—To my parents, Joseph and Natalie Bloom,
who taught me about the value of caregiving

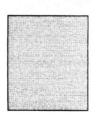

CONTRIBUTORS AND AFFILIATIONS

EDITORS

Carole T. Ferrand, Ph.D.   Dept. of Speech-Language-Hearing Sciences, Hofstra University, New York

Ronald L. Bloom, Ph.D.   Dept. of Speech-Language-Hearing Sciences, Hofstra University, New York

CONTRIBUTORS

Christine Baltaxe, Ph.D.   UCLA Neuropsychiatric Institute, Child Psychiatry Division

Andrew Blitzer, M.D., D.D.S.   Center for Voice and Swallowing Disorders Head and Neck Surgical Group, Dept. of Otolaryngology, St. Luke's/Roosevelt Hospital Center, New York; Columbia University College of Physicians and Surgeons, New York

Mitchell F. Brin, M.D.   Movement Disorders Center, Dept. of Neurology, Mount Sinai School of Medicine and the Mount Sinai Hospital, New York

Carl A. Coelho, Ph.D.   Southern Connecticut State University, New Haven, CT

Susan De Santi, Ph.D.   Milhauser Institute, New York University Medical Center

Robert A. Domingo, Ph.D.   Dept. of Speech and Hearing, Long Island University, C.W. Post Campus

Carol Flexer, Ph.D.   School of Communicative Disorders, University of Akron, Ohio

Yvonne Gillette, Ph.D.   School of Communicative Disorders, University of Akron, Ohio

Karen J. Golding-Kushner, Ph.D.   Private Practice, New Brunswick, New Jersey

Neita K. Israelite, Ph.D.   Faculty of Education, York University, Toronto

Mary Beth Jennings, M.Cl.Sc.   Canadian Hearing Society, Toronto

Jeri A. Logemann, Ph.D.   Dept. of Communication Sciences and Disorders, Northwestern University, Illinois

Louis Rossetti, Ph.D.   Dept. of Communication Sciences and Disorders, University of Wisconsin, Oshkosh, WI

Dianne C. Slavin, Ph.D.   Dept. of Speech and Hearing, Long Island University, C.W. Post Campus

Celia Stewart, Ph.D.   Dept. of Speech Pathology and Audiology, New York University

Denise Wray, Ph.D.   School of Communicative Disorders, University of Akron, Ohio

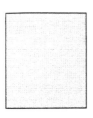

BRIEF
CONTENTS

CONTENTS

PREFACE

As the twenty-first century approaches, one is struck by the numerous changes that have occurred in the field of speech-language pathology within the last two decades. Changes are apparent in the expanding scope of practice, in service delivery models, and in the mainstreaming of individuals with medically-related communication disorders into regular educational and work settings. Several of these changes have grown out of the advances in computer technology that have provided new vehicles for studying and treating communication disorders. Others have emerged from legislation that has mandated the inclusion of persons with disabilities as full participants in society. Thus, modern practice necessitates a firm theoretical grounding, methods to apply these scientific and technological advances, and skill in translating these factors into effective clinical management objectives.

In accordance with the latest revision of scope of practice articulated by the American Speech-Language-Hearing Association (1996), speech-language pathology is viewed as a dynamic and evolving discipline. Among the newly specified procedures now included in the scope of practice are areas like cognitive-linguistic rehabilitation, swallowing disorders, and psychiatric disorders. These areas are addressed in the text, in addition to the more traditional areas of practice such as aphasia and voice disorders. Further, this book emphasizes the interdisciplinary knowledge that a speech-language pathologist brings to an educational or rehabilitation team.

This perspective on speech-language pathology serves as the underlying philosophy of this volume. Accordingly, each chapter demonstrates the integration of theory and practice called for by this approach. This text is comprehensive enough to serve as an introduction to organic and neurogenic disorders for both undergraduate students, and graduate students entering speech-language pathology from another discipline. However, the clinical practitioner will also find enough depth and breadth in this book to serve as an update of theory and practice.

We have had much success in using this approach with our own students and have field-tested most of the material presented in the book. We are therefore confident that this textbook is user friendly for both students and instructors. Students will find the information sophisticated yet accessible, as it realistically introduces them to the integration of science, theory, and practice. Instructors will find that the structure of the book is flexible. While we have organized chapters in a logical manner, instructors may easily modify the order of presentation without sacrificing the continuity of the material. Many of the chapters can stand on their own as a solid introduction to the information, or may be taught in conjunction with other chapters to allow for a more comprehensive picture. Teaching themes may be created by grouping chapters together in different ways.

The teaching aids included in this book will also benefit students. The extensive glossary at the end of the book helps to acquaint students with professional terminology contained in each chapter. Chapter summaries help the student to tie the material together and see the interrelatedness of the disorders.

We thank the undergraduate and graduate students in the department of Speech-Language-Hearing Sciences at Hofstra University, who, over the years, motivated us to compile a textbook that was current and stimulating, and which would introduce them to the modern domain of clinical practice. We appreciate our colleagues at Hofstra University, who helped to create a supportive and congenial environment in which to develop this project. In particular, we thank Professor Susan Drucker in the School of Communication at Hofstra University for her insightful commentary on the legal aspects and federal mandates relating to communication disorders. In addition, the insightful comments of the following reviewers helped us in finalizing the manuscript: Celia Hooper, University of North Carolina, Chapel Hill; Michael Trudeau, Ohio State University; and Al Bowman, Illinois State University.

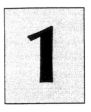

INTRODUCTION: THE SCOPE OF CLINICAL PRACTICE IN ORGANIC AND NEUROGENIC DISORDERS OF COMMUNICATION

CAROLE T. FERRAND AND RONALD L. BLOOM

T he idea for this book arose out of the editors' need, as professors, for a text that introduces organic and neurogenic disorders of communication to students in a way that is current and comprehensive, without sacrificing readability. It was the editors' experience that no existing textbook fully presented the information needed to characterize the growth and changes in the field of communication disorders over the past two decades. While this book is geared primarily toward students in communication disorders, it is also suitable for students in medical and allied health fields who need to acquire a working knowledge of medically based communication problems. This book is designed as the primary text for advanced undergraduate coursework in this area, or introductory graduate coursework. Professionals working with communicatively impaired individuals can also benefit from the in-depth and current information provided in this text.

ORGANIC AND NEUROGENIC DISORDERS

The term *organic disorders of communication* refers to any kind of anomaly in the physical structures responsible for speech production and/or language processing. Organic disorders arise from problems in respiration, phonation, articulation, hearing, and neurological functioning. Neurogenic disorders refer to those impairments stemming from damage to the central or peripheral nervous system. The distinction between organic and neurogenic disorders is not always clear, as they may coexist. They may also, however, appear independently. Organic and neurogenic disorders may be contrasted with functional disorders, in which there are no discernable physical bases for the communication problem. Organic, neurogenic, and functional disorders can be present in an individual in any combination.

Because the causes of organic and neurogenic disorders are often identifiable, treatment is typically associated with a medical model. Within the medical model the causes and symptoms of a disorder are identified and treated until they either approximate normal, or until maximum function is achieved. Consistent with the medical model, clinical management of many organic and neurogenic communication disorders tends to focus on the disease process and ways to fix the resulting

1

communication problems. It should be kept in mind, however, that while the origins of organic and neurogenic disorders of communication are often medical, the results of these disorders are often viewed and treated within a sociocultural framework. Therefore, it is necessary to view these communication disorders not only from a medical perspective, but also to appreciate that there are developmental, social, emotional, educational, and occupational consequences that must be included in the management process.

PREVALENCE OF ORGANIC AND NEUROGENIC DISORDERS

The prevalence of organic and neurogenic disorders of communication in the United States is extremely high. For instance, in 1991, approximately 42 million people in the United States were affected by some kind of communication disorder (ASHA, 1994). Of these, 28 million individuals had a hearing loss, and 14 million had a speech, voice, or language disorder. Neurological conditions account for 26 million cases of communication disorders each year. More than 1.5 million people in the United States have had some degree of acquired language disability resulting from stroke. Dementia affects 10 percent of the population over 65 years of age, and as many as 80 percent of those over 85 years of age. More than 15 million Americans have some degree of dysphagia. Aside from diseases, trauma is a major contributor to neurogenic communication disorders. More than 2 million people each year sustain head trauma, and as many as 100,000 of these endure some permanent communication disability.

These already high numbers of organic and neurogenic disorders are likely to increase for two reasons. The first is that the U.S. population is aging. More elderly people are vulnerable to disease processes that can cause communication disorders, such as stroke, hearing loss, or dementia. However, despite these diseases, more elderly people are living longer lives, and therefore require health and communication services to minimize their effects. Second, medically fragile infants who once died at or shortly after birth are now surviving, and are often at risk for the development of communication problems requiring services within the hospital, home, and educational settings.

The impact of these kinds of disorders on an individual's quality of life should not be underestimated. Communication is so fundamental to participation in society, that loss of communication skills has far-reaching consequences both for the individual and for society. The devastating effects of these problems can often be alleviated through communicative, educational, and medical services. Such services are costly, but the lack of services can prove to be even costlier to society in the long run. These kinds of services help to compensate for the lost productivity of individuals with communication disorders by helping them to become contributing members of society. Economic issues, however, are not the only considerations in the provision of services to affected individuals.

LEGAL ASPECTS OF COMMUNICATION DISORDERS

Equally important as the economic issues are the legal ramifications. Communication, and communication disorders, do not take place in a vacuum. A body of legislative enactments and administrative regulations have grown to address the rights of individuals with disorders, which are of great significance to those working with communicatively impaired persons. Federal legislation, in particular, has been evolving in a number of relevant areas within the past two decades, a time considered "recent" in terms of legal developments.

Perhaps the most sweeping articulation of societal policies with regard to a variety of disabilities is the Americans with Disabilities Act of 1990 (ADA), a civil rights statute signed into law by President George Bush. The act was designed to prohibit discrimination against people with a variety of disabilities by offering these individuals protections similar to those given to other minorities, women, and others covered by the Civil Rights Act of 1964. The stated purpose of ADA is to provide a clear and comprehensive national mandate to bring individuals with disabilities into the societal and economic mainstream of U.S. society. The law creates a central role for the federal government with regard to enforceable standards addressing discrimination against individuals with disabilities. The law specifically addresses physical disabilities affecting mobility, as well as communication (1990).

Several major pieces of federal legislation designed to provide basic educational services for children with a variety of disabilities have been enacted since 1975. The first of these was PL 94-142, signed into law by President Gerald Ford in 1975. This Education for All Handicapped Children Act has been considered a landmark of legislation for U.S. children. It is based on the principle that every child is entitled to a free public education suited to the individual's level of development. PL 94-142 mandates a free and appropriate education for all developmentally delayed and handicapped children from 3 to 21 years of age. This population includes individuals who are speech–language impaired, emotionally disturbed, mentally retarded, physically handicapped, and have multiple handicaps.

Specifically, the law requires that each of these students be placed in the "least restrictive environment" commensurate with their needs, and that they are provided the related services needed to enable them to benefit from education. Previously, speech–language and hearing programs were made available by states only when the state enacted legislation *allowing* speech and hearing services in the school, but PL 94-142 *mandated* these services. In addition, the law provided financial assistance for such services.

In 1986, PL 99-457 (ASHA Congressional Relations Division, Government Affairs Department, 1989), the Education of the Handicapped Amendments was signed into law to increase services for preschoolers, and improve support for the kinds of services offered to handicapped children ages birth to 3 years old. The law also makes provision for financial incentives to states to serve these children, who are identified as handicapped or who are at risk for developmental delay. A section of the law provides incentives for states to offer free and appropriate parent training and family services in addition to public education for eligible children with disabilities.

PL 101-476 further amended PL 94-142. The legislation called IDEA (Individuals with Disabilities Education Act) (ASHA Governmental Affairs Review, 1990) added two new categories of disability that are strongly related to communication: psychiatric disorders such as autism and traumatic brain injury. Also, the wording used to describe those individuals covered by this legislation was changed from "handicapped children" to "children with disabilities." This is consistent with current trends in the field of speech–language pathology that place the person before the label given to the disorder.

These changes in the legal environment have molded the scope of practice in speech–language pathology. The material presented in this book reflects the outcome of 20 years of expanded services. Current service delivery models now include populations who were previously underserved, as well as those who have traditionally received these kinds of services.

TECHNOLOGICAL AND THEORETICAL ADVANCES

Concurrent with these legal mandates, the field of speech–language pathology has greatly expanded its knowledge in the physiological bases of normal and disordered communication. At the same time, the availability of sophisticated instrumentation to analyze and quantify physiological and acoustic aspects of communication has increased dramatically. As a result, the scope of practice in speech–language pathology has been tremendously broadened. For instance, videofluoroscopy has facilitated the assessment and treatment of dysphagia in children and adults. Stroboscopic endoscopy utilized in the assessment of vocal problems has shed light on the normal and disordered function of the vocal folds. Brain imaging techniques such as Positron Emission Tomography

(PET) and Magnetic Resonance Imaging (MRI) have deepened our knowledge of the overlapping and interconnected neural networks involved in processing language in context. Another innovation in the field of speech–language pathology is the introduction of analytic discourse techniques used to describe subtle yet significant breakdown in communication processes.

SCOPE OF CLINICAL PRACTICE

Increasingly, students in the field of speech–language pathology are electing to work in hospitals, rehabilitation centers, acute care facilities, neonatal nurseries, and early intervention programs that focus on the communication needs of individuals with organic and neurogenic disorders. Because of the expanded scope of theory and practice in organic and neurogenic disorders, particularly as encountered in these types of settings, students in the field of speech–language pathology should have early exposure to the issues that affect these clinical groups.

Perhaps the setting most influenced by this increased scope of practice is the school. Public and private schools represent the largest work setting for speech–language pathologists. Because of the current federal mandates described above, more and more children with organic and neurogenic communication disorders are being mainstreamed into school settings where they receive support services including speech–language pathology. Thus, the speech–language pathologist working in the school system will become an integral part of the educational team dealing with children who are medically fragile, at risk for developmental delay, as well as children with autism, children with multiple handicaps, children with hearing loss, and so on. Because of the legal mandate for early intervention, preschool settings are also expanding the kinds of services provided to young children, such as feeding therapy, and intensive language intervention for those at risk for developmental delay.

Within acute care settings, speech–language pathologists may offer assessment and short-term treatment for individuals with head trauma, stroke, and laryngectomy. Often, the speech–language pathologist is called upon to evaluate and treat swallowing problems, which typically accompany acute medical conditions. A critical component of care in this kind of setting is counseling for the patient and family regarding long-term rehabilitation.

When the medical condition is no longer in its acute stage, but the patient is unable to return home, the speech–language pathologist may offer treatment in a long-term rehabilitation center. The goal of treatment in this setting is to maximize the individual's ability to communicate independently. Rehabilitation centers also focus on the individual's readjustment into society. When the patient is able to live at home, but still requires services, home health agencies employing speech–language pathologists may provide individualized treatment in the patient's home. Private practice is another area in which speech–language pathologists serve individuals with many different types of communication disorders. Services may be paid for by patients and their families, by private health insurance programs, or by federal agencies such as Medicaid.

The field of speech–language pathology has changed dramatically over the past few decades. The expansion of settings in which services are delivered is paralleled by the explosion of information and technology. As the field continues to grow, the speech–language pathologist can look forward to numerous professional challenges in a host of different clinical environments.

GOALS OF THIS TEXT

This textbook is aimed at providing students with a thorough examination of organic and neurogenic communication disorders. Several factors differentiate this book from other introductory texts. First, and most importantly, this text focuses attention on disorders that have traditionally been included in the speech–language pathologist's scope of practice, as well as on those clinical populations that reflect the expanded role of communication management in medical and educational settings. For example, attention is paid not only to aphasia, which has been within the scope of practice for many decades, but to more current issues, such as the dementia that can result from AIDS. In addition, emphasis is placed on the notion of risk, and how many different aspects of communication may be compromised by various biologic and environmental factors across the lifespan. Second, the text presents relevant anatomical and physiological information for each separate clinical population. In this way, theory is presented in the context of clinical issues and the broadened scope of practice. Third, essential information in the areas of related instrumentation, new analytic techniques, and medico-surgical advances, is highlighted. Finally, the textbook infuses a multicultural and bias-free philosophy, consonant with current legislation.

THEMES OF THE BOOK

Each chapter is written in its own unique style, reflecting the experiences and philosophy of the individual authors, but there are commonalities and unifying themes that tie the chapters together. A lifespan perspective is taken for each communication disorder, where it is appropriate. A strong element of each chapter is the central role of the multidisciplinary team in the provision of diagnostic and clinical services. The crucial role played by speech–language pathologists and audiologists is stressed.

A variety of models are inherent in the treatment approaches that are presented in the book, showing the wide diversity of modern clinical practice. While most current approaches include a strong medical component, the importance of alternative models, such as educational and sociocultural, cannot be overlooked. This is clearly apparent in the host of settings in which speech–language pathologists and audiologists are employed.

Efforts have been made in each chapter to include the most current instrumental techniques for analysis and measurement of communication behavior. Similarly, current theoretical perspectives

are presented as a basis for understanding management approaches.

PLAN OF THE BOOK

The book begins with a discussion about epidemiology, including risk factors and socio-communicative development in medically fragile children. A systems approach is used to organize subsequent chapters. First, disorders associated with the central nervous system are presented. The central nervous system disorders begin with those associated with more diffuse cognitive deficits, and progress to those resulting from more focal damage. It should be noted, however, that the demarcation between diffuse and focal disorders is not always definitive. Central nervous system disorders that are discussed cover the entire lifespan, and include the areas of mental retardation, psychiatric disorders, dementia, stroke, traumatic brain injury, and disorders of speech motor control. Disorders associated with the oral and laryngeal systems are then discussed. Again, the range of disorders that can occur across the lifespan are presented. These include craniofacial anomalies, dysphagia, voice problems, spasmodic dysphonia, and laryngectomy. Finally, disorders associated with impaired sensory systems are presented. Attention is given to children and adults with multiple disabilities. Finally, we conclude with a chapter on the deaf and hard-of-hearing populations, which explores the theory of social reconstruction as an alternative view to the medical model.

OVERVIEW OF CHAPTERS

A brief description of each chapter is provided as an overview. Dr. Rossetti, in the chapter on epidemiology, sets the stage for examining the principles and categories of risk from a biological and environmental framework. An important part of the discussion is how risk factors contribute to patterns of communication delay observed in various populations of children. Dr. Rossetti notes that those factors that contribute to mortality are the identical ones that contribute to risk for communication development. Topics discussed include babies born to teenage mothers, drug exposed infants, low birth weight infants, infants exposed to impoverished caregiving environments, and multicultural issues related to risk. Dr. Rossetti also focuses on the settings in which communication-based intervention takes place, and the efficacy of such activities.

In the first of the chapters related to disorders of the central nervous system, Dr. Domingo contrasts traditional teaching techniques based on behavioral management with more current views on the treatment of mental retardation across the lifespan. He points out how research and treatment of mental retardation now focus more on the development of social communication skills within naturally occurring contexts, rather than on language structure alone. Some of the topics addressed by Dr. Domingo include the role of "motherese" in the development of language, parent training, milieu training, and the concept of full inclusion.

Following the chapter on mental retardation, Dr. Baltaxe discusses communication handicaps associated with psychiatric disorders. She underscores the idea that mental health professionals and speech–language pathologists have much to share with respect to this patient population. Types of disorders included in the chapter are autism, disruptive behavioral disorders, emotional disorders, schizophrenias and psychoses.

Dementias in geriatric populations are described by Dr. De Santi, who distinguishes between cortical and subcortical dementias, and between those resulting from vascular etiologies and infectious diseases. Importantly, Dr. De Santi includes discussion on AIDS-related dementia in this chapter. Advances in scanning technologies are considered in relation to the various dementias. The current status of medical treatment and rehabilitation, including counseling and programs for caregivers, is addressed.

Dr. Coelho begins the next chapter with a discussion of the etiologic processes involved in Traumatic Brain Injury (TBI), and the communicative impairments that result. He discusses sequelae of TBI, including motor, speech, language, and cognitively based problems. Stages of recovery are then discussed with regard to the selection of assessment tools and focus of treatment.

Next, Dr. Bloom considers the communication disorders that result from more focal damage caused by cerebrovascular accident (CVA). Following a medical explanation of CVA, Dr. Bloom provides a brief historic overview on how brain organization has been studied. Subsequently, the chapter focuses on current neurolinguistic and neuropsychological theory and its implications for diagnosing communication impairments. The different kinds of communication handicaps that result from damage to the left and right hemispheres are reviewed next to provide a basis for differential diagnosis and clinical intervention.

A detailed discussion on motor speech disorders is presented in the next chapter by Drs. Bloom and Ferrand. They take a neuroanatomic approach to the classification of different neuromotor speech disorders. This leads logically into a systematic procedure for distinguishing among the different types of dysarthrias, and apraxia of speech. The importance of instrumentation procedures that aid in the description and classification of motor speech disorders is highlighted. Special consideration is given to individuals with cerebral palsy, and ventilator-dependent patients.

The book next presents disorders arising from the oral and laryngeal systems. First, cleft lip and palate, and other craniofacial anomalies are presented by Dr. Golding-Kushner. The chapter begins with a summary of embryonic cranial and facial development, and a common classification system for different types of clefts. Etiologies of clefts and common syndromes affecting the craniofacial complex are described, with special attention given to the syndromes that the speech–language pathologist practicing in a school or hospital setting is likely to encounter. Types of surgical and prosthetic repairs are presented. Dr. Golding-Kushner concludes the chapter with a discussion about related issues such as feeding, voice, resonance, and articulation of individuals with craniofacial disorders.

Another disorder that can result from damage to the structures of the head or neck or from lack of neuromuscular control is dysphagia. Because of the wide range of medical factors that can cause dysphagia, the frequency of swallowing disorders in children and adults is high. Dr. Logemann begins with a discussion of normal swallow physiology. Disorders of swallow physiology, presented next, are described in terms of their characteristics and symptomatology. A number of techniques utilized to study swallow disorders, such as videofluoroscopy, endoscopy, and ultrasound are discussed with respect to their advantages, limitations, and the types of populations for which they are appropriate.

The chapter on structurally related and neurogenic voice disorders by Dr. Ferrand is presented next, because it reviews laryngeal anatomy and physiology relevant to all the chapters on voice disorders. Particular attention is paid to current knowledge of vocal fold structure and function. The relationship between anatomy, physiology, and the acoustic and perceptual consequences of normal development and disordered function are emphasized. Various types of disorders across the lifespan are discussed, and behavioral and phonosurgical techniques for remediation are introduced.

Dr. Slavin extends the discussion on voice problems, by presenting information related to laryngeal cancer as well as various surgical options for removing the affected portion of the larynx. Anatomical changes resulting from the surgical extirpation of the larynx and physiological changes related to breathing, eating, and speech are outlined. Methods of alaryngeal voice production are described, and the social and emotional challenges a person may face following a laryngectomy are highlighted.

Another disorder of the laryngeal system is spasmodic dysphonia. Drs. Stewart, Brin, and Blitzer contrast past psychogenic theories of this problem with its current conceptualization as a neurogenic disorder. Two types of spasmodic dysphonia are differentiated, and the perceptual and acoustic characteristics of each of these types are

discussed. The authors emphasize the relationship between current theoretical perspectives and recent medico-surgical techniques such as botulinum toxin injection and recurrent laryngeal nerve section.

The final two chapters examine sensory deficits that give rise to organic and neurogenic problems. Drs. Flexer, Gillette, and Wray provide an overview of persons with multiple disabilities. These include deafness, blindness, multiple handicaps, orthopedic handicaps, and other health impairments. They present an overview of the disciplines involved with persons with disabilities, with a special focus on the role of the speech–language pathologist and audiologist. An appendix is provided with examples of educationally based models of intervention that utilize a functional approach to communication management. Additionally, the importance of the acoustic learning environment is a central theme of the chapter.

Finally, Dr. Israelite, with M. Jennings, presents an overview of theory, practice, and issues related to working with deaf and hard-of-hearing children and adults. The chapter opens with a discussion of theoretical perspectives. The deficit-based medical model, which has traditionally informed theory and practice in this field, is contrasted with the difference-based sociocultural model of social construction. The notion of a deaf community and culture as well as other philosophical and methodological issues arising from the tensions between the two models are introduced. This is followed by a discussion of the anatomy and physiology of hearing, the physics of sound, and individual and group amplification systems and other technical devices. Information on current technological advances, such as cochlear implants, is also provided. A section on bilingual/bicultural education describes the rationale of this approach, and considers the role of the speech–language pathologist in such a program. The final section addresses people who develop hearing loss in adulthood, including those who become hard of hearing as a natural process of aging, and those who are suddenly deafened due to trauma or disease.

Major Points of Chapter

- Demographic variables have led to an increase in the prevalence or organic and neurogenic disorders.
- Technological and theoretical advances have supported the expansion of the scope of clinical practice in speech–language pathology.
- Legal mandates have shaped the nature of service delivery, the types of patients receiving services, and the settings where services are provided.
- Treatment has broadened to include patients with different types of organic and neurogenic disorders across the lifespan.

Discussion Guidelines

1. Interview a speech–language pathologist in a school setting and ask how clinical management has changed following the passage of PL 94–142. Share the results of this interview in a class discussion.

2. Visit a speech–language and hearing center and note the instrumentation that is used to diagnose or treat various organic and neurogenic disorders. Research the clinical advantages and limitations of the instruments.

REFERENCES

ASHA Congressional Relations Division, Government Affairs Department. (1989). Current federal legislative regulatory issues: Issues of interest to speech–language pathologists and persons with communication disorders. Rockville, MD: American Speech-Language-Hearing Association.

ASHA Governmental Affairs Review. (1990). Reauthorization of EHA discretionary programs. Rockville, MD: American Speech-Language-Hearing Association.

ASHA, Legislative Council. (1994). Council report. Rockville, MD: Author.

2

EPIDEMIOLOGY OF RISK AND SOCIO-COMMUNICATIVE DEVELOPMENT IN MEDICALLY FRAGILE CHILDREN

LOUIS ROSSETTI

A nything that interferes with the child's ability to interact with the environment in a normal manner is a potential source of or contributing factor to the presence of developmental delay" (Rossetti, 1990).

In order for children to begin the process of making sense of the world, two basic factors are necessary. These are opportunity and ability. Infants enter the world uniquely predisposed to begin the process of making sense of their environment. Should anything interfere with the child's ability, or should the child be exposed to less than optimal opportunity, the risk for aberrant patterns of development is substantially increased. This chapter presents an array of issues that impact negatively on the child's overall developmental progress. These are issues that contribute to developmental delay during the preschool years and place the child at increased risk for later school failure. These factors may be biological, environmental, or a combination. Specific information relative to biological and environmental risk and subsequent developmental performance for various populations of infants will be discussed.

The efficacy of services provided for children under three depends heavily on the age at which a delay is detected. Age of identification is a key component in providing effective intervention services. Thus, early identification of children who display patterns of developmental delay, or who are at risk of doing so, is paramount. It is no surprise that professionals representing various academic disciplines are interested in the early identification of and intervention for children from birth through three years of age who either display developmental delay, or who are at risk of doing so. The range of professionals involved in early intervention is impressive, as shown in Table 2.1.

Depending on the criteria used to define language delay, the overall incidence in childhood ranges from 3 to 15 percent of all children (Silva, 1987). This estimate makes language disorders the most common developmental disability in childhood. The incidence of communication delay for various populations of infants and toddlers, specifically those presenting established risk factors, is substantially higher. It is generally accepted that communication skills demonstrate the highest pre-

9

TABLE 2.1   Professionals Involved in Early Intervention and Credentials Necessary within Each Discipline*

PROFESSION	NECESSARY TRAINING/CREDENTIALS
Medicine	Four-year medical education; internship; residency (optional); board certification in specialty (optional); state license; ongoing continuing education credits.
Physical Therapy	Undergraduate and or graduate degree in P.T.; state license.
Occupational Therapy	Undergraduate degree in O.T.; clinical training following graduation; passing grade on national examination; state license where required.
Speech–Language Pathologist	Graduate degree from accredited program; one-year clinical fellowship following graduation; passing grade on national examination; certificate of clinical competency; state license where required.
Audiology	Graduate degree from accredited program; one-year clinical fellowship following graduation; passing grade on national examination; state license where required.
Nurse	Undergraduate or graduate degree; passing grade on national examination; state license.
Psychologist	Graduate degree from accredited program; public school certification where required; state license.
Social Work	Master of Social Work (MSW) degree; national certification by National Association of Social Workers; state license where required.
Early Childhood Education Specialist	Appropriate degree; appropriate state certification/license.

*The above list reflects primary intervention disciplines.

dictive correlation with later intelligence and school performance of all childhood behaviors. Thus, it is imperative that early intervention professionals, regardless of primary academic discipline, acquire a broad understanding of epidemiologic factors related to general risk, and specifically to risk for socio-communicative delay. Those children who enter kindergarten possessing and using language well generally succeed in the early elementary grades. However, those children who do not possess age-appropriate communication skills often demonstrate a pattern of struggle during the early elementary grades that can prove quite difficult to overcome. Early identification of communication risk and delay is essential. The starting point for effective early case finding, therefore, is familiarity with risk factors.

The concept of **continuum of risk** has significant implications for the early intervention professional. This principle suggests that the be-

ginning point for delayed communication skills is not at the moment children fail to utter their first words at an age-appropriate phase in development. Rather, the child who does not demonstrate age-appropriate communication development does so due to factors that may be traced to influences relating to earlier events (biological, environmental, or both). Therefore, it is essential that the early interventionist understand the risk factors that contribute to socio-communicative delay and increased potential for school failure.

Who are these children? What specific factors contribute to increased risk for communication delay and later school failure? Are biological or environmental factors of primary importance when establishing risk status? And finally, are new populations of children emerging with whom the early interventionist must be concerned in order to provide comprehensive intervention services for these children and their families? The information that follows is intended to answer these and other questions.

ESTABLISHED AND AT-RISK CHILDREN

Established Risk Children

One helpful way to categorize children under three years who display delayed patterns of development is to view them as **established risk** versus **at risk.** Children who fall into the established risk category have known (expected) patterns of developmental delay secondary to the condition that places them in the established risk classification. In contrast, children who are placed in the at-risk classification possess various risk factors for developmental delay. However, it may not be said with certainty that they will display later delay, but only that they are at increased risk for doing so. For example, children with Down's Syndrome (the most frequent cause of mental retardation) are not considered to be "at risk" for delay. This is because the presence of the syndrome includes the established fact that some degree of mental retardation will be present. Although variation may exist in the long-term developmental performance of a child with Down's Syndrome (or any established risk child), the occurrence of a developmental delay is not unexpected. There are many genetic and metabolic syndromes and conditions in which developmental delay is expected, and in fact may be considered part of the syndrome or condition. Table 2.2 presents one classification system for viewing established risk children. This particular system is used by the state of Michigan in determining eligibility for early intervention services. The Michigan system breaks established risk into nine categories with specific conditions known to contribute to developmental delay listed under each. Although this system is not exhaustive, many of the most common established risk factors and conditions are included. Approximately 15 to 25 percent of children needing early intervention services fall into the established risk category. It is important that all members of the early intervention team become familiar with established risk factors, including genetics, neurological development, metabolic dis-

orders, and specific sensory disorders that contribute significantly to delayed development.

A variety of classification systems are available to assist in gaining a more complete understanding of the established risk child. Pediatrics, genetics, and behavioral medicine textbooks are of immeasurable value in attaining a more complete familiarity with the many established risk categories (Capute and Accardo, 1991; Batshaw and Perret, 1992; Bergsma, 1979; Blackman, 1990; Avery and First, 1989). In summary, those children who fall into the established risk classification display developmental delay secondary to the reason for their placement in the established risk group. Their delay is not unexpected, even though many factors may be present that influence the status of their development in addition to the primary risk factor.

At-Risk Children

In contrast to the child who displays established risk is the child considered to be at risk for developmental delay. A host of issues serve as contributors to increased hazard for slow maturation. The at-risk category of factors may include both biological and environmental issues. What is clear is that the environment is as powerful a factor in establishing risk status as are biological factors (Escalona, 1982). Children who match the at-risk designation are those from birth to three years of age who have an enhanced probability of displaying patterns of delayed development in the absence of early intervention services. These children are often more difficult to identify at an early age. It is mandatory that all early intervention professionals gain an adequate understanding of at-risk factors in order to enhance early case finding and subsequent referral for early intervention services, particularly since many funding agencies do not provide support for early intervention services unless the child fits an established risk category. Table 2.3 provides a list of at-risk factors that may be used in determining which infants and toddlers possess enhanced potential for delayed development. Although any of the factors listed in Table 2.3 may result in patterns of delayed development, it is generally the presence of two or

TABLE 2.2 Established Risk Factors

Chromosomal Anomalies/Genetic Disorders

Cru-du-Chat	Trisomy 21 (Down's Syndrome)
Trisomy 18	Fragile X Syndrome
Cockayne Syndrome	Laurence-Moon-Beidl-Syndrome
Warrdenberg Syndrome	Cerebro-Hepato-Renal Syndrome

Neurological Disorders

Cerebral Palsy	Kernicterus
Intercranial Hemorrhage	Wilson's Disease
Intercranial Tumors	Seizure Disorder
Head/Spinal Cord Injury	Neurofibromatosis

Congenital Malformations

Cleft Palate	Treacher Collins
Spina Bifida	Potter Syndrome
Noonan Syndrome	Microcephaly
Hypoplastic Mandible	Encephalocele

Inborn Errors of Metabolism

Hunter Syndrome	Schele Syndrome
Sly Syndrome	Sanfilippo Syndrome
Maple Syrup Urine Disease	Infant PKU
Galactosemia	Tay-Sachs Disease

Sensory Disorder

Visual Impairment	Hearing Loss
Congenital Cataract	Retinopathy of Prematurity

Atypical Developmental Disorder

Pervasive Developmental Disorder	Autistic Disorder
Failure to Thrive (Non-organic)	Reactive Attachment Disorder

Severe Toxic Exposure

Cocaine and other Drugs	Maternal PKU
Fetal Alcohol Syndrome	Lead/Mercury Poisoning

Chronic Medical Illness

Medically Fragile	Cancer
Chronic Hepatitis	Cystic Fibrosis
Diabetes	Heart Problems
Renal Failure	

Severe Infectious Disease

Cytomegalovirus (CMV)	Herpes
Syphilis	Toxoplasmosis
HIV +	Rubella
Bacterial Meningitis	Encephalitis
Poliomyelitis	Viral Meningitis

TABLE 2.3   At-Risk Factors

Serious concerns expressed by parent or primary caregiver, or professional, regarding the child's development, parenting style, or parent-child interaction

Parent or primary caregiver with chronic or acute mental illness, developmental disability, or mental retardation

Parent or primary caregiver with drug/alcohol dependence

Parent or primary caregiver with a history of loss or abuse

Family medical/genetic history characteristics

Parent or primary caregiver with severe or chronic illness

Acute family crisis

Chronically disturbed family interaction

Parent–child or caregiver–child separation

The presence of one or more of the following: parental education less than ninth grade, neither parent is employed, single parent

Adolescent mother

Parent has four or more preschool age children

Physical or social isolation and/or lack of adequate social support

Lack of stable residence, homelessness, or dangerous living conditions

Inadequate family health care or no health insurance

Limited prenatal care

Maternal prenatal substance abuse/use

Severe prenatal complications

Severe perinatal complications

Asphyxia

Very low birth weight (<1,500 grams)

Small for gestational age (<10th percentile)

Excessive irritability, crying, tremulousness on the part of the infant

Atypical or recurrent accidents on the part of the child

Chronic otitis media

more factors that results in significantly enhanced risk for slow patterns of development.

INFANT MORTALITY

Each year, approximately 40,000 U.S. infants do not reach their first birthday. Two-thirds of these infant deaths take place during the neonatal period. More than 50 percent of infant deaths take place in infants who weigh less than 1,500 grams at birth. Thus, infants who comprise less than 1 percent of all live births account for almost 40 percent of all infant deaths. Major risk factors related to infant mortality include the following (Hogue, Buehler, Strauss, & Smith, 1987):

Gender: Regardless of race, males experience higher birth-weight-specific infant mortality rates than do females.

Gestational Age: Infant mortality increases with decreasing birth weight.

Live Birth Order: Second born infants experience lower infant mortality than infants of other birth orders.

Maternal Age: Infant mortality decreases with increasing maternal age through 30 to 34 years of age, but increases for infants born to women 35 years of age and older. Optimal maternal age (childbearing) is 25 to 29 years for African-American women, and 30 to 34 years for white women.

Maternal Education: Infant mortality declines with increasing maternal education for both African Americans and whites, but declines more steeply for infants born to white women.

Prenatal Care: Infants born to mothers who obtain prenatal care beginning in the first trimester experience substantially lower infant mortality. This trend is most pronounced for infants weighing 2,500 grams or more but is also present for infants weighing between 1,500 and 2,499 grams. In 1988, only 58 percent of Native-American and Mexican-American mothers received early prenatal care. Sixty-one percent of African American and 63 percent of Puerto Rican and Central and South American mothers received early care (Mason, 1991).

Understanding Infant Mortality Statistics

One useful way of viewing the concept of risk is to become familiar with infant mortality statistics. The question can legitimately be asked, "why does one need to become familiar with infant mortality statistics?" After all, these numbers apply to children who have not survived and therefore will not be in need of early intervention services. The answer to this question is relatively simple. Because of the enormous advances in **neonatology** and pediatrics in the past decade, more infants are surviving than ever before. Although the **incidence** (new occurrences per year) of children at risk for infant mortality has not changed dramatically in the past five years, the **prevalence** (total living cases) of infants who previously might have not survived is expanding. The factors that contribute to infant–toddler mortality are the same factors that contribute to elevated risk for developmental delay for surviving children. In addition, new (expanding) populations of infants are entering the early interventionist's caseload. These include infants prenatally exposed to drugs, HIV+ babies, infants born to teenage mothers, and infants surviving at lower birth weights and younger gestational ages. Thus, it is important that early intervention professionals become familiar with infant mortality, its causes and contributing factors, and various new populations of infants and toddlers, in order to gain a full understanding of risk and long-term developmental expectations.

The infant mortality rate in the United States has declined in the past decade. In 1984 the infant mortality rate was 18.4 per 1,000 live born African American infants and 9.4 per 1,000 live born white infants. In 1990 the infant mortality rate decreased to 9.1 per 1,000 live births. In 1992 the rate was 8.5 deaths per 1,000 live births, and in 1993 the rate dropped to 8.3 per 1,000. The drop in infant mortality can be attributed to increased access to prenatal care, advances in pediatric and neonatal medicine, new drugs (surfactants), and increased ability to care for high-risk mothers. In general, those infants most likely to not survive until their first birthday are the products of single, low socioeconomic status, teenage, undereducated, African American women. These infants are at risk for infant mortality, and because more are surviving, they are at heightened risk for developmental pathology. Significant diversity exists in infant mortality statistics between various subpopulations in the United States. For early intervention professionals working in culturally diverse areas of the country, familiarity with this diversity is paramount.

LOW BIRTH WEIGHT AND PREMATURITY

One of the primary risk factors associated with developmental pathology, and specifically socio-communicative delay, is **prematurity** and **low birth weight.** The discussion that follows describes the factors surrounding low birth weight and prematurity as well as common medical complications associated with an infant being born too small and too early.

A *premature infant* is defined as a child born at or before the 36th week of gestation, one month before the estimated date of confinement/delivery. A **small for gestational age** infant (SGA) refers to a newborn whose birth weight is below the 10th percentile for gestational age. SGA babies may be premature or full term. The determining factor is whether they weighed what they should have at the time of birth. For example, a child born at 35 weeks gestation who weighs 5 pounds (2,250 grams) is considered premature, but appropriate for gestational age relative to weight. A birth weight of 2,250 grams at 35 weeks gestation places the child at the 25th percentile for weight by gestational age. However, if this same infant were born at 40 weeks gestation, it would be considered small for gestational age. At 40 weeks gestational age, the 10th percentile for weight is 5 ½ pounds (2,500 grams). The most important predictor of infant survival continues to be birth weight. Hence, risk status for later developmental delay is associated with birth weight.

Prematurity also becomes an important factor when considering risk status. Premature delivery is due to a number of factors, many of which are not fully understood. In general, however, premature deliveries account for less than 5 percent of all live births. Less than 1 percent of these infants will be infants who weigh less than 1,500 grams. Although less than 5 percent of all pregnancies occur in adolescents, they account for 20 percent of all premature births. The highest proportion of premature births take place among women of lower socioeconomic status. Non-white economically disadvantaged groups have nearly twice the prematurity rate as whites in higher socioeconomic groups. Premature infants have a higher incidence of developmental disability than the general population. The majority of premature infants, however, are free from major handicap, and as many as one-third may be developing according to age expectations.

The survival and developmental outcome of premature infants have changed dramatically in the past 15 years, due primarily to major advances in neonatal medicine. Any evaluation of premature infants' developmental outcome should be made from an historical perspective. Developmental expectations of premature infants must take into account when the infants were born and what the status of neonatal care was at that time. Present medical technology is allowing the smallest of infants increasing survival rates. Thus, infants who 5 to 10 years ago would have had no (or very minimal) chance of survival are now surviving in increasing numbers. Although the smallest of infants still display significant mortality, the survivors are currently part of long-term follow-up investigations. Definitive statements about developmental outcome for the smallest of these infants can only be made following longitudinal follow-up.

Medical Complications of Premature Low Birth Weight Infants

Many medical complications are associated with prematurity and low birth weight. Although not all infants in neonatal intensive care experience all potential complications, each possible complication contributes to risk for later developmental delay. It is the cumulative effect of a host of complications that ultimately establishes risk, and not necessarily any single factor in isolation. The discussion that follows identifies some common medical complications to which premature infants are susceptible.

Respiratory Distress Syndrome (RDS). Respiratory disorders constitute the single largest cause of death among premature/low birth weight infants. **Respiratory distress syndrome** (RDS) is a pulmonary disorder commonly encountered in premature infants. It is among the most frequent causes of death in premature infants as well as the most common illness in intensive care nurseries. RDS affects approximately 20 percent of premature infants during the first few days of life. It is caused by a deficiency of a material known as *surfactant.* Surfactant is needed in the lungs of the infant in order to prevent the air sacs in the lungs from closing. When an insufficient amount of surfactant is present, the air sacs of the lungs collapse, and respiratory efficiency decreases. In general, adequate amounts of surfactant are not produced until approximately 36 weeks gestational age. Consequently, the overall incidence of RDS is heavily associated with the child's degree of prematurity. For example, 60 percent of infants born prior to 32 weeks gestation are affected compared to 20 percent of infants born in the 34 to 36 week range.

RDS is relatively easy to detect within the first few hours following birth. Primary manifestations include grunting by the child on expiration, frequent breathing (panting) with increased effort, flaring of the nostrils, and retracting of the muscles between the ribs and below the rib cage. Medical management of RDS generally involves increasing the concentration of inspired oxygen. Some infants may require **continuous positive air pressure (CPAP).** In CPAP a mixture of oxygen and air under pressure is provided through tubes placed in the nose. A second method requires intubation. This procedure involves placing a tube down the infant's airway and keeping the lungs inflated through the use of a ventilator. Another approach toward the treatment of RDS is the use of surfactant replacement. Synthetic surfactant is available for administration to infants with RDS and has shown positive results when administered early. The survival rate for infants treated with surfactant is approximately 65 percent, versus 26 percent for children not treated (Long, Corbet, and Cotton, 1991). Many infants with RDS are not able to nurse or drink. They must be fed intravenously or given formula or breast milk through a tube that is passed through the mouth or nose and into the stomach. At present approximately 90 percent of infants with RDS survive. Most survivors demonstrate no long-term deficit. However, a small group demonstrate developmental delay secondary to RDS due to RDS and associated medical risk factors. Some infants may also have continuing problems with respiratory illness, especially during the first year of life (Blackman, 1990).

Bronchopulmonary Dysplasia. *Bronchopulmonary dysplasia (BPD)* is another frequently occurring disorder in premature infants. BPD, sometimes called chronic lung disease of the premature infant, is characterized by chronic lung changes including decreased lung capacity and increased risk for respiratory disease. It occurs in infants who had RDS and/or required prolonged mechanical ventilation and high concentrations of oxygen. Full-term infants with **meconium** aspiration, pneumonia, or other causes of respiratory distress may also develop BPD. The greater the degree of prematurity, the greater the likelihood of BPD. As many as 80 percent of infants born weighing less that 1,000 grams develop BPD, in contrast to 10 percent of infants weighing more than 1,500 grams. The mortality rate for infants

with BPD is about 20 percent in the first year of life.

BPD has two primary causes. It results from an initial injury to the lungs secondary to prematurity, as well as from the standard treatment for this initial injury. That is, the initial injury to the lungs is complicated further by the repeated pressures delivered by a ventilator for intubated infants. The increased level of oxygen needed to keep the infant alive can also further damage the lungs. What results is a vicious cycle, whereby continuing mechanical ventilation and supplemental oxygen are necessary, but their use further exacerbates the condition. BPD is a chronic lung disease lasting from months to years with mild-to-severe long-term manifestations. BPD contributes to a host of secondary medical complications over the course of the child's life. These include infection, kidney stones, fragile bones, abnormalities of the trachea, feeding problems, poor growth, high blood pressure, psychosocial problems, and enhanced potential for developmental risk.

Intraventricular Hemorrhage. A prominent risk associated with respiratory disease is bleeding into the fluid-filled spaces of the brain, known as *intraventricular hemorrhage* (IVH). For some infants IVH is present without any obvious explanation, while for others it is associated with respiratory distress, mechanical ventilation, or asphyxia. IVH is defined as extravascular blood within the cranial cavity. It is an increasing concern for infants at lower birth weight who are kept alive through the use of mechanical ventilation. The general incidence of IVH is reported to be 35 to 45 percent for infants less than 35 weeks gestation. Papile (1979) has provided a useful grading system for classification of IVH according to severity. This system is displayed in Table 2.4. When the extent of IVH is limited, the overall outcome for the child is generally good. However, if IVH is severe, the outcome may include mental retardation, spastic quadriplegia, and possible hydrocephalus. The most effective intervention for IVH is prevention. IVH is detected early through the use of ultrasound. The hemorrhage usually

TABLE 2.4   Grades for Degrees of Severity for IVH

GRADE	DESCRIPTION
Grade I	Isolated subependyman hemorrhage
Grade II	Intraventricular hemorrhage without ventricular dilation
Grade III	Intraventricular hemorrhage with ventricular dilation
Grade IV	Intraventricular hemorrhage with parenchymal hemorrhage

Source: Adapted from L. Papile (1979). Cerebral hemorrhage (CVH) in infants <1,500 grams: Developmental follow-up at one year. *Pediatric Research, 15,* 528.

reaches maximum severity at approximately 48 hours of age. Prevention of prematurity would virtually eliminate IVH in the newborn.

Necrotizing Enterocolitis. *Necrotizing enterocolitis* (NEC) is a serious intestinal disorder seen with some frequency in preterm infants. It occurs in approximately 10 percent of infants who weigh less than 1,500 grams at birth. Onset of the disorder is generally within the first week of life. NEC is a life-threatening condition. It is generally thought to be due to several factors, including injury to the intestinal wall, bacteria, and early formula feedings when the infant's gut is immature. Approximately 50 percent of infants with NEC will require surgery to remove the diseased section of the bowel. In approximately 10 percent of the infants who require surgery, an additional complication results known as "short gut syndrome." Because the remaining bowel length is insufficient, diarrhea and poor nutrition often result. Children with NEC often demonstrate an overall failure to thrive. They remain medically fragile, and subsequent developmental status may be affected.

Numerous other medical complications may be present in infants. Although these occur with less frequency than the conditions previously mentioned, they are contributors to patterns of developmental delay seen in at-risk children. These

conditions include patent ductus arteriosis (extra opening in the heart), apnea and bradycardia (cessation of breathing and reduction in heart rate), brain malformations, cerebral palsy, congenital heart disease, congenital infections (sepsis or cytomegalovirus), feeding problems, hearing problems, orthopedic problems (unusual head molding, joint problems), neurologic problems (hydrocephalus), seizure disorders, failure to thrive, and other sensory deficits. For additional material see relevant chapters in this text, as well as Blackman (1991) and Batshaw and Perret (1992).

NEW POPULATIONS OF INFANTS AT RISK FOR DEVELOPMENTAL DELAY

In addition to the more frequent medical complications of infancy that contribute to developmental delay, there are several new and expanding populations of at-risk infants. These include infants born to adolescent mothers, infants prenatally exposed to drugs, and HIV+ infants.

Teenage Mothers

Adolescent mothers present increased risk for delivering infants at elevated danger for developmental delay. Approximately 480,000 births take place each year in the United States to women under 19 years of age. Approximately 25 percent of adolescent women in the 1980s became pregnant (21 percent of whites and 41 percent of African American). The National Center for Health Statistics (1991) reported that teenage pregnancy among African American women under the age of 15 years has been increasing since 1983. The rate for teenagers in general, which had declined somewhat in the 1980s, has again begun to increase.

The primary concern for adolescent mothers is their higher incidence of delivering low birthweight/premature infants. Teenagers who give birth are less likely than older women to secure adequate prenatal care. Teenage mothers have a higher rate of spontaneous abortions, stillbirths, premature births, mentally retarded infants, and developmentally delayed children. The increased incidence of developmental delay is due to the increased biological risk as well as to the impoverished climate for optimal caretaking many teenage mothers experience. Babies born to teenage mothers have from 1.5 to 3.5 times the risk for infant mortality, compared to mothers between 25–29 years of age. Furthermore, African-American teenage mothers have from 1.3 to 2.2 times the risk for infant mortality than white teenagers.

In addition to the increased biological risk infants of teenage mothers face, the type of home environment the mothers are able to provide increases the risk status of the child. Sugar (1984) reported that the percentage of adequate stimulation directed toward infants by adolescent versus adult mothers was 73 percent and 85 percent, respectively. The best predictor of maternal involvement with premature infants is education. Teenage mothers in general demonstrate a lower educational level, suggesting that teenage maternal involvement is somewhat reduced in comparison to adult mothers. This provides additional risk for developmental delay.

Teenage mothers and their children suffer from both short-term and long-term difficulties. One significant long-term factor that contributes to the difficulties encountered by teenage mothers and their children is poverty. Poverty increases the risk for a number of environmental difficulties, not the least of which is having less emotional and social support than is generally available to older mothers. Living in a single parent, impoverished environment alone can contribute significant risk to developmental problems. Additional parenting risks for children of teenage mothers exist. Teenage mothers' initiation of verbal interaction and responsiveness to their children is reduced. Many teenage mothers talk very little to their children, and as might be expected, the children initiate less verbal interactions. Less sensitive and less emotionally positive interactions between teenage mothers and their children are additional factors that enhance the potential for developmental delay. These less than optimal interaction patterns often are revealed in the child's overall socioemotional development. Infants of teenage moth-

ers show increased avoidance behaviors with concurrent patterns reflecting disorders in attachment. (See Chapter 4.) These are serious issues and point to the multifaceted nature of risk associated with children of teenage mothers.

Children Prenatally Exposed to Drugs

A U.S. General Accounting Office (1990) report to Congress suggests that somewhere between 100,000 and 375,000 women each year give birth after exposing their unborn children to illicit drugs. When alcohol and nicotine are included, the number of exposed children is even higher. A rapidly growing body of research suggests that prenatal drug exposure is linked to increased health problems in the newborn, as well as to additional problems in the child's overall development. Although substance abuse crosses the boundaries of race, ethnicity, and socioeconomic status, studies reveal a higher incidence of reported use by poor, uninsured, minority women (Castro, Azen, Hobel, and Platt, 1993). In addition, the choice of drug seems to vary among ethnic groups. White women are more likely to admit having used alcohol or marijuana during pregnancy. African American women admit to having used cocaine (Frank, Zukerman, and Amaro, 1989). Recent estimates suggest that approximately 601,000 women in the childbearing years (15–44) are current cocaine users. Although no accurate data exist on how many of these women are pregnant at any point in time, estimates range from 1 to 36 percent (Gomby and Shino, 1991). The impact of cocaine on neurobehavioral development has been investigated both prenatally and postnatally. Specifically, studies have linked drug exposure in utero to infants' inability to maintain adequate behavioral state control in the neonatal period, depression of interactive behavior, and poor organizational response to environmental stimuli (Edmondson, 1994). Additional behavioral observations among infants prenatally exposed to drugs include mild-to-moderate tremulousness (tremors in the arms and legs), increased startle response (startling at simple sounds), irritability, abnormal sleep patterns, and poor feeding. In addition, temperamental and behavioral differences exist at six months of age. Longitudinal investigations also have reported attention and behavioral deficits and differences in play patterns and behaviors at three years of age (Edmondson, 1994).

Several paradigms exist to assist the early intervention professional in early identification of children at increased risk for prenatal drug exposure and subsequent developmental problems. Hicks and Wilson (1993) have provided helpful information regarding prenatal, delivery room (perinatal), and postnatal risk indicators. These are displayed in Table 2.5.

Table 2.6 describes common fetal and infant risk characteristics resulting from prenatal cocaine exposure. These characteristics are serious and have critical implications for the child's future development. Table 2.7 presents data regarding short- and long-term behavioral characteristics seen in children prenatally exposed to cocaine and other drugs.

Substance abuse during pregnancy continues to be a serious problem in the United States, placing an increasing number of infants at substantially increased risk for developmental delay. Drug use jeopardizes the health and well-being of the mother and child both prenatally and postnatally.

TABLE 2.5   Pre-Peri-Post-Natal Risk Indicators for Drug Usage

Prenatal Risk Indicators
Mother conceals or denies pregnancy
Mother unsuccessfully sought or attempted abortion
Mother seeks, then reverses the decision to relinquish the child for adoption
History of severe marital discord
Mother makes no preparation for the birth of the child
Either parent has a history of serious mental illness, institutionalization, current
    depression, or repeated foster care placement
Either parent has a history of previous abuse/neglect of another child in the family
Mother consistently misses appointments and is noncompliant

Perinatal Risk Indicators
Mother displays hostile reaction following birth
Mother avoids verbal/nonverbal interactions with staff
Mother avoids or makes no eye contact with infant
Mother is disappointed over the sex or appearance of child
Negative interaction is observed between mother and baby

Postnatal Risk Indicators
Mother displays lack of behaviors indicating maternal attachment
Mother is reluctant to hold, feed, or name the infant
Mother avoids eye contact or touch with the infant
Mother makes negative comments about the infant
Mother cares for the infant in an inappropriate manner
Mother tries to have the infant discharged from the hospital against medical advice
Mother departs from the hospital under suspicious circumstances
Mother visits infrequently if she goes home before infant
Mother is reluctant to come for the child when the child is discharged from the hospital

Source: Adapted from B. Hicks and G. Wilson (1993). *Kids, crack and the community: Reclaiming drug-exposed infants and children.* National Education Service: Bloomington, IN.

TABLE 2.6 Prenatal Exposure to Cocaine: Risks for the Fetus and the Infant

FETAL RISK	INFANT RISK
Decrease in blood/ oxygen flow	May display physical withdrawal
Intrauterine growth retardation	Irritability
Stroke (irreversible brain damage)	Jitteriness
Miscarriage	Disorganization
Abrupto placentae	Seizures
Neonatal neuro- behavioral dysfunction	Small head size
Meconium staining	Premature birth
Hyperactivity	Respiratory problems
Hepatitis and HIV + from mother	Poor interaction ability

Source: Adapted from *Alcohol and other drugs: Impact on women and their families* (1992). Illinois Department of Alcohol and Substance Abuse. William T. Atkins, Director. Springfield, IL.

Children prenatally exposed to illegal substances are arguably the most expensive group of children with special needs who will enter the education system. This cost relates to actual dollars, as well as the amount of time needed to identify and effectively plan constructive treatment and intervention strategies.

Pediatric HIV Infection (AIDS)

The first cases of AIDS in adults were reported in 1980. AIDS in children was reported one year later. In the years from 1981 to 1989, more than 2,700 cases of childhood AIDS were reported in the United States (Centers for Disease Control, 1991). It is believed that for every child diagnosed with AIDS, at least 10 others are infected with the HIV virus (Gwinn, Pappaioanou, and George, 1991). In 1987 pediatric AIDS was the ninth leading cause of death in children 1 to 4 years, and the 12th leading cause of death for children 5 to 14

TABLE 2.7 Age-Related Behavioral Characteristics of Drug–Exposed Children

Birth to 2 Years
   Lack of oral language abilities
   Inappropriate use of gesture
   Limited or no expressive language
   Attention deficits
   Unusual behavior patterns
   Decreased problem-solving
   Low muscle tone
   Rapid mood swings
   Difficult to console

2 to 4 Years
   Word retrieval problems
   Problems identifying colors
   Difficulty with concept formation
   Use of disorganized sentences
   Deficient pragmatic skills
   Detached socially
   Hyperactive with decreased attention
   Difficulty in shifting from task to task
   Decreased cooperative activity

4 to 6 Years
   Limited vocabulary skills
   Difficulty with abstract concepts
   Primary use of simple vs. complex sentences
   Difficulty interacting with peers
   Reduced attention span
   Easily distracted
   Difficulty in shifting tasks
   Easily overloaded

6 Years and Older
   Difficulty with word retrieval
   Disorganized sentence construction
   Short attention span
   Difficulty staying on task
   Low tolerance for change
   Multiple articulation problems
   Poor interaction with other children

Source: Adapted from K. Rivers (1992). Language and behavioral concerns for drug-exposed infants and toddlers. In L. Rossetti, (Ed.), *Developmental problems of drug-exposed infants.* San Diego: Singular Press.

years. AIDS is likely to be among the top five causes of death for infants and young children within the next decade. Approximately 60 percent of children infected by their mothers develop symptoms in the first year of life, and almost 80 percent by 2 years of age. This is a much shorter incubation period than is present for adult infections. The usual onset of symptoms in perinatally infected children occurs between 3 and 10 months of age. A variety of symptoms are reported when the child is initially diagnosed. The child generally appears to be chronically ill with symptoms that include failure to thrive, intermittent fever, recurrent diarrhea, and weight loss. In approximately 10 to 15 percent of cases of pediatric AIDS, loss of developmental abilities is the sole initial complaint (Bellman, Diamond, and Dickson, 1988).

Developmental problems for HIV/AIDS babies appear in approximately 75 to 90 percent of children with HIV infection (Butler, Hittleman, and Hauger, 1991). These deficits include mental and motor delays, loss of previously attained developmental milestones, acquired microcephaly, short-term memory problems, cognitive deficits, fine and gross motor delay, communicative delay, visual spatial deficits, problems with social and adaptive behavior, and attentional difficulties in older children. This pattern of developmental delay is confounded by additional biological factors that may include prenatal drug exposure, prematurity, low birth weight, and general failure to thrive. Long-term hospitalization, chaotic family environments, and understimulation also contribute to the pattern of developmental delay. Infants and toddlers with pediatric AIDS present the early intervention team with a significant and multifaceted challenge. Environmental and biological factors contribute equally to the pattern of delay noted in an overwhelming percentage of HIV/AIDS babies.

The key element in any intervention program for HIV/AIDS babies is early identification. Developmental assessment at regular intervals is paramount. Once a pattern of delay is confirmed, children with HIV who are younger than three years should be enrolled in an appropriate early intervention program. Three- to five-year-old children should be referred to the local schools for appropriate educational intervention. It is imperative that all early intervention professionals keep abreast of changes in identification and management, both medical and educational, for HIV/AIDS infants and toddlers. This is an emerging area in early intervention, and one which promises to vary over time.

DEVELOPMENTAL EXPECTATIONS FOR AT-RISK/ESTABLISHED RISK INFANTS AND TODDLERS

The information presented thus far was introduced in a categorical fashion. In reality, it is quite difficult to determine developmental risk attributable to each condition previously described. Rarely is an infant at risk due to the occurrence of a single risk factor. Rather, the general pattern is that the infant displays risk, or patterns of established delay, due to a combination of factors that may change over time. In essence, any combination of the factors described previously may apply for a given child. This makes it difficult for the early interventionist to determine developmental expectations for a given population of children. Conscientious review of carefully conducted investigations regarding the populations of infants described above is instructive regarding developmental performance in the long- and short-term. Table 2.8 presents a summary of developmental follow-up studies utilizing various populations of infants and toddlers. It is crucial that early intervention professionals become familiar with information such as is presented in Table 2.8. This knowledge will enhance early case finding and thereby strengthen developmental outcomes for infants and toddlers.

EARLY INTERVENTION SERVICES

The follow-up data presented in Table 2.8 clearly indicates that socio-communicative development is the single most important developmental

TABLE 2.8 Developmental Expectations for At-Risk Infants

DATE	AUTHORS	POPULATION	OUTCOME
1987	Schraeder et al.	VLBW infants <1500g	More that 1/2 of variance relative to performance at 36 months of age due to biological factors
1989	Clark	Established risk and at-risk babies	Problems in speech and language development observed
1990	Largo et al.	118 pre-term and 78 mentally retarded infants followed to age 9 years	Language scores prior to two years was the strongest predictor of later performance
1986	Largo, et al.	114 pre-term infants followed to age 5	Language development delayed
1988	Greenberg, et al.	30 pre-term infants followed to age 2	Pre-term infants significantly lower in motor skills
1985	Forslund, et al.	46 pre-term infants followed to age 18 months	Motor, neurological, and language development were delayed
1991	Booth, et al.	18 high-risk infants followed to age 4	Attachment problems and increased aggressiveness noted
1991	Wille	18 premature, low SES infants followed to 12 months on measures of attachment	Infants were found to demonstrate insecure attachment—prematurity and low SES accounted for differences observed
1983	Wright	70 premature infants followed to age 3.5 years	Differences observed in language expression and comprehension compared to matched peers
1991	Blackman	Review of world's literature on low birth weight infants at school age	General cognitive ability within normal range; specific areas of weakness noted; underachievement, grade retention, and a need for special education more likely
1991	Hack, et al.	Outcome measures on infants between 1250g and 1500g at birth	21 percent of infants followed demonstrated developmental complications
1990	Schraeder, et al.	37 infants <1500g followed to age 4 years	More behavior problems than would be expected in the general population
1986	Eilers, et al.	43 infants <1250g followed into school	Over half (51.5 percent) of infants followed required special education
1992	Cusson	43 high-risk low SES infants followed to 26 months	No relationship between developmental outcome and severity of neonatal complications found—mean mental and motor scores within normal limits by age 2
1987	Macey, et al.	Pre-term infants followed to age 12 months	Infants showed less exploratory play and stayed closer to mother during free play
1991	Oberklaid, et al.	126 pre-term infants followed into school	No differences observed on temperament measures at 5 years of age
1990	Williamson, et al.	61 infants <1500g followed to age 1 and compared to healthy infants	Differences observed in fine motor skills—global developmental scores infants are not adequate in following high-risk
1991	Aram, et al.	249 infants <1500g compared with 363 normal birth weight infants at 8 years of age	Speech and language skills significantly lower for LBW children—language deficit and general developmental problems more prevalent
1982	Bhargave, et al.	40 small-for-date infants compared to 40 term infants at age 1 year	Widening of gap between groups with advancing age–language differences observed between groups

TABLE 2.8   Continued

DATE	AUTHORS	POPULATION	OUTCOME
1987	Hubatch, et al.	10 pre-term infants compared to 10 full-term infants on language skills	Superior language skills observed in term infants
1991	Ornstein, et al.	25 studies of low birthweight children reviewed	Age-appropriate IQ noted; increased need for special education, visual motor problems noted, behavioral difficulties present, fine and gross motor incoordination present
1992	McCormick, et al.	Infants <1500 g followed to age 8–10 years	Children born at lower birth weights experience increased morbidity at school age
1991	Escobar, et al.	Review of 111 studies of LBW infants	Median incidence of disability was 25 percent
1991	Veen, et al.	1338 low birth weight children from the Netherlands followed to age 5 years	Prevalence of disability was 27 percent
1990	Grunau, et al.	Infants <1000g followed to age 3 years	Language outcome below that of healthy infants
1988	Vohr, et al.	50 infants <1500g at birth	Lower scores obtained on language tests
1993	Byrne, et al.	71 low birth weight infants followed to age 2 years	Overall language scores lower than peers

domain that differentiates no-risk from at-risk infants and toddlers. This is significant because children with early communication delay are at high risk for developing learning problems once the child reaches school age. Early detection and intervention are critical for academic and emotional health. Data of this nature suggests one important concept in early intervention: those children who enter school possessing and using the language competently generally do well in kindergarten. In contrast, those children who do not enter school with age-appropriate socio-communicative ability are at substantial risk for school failure. At-risk children, regardless of the specifics of their risk status, display delayed communication skills more frequently than any other developmental deficit. Communication skills are the single best predictor of future cognition and subsequent school performance. Hence, it becomes compulsory that care be directed toward early identification, assessment, and intervention for infants with established or at-risk status. The following discussion describes a variety of issues relative to communication-based early intervention services and the efficacy of such efforts.

Communication-Based Early Intervention

An increasing number of early intervention providers (including all the disciplines mentioned earlier in this chapter) are involved in delivering intervention services for children from birth. Clinicians involved in service provision from the earliest days of the child's life are generally employed in hospital settings, specifically in the neonatal intensive care nursery (NICU). A variety of publications exist which describe the nature of the intensive care nursery (Rossetti, 1995).

The specific academic disciplines that deliver NICU-based developmentally appropriate care vary. No specific model demonstrating superior efficacy has emerged. Hence, any one of the traditional early intervention disciplines may provide care in the NICU. Clinicians working in the NICU have basically three avenues of service delivery available to them. These include services delivered to the child, the parents, or the NICU staff. The efficacy of NICU-based intervention has been established, and a majority of NICUs pay particular attention to providing developmentally appropriate care (Brown, Thurman, and Pearl, 1993). The actual services provided include modifying the environment of the nursery to reduce environmental stressors, providing parents with information designed to enhance their attachment to the infant and alert them to the increased risk their child displays as a result of prolonged hospitalization, and providing the medical staff with necessary ongoing data to assist them in gaining a more complete understanding of how the nursery impacts upon later development. Any member of the early intervention team can be involved in providing information of this nature. However, the speech–language pathologist possesses a wealth of information regarding communication development that must be shared with the early intervention team. The result will be enhanced familiarity with issues related to socio-communicative skills on the part of all team members.

Careful discharge planning must take place as the time for the child's dismissal from the hospital nears. Once the child transitions to the home, early intervention services continue and become essentially home-based. In fact, a majority of community-based early intervention agencies are providing services in the home predominantly for children under one year. As the child nears one year of age, both home-based and center-based services are delivered. There are distinct advantages to a home-based model of service delivery. However, as the child matures, a variety of advantages to center-based services emerge (Table 2.9). Once the child reaches age three, services are delivered primarily in the school setting.

During the earliest stages of communication-based intervention, professionals direct the majority of attention to the parents. It is essential that parents become acquainted with the way babies transmit communicative signals. The child's communicative signals, although initially nonverbal (prelinguistic) in nature, and the parent's ability to identify and respond to these signals, form the basis for early communication-based intervention. (See Chapter 14.) Professionals working on communication-based intervention, regardless of primary academic discipline, normally spend a great deal of time demonstrating to parents and other caregivers how the infant communicates, as well as how the parents might enhance the child's communicative capability. A careful review of existing literature relative to how mothers and babies interact suggests that mothers utilize seven basic strategies when talking to their babies. These are listed in Table 2.10. These ingredients form the basis for

---

TABLE 2.9   Advantages of Home- and Center-Based Intervention Services

Home-Based Intervention
Parents and children feel more comfortable in their own home.
Children are more likely to respond optimally in their home. It affords a more naturalistic setting.
The health of the child is better protected. This is important for medically fragile children.
Parent and child routines are not interrupted. As a result a more accurate sample of parent/child interaction may be obtained.
There is a greater likelihood of gaining helpful insights as a result of other family members being present.

Center-Based Intervention
Parents and children have greater access to staff and more services, if needed.
Parents are afforded the opportunity to meet and interact with other parents of children with special needs. This benefit should not be underestimated. It is quite supportive to have parents meet other parents with whom they might share frustrations, and other experiences.
Should any specialized services be needed, they may be more readily available to the child.

TABLE 2.10 Characteristics of Mother–Infant Communication

MOTHERS UTILIZE...

Short utterance length with simplified syntax
Small core vocabulary that is object-centered
Topics are initially limited to the here and now
Heightened facial expression and gesture
Frequent questioning and greeting
Meaningful responses with turn-taking and
  prolonging of interactions
Frequent verbal rituals

early communication-based intervention. Once the child moves from the prelinguistic stage to the linguistic stage of communication, a more traditional approach toward vocabulary building, sentence structure, and increasing the length of utterance is generally adopted by the speech–language pathologist. Efforts of this nature are essential if established and at-risk infants and toddlers are to reach optimal communication status, thereby increasing their potential for school success. A variety of materials exist which provide detailed suggestions regarding prelinguistic and postlinguistic communication-based intervention (Weitzman, 1992; Manolson, 1992; Rossetti, 1995).

The Efficacy of Early Intervention

The **efficacy** of early intervention is a very important topic. Professionals from a variety of academic disciplines are required to demonstrate the effectiveness of the services they provide. Is early intervention effective? This question must be answered by all involved in providing early intervention services, regardless of employment setting or the nature of services provided. Efficacy depends in large measure on two factors, each of which is important for the early interventionist to understand.

The first element in effective early intervention is the age at which the child's delay, or risk status, is detected. In other words, children who are recognized early as presenting confirmed developmental delay, or who are at risk of displaying later delay, do better than those who are identified at later ages. The bulk of this chapter presents issues that relate to established and at-risk principles for a variety of infants and toddlers. New populations of infants will emerge over time, and it is imperative that professionals, including speech–language pathologists, remain current relative to these new risk criteria. Ongoing familiarity with these matters can lower the age at which infants and toddlers with or at risk for developmental delay are recognized.

The second factor that significantly contributes to the effectiveness of early intervention services is the involvement of the parents/caregivers. Infants and toddlers whose parents are involved do better than those whose parents are uninvolved. Professionals working with at-risk children must do all that is possible to increase the likelihood that parents will feel fully involved in all early intervention activities (see Rossetti, 1995).

Early identification of children with established risk, and those at-risk, as well as increased caregiver involvement in early intervention, will serve to improve overall child outcome. The result will be that more children will be ready for kindergarten at the appropriate age. Recall that the single best predictor of school success is communication skills. Hence, communication-based intervention, whether provided primarily by the speech–language pathologist or another member of the early intervention team, must be the primary focus. Age-appropriate communication performance is the overall goal of infant-toddler intervention. Although other areas of developmental performance are important, school success depends heavily on effective communication skills.

SUMMARY

Effective early intervention begins with an enhanced ability to identify, as early as possible, those children in need of services. This cannot happen until all intervention providers become familiar with the concepts of established risk and at-risk. It is imperative that all early interventionists, including speech–language pathologists, remain current relative to advances in medical technology that will allow new populations of infants and toddlers to survive, thus increasing the incidence of at-risk children. Complete familiarity with established and at-risk factors, from both a biological and environmental standpoint, is never possible. Rather, the student should view the process as ongoing. Early intervention professionals must dedicate themselves to do all that is possible to improve the health and emotional status of these children, and their families. To do less is to lose sight of the significant positive effect that can result from early identification and intervention.

Major Points of Chapter

- There are differences between children who are at risk and those who have established risk factors for developmental communication problems.
- Numerous biological and environmental factors increase risk for developmental problems.
- A link exists between infant mortality and risk factors associated with developmental pathology.
- There are several new and expanding populations of at-risk infants including those born to teenage mothers, drug-exposed infants, and HIV+ infants.
- Children with early communication delay are at high risk for developing later learning problems.
- Early intervention is crucial for minimizing the effects of developmental delay.

Discussion Guidelines

1. List and give a brief description of the risk factors related to infant mortality. Discuss the implications of this list for an early intervention team.
2. Describe what is meant by the term "continuum of risk," and provide an explanation for each of the categories of risk in the chapter.
3. Teenage mothers and their children suffer from both short-term and long-term difficulties. Describe what these difficulties are, and

how they may be prevented or overcome. Present this information in a workshop format to your classmates.

REFERENCES

Aram, D., Hack, M., Hawkins, S., Weissman, B., & Clark, E. (1991). Very low-birthweight children and speech and language development. *Journal of Speech & Hearing Research, 34,* 1169.

Avery, M., & First, L. (1989). *Pediatric medicine.* Baltimore, MD: Williams and Wilkins.

Batshaw, M., & Perret, Y. (1992). *Children with disabilities: A medical primer.* Baltimore, MD: Brookes Publishing.

Bellman, A., Diamond, G., & Dickson, D. (1988). Pediatric acquired immunodeficiency syndrome: Neurological syndromes. *American Journal of Diseases of Children, 142,* 29.

Bergsma, D. (1979). *Birth defects compendium.* New York: Alan R. Liss.

Bhargava, S., Datta, I., & Kumari, S. (1982). A longitudinal study of language development in small-for-dates children from birth to five years. *Indian Pediatrics, 19,* 123.

Blackman, J. (1990). *Medical aspects of developmental disabilities in children birth to three.* Rockville, MD: Aspen.

Blackman, J. (1991). Neonatal intensive care: Is it worth it? *Pediatric Clinics of North America, 6,* 1479.

Brown, W., Thurman, K., & Pearl, L. (1993). *Family centered early intervention with infants and toddlers.* Baltimore, MD: Brookes Publishing.

Butler, C., Hittelman, J., & Hauger, S. (1991). Approach to neuro-developmental and neurologic complications in pediatric HIV infection. *Journal of Pediatrics, 119,* 41.

Byrne, J., Ellsworth, C., Bowering, E. & Vincer, M. (1993). Language development in low birthweight infants: The first two years of life. *Journal of Developmental and Behavioral Pediatrics, 14,* 21–27.

Capute, A., & Accardo, P. (1991). *Developmental disabilities in infancy and childhood.* Baltimore, MD: Brookes Publishing.

Castro, L., Azen, C., Hobel, C., and Platt, D. (1993). Maternal tobacco use and substance use: Reported prevalence rates and associations with delivery of small-for-gestational-age neonates. *Obstetrics and Gynecology, 81,* 396.

Centers for Disease Control. (1991). The HIV/AIDS epidemic: The first 10 years. *Journal of the American Medical Association, 265,* 3228.

Clark, D. (1989). Neonates and infants at risk for hearing and speech-language disorders. *Topics in Language Disorders, 10,* 1.

Cusson, R. (1992). Developmental outcome in high risk preterm infants throughout the first two years of life. *Neonatal Network, 11,* 69.

Edmondson, R. (1994). Drug use and pregnancy. In R. Simeonnson (Ed.), *Risk resilience and prevention: Promoting the well-being of all children.* Baltimore, MD: Brookes Publishing.

Eilers, B., Desai, N., Wilson, M., & Cunningham, D. (1986). Classroom performance and social factors of children with birth weights of 1,250 grams or less: Follow-up at 5 to 8 years of age. *Pediatrics, 77,* 203.

Escalona, S. (1982). Babies at double hazard: Early development of infants at biologic and social risk. *Pediatrics, 70,* 5.

Escobar, G., Littenberg, B., & Petitti, D. (1991). Outcome among surviving very low birthweight infants: A meta-analysis. *Archives of Disease in Children, 66,* 204–211.

Forslund, M., & Bjerre, I. (1985). Growth and development in preterm infants during the first 18 months. *Early Human Development, 10,* 201.

Frank, D., Zuckerman, B., and Amaro, H. (1989). Cocaine use during pregnancy: Prevalence and correlates. *Pediatrics, 82,* 888.

Gomby, D., and Shino, P. (1991). Estimating the number of substance-exposed infants. *The Future of Children, Drug Exposed Infants, 1,* 17.

Greenberg, M., & Crnic, K. (1988). Longitudinal predictors of developmental status and social interaction in premature and full-term infants at age two. *Child Development, 59,* 554.

Grunau, R., Kearney, S., & Whitfield, M. (1990). Language development at 3 years in pre-term children of birthweight below 1000g. *British Journal of Disorders of Communication, 25,* 173–182.

Gwinn, M., Pappaioanou, M., and George, J. (1991). Prevalence of HIV infection in women in the United States: Surveillance using newborn blood samples. *Journal of the American Medical Association, 265,* 1704.

Hack, M., Horbar, J., Malloy, M., Tyson, J., Wright, E., & Wright, L. (1991). Very low birth weight outcomes of the National Institute of Child Health and Human Development neonatal network. *Pediatrics, 87,* 587.

Hicks, B., and Wilson G. (Eds.). (1993). *Kids, crack and the community: Reclaiming drug-exposed infants and children.* National Education Service: Bloomington, IN.

Hogue, C., Buehler, J., Strauss, L., and Smith, C. (1987). Overview of the National Infant Mortality Surveillance (NIMS) project: Design, methods, results. *Journal of the U.S. Public Health Service, 102,* 126.

Hubatch. L., Johnson, C., Kistler, D., Burns, W., & Moneka, W., (1985). Early language abilities of high risk infants. *Journal of Speech & Hearing Disorders, 50,* 195.

Largo, R., Graf, S., Kundu, S., & Hunzicker, U. (1990). Predicting developmental outcome at school-age from infant tests of normal, at-risk, and retarded infants. *Developmental Medicine & Child Neurology, 32,* 30.

Largo, R., Molinari, L., Pinto, L., & Weber, M. (1986). Language development of term and preterm children during the first five years of life. *Developmental Medicine and Child Neurology, 28,* 333.

Long, W., Corbet, A., and Cotton, R. (1991). A controlled trial of synthetic surfactant in infants weighing 1550 grams or more with respiratory distress syndrome. *New England Journal of Medicine, 325,* 1696.

Macey, T., & Harmon, R. (1987). Impact of premature birth on the development of the infant in the family. *Journal of Consulting & Clinical Psychology, 55,* 846.

Manolson, A. (1992). *It takes two to talk.* Toronto: The Hanen Center.

Mason, J. (1991). Reducing infant mortality in the United States through "Healthy Start." *Public Health Reports,* 479.

McCormick, M., Brooks-Gunn, J., Workman-Daniels, K., Turner, J., & Peckham, G. (1992). The health and developmental status of very low birthweight children at school age. *Journal of the American Medical Association, 267,* 2204–2208.

National Center for Health Statistics. (1991). *Monthly Vital Statistics Report, 40,* 8.

Oberklaid, F., Sewell, J., Sanson, A., & Prior, M. (1991). Temperament and behavior of preterm infants: A six year follow-up. *Pediatrics, 87,* 854.

Ornstein, M., Ohlsson, A., Edmonds, J., & Asztalos, E. (1991). Neonatal follow-up of very low birthweight/extremely low birthweight infants to school age: A critical overview. *Acta Pediatrica Scandinavia, 80,* 741–748.

Papile, L. (1979). Cerebral intraventricular hemorrhage (CVH) in infants <1,500 grams: Developmental follow-up at one year. *Pediatric Research, 15,* 528.

Rossetti, L. (1990). *Infant toddler assessment: An interdisciplinary approach.* Austin, TX: Pro-Ed.

Rossetti, L. (1995). *Communication intervention: Birth to three.* San Diego: Singular Press.

Schraeder, B., Herverly, M., & Rappaport, J. (1990). Temperament, behavior problems, and learning skills in very low birth weight preschoolers. *Research in Nursing & Health, 13,* 27.

Schraeder, B., Rappaport, J., & Courtwright, L. (1987). Preschool development of very low birthweight infants. *Journal of Nursing Scholarship, 19,* 174.

Silva, P. (1987). Epidemiology, longitudinal course and some associated factors: An update. In W. Yale & M. Rutter (Eds.), *Language development and disorders* (pp. 1–15). Philadelphia: J. B. Lippincott.

Sugar, M. (1984). *Adolescent parenthood.* New York: S. P. Medical and Scientific Books.

U. S. General Accounting Office. (June 1990). *Drug exposed infants: A generation at risk.* (Report to the Chairman, Committee on Finance, US Senate). Washington, D.C.: U.S. Government Printing Office.

Vohr, B., Garcia-Coll, C., & Oh, W. (1988). Language development of low birthweight infants at 2 years. *Developmental Medicine & Child Neurology, 30,* 608–615.

Weitzman, E. (1992). *Learning language and loving it.* Toronto: The Hanen Center.

Williamson, D., Wilson, G., Ligschitz, M., & Thurber, S. (1990). Nonhandicapped very-low-birth-weight infants at one year of age: Developmental profile. *Pediatrics, 30,* 405.

Willie, D. (1991). Relation of preterm birth with quality of infant-mother attachment at one year. *Infant Behavior & Development, 14,* 227.

Wright, N. (1983). The speech & language development of low birth weight infants. *British Journal of Disorders of Communication, 18,* 187.

3

THE LIFELONG DEVELOPMENT OF COMMUNICATION SKILLS IN PEOPLE WITH MENTAL RETARDATION

ROBERT A. DOMINGO

What is mental retardation? The problem of defining retardation has generated an ongoing debate regarding the specific parameters to be included in the definition. At any given time, intelligence, social competence, biological bases, duration into adulthood, learning capacity and/or curability have each been factored into the definition. This should not be viewed as an impediment to the work of definition and classification of mental retardation, but rather as a reflection of a dynamic process that reassesses the ability of people to fit into an ever-changing world.

In 1959, a group of medical, psychological, therapeutic and educational professionals, collectively known as the *American Association on Mental Deficiency (AAMD)* pooled their resources to arrive at an acceptable definition of retardation. Since that time, the AAMD definition periodically has been revised to reflect current trends. A direct outcome of the ongoing work of this group to operationally define retardation has been an official name change. The group is currently known as the *American Association on Mental Retardation, or AAMR.* This shift in naming reflects a change in the way the Association has come to view the

population of mentally retarded persons more positively, and not as persons with "deficiencies."

In each of the revisions of the AAMR definition (1992), three key elements of the definition have remained consistent. These include: (1) low general intellectual functioning; (2) problems in adaptation; and (3) chronological age. In its present form, the definition of mental retardation maintains the language of these elements while emphasizing "abilities, environments, support networks and empowerments" (AAMR, 1992). According to the most recent AAMR position statement, "Mental retardation refers to substantial limitations in present functioning. It is characterized by significantly subaverage intellectual functioning, existing concurrently with related limitations in two or more of the following applicable adaptive skill areas: communication, self-care, home living, social skills, community use, self-direction, health and safety, functional academics, leisure, and work. Mental retardation manifests before age 18."

The change in perspective is reflected in the research on communication that has been conducted over the past two decades. Early research in the 1960s and 1970s focused predominantly on identifying either phonological or grammatical aspects of mentally retarded individuals' speech and language skills (Blount, 1968; Schiefelbusch, 1972). Current investigations, however, look to examine interactive abilities and the development of social skills and functional communication within more naturalistic contexts, such as residential, educational, and work settings (e.g., Linder, 1978; Anderson-Levitt & Platt, 1984; Warren & Kaiser, 1986; Kernan & Sabsay, 1987; Goetz & Sailor, 1988; Brinton & Fujiki, 1993).

This chapter begins with a synopsis of the prevalence of mental retardation in the United States, followed by discussion focusing on early detection, cognitive skills critical to learning, and the development of functional communicative skills in people with mental retardation across the lifespan. The speech–language pathologist's role as an integral member of the transdisciplinary team is also presented. "Traditional" teaching techniques based on principles of behavior management will be reexamined in light of their failure to create optimal environments for the development of functional communication skills. Finally, alternative approaches that optimize the acquisition of pragmatic language functions are discussed, as well as the community integration of people with retardation.

THE PREVALENCE OF MENTAL RETARDATION

Prevalence of retardation can be defined as the total number of retarded persons in a population divided by the total number of people in that population. Based on numerous studies, Mac-Millan (1982) concluded that the prevalence of mental retardation in the general population of America is less than 1 percent. He noted that mental retardation is not uniformly distributed throughout the population, but varies with age, IQ, sex, community, state, social class, and race. He also pointed out that despite scientific advances in discovering genetic and environmental causative factors, "in at least 75% of the cases of retarda-

tion, nothing can be confidently pinpointed as the cause of the condition" (p. 83).

The population of people with mental retardation in the United States can be categorized into two groups, based on IQ. The vast majority of cases, around 75 percent, fall into an IQ range of 50/55 to 70/75 (traditionally labeled *mildly retarded*), and consist largely of individuals from lower socioeconomic groups, with many from ethnic minorities. For the most part, this group appears to be neurologically "normal," in that they exhibit no easily detectable clinical or physical signs. These individuals typically are not diagnosed until they reach school age, at which time difficulties in learning abstract concepts set them apart from their peers without retardation. In the remaining 25 percent of the "clinically" mentally retarded cases (IQ scores of 50 to 55 and under, labeled *moderate, severe* or *profound*), some central nervous system pathology persists with associated physical handicap. This group is frequently diagnosed between birth and early childhood, when behavioral repertoire consists largely of reflexive responses to environmental stimuli. This population may exhibit intellectual and physical limitations resulting from major chromosomal anomalies or brain damage.

The use of labels to attribute status or level of disability to people with retardation has been practiced for some time. In 1876, the American Association for the Study of the Feeble-Minded, an ancestor of the present-day AAMR, referred to mild, moderate and severe-profound levels of retardation as *moron, imbecile,* and *idiot,* respectively. While these labels were initially employed as diagnostic categories, they have since degenerated into insults. Blatt (1985) argued that the use of labels often does more harm than good. He posited that people with mental retardation or learning disability actually became what the name implied by virtue of the professionally attached name. He further asserted that terms such as *MR, LD,* and *MI* (mental illness) are merely inventions; the only thing that makes a person "retarded" or "disabled" is the agency or official body designating that person as such.

The current practice of professionals in the field of developmental disabilities regarding labels is to put the person first. Thus, terms such as *adult with mental retardation* or *child with autism* are the preferred means of reference, as opposed to using *retarded* or *handicapped* as an adjective describing the individual.

EARLY IDENTIFICATION AND THE TRANSDISCIPLINARY APPROACH

Signs and symptoms of a child at risk for mental retardation can be identified by the child's primary care physician or pediatrician. (For detailed information on risk factors, see Chapter 2.) These include structural anomalies or dysmorphisms (body malformations that are associated with various syndromes), metabolic abnormalities, neurologic signs, and/or gross motor delays (Shapiro, Palmer, & Capute, 1987). Delays in early receptive and expressive language also help physicians in diagnosing developmental disabilities such as mental retardation or cerebral palsy within the first year of life (Farber, Shapiro, Palmer, & Capute, 1985).

In the absence of observable signs or symptoms that may accompany an adverse birthing situation, parents of children at risk may begin to notice delays in the development of speech, problems with toilet training, ambulation difficulties, and/or lack of ability to interact with others in a socially appropriate manner. Typically, these problems are of sufficient magnitude that parents will seek out explanations or medical guidance. Subsequent consultations with the pediatrician often help to confirm parental misgivings that something is not quite right. Allen, Rapin and Wiznitzer (1988) concurred that primary physicians play a crucial role in making early diagnoses and implementing remedial action and/or referral to the appropriate clinical specialists as soon as detection occurs.

In some cases, however, pediatricians may opt for a more conservative approach when making a diagnosis of a child with questionable developmental progress. In such cases it is often the allied developmental or habilitative specialists, such as a special education teacher, a speech–language pathologist or audiologist working with developmentally disabled children, who make the initial observation and recommendation to the parent that their child be seen by a physician for additional testing.

The need for a **transdisciplinary approach** in the identification and treatment of mental retardation must be present from the outset. As children with established risk or at risk are born and mature, they are entitled by law to develop to their potential in terms of physical, educational, psychological, mental, and emotional health in the least restrictive environment. Laws such as *PL 94–142*, the *Education for All Handicapped Children Act; PL 95–457*, the *Education for the Handicapped Act* (which includes children from ages birth to three); *PL 95–602*, the *Developmentally Disabled Assistance Act;* and *PL 101–476*, the *Individuals with Disabilities Education Act*, recognize the rights of disabled people to receive the same educational and habilitative treatment as their normally developing peers. Professionals from diverse disciplines must be prepared to play crucial roles to aid in the development of skills in persons with developmental disabilities: physicians, teachers, speech–language pathologists, audiologists, physical and occupational therapists, social workers, nutritionists, lawyers, and legislators. Specialists from these groups and the child's parents must function as a transdisciplinary team, working within their own specialty areas as well as contributing input across disciplinary lines to guarantee the rights of the disabled to develop to their potential. (See Chapter 14 for more information on transdisciplinary teams.)

MENTAL RETARDATION ACROSS THE LIFESPAN

Developmental specialists must strive to provide habilitative services to people with retardation throughout life—not only during childhood—but also through adolescence and later adulthood. By providing ongoing learning experiences, parents and educators help ensure the continuation of intellectual development throughout the years following early childhood, as children learn to adjust to a more complex world.

Falvey, Bishop, Grenot-Scheyer and Coots (1988) advocated long-term systematic planning and coordination between school and post–school programs for retarded adolescents. Functional academic and adaptive skills learned in the classroom should be maintained beyond the school environment, thus facilitating "continued acquisition of skills leading to increased integration of the individuals into the community" (p. 53).

Other researchers have concluded that **career education** programs for adults with mental retardation are needed to facilitate placement for those not easily or quickly transitioned into the community. The ultimate goal of this type of program is "independence." Knapczyk, Dever and Scibek (1982) defined independence as the ability to live one's life without having to depend on the assistance of social service agencies to make ordinary day-to-day decisions. Learning the necessary adaptive living skills to function within a community provides some adults with mental retardation with the capability to make it on their own.

The education of persons with mental retardation should neither be confined to academic endeavors nor discontinued when school ends. Rather, training should be considered an ongoing and dynamic process throughout the lives of persons with retardation. Ideally, intervention should consist of transdisciplinary training of real life skills that lead the individual to greater independence within the community.

MODELS OF LEARNING AND LANGUAGE ACQUISITION

Individuals with mental retardation are for the most part considered "slow" learners, though not all people with retardation operate at the same delayed rate of acquisition. The degree to which knowledge is attained depends on a number of factors, including (1) the degree of severity of retardation in the individual (mild-moderate-severe-profound); (2) the subject material being learned (concrete versus abstract task); (3) the

person or persons serving as instructor (parent, teacher, therapist); and (4) the extent to which the material being taught impacts on the person's ability to function in particular settings (functional outcome).

In considering how people with retardation learn, it is important to note that different types of material are best learned in different ways. While particular concrete skills (e.g., learning how to button a shirt) may be learned through repetition and practice, more abstract concepts (e.g., learning how to budget one's finances accordingly) may require active problem-solving and deductive reasoning in order to be acquired. Intervention must therefore focus on developing specific learning strategies that reflect the varied skills people with retardation will need to function in society.

Operant Behaviorism

Operant behaviorism, which stresses the role of environmental stimuli in eliciting an individual's response, appears to be the learning model of choice when teaching concrete tasks that can be readily sequenced (e.g., tying one's shoes or cooking a three-minute egg). In teaching such fundamental tasks, instructors provide an initial discriminative stimulus (i.e., a specific instruction or direction about the task at hand) that makes a desirable response more probable following that stimulus. When desirable or appropriate responses result from instruction, these responses need to be encouraged through positive reinforcement, which is the scheduled consequence for responding in a desired manner. In contrast, undesirable or inappropriate responses to stimuli elicit an opposite consequence or negative reinforcement. In addition, operant behavioral instruction uses contingencies that take into account the environmental setting. By controlling the setting, the stimuli, and the consequences (either positive or negative), instructors employing behavioral strategies attempt to shape the desired response. Thus, through operant conditioning, people with mental retardation are able to learn self-help skills; and/or have been able to terminate undesirable and self-destructive behaviors.

Cognitive–Developmental Theory

Cognitive theorists view learning in a somewhat different light. Rather than looking solely at the ability of individuals to respond to planned stimuli in order to effect changes in behavior, proponents of the **cognitive–developmental theory** view people (with or without retardation) as active participants in the learning process. Individuals are considered capable of performing higher-order mental processes that allow generalizations and inferences to occur during learning. In this approach, greater emphasis is placed on the environment as the means by which more self-directed learning can occur (e.g., learning the names of things and how they are used within the appropriate setting, such as the name and function of utensils or appliances while cooking in the kitchen). Thus, strategies based on cognitive theories (e.g., **Piagetian developmental theory;** Ginsburg & Opper, 1979) may be more useful in developing abstract ideational representations, such as the development of language, in persons with mental retardation.

According to Piagetian cognitive developmental theory, children must initially "map," or form mental representations of life's experiences in memory, in order to become efficient learners. Once accomplished, children must then assimilate or accommodate new life experiences and compare novel or new input with stored information. **Assimilation** refers to children's ability to adapt their growing perception of the world to their existing system. **Accommodation** refers to their ability to adapt existing mental structures to the reality they encounter every day. Both assimilation and accommodation operate simultaneously in every intellectual act to broaden existing mental structures. In addition, these processes force the individual to develop new mental structures when those that are present are not able to account for new experiences (Inhelder, 1968).

Weisz and Zigler (1979) reviewed a body of research that applied the Piagetian learning model to individuals with mental retardation. They concluded that mentally retarded individuals attained the same developmental stages as nonretarded persons, though in delayed fashion. Individuals' ability to advance through developmental levels is determined by the severity of retardation they demonstrate. In general, the more pronounced the retardation, the longer the time frame for acquisition of skills. Weisz and Zigler stressed the importance of providing people with retardation with environmental opportunities to interact with objects on a level commensurate with their stage of development. This kind of interaction allows cognitive skills to develop through active problem-solving strategies.

Language Acquisition

Other researchers have specifically considered the difficulties that children with and without retardation have with the acquisition of language. Snyder and McLean (1977) proposed that linguistic acquisition results largely from an interactive process that takes place externally between the child and the environment, and internally between the child's cognitive capacities and processes. Thus, children are seen as active participants who use information-gathering and information-processing strategies they have at their disposal, to make sense of incoming signals, and to formulate ideas and thoughts into expressible speech. For example, children first learning language *overextend* their vocabulary use and apply the same name to a variety of animals (e.g., "doggie" to name dogs, cats, sheep, and so on), because of the semantic features that members of the group share, such as four-leggedness. Adults assist in this active learning process by using questions or contingency responses that are tied to prior utterances made by the child (i.e., making corrections or modeling/ expanding the child's naming response when an overextension occurs). This model of language acquisition includes both linguistic and non-linguistic contexts, that is, the language and the environmental setting in which it occurs. In terms of this model, any difficulty that children with retardation have in acquiring language is attributed to specific process deficits they demonstrate in one or more of these three interactive strategies, including information-gathering, information-processing, and adult-directed facilitation.

Hamblin and Hamblin (1984) also considered the effects of linguistic and nonlinguistic variables on learning across different settings and different speakers with retardation. They examined the functioning of orphaned infants with retardation who were grouped together with adolescent children with retardation in the orphanage setting. Significant improvements in the functioning of the infants resulted from the increased interactions they had with the older children. The younger group also demonstrated faster language learning when certain nurturing staff members interacted with them at critical times during their infancy and early childhood.

Communication is considered both social and interactive in nature. Language develops in a naturalistic manner as speakers and listeners engage in topics that make sense in different settings (e.g., talking about food at mealtime or about what to buy while at the mall). These kinds of functional communicative interactions help people with retardation meet their environmental and social needs. Operant models may be useful in helping a person with retardation learn concrete tasks that can be easily broken down into component parts via a step-by-step task analysis. However, the ability to communicate with a variety of speakers across many contexts is a far more complex task to accomplish, and thus may not be attained within the scope of operant procedures. Strategies for facilitating the development of functional communication skills in people with retardation are more effective when based on cognitive learning models. These are the models of choice when the task to be learned is a social and interactive one.

THE DEVELOPMENT OF FUNCTIONAL COMMUNICATION SKILLS

The following section examines the development of **functional communication skills** in children and adults with developmental disabilities from the cognitive–developmental perspective. As noted, providing opportunities throughout life to learn functional skills through active problem-solving often involves the manipulation of linguistic and nonlinguistic variables within the environment, including the interlocutor and/or the setting. These factors operate in an integrative manner to foster the development of communication skills in persons with retardation (Domingo, 1994).

The Role of Mothers and Other Caregivers

Many studies have examined the influence of mothers and other early care providers in facilitating social and communicative skills in infants and preschoolers with developmental disabilities. These studies overwhelmingly support the early implementation of interactive learning models when a diagnosis is initially made of a child who is at risk for developmental problems. Early intervention strategies typically call upon parents and/or early care providers to serve as the "first line of defense" when it comes to interacting functionally or naturalistically with children with developmental disabilities.

Mothers and other caregivers tend to show sensitivity to the child's linguistic level, and employ simplified language when communicating with their young child. This practice of using age-appropriate vocabulary, simpler sentences, and more pronounced intonational patterns in language used with children is known as "motherese" (see Snow, 1972; 1977 for a detailed description of the term). Motherese has been found to play an important role in facilitating language development. This is true for both developmentally delayed and non-delayed children.

In the case of children with mental retardation, a link has been established between making substantial gains in the areas of cognition and receptive and expressive language, the age that early intervention began, the severity of the disorder, and the extent to which parents of high-risk infants interacted with their children in "normal" (i.e., naturalistic and functional) interactions (Maisto & German, 1979). Researchers, therefore, have emphasized the importance of the parent–child relationship in fostering intellectual and linguistic development of children with mental retardation (Rondal, 1980).

However, parents of children with disabilities are not always able to adopt an interactive style that matches the child's linguistic or cognitive limitations. In some cases, parents tend to be more directive and controlling in their communicative styles. This increased structure is not necessarily effective in obtaining compliance from children with disabilities (Lemanek, Stone, & Fishel, 1993). Handicapped children with disabilities whose parents tend to be highly structured and directive in their verbal interactions are less able to develop self-initiated communicative routines (Bailey & Slee, 1984).

Parents of children with developmental disabilities may operate under certain a priori assumptions regarding limitations in their children's learning potential. This may help explain why they often do not alter their speaking from a directive to a more facilitative style when presented with the opportunity. When limitations in parental speaking style based on preconceptions of their children's ability are noted, it must become the responsibility of the speech–language pathologist to model different ways of talking to children. They must help mothers and fathers of children with disabilities to develop different patterns of relating to their children that encourage communicative interactions. With observation and training, mothers and other caregivers may learn to rely less on direction-giving and work to foster active participation and linguistic growth in their children with special cognitive and communicative needs.

Parent Training

Several studies have concluded that a need exists for parent training, for those caregivers who are less than optimally prepared to deal with the range of problems that accompany developmentally disabled offspring. Parents may need to be taught how to provide optimal stimulation for their children at home, or to be prepared to seek services elsewhere when home resources are insufficient to address the child's various needs. Several different training techniques have been compared, to determine which are the most effective.

In one study (Feldman, Sparks, & Case, 1993), mothers with mental retardation were provided with appropriate instruction in how to work with high-risk infants. These mothers were provided with either interactive training (that included verbal instruction, modeling, feedback, and reinforcements designed to improve mother–child interactions and child verbalizations) or attention-control training (that included safety and emergency procedures). These groups were compared to one another in terms of how quickly their children began to communicate. Results indicated that speech emerged significantly sooner in the children whose mothers received interaction training, as compared to the control group of mothers who received attention-control training only.

Further, parents who received instruction on how to be facilitative with their preschool-aged children with developmental delays became more responsive, less directive, and provided clearer linguistic models than did parents of preschoolers who did not receive similar training. These positive changes were accompanied by concomitant increases in the children's use of vocal turns (Tannock, Girolametto, & Siegel, 1992).

Modeling techniques to teach children with retardation and their nonretarded parents new ways of interacting with one another were emphasized by Seitz and Hoekenga (1974). Modeling techniques included the use of lexical prompts to provide essential vocabulary items, **expansion** to elicit phrases and sentences of increased length, and redirection to the topic (all key elements of "motherese"). These techniques helped to facilitate an increase in the children's use of verbal communication.

Findings on parent training programs suggest that language intervention based on social interaction can be a useful adjunct to other intervention strategies in facilitating communication skills in children with retardation. In some cases, however, parents and early care providers may not possess the resources necessary to effectively carry out early intervention strategies at home. When conditions at home are inadequate to meet the cognitive and linguistic challenges of children with developmental disabilities, parents may need to consider special programs outside the home environment to address these developmental concerns.

Early Intervention Centers

Children who are enrolled in a child-centered prevention-oriented program have been shown to score consistently higher than children who remain at home (Ramey & Campbell, 1984; Ramey & Gowen, 1984). Language, cognitive, social, and perceptual–motor development are typically stressed in early intervention programs. Thus, these studies strongly support the need for early intervention in daycare settings.

As the early detection of children with developmental problems continues to improve (aided by advances in medical science and educational resources), a greater need emerges for securing appropriate services for preschool children as soon as a diagnosis is made. Parents of children with problems must realize that new rules now pertain. Merely talking to their at-risk child as they might to children without delays will not necessarily result in the same developmental or linguistic outcomes. In the interim, parents may need to seek help from habilitative specialists in the areas of parental training and home treatment. Further support in the form of an early intervention center may be warranted if at-home resources prove to be insufficient to the task.

Milieu Training

Investigations have also looked at how children with mental retardation learn to become effective communicators through formal instruction in individual and group therapy settings. Much research has been conducted in the areas of incidental teaching (Hart & Risley, 1968), the mand-model technique (Rogers-Warren & Warren, 1980), and the delay procedure (Halle, Baer, & Spradlin, 1981). Collectively referred to as **milieu training,** these naturalistic intervention strategies encompass the training of both *formal* (syntactic/morphologic) and *functional* aspects of language, by using "various prompting techniques, natural consequences, and some degree of environmental engineering" (Goetz & Sailor, 1988, p. 44) in informal contexts.

Incidental language teaching is defined as those interactions between adults and children that arise naturally in an unstructured situation, transmit new information, or give the child practice in developing communication skills (Warren & Kaiser, 1986). Since 1986, Warren and Kaiser and others have worked to develop and refine the incidental milieu training approach. For instance, Warren and Bambara (1989) investigated the syntactic and pragmatic effects of milieu language intervention to teach the action–object form (e.g., "drink milk") to children with moderate to borderline mental retardation (IQ range 40 to 90). Each child received three to four training sessions per week in a small group interactive play situation. Milieu training procedures were found to be useful in enhancing the children's acquisition and use of basic syntactic–semantic forms. It was also suggested that systematic adult commenting, spontaneous imitation, and child conversational scaffolding (Bruner, 1983) played significant roles in this teaching approach. **Scaffolding** refers to the adult practice of reducing linguistic input and instruction gradually as the child gains competence with the language construct being taught.

Milieu language training has also been employed to train individuals with mild mental retardation in the use of early relational (e.g., "more," "no") and substantive (e.g., "baby," "mommy") lexical forms (Warren & Gazdag, 1990), as well as in the acquisition and use of common nouns (e.g., names of food or toys) and action verbs (e.g., "eat," "drink," "play"). The research has demonstrated that not only do children show substantial increases in their productive use of words in the play training sessions, but 80 percent of the children generalized the use of common nouns and verbs into speaking contexts outside the training situation.

Recently, milieu training has been further modified and refined. Enhanced milieu teaching (EMT) is a "hybrid" naturalistic strategy that blends key aspects of milieu teaching with a responsive conversational style (Kaiser & Hester, 1994). It provides verbal models of language in a naturalistic and interactive setting. Kaiser and Hester examined the primary and generalized effects of EMT with preschool children with significant language delays and accompanying conditions of either autism, Down syndrome, cerebral palsy, developmental apraxia and/or general developmental delay. During training, the children systematically increased the frequency of targeted language skills (two to three word utterances incorporating the semantic notions of agent/action/object, e.g., "Boy eat cookie," "Mommy drive car"; or use of the present progressive morphological inflection, e.g., "playing," "cooking"). The children also maintained these newly learned skills once treatment was discontinued. In fact, the children were able to generalize use of trained language forms to different teachers, peers, and parents.

A major contribution to our current understanding of the development of functional language through naturalistic means has been realized through the work conducted in milieu or incidental teaching. Intervention strategies that focus on learning in real life situations encourage persons with developmental disabilities to achieve a level of communicative competence that serves their daily living needs.

FROM INSTITUTION TO INCLUSION

Jorgensen and Calculator (1994, p. 1) stated that an "evolution of best practices in educating students with severe disabilities" has been ongoing since the 1960s and 1970s when deinstitutionalization first began in the United States.

Historical Perspective

Over the past century, the care that has been provided to individuals with mental retardation has undergone major change. Gone are the days of massive institutionalization, in which people with disabilities were removed from mainstream society and given minimum provisions of food and shelter, provided they followed the rules. In such places, beatings, seclusion, and/or the withholding of the barest essentials were common forms of punishment for noncompliant behaviors (Scheer-

enberger, 1983). The chance of obtaining an education, or any form of training that could potentially serve to integrate the person into the outside world was unthinkable.

Laws such as PL 93-112, the *Rehabilitation Act,* and PL 101-336, the *Americans with Disabilities Act,* mandated humane treatment and civil rights for all disabled persons. In addition to having health and other custodial needs met, people with disabilities also obtained the right to educational training and rehabilitation under the improved legislative climate. These developments came about largely through the efforts of Wolfensberger (1972, 1974) and others, who argued that individuals with developmental disabilities should not be denied the opportunity to function within a deinstitutionalized or "normalized" environment. Thus, in order to guarantee that individuals with special needs experience success in the community, appropriate education for all is clearly mandated.

The passage in 1975 of the landmark *Education for All Handicapped Children Act, PL 94-142,* changed the way educators viewed the instructional needs of persons with mental retardation. Traditional views of teaching have expanded to keep pace with a growing awareness that, in order to succeed in the community, individuals need to possess more than a requisite academic background. They must also possess appropriate communication, social, domestic, financial, recreational, and self-preservational skills to exhibit functional independence. As a result of PL 94-142 and other laws, special education programs that exist today span a wide continuum. On the one hand, mainstream and/or integrated programs exist for those individuals with mild to moderate impairments: lessons and activities are conducted largely within nonhandicapped classrooms to enhance greater levels of learning, socially appropriate behavior, and independence for the special needs student. Other programs may consist of institutional or day treatment facilities for those with severe to profound cognitive and physical handicaps. In these settings, an educationally and clinically oriented program is conducted to facilitate basic skill maintenance. As

Das (1980, pp. 92–93) pointed out in response to the question of the kinds of skills schools should be teaching the child with mental retardation, "We want the child to grow up to be an individual who can plan, create, and make decisions . . . and to act in a manner that will preserve man's cultural gains and advance human civilization."

Inclusionary Model

Jorgensen and Calculator (1994) most strongly called for an instructional model based on full inclusion. Such a model challenges both special and regular classroom educators and administrators to reform existing educational curricula. In their model, *all students* with special needs should be included in *all* regular classroom curricular and social activities, without exception. The educational restructuring that they call for is consistent with the concept of "effective schooling" for all. *Effective schooling* is characterized by a number of key principles, including: (1) a curriculum driven by a small set of desired student outcomes; (2) teacher empowerment; (3) site-based management; (4) active involvement of students in the learning process; (5) increased reliance on collaboration among staff; (6) the use of coaching as the dominant teaching style; (7) the use of nontraditional evaluative processes; and (8) individualization in teaching methods based on students' learning styles and needs (Jorgensen & Calculator, 1994).

Implementation of these principles would significantly change the way classrooms are run. Traditional curricula for different grades and age groups would give way to individualized needs. Teachers would act on stated recommendations on-site without waiting for administrative clearance to enact such changes. Revisions in the way students are taught and evaluated would evolve, since formal educational assessments and teaching approaches that currently exist are biased against students with physical or mental impairments. Students themselves would be empowered to play a greater role in determining their own school agendas, assisting the teacher in determining an appropriate course of study based on individual needs and strengths.

Full inclusion has not been implemented in all settings across the country due to logistics, and perhaps a strong sense from the administrative and educational communities that this concept needs more careful consideration. The notion of full inclusion may have limitations. One principle concern is that the child without impairments might receive a poorer education, as the primary focus would be on the handicapped learner. This concern has kept many school districts in the "planning stage."

Mainstreaming in the Classroom

While full inclusion is not yet a reality, mainstreamed integrated classrooms are excellent settings that provide learning experiences to a heterogeneous student mix (i.e., students from different educational and/or functional levels who are grouped together). For the child with an impairment, the integrated class provides for the development of active problem-solving and increased socialization through incidental language instruction. For the child operating at a higher functioning level, the integrated class serves as an area where a nurturing attitude and interpersonal social skills can develop, as well as the ability to develop and display communicative competence.

Children with mental retardation, motor delays, or language impairments have been reported to exhibit steady increases in positive social interactions over time within an integrated setting (Beckman & Kohl, 1987). Interestingly, both the handicapped and nonhandicapped children engaged less in primitive mouthing responses and/or generalized play strategies, such as throwing or banging. These play findings reflect improved cognitive abilities across both groups. Thus, having a person in class with special needs appears to create greater opportunities for socialization to develop in the nonhandicapped children as well. The integrated classroom is a more socially stimulating and cognitively challenging place for children with and without preexisting conditions.

Integration has also been shown to benefit different levels of children with retardation who are brought together in the same classroom. Masters and Pine (1992) examined the influence of incidental language in both verbal and preverbal children with retardation. Following a six-week incidental language intervention program, all children demonstrated an increase in the use of verbal and gestural acts. The preverbal children made even greater gains than the verbal children, indicating that the verbal children provided the preverbal children with useful communicative models. Further, verbal children with retardation were provided with opportunities to display competence in the use of the language models they provided.

Thus, while the reality of inclusion may still be a long way off in terms of total implementation, the value of integrating different levels of students within a single classroom setting cannot be ignored. As the previous discussion suggests, benefits may be realized by all children within an integrated classroom, regardless of educational or functional background. More research into the inclusional model of education as it relates to the development of functional communication, socialization, and real life skills in children with and without developmental disabilities is necessary. This research will help determine what specific skills are needed to meet all children's environmental and communicative needs.

FUNCTIONAL COMMUNICATION AND AUGMENTATIVE STRATEGIES

The role that communication plays in classroom activities is very clear. However, not all people who are developmentally disabled possess either vocal or verbal abilities to convey messages. This can be a problem for the nonverbal person with physical, cognitive, or neurological problems who has something to say. Under this condition, it becomes the responsibility of speech–language pathologists to develop augmentative communication strategies that assist both nonverbal people and their significant others to communicate in a functional manner. The role that significant others play in making up a support network is very important. The support network helps to ensure success with an augmentative communication system.

According to Mirenda and Mathy-Laikko (1989), success with an augmentative communication system is contingent on a number of key factors, including: (1) the committment of family members and peers to provide life-long assistance to the person using augmentative communication; (2) the need for a well-coordinated transdisciplinary team approach to expedite the treatment of coexisting problems (see Chapter 14 for a detailed discussion of the transdisciplinary approach); and (3) information about augmentative communication options. These factors are significant in that their focus is not on the communicative limitations of the person with developmental disabilities per se, but rather on the **support network** of the potential augmentative communication user. This network includes family members, friends, and professionals who interact with the nonspeaker throughout life. Without a consideration of the network, any discussion of augmentative communication potential would be incomplete, since both givers and receivers of messages are necessary for communication to occur.

Aided Augmentative Communication Systems

Aided augmentative communication systems are defined as nonspeech systems that involve some device or picture display to aid the nonverbal user in communicative interactions. Electronic and/or homemade communication boards with or without voiced outputs are examples of aided nonspeech communication systems. Such nonspeech communication devices can only be as functional to the user as the displayed **lexigrams** (symbols/pictures) allow. Most likely, the individual who uses a nonspeech communication system possesses limited physical or cognitive capabilities. This person would therefore be unable to express a thought spontaneously unless a corresponding symbol or picture representing the idea was displayed. Careful consideration must be given to what pictures or symbols to include on an augmentative picture array. Space is usually limited, and should be utilized contingent on that user's particular needs. While concrete items (e.g., food or clothing preferences) are easily produced in picture form, more abstract ideas (e.g., concepts like beauty or frustration) are more difficult to depict, as such notions are subject to individual variation and opinion.

Adamson, Romski, Deffebach and Sevcik (1992) explored this issue of what picture or word choices to provide to nonspeech communication users. They found that as soon as certain social–regulative symbols were introduced into the computerized speech output devices of users with moderate to severe mental retardation and severe expressive language disabilities, users learned and began using the symbols in appropriate, functional ways. These symbols included words/phrases such as "please," "thank you," "I'm finished," and other social–regulative expressions. While nouns (pictures of people, places, and things) make up the majority of selections available to nonspeech communicators (given that they are the easiest to obtain and categorize), the authors opted for a more diverse vocabulary. This proved to be useful in facilitating increased social and regulative language functions.

Romski and Sevcik (1989) found that individuals with retardation exhibited patterns of acquisition that were similar to those of nonretarded children who first acquire a beginning vocabulary. That is, subjects with retardation exhibited symbol overextensions as they learned to use the symbols displayed on their respective picture boards. In one type of overextension, children used a lexigram to represent a related topic or idea for which there was no other symbol available (e.g., "apple" used in place of "knife"). Children also used lexigrams in place of related ones that were represented and available for their use (e.g., using "milk" in place of "glass"). Thus, symbols can function in the same way as words to represent thought.

Electronic devices have also been used to augment the educational skills of persons with retardation once they enter a school setting (Osguthorpe & Chang, 1988). Students from different day schools and residential facilities for multiple disabilities were provided with instruction on the use of computerized symbol processors, and their receptive and expressive language skills were

measured and compared against a control group of children who received classroom instruction only (without augmentative supports). Individuals who received augmentative training showed improvements in writing skills, as well as significantly better language comprehension scores and symbol recognition than those who received classroom instruction only. Students exhibited an overall positive attitude towards the technology, with the system appearing to be positively correlated with measures of self-esteem, socialization, and increased verbal output.

Abrahamsen, Romski and Sevcik (1989) also presented evidence that successful participation in an augmentative communication program can foster developmental changes that extend beyond the scope of the instruction being provided. They placed 10 matched pairs of individuals with severe mental retardation into either a lexigram condition in which instruction in the use of symbols was provided, or a control condition which provided the subject with social stimulation without lexigram training. Besides the fact that students learned symbol usage, individuals from the lexigram group also exhibited positive changes in their attention to task, intentional communication, and social ability. Students from the control condition acquired improved socialization skills, but exhibited no carryover into intentional communication or attentional ability.

Unaided Augmentative Communication Systems

Unaided augmentative communication systems are defined as those nonspeech systems that do not require any additional augmentative device other than the communicator in the conveying of messages. Sign language is an example of an unaided nonspeech communication system. Signing is sometimes used as an augmentative or alternative choice for persons with retardation who possess inadequate verbal skills and/or intelligibility. As Kiegsmann, Gallaher and Meyers (1982) pointed out, any decision to implement signing with severely language-delayed children must be contingent on the child's developmental, cognitive, and communicative abilities, as well as on the support network that is made up of the child's family and school environment. If care is not taken during the planning stages of therapy to include essential components that might contribute to the program's success, mismatches could occur. These mismatches between what the signer needs to know and what the trainer provides by way of instruction could lead to failure on the part of the child to learn necessary signs, and/or concomitant failure on the part of the support network to provide the appropriate therapeutic intervention for the child.

Bryen, Goldman, and Quinlisk-Gill (1988) pointed out that the decision to select signing as an intervention strategy in 12 different training facilities was not always based on a full consideration of prognostic factors that indicated its potential success as a therapy tool. They noted that despite the "common practice" of facilities to adopt a sign program, signing is not always an effective communicative alternative for school-aged students with severe–profound mental retardation.

For many individuals with developmental disabilities, however, manual communication is the most effective and appropriate nonspeech communication system. Gaines, Leaper, Monahan, and Weickgenant (1988), for example, reported that 21 children with autism and/or mental retardation were able to learn single-word or multiple-word phrases following a training period where a **total communication** (signed and spoken) program was conducted. Success for individual children was strongly correlated with several factors, including their gestural imitation abilities, playing style, language age, developmental age, and fine motor skills during the training period.

Further, Schuebel, and Lalli (1992) implemented a manual communication system with a 39-year-old male with retardation who had never before exhibited vocal communication. The researchers employed a modified incidental sign teaching approach, combining models, verbal prompts, physical guidance, positive reinforcement, and naturally occurring reinforcers within the client's daily environment. Results showed that the subject could use manual signs independently during structured interactions and could maintain his level of performance in subsequent evaluative sessions conducted at regular intervals.

The positive effects of employing either an aided augmentative communication system (e.g., electronic or homemade picture board) or unaided system (e.g., sign language) to assist in the acquisition of functional communication skills in nonverbal persons have been well documented. However, as noted above, great care must be exercised in selecting the appropriate system for an individual user. In addition, one must consider the effect that the selected system has in meeting the communicative needs of the nonverbal user across different settings and with different interactants. For additional readings in the areas of decision-making and the selection of nonspeech communication systems that constitute a "best fit" for individuals with developmental disabilities, the reader is referred to Musselwhite and St. Louis (1982), Calculator (1988), Beukelman and Mirenda (1992), or Silverman (1994).

COMMUNITY INTEGRATION AND ADULTS WITH MENTAL RETARDATION

With deinstitutionalization, a steady decline in the number of people with mental retardation residing in large, state-run facilities has been noted. A correspondingly steady increase has occurred in the number of these people living in the community and working in vocational training sites (ASHA, 1989). In short, there are more people with developmental disabilities living and working in local communities than ever before. In most cases, these people require ongoing counseling, vocational training, and assistance with real life skills to ensure their successful integration within the community.

Real Life Skills

As is evident in today's society, community success for people with developmental disabilities is not automatically guaranteed. It is predicated on a number of conditions that, if not met, often lead to reinstitutionalization or altered community placements for the individual who has difficulty in adjustment. Schalock, Harper, and Genung (1981) reported that successful residential placement was associated with appropriate sensorimotor and work skills, appropriate social–emotional behavior, gender, and family acceptance of the placement. Success in a residential placement was further associated with active involvement of the individual with the transdisciplinary team of habilitation specialists who are concerned with therapeutic issues. Success within a vocational or work setting was contingent on the person's language and psychomotor skills, education received prior to program placement, community and institution size, as well as family involvement.

If a person with retardation is not successful in a residential placement, it might be related to poor money management, apartment cleanliness, social behavior, and/or problems with meal preparation. Difficulties with vocational or work placement might be related to inappropriate behavior on the job or the need for additional training (Schalock & Harper, 1978).

Neville-Smith (1985) reported that a possible reason why young "intellectually retarded" adults had trouble adjusting into the community may have been that the "body movements of such subjects tend to be jerky and their posture tends to be wooden, while their speech itself can often be slurred and/or abrupt" (p. 559). The author suggested that these physical characteristics might have been perceived as hostile by members of the community in which people with retardation were being integrated, and so induced an unreasonable fear reaction.

Appropriate Communication in the Community

In addition to behavior, cleanliness, and work habits, a major factor contributing to successful tenure in a community residential or vocational setting is appropriate communication. As adults with mental retardation enter the community and integrate more completely into the fabric of society, their ability to communicate in a functional manner serves as a common denominator between themselves and other (nonretarded) citizens. As such, their **communicative competence** has been the subject of intense scrutiny over the past two decades, with studies focusing on a number of different fronts.

Rosenberg and Abbeduto (1993) provided an historical perspective by pointing out the failure of operant practices during the 1960s and 1970s to produce speech and language results that were generalizable from training sessions to more informal, conversational settings. They urged that increased efforts be made in pragmatics (language as it is used in natural situations), given the current climate in the community integration movement.

Goetz and Sailor (1988) called for a "new direction" in the training of functional communicative skills within more naturalistic surroundings. The new direction they suggested incorporates two distinct themes, both considered critical to functional language acquisition. They include: (1) the role of language context to encourage generalization and spontaneous language production; and (2) the role of language content to attain spontaneous and generalized language use.

Throughout the 1980s and continuing into the present, many studies of language context (settings in which language occurs and with whom) have been conducted. Some have examined locale (e.g., group homes, sheltered workshops, institutions), while others have looked at the roles that various interlocutors play (e.g., teachers, parents, children, or peers). In terms of content (what language consists of), the pragmatics of turn-taking, topic maintenance, speech acts, conversational control, and narrative discourse rules have been examined. In general, the studies of context and content have determined that speakers with retardation possess the necessary linguistic skills to achieve the communicative competence necessary for community integration. These skills enable them to "initiate and maintain social relationships, exchange information, negotiate misunderstandings, and direct the behavior of others" (Brinton & Fujiki, 1993, p. 10).

In 1979, Bedrosian found that the communicative intentions of topic initiations made by adults with retardation varied as a function of the speaker involved in the interaction. For example, some initiations made with peers (e.g., name calling) were not found in topic initiations made with parents, which reflected what the author called *appropriate adherence* to discourse rules, or knowing how and what to say to whom in given situations. Most initiations made with parents consisted of informatives (i.e., the giving of information), while more requests were used to initiate topics with peers. Based on these and later findings, Bedrosian (1993) pointed out that a careful analysis of topic difficulties in adult speakers with retardation could aid in the design of appropriate and effective intervention programs, such as the systematic manipulation of speaker or setting in context to elicit appropriate topic use, or content.

In a study of language style in people with mild to moderate retardation across community and institutional settings, Brinton and Fujiki (1993) found that the ability of community-based speakers with retardation to formulate utterances and make linguistic contributions that take a listener's perspective into account was a valued and useful tool that aided in community integration. These speakers' responsive (versus assertive) style constituted a more appropriate fit, given the social nature of conversational interactions. The community-based speakers asked fewer questions and were more appropriate in their responses to questions. Their conversational repairs evaluated the conversational needs of the listener more, and they spent less time on inappropriate topics. Institutionalized subjects, on the other hand, were more assertive and less responsive in their conversational dealings with others. More of their utterances consisted of inappropriate topics, and they provided fewer repairs that contained added information for the listener's benefit. These communicative limitations created greater adjustment problems for the institutionalized individuals, and made community integration more difficult.

The influence of the linguistic setting also determines how speech acts are formulated by adult speakers with retardation. Anderson-Levitt and Platt (1984) looked at language use in two recurrent social settings: dinnertime in a group home, and weekly discussion groups for adults in a sheltered workshop. The difference in language use between the two settings was attributed in part to the relative degree of seniority each participant possessed in the respective setting. In the residential setting, senior members used language to define who they were within the "pecking order," which allowed them to display a more superior attitude towards newer group members. Thus, the majority of speech acts found in this setting had to do with making announcements about chores, and challenging the announcements made by others.

In contrast, discussion groups held in the sheltered workshop were arenas where members of the group could work out their own personal problems with minimal staff intervention. Adults were provided a setting where they could enjoy respite from staff regulation and monitoring. The majority of speech acts found in this setting involved the statement of problems, attribution of blame, and occasional contesting of blame through use of challenges. Speakers with retardation in the workshop setting often formed alliances and banded together when blames or challenges were made, to solve problems or display solidarity.

Turn-taking was also examined by Anderson-Levitt and Platt (1984) in both settings. In the dinnertime context, turn overlaps were noted as group home residents vied for attention and interactional control. In contrast, turn-taking in the group meeting context was more often prearranged than spontaneous, i.e., not all turns were allocated through mutual negotiation in the course of the meeting. A number of systems for controlling the interaction and gaining the floor applied, such as members of the group "reserving" a future turn to talk, prearranging among themselves who would take turns to talk (and/or who would serve as the "representative" speaker); the use of "announcements" to gain the conversational floor; or gaining entrance to talk in a manner consistent with that found in normal discourse, i.e., by stepping in at the appropriate time while making reference to the prior speaker's topic.

A natural extension of this work on the communicative skills of adults with mental retardation is an examination of the communicative competence found in a more elderly retarded population. Current advances in medical technology lengthen life expectancy. Consequently, any "lifespan" discussion would be incomplete without mention of the language of senior citizens with mental retardation. Fujiki and Brinton (1993) compared groups of young and elderly subjects with retardation to determine how the groups would function on certain cognitive and social tasks. The young group consisted of 20 adults with retardation between the ages of 20 and 36, while the elderly group consisted of 20 adults between the ages of 55 and 77. All individuals resided within community-based settings. For the most part, both age groups performed comparably on tasks that required cognitive resources (e.g., memory) in the recollection of either lists of facts or details from stories. On social interactional tasks, the elderly adults were better able to respond to listener feedback and were more assertive in controlling aspects of the conversation than the younger individuals. Fujiki and Brinton suggested that the older adults may comprise a group of survivors whose long histories with institutionalization and lack of formal education helped to form them into robust individuals with the capacity to overcome many odds. Future research is needed to determine whether this hardiness of character will also be represented in the next generation of adults as they age.

Problems in Communicative Design

From the above discussion it is clear that people with retardation are competent in their language use across contextual and content boundaries. However, the fact remains that many speakers with retardation often bring attention to themselves through the inappropriate use of speech and language, and so are stigmatized (Edgerton, 1967) as a result. This remains true despite their reported skill in communicative function. A common observation made by nonretarded people who have conversed with a person with retardation is that something appears to be "not quite right" with the interaction. While persons with retardation are shown to be competent communicators (as the above studies suggest), their consistency in employing adequate skills may be called into question. Their ultimate success with communication may be predicated on a number of variables, such as: (1) their ability to demonstrate background knowledge; (2) their knowledge of discourse rules; (3) their ability to self-regulate during conversations; as well as (4) preconceived notions of competence or inadequacy.

Sabsay and Kernan (1983) observed that adults with retardation exhibited limitations in **communicative design,** or the ability to take into account the informational needs of the listeners in order to construct a meaningful dialogue. Speakers with mild-to-moderate retardation at times failed to take aspects of the total speech situation into account, such as the linguistic, social, and interpersonal setting. In so doing, these speakers failed to utilize the rules of speaking that pertain in given situations (e.g., speaking softly in a restaurant, or not speaking about personal or hygienic concerns to strangers).

Problems have also been noted in **discourse** abilities. Speakers with retardation sometimes begin to say something then change their minds about the narrative's form and start over again; or, they change what they initially started talking about rather than rephrase the original narrative (Kernan & Sabsay, 1982). These individuals demonstrated a lack of cohesion between sentences and inappropriate use of cohesive devices (e.g., personal pronouns or conjunctions) that create coherent dialogue. Conversations thus appear disjointed or discontinuous; ideas expressed in one sentence are not related to subsequent mentions of the same idea in later discourse (Halliday & Hasan, 1976).

Learned Helplessness

Despite these reported limitations, it has been noted that speakers with retardation have an existing underlying ability to sometimes perform communicative design, depending on the situation (Sabsay & Kernan, 1983; Abbeduto, 1991; Abbeduto & Rosenberg, 1992). Their inconsistency in doing so at all times may be due to the necessity for some form of external guidance. This structured guidance is provided in the form of some nonretarded speaker who helps to monitor and regulate the construction and flow of information for the retarded speaker in speaking contexts. Sabasay and Kernan reported that it is fairly easy to take over and control an interaction that involves a person with retardation. It is also a fairly common phenomenon that occurs throughout the life of the retarded person.

Edgerton (1967) referred to this reliance on others to help as *learned helplessness,* a notion that depicts persons who are retarded as dependent and passively compliant members of society. Edgerton found that people with retardation often managed their verbal routines by relying on other-regulatory (or what he called *compensatory*) devices in interactions with nonretarded speakers. For example, his observations showed that the adults who were recently released from an institution spoke as minimally as possible, to control for possible misunderstandings that they felt might occur between themselves and others in the community.

Linder (1978) also examined the notions of passivity and dependence on other-regulation, but from the nonretarded speaker's point of view. He claimed that nonretarded speakers held preconceived assumptions about the incompetence of speakers with retardation. Nonretarded speakers felt that people with retardation were unable to carry out conversations adequately. They also mentioned their need to manage the conversations they had with retarded speakers in order to minimize perceived differences between them. Nonretarded speakers therefore chose to speak of mundane topics that were of little interest to either party, used repetitive questions and reformulations, and employed simple syntactic constructions. Ironically, in their attempt to avoid potential mismatches between conversational partners, the nonretarded speakers managed only to highlight differences between themselves and speakers with retardation through their simplification of language.

Community integration requires a variety of real life skills, including money management, meal preparation, appropriate social–emotional behavior, and communicative competence. With respect to communication, much research has been conducted in the pragmatics of language, to ensure that individuals with retardation are given the opportunity to acquire functional communication skills in naturalistic settings. Studies of the context and content of language have indicated that, while speakers with retardation rely to some degree on the influence of others to monitor and regulate conversations for them, they also are able in a variety of situations to independently exhibit communicative competence. As the move to deinstitutionalize people from large residential facilities continues, and as community integration efforts continue to grow, the identification and development of skills that are needed for people with retardation to succeed continue to be of primary importance.

SUMMARY

Over the last twenty years, an information explosion has occurred that has changed the way we look at and treat people with developmental disabilities. For one thing, laws now mandate that people with developmental disabilities (including mental retardation, learning disabilities, cerebral palsy, and autism) are entitled to the same rights and privileges as all others in society. These include the right to live and work in the mainstream, and to enjoy all the comforts that society can provide.

A major focus of the current work in developmental disabilities is in the area of facilitating communicative competence across the life span. The number of people with disabilities being integrated into the community continues to grow each year. It becomes increasingly important for professionals to work in a transdisciplinary manner to establish appropriate guidelines that will foster the development of real life skills and functional communication for these individuals.

Facilitation of functional communication in a naturalistic setting includes both linguistic (i.e., content) and nonlinguistic (i.e., context) aspects of the language. Parents, teachers, speech–language pathologists, and others concerned with the communication skills of people with developmental disabilities must strive to create an environment (at home, in school, at work, in the park, at the store) where language is central to, and a natural outcome of, ongoing daily events. Words, signs, pictures, or symbols need not be spoken, gestured, or pointed to for the sake of naming or for the appeasement of the parent, teacher, or speech–language pathologist who is concerned with attaining some quantitative measure of success. Rather, the use of verbal or nonverbal symbols should be reserved for those times when a person needs to communicate an essential thought or re quest, like giving the punchline to a joke or requesting a tissue or a second slice of pizza.

The speech–language pathologist plays a central role in fostering the development of functional communication skills throughout the lifespan of persons with retardation. Through early detection and assessment, the speech–language pathologist provides valuable information to parents and pediatricians regarding the course of normal cognitive and prelinguistic development, and indicates when and if an infant may be at risk for developmental language delays. During preschool and school-age periods, the speech–language pathologist serves as an essential classroom resource and provides information on phonologic, morphologic, syntactic, semantic, and pragmatic aspects of language development that should occur at certain times in a child's life. Later, as the individual with developmental disabilities matures into adulthood, the speech–language pathologist provides input to maximize communication in different settings, and with different interlocutors, to ensure the integration of the adult into residential or vocational placements.

As progress in early intervention, educational inclusion, and community integration continues, speech–language pathologists and others within the transdisciplinary support network must extend their professional expertise to people of all ages with developmental disabilities. Success in the area of functional communication development is a critical component of the education and health of individuals with mental retardation.

Major Points of Chapter

- Changes in the definition of mental retardation reflect society's changing attitudes towards people with mental retardation.
- The communication abilities of people with mental retardation are presently viewed from a sociocultural framework rather than a strictly linguistic one.
- A transdisciplinary approach to mental retardation provides an optimal environment to support communicative and social development across the entire lifespan.
- Community integration beyond the school age years is the ultimate goal of transdisciplinary treatment.
- The clinical utility of operant learning models is contrasted with cognitive learning theory in the development of communication.
- Functional communication is often facilitated in naturalistic communication settings.

Discussion Guidelines

1. Discuss what is meant by "inclusion" from the perspective of a classroom teacher who must accommodate a variety of different skill levels into a common curriculum. How does the concept of inclusion differ from mainstreaming?

2. Describe why operant conditioning as a training methodology fails to foster the development of pragmatic communication skills in people with developmental disabilities. Contrast operant conditioning with an interactive problem-solving approach to teaching those with mental retardation.

REFERENCES

Abbeduto, L. (1991). The development of linguistic communication in persons with mild to moderate mental retardation. In N. Bray (Ed.), *International Review of Research in Mental Retardation.* New York: Academic Press.

Abbeduto, L. & Rosenberg, S. (1992). The development of linguistic communication in persons with mental retardation. In S. Warren & J. Reichle (Eds.), *Perspectives on Communication and Language Intervention.* Baltimore, MD: Brookes Publishing.

Abrahamsen, A., Romski, M., & Sevcik, R. (1989). Concomitants of success in acquiring an augmentative communication system: Changes in attention, communication and sociability. *American Journal on Mental Retardation, 93*(5), 475–496.

Adamson, L., Romski, M., Deffebach, K., & Sevcik, R. (1992). Symbol vocabulary and the focus of conversations: Augmenting language development for youth with mental retardation. *Journal of Speech and Hearing Research, 35,* 1333–1343.

Allen, D., Rapin, I., & Wiznitzer, M. (1988). Communication disorders of preschool children: The physician's responsibility. *Journal of Developmental and Behavioral Pediatrics, 9*(3), 164–170.

AAMR: American Association on Mental Retardation (1992). *Mental Retardation: Definition, Classification, and Systems of Supports* (9th ed.). Annapolis Junction, MD: AAMR Publications Ctr.

ASHA: American Speech–Language–Hearing Association, Committee on Mental Retardation and Developmental Disabilities (1989). Deinstitutionalization: Its effect on the delivery of speech–language–hearing services for persons with mental retardation and developmental disabilities. *ASHA, 31,* 84–87.

Anderson-Levitt, K., & Platt, M. (1984). The speech of mentally retarded adults in contrastive settings, *Working Paper No. 28.* Socio-Behavioral Group, Mental Retardation Research Center, University of California, Los Angeles.

Bailey, L., & Slee, P. (1984). A comparison of play interactions between non-disabled and disabled children and their mothers: A question of style. *Australia and New Zealand Journal of Developmental Disabilities, 10*(1), 5–10.

Beckman, P., & Kohl, F. (1987). Interactions of preschoolers with and without handicaps in integrated and segregated settings: A longitudinal study. *Mental Retardation, 25*(1), 5–11.

Bedrosian, J. (1979). *Communicative performance of mentally retarded adults: A topic analysis.* Paper presented at the American Association on Mental Deficiency Annual Convention, Miami Beach, Florida.

Bedrosian, J. (1993). Making minds meet: Assessment of conversational topic in adults with mild to moderate mental retardation. *Topics in Language Disorders, 13*(3), 36–46.

Blatt, B. (1985). The implications of the language of mental retardation for LD. *Journal of Learning Disabilities, 18*(10), 625–626.

Blount, W. (1968). Language and the more severely retarded: A review. *American Journal of Mental Deficiency, 1,* 21–29.

Brinton, B., & Fujiki, M. (1993). Communication skills and community integration in adults with mild to moderate retardation. *Topics in Language Disorders, 13*(3), 9–19.

Bruner, J. (1983). *Child's talk: Learning to use language.* New York: W.W. Norton.

Bryen, D., Goldman, A., & Quinlisk-Gill, S. (1988). Sign language with students with severe/profound mental retardation: How effective is it? *Education and Training in Mental Retardation, 23*(2), 129–137.

Buekelman, D., & Mirenda, P. (1992). *Augmentative and alternative communication: Management of severe communication disorders in children and adults.* Baltimore, MD: Brookes Publishing.

Calculator, S. (1988). Teaching functional skills in nonspeaking adults with mental retardation. In S. Calculator & J. Bedrosian (Eds.), *Communication assessment and intervention for adults with mental retardation.* Boston, MA: College-Hill Press.

Das, J. (1980). On cognitive competence and incompetence: A cross-cultural perspective. *Mental Retardation Bulletin, 8*(2), 81–95.

Domingo, R. (1994). The expression of pragmatic intentions in adults with mental retardation during instructional discourse. In R. Bloom, L. Obler, S. DeSanti & J. Ehrlich (Eds.), *Discourse analysis and applications: Studies in adult clinical populations.* Hillsdale, NJ: Lawrence Erlbaum Associates.

Edgerton, R. (1967). *The cloak of competence: Stigma in the lives of the retarded.* Berkeley, CA: University of California Press.

Falvey, M., Bishop, K., Grenot-Scheyer, M., & Coots, J. (1988). Issues and trends in mental retardation. In S. Calculator & J. Bedrosian (Eds.), *Communication assessment and intervention for adults with mental retardation.* Boston, MA: College-Hill Press.

Farber, J., Shapiro, B., Palmer, F., & Capute, A. (1985). The diagnostic value of the neurodevelopmental examination, *Clinical Pediatrics, 24*(7), 367–372.

Feldman, M., Sparks, B., & Case, L. (1993). Effectiveness of home-based early intervention on the language development of children of mothers with mental retardation. *Research in Developmental Disabilities. 14*(5), 387–408.

Fujiki, M., & Brinton, B. (1993). Growing old with retardation: The language of survivors. *Topics in Language Disorders, 13*(3), 77–89.

Gaines, R., Leaper, C., Monahan, C., & Weickgenant, A. (1988). Language learning and retention in young language-disordered children. *Journal of Autism and Developmental Disabilities, 18*(2), 281–296.

Ginsberg, H., & Opper, S. (1979). *Piaget's theory of intellectual development* (2nd ed.). Englewood Cliffs, NJ: Prentice-Hall.

Goetz, L., & Sailor, W. (1988). New directions: Communication development in persons with severe disabilities. *Topics in Language Disorders, 8*(4), 41–54.

Halle, J., Baer, D., & Spradlin, J. (1981). An analysis of teacher's generalized use of delay in helping children: A stimulus control procedure to increase language use in handicapped children. *Journal of Applied Behavior Analysis, 14*, 389–409.

Halliday, M., & Hasan, R. (1976). *Cohesion in English.* London: Longman Publishing.

Hamblin, R., & Hamblin, J. (1984). Language acquisition and intelligence: Experimentally effective strategies. *Acta Paedologica, 1*(1), 1–22.

Hart, B., & Risley, T. (1968). Establishing use of descriptive adjectives in the spontaneous speech of disadvantaged preschool children. *Journal of Applied Behavior Analysis, 8*, 411–420.

Inhelder, B. (1968). *The diagnosis of reasoning in the mentally retarded.* New York: John Day Publishing.

Jorgensen, C., & Calculator, S. (1994). The evolution of best practices in educating students with severe disabilities. In S. Calculator & C. Jorgensen (Eds.), *Including students with severe disabilities in schools: Fostering communication, interaction, and participation.* San Diego, CA: Singular Publishing Group.

Kaiser, A., & Hester, P. (1994). Generalized effects of enhanced milieu teaching. *Journal of Speech and Hearing Research, 37*(6), 1320–1340.

Kernan, K., & Sabsay, S. (1982). Semantic deficiencies in the narratives of mildly retarded speakers. *Semiotica, 42*, 169–193.

Kernan, K., & Sabsay, S. (1984). Getting there: Directions given by mildly retarded and nonretarded adults. In R. Edgerton (Ed.), *Lives in Process: Mildly Retarded Adults in a Large City.* Washington, DC: AAMD Monograph, No. 6.

Kernan, K., & Sabsay, S. (1987). Referential first mention in narratives by mildly retarded adults. *Research in Developmental Disabilities, 8*, 361–370.

Kiegsmann, E., Gallaher, J. & Meyers, A. (1982). Sign programs with nonverbal hearing children. *Exceptional Children, 48*(5), 436–445.

Knapczyk, D., Dever, R., & Scibak, J. (1982). Career education for institutionalized severely handicapped persons. In A. Fink & C. Kokaska (Eds.), *Career education for the behaviorally disordered.* Council on Exceptional Children (CEC) Monograph.

Lemanek, K., Stone, W., & Fishel, P. (1993). Parent-child interactions in handicapped preschoolers: The relation between parent behaviors and compliance. *Journal of Clinical Child Psychology, 22*(1), 68–77.

Linder, S. (1978). The perception and management of "trouble" in "normal-retardate" conversations. *Working Papers No. 5.* Socio-Behavioral Group, Mental Retardation Research Center, University of California, Los Angeles.

MacMillan, D. (1982). *Mental retardation in school and society* (2nd ed.). Toronto: Little, Brown and Co.

Maisto, A., & German, M. (1979). Variables related to progress in a parent training program for high-risk infants. *Journal of Pediatric Psychology, 4*(4), 409–419.

Masters, J., & Pine, S. (1992). Incidental group language therapy: Verbal and preverbal children. *Child Language Teaching and Therapy, 8*(1), 18–29.

Mirenda, P., & Mathy-Laikko, P. (1989). Augmentative and alternative communication applications for persons with severe congenital communication disorders: An introduction. *Augmentative and Alternative Communication, 5*(1), 3–13.

Musselwhite, C., & St. Louis, K. (Eds.), (1982). *Communication programming for the severely handicapped: Vocal and non-vocal strategies.* San Diego, CA: College-Hill Press.

Neville-Smith, C. (1985). Young intellectually retarded adults. *British Journal of Psychiatry, 146,* 559.

Osguthorpe, R., & Chang, L. (1988). The effects of computerized symbol processor instruction on the communication skills of nonspeaking students. *Augmentative and Alternative Communication, 4*(1), 23–34.

Ramey, C., & Campbell, F. (1984). Preventive education for high-risk children: Cognitive consequences of the Carolina Abecedarian Project. *American Journal of Mental Deficiency, 88*(5), 515–523.

Ramey, C., & Gowen, J. (1984). A general systems approach to modifying risk for retarded development. *Early Child Development and Care, 16,* 9–26.

Rogers-Warren, A., & Warren, S. (1980). Mands for verbalization: Facilitating the display of newly trained language in children. *Behavior Modification, 4,* 361–382.

Romski, M., & Sevcik, R. (1989). An analysis of visual-graphic symbol meanings for two nonspeaking adults with severe mental retardation. *Augmentative and Alternative Communication, 5*(2), 109–114.

Rondal, J. (1977). Maternal linguistic environment and mental retardation. *Enfance, 1*(1), 37–48.

Rondal, J. (1980). The interactive point of view in language development, disorders, and intervention. *Psychologica Belgica, 20*(2), 185–204.

Rosenberg, S., & Abbeduto, L. (1993). *Language and communication in mental retardation: Development, processes, and intervention.* Hillsdale, NJ: Lawrence Erlbaum Associates.

Sabsay, S. (1979). *Communicative competence in Down's syndrome adults.* Unpublished doctoral dissertation, University of California, Los Angeles.

Sabsay, S., & Kernan, K. (1983). Communicative design in the speech of mildly retarded adults. In K. Kernan, M. Begab & R. Edgerton (Eds.), *Environments and behavior: The adaptation of mentally retarded persons.* Baltimore, MD: University Park Press.

Schalock, R., & Harper, R. (1978). Placement from community-based mental retardation programs: How well do clients do? *American Journal of Mental Deficiency, 83*(3), 240–247.

Schalock, R., Harper, R., & Genung, T. (1981). Community integration of mentally retarded adults: Community placement and program success. *American Journal of Mental Deficiency, 85*(5), 478–488.

Scheerenberger, R. (1983). *A history of mental retardation.* Baltimore, MD: Brookes Publishing.

Schiefelbusch, R. (Ed.). (1972). *Language of the mentally retarded.* Baltimore, MD: University Park Press.

Schuebel, C., & Lalli, J. (1992). A program for increasing manual signing by a nonvocal adult within a daily environment. *Behavioral Residential Treatment, 7*(4), 277–282.

Seitz, S., & Hoekenga, R. (1974). Modeling as a training tool for retarded children and their parents. *Mental Retardation, 12*(2), 28–31.

Shapiro, B., Palmer, F., & Capute, A. (1987). The early detection of mental retardation. *Clinical Pediatrics, 26,* 215–220.

Silverman, F. (1994). *Communication for the speechless* (2nd ed.). Englewood Cliffs, NJ: Prentice-Hall.

Snow, C. (1972). Mother's speech to children learning language. *Child Development, 43,* 549–565.

Snow, C. (1977). The development of conversations between mothers and babies. *Journal of Child Language, 4,* 1–22.

Snyder, L., & McLean, J. (1977). Deficient acquisition strategies: A proposed conceptual framework for analyzing severe language deficiency. *American Journal of Mental Deficiency, 81*(4), 338–349.

Tannock, R., Girolametto, L., & Siegel, L. (1992). Language intervention with children who have developmental delays: Effects of an interactive approach. *American Journal on Mental Retardation, 97*(2), 145–160.

Warren, S., & Bambara, L. (1989). An experimental analysis of milieu language intervention: Teaching the action-object form. *Journal of Speech and Hearing Disorders, 54*(3), 448–461.

Warren, S., & Gazdag, G. (1990). Facilitating early language development with milieu intervention procedures. *Journal of Early Intervention, 14*(1), 62–86.

Warren, S., & Kaiser, A. (1986). Incidental language teaching: A critical review. *Journal of Speech and Hearing Disorders, 51*(4), 291–299.

Weisz, J., & Zigler, E. (1979). Cognitive development in retarded and nonretarded persons: Piagetian tests of the similar sequence hypothesis. *Psychological Bulletin, 86,* 831–851.

Wolfensberger, W. (1972). *The principle of normalization in human services.* Toronto: National Institute on Mental Retardation.

Wolfensberger, W. (1974). Social role valorization: A proposed new term for the principle of normalization. *Mental Retardation, 21,* 234–239.

4

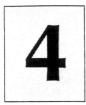

COMMUNICATION BEHAVIORS ASSOCIATED WITH PSYCHIATRIC DISORDERS

CHRISTINE A. M. BALTAXE

Communication specialists as well as mental health professionals are only now beginning to become more sensitized to the unusually close association between communication disorders and psychiatric disorders. This growing awareness is largely due to a number of large scale studies over the past decade that have shown that children and adolescents with communication disorders are at serious risk for psychiatric disorder (Beitchman, Nair, Clegg, Ferguson, & Patel, 1986a, 1986b; Beitchman, Peterson, & Clegg, 1988; Beitchman, Hood, Rochon, & Peterson, 1989a, 1989b; Cantwell & Baker, 1977, 1985, 1987a, 1987b, 1991a; Cantwell, Baker, & Mattison, 1979, 1980). From these studies, it is estimated that at least 50 percent of children and adolescents with a primary diagnosis of a communication disorder will also have diagnosable emotional, behavioral, or other psychiatric disorders. In other words, one-half of the children seen for speech–language diagnosis will also have a psychiatric disorder.

Communication problems of equal or even greater magnitude have also been identified in several recent studies where the primary diagnosis was a psychiatric disorder, with prevalences ranging from 24 to 93 percent (Baltaxe & Simmons, 1988a, 1990, 1992a; Camarata, Hughes, & Ruhl, 1988; Chess & Rosenberg, 1974; Cohen,

Davine, Horodesky, Lipsett, & Isaacson, 1993; Grinnell, Scott-Hartnett, & Larson-Glasier, 1983; Gualtieri, Koriath, Von Bourgondien, & Saleeby, 1983; Trautman, Giddan, & Jurs, 1990). These studies show that deficits in language are pervasive, while speech difficulties play a minor role. Earlier, small scale studies and case reports had suggested a relationship between communication disorders and psychiatric disorders (Affolder, Brubaker, & Bischofberger, 1974; Fundudis, Kolvin, & Garside, 1979; Solomon, 1961; Stevenson & Richman, 1976, 1978). This association between language and speech disorders and psychiatric disorders is far greater than would be expected from estimates of prevalence for childhood speech and language disorders in the general population, which range from less than 1 percent to more than 33 percent for speech, and from 1 percent to 17 percent for language. (For reviews see Beitchman et al., 1986a; and Cantwell & Baker, 1977, 1991a.) Nevertheless, communication impairment in psychiatrically ill youngsters and psychiatric disability in communication handicapped youngsters often goes unrecognized (Alessi & Loomis, 1990; Cohen et al., 1993; Love & Thompson, 1988).

When a child has a communication handicap and a psychiatric disorder, both disorders require

51

attention and intervention. It is clear that cooperation and the exchange of information between the treating mental health professional and the treating communication disorders specialist benefit the child not only with respect to diagnostic identification, but also with respect to optimal intervention for both disorders. The coexistence of communication handicaps and psychiatric disorders underscores the need for interdisciplinary and transdisciplinary training and cooperation between mental health professionals and speech–language pathologists. It also calls for at least a rudimentary understanding of each discipline's realm of knowledge and tools of trade by members of the other discipline. Clinical experience has shown that the diagnosis and treatment of one or both types of disorders in a child will depend on referral patterns, that is, what type of services are sought first—speech–language services or medical or psychiatric services. But it will also depend on the training and sophistication of the professionals involved in evaluating and treating the child, as well as the existing biases of the discipline first consulted. Ignoring the psychiatric disorder or the communication disorder in treatment could have far-reaching negative consequences, such as an impact on the child's self-concept, school achievement, and interpersonal relations, as well as the regulation of behavior. Because of the possible interactive consequences of these two disorders on each other, nontreatment could also contribute to the development, persistence, or worsening of one or both conditions (Baker & Cantwell, 1987a, 1987b; Prizant, Audet, Burke, Hummel, Maher, & Theodore, 1990).

Major psychiatric disorders and communication handicaps often last a long time, and may be lifelong. However, when children with such disorders begin treatment early, their skills and abilities, and adjustment to the demands of daily living, typically improve. Comprehensive treatment may include psychotherapy, medication, special schools or hospitals, special school programs and therapy programs (e.g., speech and language therapy, social skills training, and behavior programs), and active involvement of the family.

This chapter provides an introduction to terminology associated with psychiatric parlance, and a brief identification of the primary classes of psychiatric disorders associated with communication deficits as identified in the *Diagnostic and Statistical Manual of Mental Disorders IV (DSM-IV)* (American Psychiatric Association, 1994). Some of the behavioral, developmental, and linguistic characteristics in children and adolescents that may serve as red flags for psychiatric disorder will then be discussed. Following that, a description of predisposing factors and risk factors for psychiatric disorder and communication handicap and a summary of the cause and effect relationships that may link the two types of disorders are presented. The chapter concludes with a description of the role of the speech–language pathologist in a psychiatric setting.

EMOTIONAL, BEHAVIORAL, AND OTHER PSYCHIATRIC OR MENTAL DISORDERS AND THE *DIAGNOSTIC AND STATISTICAL MANUAL OF MENTAL DISORDERS IV (DSM-IV)*

Speech–language pathologists currently use the terms "emotional disorder" and "behavior disorder." However, the definitions of these terms differ from those used in the mental health community. Speech–language pathologists often use the term *emotional disorder* synonymously with *psychiatric disorder,* while *behavior disorder* is generally not even considered a mental illness. To the mental health professional, the terms *emotional disorder* and *behavior disorder* have specific connotations and specific criteria that must be met in order to make these diagnoses. Emotional and behavior disorders constitute two subgroups among a variety of psychiatric disorders described in the *DSM-IV.*

The *DSM-IV* is a descriptive, multiaxial, diagnostic framework that identifies and lists the essential features that must be present for a diagnosis of a particular disorder to be made. One or more clinical conditions shown by the patient, the psychosocial and environmental stressors, together with a rating of global functioning, are coded on five separate axes. The diagnosis of a mental disorder carries with it the notion that the disorder is a "manifestation of a behavioral, psychological, or biological dysfunction in the individual" (APA, 1994, pp. xxi–xxii). According to *DSM-IV*, all emotional, behavioral, and other psychiatric disorders are mental disorders. The *DSM-IV* defines a mental disorder as "...a clinically significant behavioral or psychological syndrome or pattern that occurs in an individual and that is associated with present distress (e.g. painful symptom) or disability (i.e. impairment in one or more important areas of functioning) or with a significantly increased risk of suffering death, pain, disability, or an important loss of freedom" (APA, 1994, p. xxi).

In psychiatric parlance, emotional disorders are sometimes called *internalizing disorders,* because they are disorders that cause pain or distress to the individual. Emotional disorders contrast with *behavior disorders,* which have also been called *externalizing disorders*—that is, causing pain, distress, or discomfort to others. The identification of one or the other of these disorders depends on the presence of specific symptoms. For example, in order for a youngster to be diagnosed as having separation anxiety disorder (an emotional disorder), or conduct disorder (a behavior disorder), the *essential* characteristics for these diagnoses listed in *DSM-IV* must be met. Additional commonly *associated* characteristics may also be present. Since communication disorders may or may not occur with emotional or behavior disorders, communication impairments may be considered associated features of these disorders. In other psychiatric disorders, communication problems may be inherent features of the disorder itself and considered an essential feature of the diagnosis. This means that the clinical diagnosis of these disorders can only be made when specific characteristic features of language and communication are present. Such disorders include, in particular, the pervasive developmental disorders such as autism and Asperger's disorder (APA, 1994).

According to the *DSM-IV*, psychiatric or mental disorders consist of two types: those usually first diagnosed in infancy, childhood, or adolescence, and those more commonly diagnosed in late adolescence or adulthood. The prevalence of these psychiatric disorders in the general population varies as does age of onset, role of gender, **comorbidity** with other psychiatric or medical conditions, as well as co-occurrence with communication disorders. Almost all of the mental disorders first diagnosed in infancy, childhood, and adolescence are commonly associated with some type of communication deficit or have essential features of language disability (Baltaxe & Simmons, 1988a, 1988b, 1990, 1992a, 1992b; Beitchman, Nair, Clegg, & Patel, 1986; Cantwell & Baker, 1987; 1991a; Trautman et al., 1990).

Disorders diagnosed in childhood include the **pervasive developmental disorders** (autism, Asperger's syndrome, **Rett's syndrome,** and **childhood disintegrative disorders**), the behavior disorders (attention deficit hyperactivity disorder, oppositional defiant disorder, and conduct disorder), the emotional disorders (e.g., anxiety disorders, adjustment disorders, post-traumatic stress disorder, elective mutism), the tic disorders (e.g. Tourette's disorder, transient tic disorder), mental retardation, communication disorders, and learning disabilities, as well as a group of problems that do not constitute diagnoses in themselves, but rather may be characterizations of family conflict (e.g., a parent–child problem). Disorders typically diagnosed in adulthood include the schizophrenias and psychoses, the mood disorders (e.g., depression and bipolar disorder) and the personality disorders (e.g., schizotypal and schizoid personality disorder) (Baltaxe & Simmons, 1987, 1990, 1992b, 1995, Grinnel et al., 1983; Gualtieri et al., 1983; see Appendix B).

The division of psychiatric disorders into those with onset in the early years and those with onset in adulthood must not be taken as absolute. Thus, attention deficit hyperactivity disorder (ADHD) may not be diagnosed until adulthood, although earlier clinical signs may be present. It is also not uncommon for the age of onset of an adult-type disorder to occur in the middle childhood years, prepuberty, or early adolescence.

When this happens, the prevalence of communication handicaps in these disorders tends to be quite high (Baltaxe & Simmons, 1987, 1995).

Behavioral and emotional disorders are the most common psychiatric disorders of childhood and adolescence and in the general population, but prevalence rates depend on type of disorder. Large scale epidemiological studies' prevalence estimates in the general population for attention deficit hyperactivity disorder (ADHD) have ranged between 2.2 percent and 9.9 percent, for oppositional defiant disorder from 5.7 percent to 9.5 percent, and for conduct disorder from 1.5 percent to 9.5 percent (Anderson, Williams, McGee, & Silva, 1987; Bird, Gould, Yagert, Staghezza, & Canino, 1989; Costello, Costello, & Edelbrock, 1988; Velez, Johnson, & Cohen, 1989). Behavior disorders and emotional disorders are also the psychiatric illnesses most likely to be seen in children and adolescents with speech and language disorders in community and psychiatric hospital settings (Cantwell & Baker, 1991a; Beitchman et al., 1986a, b; Camarata et al., 1988; Baltaxe & Simmons, 1988a, 1988b, 1990, 1992a).

In addition to the behavior, emotional, and pervasive developmental disorders, there are still other psychiatric conditions in which communication handicaps can be expected. These conditions are generally seen with lesser frequency in speech and hearing centers or in school populations, but are frequently seen in hospital populations. Psychiatric disorders under this rubric include the schizophrenias and psychoses, personality disorders, mood disorders, and tic (movement) disorders.

SIGNS AND SYMPTOMS OF PSYCHIATRIC ILLNESS IN CHILDREN AND ADOLESCENTS

Psychiatric illness in a child must be considered a serious condition that may affect several areas of development and functioning in the child's life. These areas may include emotional, social, and intellectual development and abilities, as well as the development and use of linguistic skills. A careful medical, family, school, and social history along with direct observation and personal interaction with the child, and a mental status examination by a psychiatrist are necessary to diagnose a possible mental illness. Important questions to be answered in the diagnostic process must include those addressing the child's overall function and development, development in specific areas (e.g., motor, cognitive, and language), the child's emotional state, current language skills, thought processes, school and play behaviors and performance, eating and sleeping patterns, friendships, peer and family relationships, and family history of specific disorders.

When a child is suspected of having a major psychiatric disorder, there are signs and symptoms that may be indicative of specific psychiatric conditions. These include: failure to look or smile at parents or others; lack of or restricted facial expression; facial expression and body language that are incongruous to what the child communicates; odd ways of speaking; odd or repetitive movements; lack of interest in, or awareness of, other people; strange and unusual actions or appearance; intense anxiety and panic in response to a change in surroundings; breaking of rules; and disregard for other people's rights and property.

In young children signs and symptoms of psychiatric disorder may also include failing at school or a drop in grades, excessive worrying, refusal to go to school or go to sleep or to take part in activities that are normal for the child's age. Other warning signs or red flags may include avoidance of, or withdrawal from, specific people or situations, lack of stranger anxiety, perseveration on activities or topics, constant hyperactivity, fidgeting, constant movement, persistent nightmares, an apparent lack of following verbal directions, persistent disobedience or aggression, provocative opposition to authority figures, and frequent and unexplainable temper tantrums, as well as lying, stealing, and cruelty to animals.

These symptoms may also be present or persist in the preadolescent and adolescent. At that time red flags may include: a marked change in school performance; dropping out of school; abuse of alcohol and/or drugs; an inability to cope with problems and daily activities; frequent outbursts of anger; marked changes in sleeping and/or eating habits; moodiness and mood swings; many complaints of physical ailments; aggressive and nonaggressive consistent violation of rights of others; opposition to authority; truancy; theft and vandalism; an intense fear of becoming obese with no relationship to actual body weight; depression as evidenced by sustained, prolonged, negative mood and attitude often accompanied by poor appetite, difficulty sleeping, and thoughts of death. Since there are many different kinds of psychiatric disorders, the specific diagnosis will depend on the combination of symptoms in conjunction with other history and family information.

THE ASSOCIATION BETWEEN COMMUNICATION PROBLEMS AND PSYCHIATRIC DISORDERS

Two approaches have been used to examine the relationship between psychiatric disorders and communication handicaps. One approach studies psychiatric illness in communication disordered youngsters; a second approach studies communication handicaps in psychiatrically ill youngsters. These studies have used different approaches to determine the presence of psychiatric symptoms and conditions and the presence of speech and language deficits. Methods have included chart review; psychiatric and parental interviews; observational methods, including behavior ratings, teacher ratings, and questionnaires; as well as standard scores on more formal testing.

Studies have shown that there is a significant relationship between communication disorders and psychiatric symptomatology and that children with communication disorders are often at risk for psychiatric disorder. For instance, Aram and Nation (1980) studied 20 language disordered teenagers between the ages of 13 and 16 years using a parental questionnaire. They found that the language disordered teenagers were significantly

more schizoid, immature, obsessive-compulsive, hostile, and withdrawn compared to the norm. Silva, Justin, McGee, and Williams (1984), in a study of 57 language delayed three year olds, found that the language delayed children had significantly more behavior problems according to teacher and parent reports than did the control subjects. Tallal, Dukette and Curtiss (1989), using parent behavioral ratings, compared 81 four year old language delayed children with 49 controls and found that the language delayed group had significantly higher mean total symptoms and internalizing disorder scores than did the control group.

The studies showed considerable variations in the prevalence of psychiatric symptoms and disorders. The studies focused primarily on early- and mid-childhood years, with some excursions into the later years. It is difficult to identify the full range of psychiatric diagnoses because of the looseness and ambiguities of psychiatric descriptors used in these studies. It is also difficult to identify the specific nature of the communication characteristics. More recent studies have provided specific data regarding the relationship between speech, language, and psychiatric disorder.

The largest study of psychiatric symptoms and disorders in children with communication difficulties was conducted by Cantwell, Baker and colleagues in a series of investigations between 1977 and 1992 involving 600 children with communication problems between the ages of 1.7 years and 15.9 years (mean age 5.6 years) in a community speech and hearing clinic. The authors concluded that approximately 50 percent of their subjects had diagnosable psychiatric disorders. Using *DSM-III* and *DSM-III-R* (APA, 1980, 1987) criteria, they found that behavior disorders were the most frequent in occurrence (26 percent) and among these, attention deficit hyperactivity disorder (ADHD) was the most common (19 percent). Oppositional and/or conduct disorders were found in an additional 7 percent of children. Emotional disorders (such as anxiety disorders and post-traumatic stress disorders) were diagnosed in another 20 percent and 4 percent also had an affective or mood disorder (Cantwell & Baker, 1991a, 1991b; Baker & Cantwell, 1985). Thus, the psychiatric diagnoses of behavior disorders and emotional disorders occurred at the highest rate and also at a significantly higher rate in the group with communication disorders than in the general population (Szatmari, 1992). Less than 2 percent of the sample had a diagnosis of pervasive developmental disorder, while 6 percent had a diagnosis of mental retardation. Interestingly, these studies also showed that psychiatric disorders were more significantly associated with a language problem (with or without speech problem) compared to a speech only disorder such as articulation, fluency, or voice (Baker & Cantwell, 1985; Cantwell & Baker, 1985; Cantwell, et al., 1979, 1980). About one-half of the children with concurrent speech and language disorders and two-thirds of the children with a language disorder alone had a diagnosable psychiatric disorder, while this was true for only one-third of the children with speech disorder only.

Severity of psychiatric symptomatology also varied for speech disorders and language disorders. Children with speech disorders alone had the least severe symptoms of psychiatric disorder, while children with language disorders showed more serious psychiatric impairment. Although the relationship was not exclusive, speech disorders appeared more closely associated with the presence of an emotional disorder, such as overanxious disorder, reactive attachment disorder, post-traumatic stress disorder, or adjustment disorder. On the other hand, the most common psychiatric symptoms associated with a language disorder were behavior disorders. Of these, ADHD occurred most frequently, followed by oppositional and conduct disorder (Cantwell & Baker, 1985, 1987a, 1987b, 1991a; Cantwell et al., 1980). As noted above, ADHD was also the disorder that occurred with the highest frequency in the total sample of children. The Cantwell and Baker studies show a strong link between language impairment and ADHD. These findings led

Cantwell and colleagues to conclude that the children most at risk for psychiatric disorder are the ones with language disorders, while those with least risk for psychiatric disorder are the ones with speech disorder only.

Communication Problems in Children and Later Psychiatric Disturbance

Severity of communication disorder may be related to later psychiatric disturbance. Lerner, Inui, Trupin, and Douglas (1985) followed up 88 preschoolers 11 and a half years after initial assessment, and found that the presence of a speech/language problem at ages three to five was a strong predictor of psychiatric illness at follow-up. Cantwell and Baker (1991) noted that while psychiatric symptoms disappeared in some children, almost one-fourth of the entire sample that initially had been healthy psychiatrically had become psychiatrically ill on follow-up. The majority were diagnosed with disruptive behavior disorders, which increased from an initial 26 percent to 45 percent on follow-up. ADHD occurred with greatest frequency (38 percent). In addition, 18 percent also had some type of emotional disorder (4 percent with mood disorder and 14 percent with anxiety disorder). The authors concluded that although differences in the time of onset of certain psychiatric disorders may account for some of this increase in psychiatric disorder, the emergence of psychiatric disorders in initially psychiatrically healthy children appeared to be correlated with whether or not a language disorder was present at the time of initial evaluation.

The presence of ADHD and language delay was also strongly linked to the presence of a learning disability, such as a deficit in reading, writing, or mathematics. Rutter (1974) noted earlier that children with learning disorders were more likely to have behavior disorders than emotional disorders. Several other studies have also linked learning disabilities with language disorders (Baltaxe & Simmons, 1987; Rudel, Denckla, & Browman, 1981; Wiig & Semel, 1973, 1975).

Communication Disorders with Psychiatric Disorders as the Index Problem

The association between communication problems and psychiatric disorders is even higher in studies of psychiatrically ill children, although reported prevalence rates vary. In addition, the range of psychiatric disorders associated with communication disorders also widens in these generally hospital based studies of psychiatrically ill children and adolescents. Behavior disorders, in particular ADHD, and emotional disorders, such as anxiety disorders, have been the major psychiatric disorders represented in the above studies of children with communication disorders discussed earlier. Although disruptive behavior disorders, in particular ADHD and emotional disorders, remain at the top of the list in frequency in studies of psychiatrically ill children, several other classes of psychiatric disorder also emerge as highly associated with communication disorders. In addition, the severity and pervasiveness of both the communication disorder and the psychiatric disorder in these psychiatric hospital settings appear to be greater. In a study of 104 four-to-twelve-year olds with psychiatric disorders, Weber (1965) found that more than 75 percent of the children also had speech and language problems. On the other hand, Chess and Rosenberg (1974) found an incidence of speech/language problems of only 24 percent in a sample of 563 children seen in child psychiatric practice, based on patient records and speech and language tests.

Speech–language disorders may occur across all *DSM* diagnoses, although they are not necessarily associated with seriousness of mental illness. Patients with gross neurological symptoms or schizophrenic diagnoses frequently show relatively intact language ability while borderline and behavior-disordered children are likely to show more serious language disabilities. For example, Camarata et al. (1988) studied 38 behavior-disordered students enrolled at least part time in special education classes in a school setting. Based on formal language testing, 97 percent fell below the mean on standardized tests of language.

Representing the collaboration between a communication specialist and a child psychiatrist, and using measures of known reliability and validity, Baltaxe and Simmons investigated the relationship between psychiatric disorders and communication disorders in children and adolescents seen in the inpatient and outpatient services of an acute care psychiatric facility (Baltaxe & Simmons, 1988a, 1988b, 1990, 1992a, 1992b, 1995a, 1995b). The authors concluded that out of 125 psychiatrically ill preschoolers, about one-fourth (27 percent) of the group had mental retardation, one-fourth (25 percent) had pervasive developmental disorders such as autism, and one-fifth (20 percent) had disruptive behavior disorders including ADHD and conduct disorder. Emotional disorders were present in another 6 percent, and parent–child problems in another 9 percent. Other diagnoses occurred with lesser frequency. Language problems were pervasively present in 90 percent of the group.

Language impairment in the children with mental retardation was significantly greater than expected based on their overall IQ. Language impairment in children with pervasive developmental disorders was seen across all or most language areas, as well as in pragmatics. This was not the case in children with parent–child problems, who presented with a more scattered language profile.

Baltaxe and Simmons (1990), Baltaxe (in press) have also reported that communication disorders occurred at a rate of 99 percent in the developmental disorders (mental retardation and the pervasive developmental disorders), 66 percent in the disruptive behavior disorders including ADHD, and 63 percent in the emotional disorders. Communication disorders also occurred at a rate of 63 percent in the category of parent–child, family circumstances, and psychosocial stress problems, and 59 percent in personality disorders, especially in schizoid, schizotypal, borderline, and obsessive–compulsive personality disorder. In addition, 58 percent of the children and adolescents in their study diagnosed with schizophrenia and psychosis had communication disorders, as did 40 percent of the youngsters diagnosed with mood disorders such as depression and bipolar disorders and 91 percent of the children with organically based mental disorders and movement (tic) disorders. Seventy-seven percent of the children with elimination disorders such as bedwetting also had communication disorders, as did 26 percent of the adolescents with a history of substance use, although these last three diagnostic categories (organically based mental disorders and movement disorders, elimination disorders, and substance use) were represented in lesser numbers.

This study shows a broader range of specific classes of psychiatric disorders associated with communication disorders when a wider age range, larger sample size, psychiatric versus nonpsychiatric setting, and more formal measures are utilized. However, except for the pervasive developmental disorders, such as autism, the cooccurrence of communication disorders with psychiatric disorders cannot be predicted from type of psychiatric disorder. The study suggests, however, that some psychiatric disorders appear more "at risk" for the presence of a communication disorder. The dichotomy between speech versus language problems was also apparent in the study. Thirteen percent of the communication-impaired sample had pure speech disorders, while 87 percent had language problems with or without additional speech problems. More than one-third of the language-impaired group was globally impaired in all receptive and expressive language areas (receptive and expressive vocabulary, grammar, and **abstract language**) as well as in auditory language processing. Expressive language impairments without receptive impairments were identified in 11 percent of the sample, and receptive impairments without expressive impairments were identified in 4 percent of the sample.

Clearly, when communication disorders associated with psychiatric disorders are studied in hospital settings, language problems increase even more and the category of pure speech disorders shrinks when compared to community-based studies. Additionally, there seems to be an age-related decrease in speech disorders, while language disorders persist across the various age groups.

PREDISPOSING FACTORS AND RISK FACTORS FOR PSYCHIATRIC DISORDER AND LANGUAGE PROBLEMS

A variety of general risk factors for the development of both psychiatric disorders and communication problems have been identified (Baltaxe & Simmons, 1988a, 1988b, 1990, 1992a, 1992b; Baker & Cantwell, 1987a; Beitchman, 1985; Beitchman, Hood, & Inglis, 1990; Cantwell & Baker, 1991a; Prizant et al., 1990; Rutter, 1971; Theodore, Maher, & Prizant, 1990). These risk factors include perinatal complications and premature births; delays in the areas of linguistic, cognitive, motor, and sensory development; central nervous system dysfunction; general medical condition; and male gender. (Refer to Chapter 2 for a more detailed discussion.)

For the development of psychiatric disorders in children with or without communication problems, risk factors also include parental mental illness and low socioeconomic status. Psychosocial stress can also contribute to risk, including adverse environmental and family conditions, physical and sexual abuse, and other stressful life events. When a communication problem is present, the type of communication impairment also plays a role in the development of a psychiatric disorder. In addition, the communication-handicapped child, and in particular the language-impaired child, is at risk for the development of specific types of psychiatric disorders.

Risk Factors Associated with Lower IQ, Developmental Delays, Central Nervous System Dysfunction, and other Medical Conditions

Intelligence.   **Epidemiological** and other investigations have shown that psychiatric disorders and communication problems are more frequent in children and adolescents with lower IQ than in those with higher IQ (Cox, Rutter, & Yule, 1977; Miller, 1981; Rutter, Tizard, & Whitmore, 1970). This trend is greatest in the lowest IQ groups, although it can be found throughout the IQ distributions. Mental retardation is a common co-morbidity factor in children with pervasive developmental disorders such as autism, Retts syndrome, and disintegrative psychosis. A general deterioration in cognitive function and language abilities can also be expected with the development of some psychiatric disorders, such as the psychoses and the schizophrenias and, in some instances, autism (APA, 1994; Baltaxe & Simmons, 1983, 1992b, 1995). A somewhat lowered IQ, especially verbal IQ, can also be a risk factor for ADHD and the disruptive behavior disorders, although for the most part IQ level does not show any connection to specific psychiatric syndromes (Rogeness, 1994; Shaffer, 1986).

Developmental Delays. Delays or abnormalities in all areas of development and behavior, including language, are frequently linked to an increased incidence of perinatal complications; central nervous system dysfunction; and such medical conditions as encephalitis, **neoplasms,** prenatal trauma, and seizure disorders (Baltaxe & Simmons, 1995). Such delays and abnormalities as well as the presence of organic factors such as **metabolic disease,** may also play a role in the development of psychiatric disorders. Baltaxe and Simmons (1987, 1992b) found developmental language delays or disturbances in 80 percent of the 20 children they studied with prepubertal onset schizophrenia or schizotypal personality disorder. McGee, Partridge, Williams, et al. (1991) suggested that early language delays and hyperactivity may be a possible risk factor for the development of ADHD in early life. Baumeister, Canino, and Bird (1994) noted that preschool behavior problems constitute a strong risk factor for antisocial disruptive disorders at age 11.

Organic Factors and Central Nervous System Dysfunction. With respect to organic factors, Wilcox and Nasrallah (1987) reported an increased incidence of head trauma before the age of 10 for individuals with early onset schizophrenia. O'Callaghan, Larkin, and Waddington (1990) noted an excess of obstetric complications in the

histories of patients with schizophrenia. Previous head trauma is a common finding in the histories of individuals with other psychiatric disorders as well.

Chronic brain syndromes may also place children and adolescents at greater risk for psychiatric disorder (Steinberg, 1985). **Seizure disorders** have long been known to be associated with psychiatric disorders and communication disorders. Shaffer (1986) noted that children suffering from uncomplicated idiopathic epilepsy were about four times as likely to have a psychiatric disorder, and children with structural abnormality were about five times as likely. Children with both structural damage and epilepsy had an even greater prevalence of disturbance. Baltaxe and Simmons (1992a) found that approximately one-third of 600 inpatient children with both language disorder and psychiatric disorder also had seizure disorders or other evidence of organicity. A high incidence of seizure disorders was also reported for children and adolescents diagnosed with psychoses and schizophrenias (Graham, 1986; Shaffer, 1986; Slater, Beard, & Clithero, 1963) and has been documented for autism (Volkmar & Cohen, 1994; Volkmar & Nelson, 1990). Exposure to toxic substances may also affect the child's brain and behavior and can produce psychiatric symptoms. Thus, children with lead exposure may appear hyperactive, inattentive, and irritable. They may also have problems with language, learning, growth, and be susceptible to hearing loss.

Medical Conditions. Hagerman and Falkenstein (1987) associated frequency of otitis media in childhood with later onset of hyperactivity. Hindley, Hill, McGuigan, and Kitson (1994), in their study of deaf and hearing-impaired youngsters found the prevalence of psychiatric disorder to be close to or over one-half (42 to 60 percent). Earlier studies also pointed to the high prevalence rate of psychiatric disorders in the deaf and hearing impaired (Rutter, Tizard, & Whitmore, 1970; Fundudis et al., 1979). Recurring otitis media and hearing impairment frequently also are associated with language delays or disturbances.

Risk Factors Associated with Psychosocial Stressors, Adverse Family Conditions and Parental Mental Illness, and Genetic Predisposition

A high incidence of **psychosocial stressors,** such as turbulent family conditions, have been associated with children with both a communication disorder and a psychiatric disorder (Baltaxe & Simmons, 1988a, 1988b, 1990, 1992a; Beitchman et al., 1986a; Cantwell & Baker, 1991a). Cantwell and Baker (1991a) reported the presence of significant psychosocial stressors in almost two-thirds (65 percent) of psychiatrically ill children with communication problems. Difficulties in parent–child relations were also an indicator of psychosocial stress in the Baltaxe and Simmons studies. Esser, Schmidt, and Woerner (1990) found that in addition to hyperkinetic symptoms, adverse family relations, a learning disability at age 8, and the number of stressful life events experienced in the preceding five years, all were found to predict conduct disorder at age 13.

Familial Factors. Parental mental illness has also been associated with the presence of psychiatric symptoms and communication difficulties. Wolff, Narayan, and Moyes (1988) found that a schizoid personality is common in mothers and fathers of children with autism. The risk for increased mental illness in the offspring is particularly strong when the parent's illness is manic–depressive illness, major depression, schizophrenia, alcoholism, or other drug abuse. When both parents are mentally ill, the risk for psychiatric illness in the offspring is even greater. While some of the risk for the offspring may accrue from the parents' behavior or moods and a concomitant inconsistent, unpredictable family environment, it is generally assumed that risk for psychiatric disorder is inherited. Other studies have also shown familial genetic factors. A very high concordance rate for autism among monozygotic twins (but not for dizygotic same-sex twins) has been identified in a series of population-based studies (Folstein & Rutter, 1977; Steffenburg, Hellgren, Andersson, Gillberg, Jakobsson, & Bohman, 1989). Gillberg,

Gillberg, and Steffenburg (1992) found a familial clustering of autism spectrum problems in families with autism or Asperger's disorder. They identified significant association between autism and Asperger's disorder in first degree relatives. Bolton and Rutter (1990) noted that autism was 50 times more common in siblings of children with autism than was expected on the basis of general prevalence for the autistic disorder. There also appeared to be a increased familial incidence of language-learning and social disabilities. The most convincing and consistent data also indicate that genetic etiological factors are at work in the development of ADHD (Castellanos & Rapoport, 1992). All of the above disorders are significantly associated with communication problems. It is not clear, however, to what degree genetic predisposition plays a specific role with respect to language dysfunction.

Risk Factors Associated with Gender, Type of Communication Disorder, and Type of Psychiatric Disorder

Gender. Differential vulnerabilities to communication disorders for males and females exist. Many studies have demonstrated that a greater number of males than females have developmental communication deficits (Gillespie & Cooper, 1973; Hull, Mielke, Timmons, & Willeford, 1971; Ludlow & Cooper, 1983; Neils & Aram, 1986; Stewart, 1981; Stewart & Spells, 1983). Reported male:female ratios in these studies have varied, ranging from 1.7:1 to 4.1:1 (Hier & Kaplan, 1980, Millisen, 1971). Similarly, greater male vulnerability also exists for most psychiatric disorders of childhood and adolescence (APA, 1994; Earls, 1987; Gould, Wunsch-Hitzig, & Dohrenwend, 1980). The reported male:female ratios for vulnerability in psychiatric disorders have also varied, depending on the study and psychiatric disorder examined (Anderson, Williams, McGee, & Silva, 1987; Crowther, Bond, & Rulf, 1981; Rutter, Cox, Tupling, Berger & Yule, 1975), but most psychiatric disorders are male dominated.

When communication problems occur in children and adolescents with psychiatric disorders, male prevalence also increases (Baltaxe, & Simmons, 1992; Chess & Rosenberg, 1974). However, it is not clear to what extent the gender role is affected by the interaction of the two types of disorders because communication disorders in children and adolescents with psychiatric problems often go unreported. When gender ratios are included in studies of communication disorders in psychiatric populations, the male:female ratio is reported to be close to 3:1 (Baltaxe, & Simmons, 1988a; Chess & Rosenberg, 1974; Gualtieri et al.,1983), although in some cases the male:female ratio is even higher (Camarata et al., 1988; Trautman et al., 1990). Variables known to play a role in the gender ratio are type of psychiatric disorder (Anderson et al., 1987; Costello et al., 1988); type of communication disorder (Stewart, 1981); age of child (Offord et al., 1987; Baltaxe & Simmons, 1991; Cantwell & Baker, 1991a); and the criteria used in the identification of a communication disorder (Beitchman et al., 1986a). For example, general population studies have found a higher incidence of ADHD and behavior disorders in boys than in girls (Crowther et al., 1981; Offord et al., 1987). Cantwell and Baker (1991a) reported a greater incidence of behavior disorders among boys in their sample, with more than twice as many boys so identified as girls, while for emotional disorders (anxiety disorders in particular), almost three times as many girls were identified as compared to boys.

The reasons for the greater male vulnerability to developmental communication disorders and psychiatric disorders currently is not well understood. However, the role that genetically predisposing factors and hormonal differences play in contributing to the higher frequency of these disorders in males during development has been questioned (Beitchman, 1986a; Earls, 1987; Graham, 1986; Ludlow & Cooper, 1983; Ounsted, Moar, & Scott, 1986).

While earlier studies of communication problems in individuals with psychiatric disorders have noted a general male prevalence, those studies have not focused on other differences that may exist between males and females. These include possible differences with respect to specific types of communication problems, differences in the pattern and severity of communication problems, and differences due to other diagnostic or medical factors associated with gender.

Baltaxe and Simmons (1992a) examined the variables related to gender in 600 children and adolescents who had both a psychiatric disorder and a communication problem. As expected, males showed a greater incidence of communication problems compared to females, at a ratio of 3:1. However, while the same types of speech and language deficits were identified in male and female children, significantly more females than males were impaired in all of the areas tested (receptive and expressive vocabulary, syntax, abstract language, and auditory language processing). No such gender differences were found for the areas of speech which, included articulation, voice, fluency, and prosody. Earlier studies found language represented a more severe and serious communication problem than speech (Baltaxe & Simmons, 1988a, 1990, 1991; Cantwell & Baker, 1987a, 1987b, 1991a). Further analysis showed that significantly more males had pure speech disorders—that is, males were impaired only in the areas of speech, for example, articulation, voice, or fluency. In contrast, significantly more females had pure language disorders—that is, vocabulary, grammar, and abstract language. Females also showed a greater severity of language problems. Significantly more females than males showed global impairment in all the language areas tested.

With respect to psychiatric disorders, significantly more females had emotional disorders (such as anxiety disorders, adjustment disorders) while significantly more males had disruptive behavior disorders and mood disorders. In addition, a greater proportion of females were diagnosed with mental retardation, seizure disorders, and organic brain disorders, but analysis showed that severity of language disorder in the females was affected neither by psychiatric nor medical diagnosis.

The findings of greater vulnerability but lesser severity in males and lower vulnerability but greater severity in females parallels gender distributional patterns in other developmental, psychiatric, and physical disorders such as autism, ADHD, stuttering, reading disability, Down syndrome, and cerebral palsy. The above results are consistent with a differential genetic loading for these disorders in males and females (Baltaxe & Simmons, 1992a).

Type of Communication Disorder. As the above studies have shown, communication handicaps of all types can co-occur with psychiatric disorders. However, results of these studies overwhelmingly indicate that delays and disturbances in the area of language (rather than in speech) carry a greater risk for psychiatric disorder. Language problems tend to persist into adolescence, and there may be a continuing increased risk for development of a psychiatric disorder in these language-disordered children through adolescence (Baker & Cantwell, 1987).

When individual areas of language have been examined, the highest prevalence of language deficits in psychiatric disorders are in abstract language and in **auditory language processing skills,** followed by impairment in vocabulary and grammatical skills (Baltaxe & Simmons, 1990, 1992a). Language usage or pragmatics is often seriously impaired, although the specific pragmatic deficits depend on type of psychiatric disorder. (Baltaxe, 1993). Pragmatic deficits occur in a wide range of areas. These include providing irrelevant information to the listener; not syntactically distinguishing between old and new information; inappropriate topic initiation and maintenance; inappropriate turn-taking (e.g., overlapping with and interrupting the speaker, refusal to yield the floor or lack of response); inappropriate use of register (e.g., using formal language in a conversational setting); and use of body language, facial expressions, or prosodic features that are incongruent with the content of what is said.

Deficits in pragmatics also include specific features that are diagnostic for individual psy-

chiatric disorders themselves. For example, the autistic child, or the child with schizotypal personality disorder, schizophrenia, or psychosis, may not be able to use or interpret the required prosodic signals to communicate or evoke certain emotions in the listener. Children and adolescents with these disorders may also have difficulties with the use of or interpretation of secondary or derived meanings, abstract language, and with taking the listener's perspective, thus creating serious social-communication handicaps. Children with reactive attachment disorder (an emotional disorder) may not differentiate their social use of language regardless of whether the listener is a familiar person or a stranger. The child's verbal and nonverbal behaviors may be overfamiliar and inappropriate for strangers. On the other hand, children with an anxiety disorder (a different emotional disorder) may shrink from social contact with strangers and their pragmatics will reflect this as well, while a child with a behavior disorder (such as a conduct disorder) may violate the principles of politeness in a social situation.

Severity and pervasiveness of general language disability have also been correlated with severity and pervasiveness of psychiatric disorder in some studies. Thus, children with a more severe and pervasive language disability may also be at risk for a more severe and pervasive psychiatric disorder.

Language plays an important role in all aspects of a child's development including concept formation, play, reasoning, problem-solving, academic achievement, the acquisition of interpersonal skills, and the development of a self-image. Language also plays a role in regulating the child's own behavior and controlling and manipulating the behavior of others. Prizant et al. (1988) suggest that children with language disorders often do not develop the communicative competence needed for mutual and self-regulation. Competence in self-regulation allows a child to use language to modulate internal emotional states and level of arousal. When language development is delayed, impaired, or arrested, it may be among the most disruptive factors in a child's development. As a result, communication failures may also lead to secondary psychiatric difficulties.

Type of Psychiatric Disorder.   The results of the previously discussed studies indicate that a wide range of psychiatric disorders co-occur with language disorders. However, some psychiatric disorders may carry a greater risk for communication problems and for language disorder in general. These include pervasive developmental disorders, ADHD and disruptive behavior disorders, emotional disorders, schizophrenias and psychoses, personality disorders, and mood disorders.

Pervasive Developmental Disorders.   The pervasive developmental disorders are characterized by uneven development in separate areas of growth. Communication deficits are an integral part of these disorders and must be present in order for the diagnosis to be made. Pervasive developmental disorders include autism, pervasive developmental disorder not otherwise specified (PDD NOS), Rett's disorder, Asperger's disorder, and disintegrative psychosis of childhood. The most extensive studies of language disorders associated with psychiatric disorders have centered on autism, which has a prevalence in the general population of about 5 in 10,000 (APA, 1994). For autism to be diagnosed, characteristics of the disorder have to be present by the age of 3 years. About 75 percent of children with autism have an IQ below 70. Asperger's disorder is defined as high-functioning autism without the early developmental abnormalities in language inherent in the autistic disorder (i.e., language development is normal, not delayed). The diagnosis of Asperger's disorder is limited to individuals with a normal IQ. The diagnosis of childhood disintegrative disorder is applicable to those individuals with the symptomatology of autism but presenting with a regression after a prolonged period (2 to 10 years) of normal development (Minshew, 1995). Seizure disorders (Volkmar & Nelson, 1990), **fragile X syndrome** (Goldson & Hagerman, 1992), **tuberous sclerosis** (Baltaxe & d'Angiola, in press), Tourette's disorder, and mental retardation pro-

vide frequent comorbidity factors in autism. Communication abilities, social skills, intervention, and the presence of other medical conditions all are significant outcome variables.

Autism has been the most thoroughly studied of the pervasive developmental disorders and may be the most frequent in occurrence. It is characterized by a qualitative impairment in social relationships. The autistic child does not develop friendships with other children and has difficulties with peer relationships in general. There may be a general lack responsiveness in social situations. A lack of, or restricted, eye contact is generally part of the diagnostic picture. The autistic child may also adhere to restricted, repetitive, and stereotyped patterns of behavior, interests, and activities. There may be stereotyped and repetitive motor mannerisms and inflexible adherence to specific rituals and routines. For example, play behavior may be limited to the repetitive lining up of blocks, interest may be limited to observing spinning objects such as ceiling fans, a strict sequence in bathroom or dressing routines may have to be observed to avoid temper tantrums, and the child may demonstrate hand flapping and other motor mannerisms. The autistic child may also prefer inanimate objects to animate objects, and may prefer parts of objects to the whole object. Food preferences may also be limited. Unusual attachment to and interest in objects, such as a piece of paper, may also be seen. Restricted interests in the higher-functioning autistic child may include such areas as computers and computer games or number calculations to the exclusion of all other interests. However, the most striking characteristics are associated with communication behaviors.

Communication profiles of autistic children come in a number of forms and vary with the presence of other cognitive deficits and age of the child. Only 50 percent of autistic children do not develop communication. Of those who do, 25 percent develop rudimentary and abnormal verbal and nonverbal communication, while the remainder make better progress. There may be a qualitative impairment in communication, ranging from a total lack of or delayed development of spoken language and difficulties in sustaining conversations, to stereotyped repetitive use of language or idiosyncratic language. In those children who develop speech, the development of the sound system appears to be the least disturbed, although developmental delays and abnormalities of articulation have also been reported (Baltaxe & Simmons, 1981a, 1981b), and there may be problems with intelligibility.

Prosodic deficits in autistic children have been described consistently as an integral part of the speech and language disorder in autism (APA, 1994; Baltaxe, 1984; Baltaxe & Guthrie, 1987; Baltaxe & Simmons, 1981b, 1985; Baltaxe, Simmons, & Zee, 1984; Kanner, 1943). Such deficits still remain evident in children who show considerable improvement in language skills (Baltaxe & Simmons, 1983; Rutter & Lockyer, 1967). When language develops, pitch, intonation, rate, and rhythm may be abnormal (Baltaxe & Simmons, 1985). The autistic child's speech has often been described as dull, wooden, improperly modulated, or having a singsong quality with overprecision in articulation (Goldfarb, Goldfarb, Braunstein, & Lorge, 1972).

Disfluency in the form of false starts, reformulations, repetitions of parts of words, whole words, and utterances are characteristic of the higher-functioning verbal autistic individual (Baltaxe & Simmons, 1977, 1981a 1983). Autistic children may also have a variety of voice problems including hypo- and hypernasality (Baltaxe & Simmons, 1981a). Apraxia has also been reported as a characteristic of some autistic individuals (Minshew, 1995).

Echolalia is a prominent feature in the speech production of many autistic children. Echolalia can occur immediately after the linguistic stimulus occurs or or may be delayed in time. It can consist of a complete repetition of what the child heard or only a partial repetition. These forms of echolalia play an important role in language acquisition (Baltaxe, & Simmons, 1975; Prizant, 1983; Schuler & Prizant, 1985). An estimated 75 percent of all autistic children who develop communicative speech have been reported to go through an echolalic phase (Ricks & Wing, 1975; Rutter, 1974b).

Deficits are also noted in semantics. Autistic children may have idiosyncratic meanings for individual words, and peculiar word choices in general. They may also have difficulty with multiple meanings and abstract meanings as well as with generalizing meaning across different settings. Grammatical structures may be those expected of a younger child (Pierce & Bartolucci, 1977; Swisher & Demetras, 1985). Special grammatical classes such as prepositions, adjectives, and verbs tend to be difficult for autistic children. The language productions of an autistic individual may be overly abstract or overly concrete or idiosyncratic. The rules of syntax and morphology may be violated inconsistently, and there may be residual use of echolalia. Comprehension may be impaired in the presence of an adequate auditory memory. Even in higher functioning individuals (Asperger's disorder), there are still problems in comprehension, semantics, and speech production, and difficulties with the fine nuances of language (Baltaxe & Simmons, 1981a, 1992b).

It is social communication, however, in its verbal and nonverbal form, that remains the most seriously impaired area in autism, even in the higher-functioning individual. The autistic child has difficulty understanding the facial expression, body language, and intonation of others. Although to date no single study has fully identified the range of pragmatic disabilities in the disorder, the deficits appear to be heterogeneous and depend on age and overall cognitive function of the child.

The young autistic child may show poor eye contact, difficulties with mutually shared points of reference, and difficulties with reciprocal social play. Later problems with pragmatics include general discourse features such as not providing sufficient background information to the listener, not taking the listener's perspective when incorporating new and old information in a linguistic interchange, lack of monitoring the face of the conversational partner for cues to understanding, and/or poor, insufficient, or inappropriate referencing deficits relating to topic development and sequencing, including perseveration and redundancy of topics (Baltaxe & d'Angiola, 1992, 1996; Baltaxe & Simmons, 1992b, 1995).

The older verbal child may have difficulties initiating and sustaining a conversation. Turntaking may also be difficult. Problems can also arise in switching register or adjusting one's language to a particular social situation, such as using vocabulary and syntax that are too formal or not formal enough. Difficulties may exist with following social cues and observing the rules of politeness under varying social conditions, expressing appropriate emotions in a given context, taking the listener's perspective when incorporating new and old information in a linguistic interchange, and performing simple and complex verbal problem-solving tasks (for reviews see Baltaxe & Simmons, 1992b; Baron-Cohen, 1988; Watson, 1988). Some of these problems have been interpreted as the autistic individual's difficulty with conceptual thinking and the ability to make inferences (Rumsey, Andreason, & Rapoport, 1986). Nonverbal parameters of communication such as eye contact, facial expression, and body language are also impaired in autism, even in the higher-functioning individual (Tantam, Holmes, & Cordess, 1993).

Autistic children sometimes have an unusual scatter of skills. An autistic individual may perform well on auditory memory tasks and on visual spatial tasks, while doing poorly on other tasks, such as linguistic or gross motor tasks. When there is an area of function in which the autistic individual does unusually well compared to other areas, that area is termed a *splinter skill.* Splinter skills may consist of an unusual ability for drawing, mathematical calculation, or musical abilities. Another one of these splinter skills is hyperlexia—a special ability to read—though generally without much comprehension (Huttenlocher & Huttenlocher, 1973; Ross, 1979).

Mental Retardation. In order for a child to be diagnosed as mentally retarded, the child has to have both a significantly low IQ and considerable problems in adapting to everyday life. Mental retardation may be complicated by physical, behavioral, and/or emotional problems. Communication problems are a commonly associated feature of mental retardation. Mental retardation results in delays in language development. However, because mental retardation may be associated with a variety of underlying causes, additional language problems can also be expected beyond the delay associated with a lower mental age (Miller, 1981).

Attention Deficit Hyperactivity/Disruptive Behavior Disorders. This group of disorders includes attention deficit hyperactivity disorder (ADHD)—the most highly represented disorder—as well as oppositional defiant disorder and conduct disorder. ADHD and its subtypes, as noted earlier, are among the most common psychiatric disorders of childhood, in addition to oppositional disorder (Szatmari, 1992). Attention deficit hyperactivity disorder appears to be the disorder most commonly seen in speech–language clinics and psychiatric settings and has received the most recent attention. While hyperactivity can be a symptom of other disorders or a dimension of personality (Werry, 1992), the key symptoms of ADHD are hyperactivity, short attention span, distractability, and impulsivity. The peak age range for referral for children with ADHD is from 7 to 9 years, although it is generally believed that the disorder arises during the preschool years (APA, 1994; McGee, Williams, & Feehan, 1992). The disorder is 10 times more common in boys than in girls. The child with ADHD appears developmentally immature, has difficulty organizing work, and gives the impression of not having heard instructions; is easily distracted, makes careless, impulsive errors; has difficulty with turn-taking in school; fails to follow through on requests of parents and teachers; and has difficulty understanding or following the rules of a game (APA, 1992). At least 50 percent of children with hyperactivity also have problems with peers, due to some of the above problems. The child with ADHD often has severe deficits in language usage or social communication (Baltaxe & Simmons, 1987; Whalen

& Henker, 1992). This impairment in language usage is considered by some the most severe aspect of the disorder (Hinshaw, 1992).

Comorbidity of ADHD is frequent with both conduct disorder and oppositional disorders (Biederman, Faraone, & Lapey, 1992; Werry, 1992). ADHD is also increasingly being recognized as a heterogeneous disorder (Biederman et al., 1992).

Conduct disorders are the most serious of this group of disorders and have the most serious implications. Children and adolescents with these disorders have great difficulty following rules and behaving in a socially acceptable way. They are often aggressive (both physically and verbally) with other children and adults. They may lie, steal, destroy property, and misbehave sexually. Children, adults, and social agencies often view them as bad, or delinquent, rather than mentally ill. Many factors may lead to a child developing a conduct disorder, including brain damage, child abuse, defects in growth, school failure, and negative family and social experiences.

A verbal IQ of close to 10 points below average as well as lower scores on reading and spelling have been reported as commonly associated with both ADHD and conduct disorder (Hodges & Plow, 1990; Rogeness, 1994). However, communication problems in these disorders often go undetected because they may be subtle in nature (Cohen et al., 1993). In youngsters diagnosed with these disorders who are also language impaired, auditory processing problems and abstract language deficits in particular are deficient, but there are also problems in receptive and expressive vocabulary and syntax.

Emotional Disorders. Emotional disorders include a variety of psychiatric disorders such as anxiety disorders, adjustment disorders, phobias, and post-traumatic stress disorder. Among the emotional disorders, anxiety symptoms and disorders are common in children and adolescents with an overall prevalence rate of approximately 8 percent to 10 percent (Bell-Dolan & Brazeal, 1993). Among these, overanxious disorder and separation anxiety disorder are the most common. The

anxiety disorders are characterized by excessive and unrealistic anxiety, subjective distress, and a maladaptive reaction to feared stimuli or situations. While transient anxiety or distress is normal in healthy children, when anxieties become severe and begin to interfere with the daily activities of childhood such as separating from parents, attending school, and making friends, a more serious mental disturbance may be present. Children with separation anxiety, for example, may show the following symptoms: constant thoughts and fears about safety of self and parents, refusing to go to school, frequent physical complaints, overly clingy behavior at home, panic or tantrums at time of separation from parent, and extreme worries about sleeping away from home. Children with anxiety disorders may be afraid to meet or talk to new people, or may have difficulty making friends outside the home. Anxious children may be overly uptight and tense. They may have many worries about things before they happen, and there may be a constant concern or worry about school, friends, or sports. Because anxious children may be quiet, compliant, and eager to please, their difficulties may be overloaded. Early intervention is necessary to prevent failures in friendships, self-esteem, and schoolwork.

Panic disorder is another common emotional disorder in children. Children with panic disorder have unexpected and repeated episodes of intense fear or discomfort, along with physical symptoms such as a racing heartbeat or shortness of breath. Panic attacks can interfere with relationships, schoolwork, and normal development. Some of the symptoms of panic disorder include intense fearfulness; racing or pounding heartbeat; dizziness or lightheadedness; shortness of breath or a feeling of smothering, trembling or shaking; a sense of unreality; and a fear of dying, losing control, or going crazy.

Other types of emotional disorders, including post-traumatic stress disorder, may occur in children who have been physically or sexually abused. Children who have been physically abused may display a poor self-image; an inability to depend on, trust, or love others; aggressive and disruptive behavior; passive and withdrawn behavior; fear of entering into new relationships or activities; school failure; and/or serious drug and alcohol abuse. Children who have been sexually abused may display an unusual interest in or avoidance of all things of a sexual nature; sleep problems; nightmares; depression or withdrawal from friends or family; seductiveness; statements that their bodies are dirty; secretiveness; refusal to go to school; delinquency; aspects of sexual molestation in drawings, games, and fantasies; unusual aggressiveness; suicidal behavior; and other severe behavior changes.

About two-thirds of all children with emotional disorders also have communication problems. As with the behavior disorders, pragmatics, auditory language processing, abstract language, and receptive and expressive grammar and vocabulary can be impaired (Baltaxe, 1993; Baltaxe & Simmons, 1990, 1991, 1995).

Personality Disorders. The characteristics of personality disorders are inflexibility, maladaptive personality traits, and excessive functional impairment or distress (APA, 1994). Of the personality disorders, schizotypal personality disorder (SPD) and schizoid personality disorder are associated with communication impairments. Personality disorders typically have an onset in adolescence or early adulthood, but they can also occur in preadolescence. Individuals with these two disorders frequently have no close friends or confidants. They also have what has been described as peculiar ideas, unusual perceptual experiences, odd speech, inappropriate **affect,** and odd behaviors (APA, 1994). Odd speech has been further characterized as impoverished, digressive, vague, or inappropriately abstract speech. This type of speech points to major pragmatic deficits in children and adolescents diagnosed with these disorders. While deficits in other areas of language disorders occur, their co-occurrence with personality disorders is more scattered, and the overwhelming area of deficit is the pragmatic domain.

Schizotypal personality disorder and schizoid disorder have been discussed in relation to As-

perger's syndrome and high-functioning autism (Baltaxe, Russell, D'Angiola, & Simmons, 1995; Baltaxe & Simmons, 1992b). All of these disorders have been characterized as social–communication spectrum disorders (Baltaxe, 1993; Baltaxe & Simmons, 1992b; Tanguay, 1990). A diagnosis of schizotypal personality disorder is frequently used for an individual who, by symptomatology, falls between autism and schizophrenia (Baltaxe & Simmons, 1992b). As with autism and pervasive developmental disorders, the area of pragmatics is particularly relevant in diagnosing schizotypal personality disorder. While pragmatics has been studied extensively in autism, pragmatics in personality disorders has not been explored thoroughly.

Schizophrenias/Psychoses.   Schizophrenia with onset in childhood or adolescence is a relatively rare disorder, affecting approximately 3 in 10,000 youngsters and is hard to recognize in its early phases. The diagnosis of schizophrenia in childhood and adolescence has not been uniquely defined and may differ in presentation from adult schizophrenia. Some of the early warning signs include trouble telling dreams from reality; seeing things and hearing voices that are not real; confused thinking; vivid and bizarre thoughts and ideas; extreme moodiness; odd behavior; ideas that people are out to get them; behaving like a younger child; severe anxiety and fearfulness; confusing television with reality; severe problems in making and keeping friends; delayed or abnormal language development; and strange body posturing and upper extremity movements.

For the diagnosis of schizophrenia to be made in childhood, adult diagnostic criteria must be fulfilled. These include the presence of a **thought disorder,** hallucinations, motility disturbances, and disturbances in social relationships. In childhood, thought disorders and hallucinations are among the main differential criteria that distinguish schizophrenia from other psychiatric conditions, particularly from autism, pervasive developmental disorder not otherwise specified (PDD NOS), and schizotypal personality disorder. Additional considerations in differentiating schizophrenia from these other conditions involve the age at onset (APA, 1994; Rutter & Schopler, 1987).

Because a thought disorder manifests itself in expressive language, the characteristics of language have always been among the key diagnostic features of schizophrenia (Andreason, 1979a, 1979b; Bleuler, 1911/1950; Kraepelin 1919/ 1971). The linguistic manifestations of thought disorder in adults and children have been studied through instruments with known validity and reliability such as the Thought Disorder Scale and the Thought Disorder Index (Andreason, 1979a, 1979b, Arboleda & Holzman, 1985; Caplan, 1994a, 1994b; Caplan, Purdue, Tanguay, & Fish 1990), as well as through formal discourse analysis as an aspect of pragmatics (Rochester & Martin, 1979). From a pragmatic perspective, most manifestations of thought disorder in persons with schizophrenia have been identified as a dysfunction in a speaker–hearer role relationship. Schizophrenic speakers do not put themselves into the listener's shoes, so information provided to the listener may be vague, and may miss the point or almost miss the point. Too much or not enough information may be provided, or the discourse may not make any sense (Baltaxe & Simmons, 1987; Rochester & Martin, 1979). Translated into psychiatric parlance, characteristics of a formal thought disorder include tangentiality, derailment, circumstantiality, and incoherence. The emergence of these impairments in communication is assumed to coincide with the onset of the schizophrenic disorder (APA, 1994).

A significant number of children and adolescents who are diagnosed as schizophrenic, in addition to delays and abnormalities in behavioral, emotional, and motor development, also have delays and abnormalities in language development (Beitchman, 1985b; Graham, 1986). In fact, Baltaxe and Simmons (1992a) suggest that language dysfunction may be an early neurodevelopmental indicator of schizophrenia. However, there are currently no studies addressing speech and language behaviors in adults with onset of schizophrenia in childhood.

Mood Disorders. Mood disorders, and in particular depressive disorders, do not only occur in adults but also in children and adolescents. According to the American Psychiatric Association (APA, 1992), depression exists in about 5 percent of children and adolescents in the general population, although estimates vary from between 1.8 percent (Anderson et al., 1987) to 5.9 percent (Bird et al., 1989). Children who are under stress, who experience loss, or who have attentional, learning, or conduct disorders are also at high risk for depression. Signs of depression in children include persistent sadness, an inability to enjoy previously favorite activities, increased activity or irritability, frequent complaints of physical illnesses such as headaches and stomach aches, frequent absences from school or poor performance in school, persistent boredom, low energy, poor concentration, or a major change in eating and/or sleeping patterns. McCauley and Meyers (1992) also noted that school failure is common, particularly in adolescents.

There are few studies of communication problems associated with mood disorders. Baltaxe and Simmons (1990) found that 40 percent of children and adolescents diagnosed with mood disorders (primarily depressive disorder) also had speech and language problems, and there was a significant subgroup of children in their sample of 600 who had both a mood disorder and a communication problem. While the strengths and weaknesses of the psychosocial functioning of depressed youngsters is currently not well understood, there is preliminary evidence that the domain most impacted is interpersonal relatedness, thus implicating the area of pragmatics. Deficits seen in pragmatics with respect to mood disorders relate to general discourse features, such as failure to orient listener, difficulty relating a coherent narrative; difficulty initiating or perseverating on a topic; paucity of speech; difficulties with lexical selection; poor eye contact; monotonous prosody, including more pausing, less pitch modulation, and slower rhythm; paucity of responses; lack of facial expression; restricted body movement; and a general lack of interest in being a conversational partner (Baltaxe & Simmons, 1990).

PSYCHIATRIC DISORDERS AND COMMUNICATION DISORDERS IN THE MIDDLE AND LATER YEARS

The *DSM-IV* differentiates between disorders usually first diagnosed in infancy, childhood, or adolescence and those diagnosed in adulthood. Autism, pervasive developmental disorder, Asperger's syndrome, mental retardation, ADHD, and disruptive behavior disorders are among the first type of disorders to be diagnosed. Other disorders including the schizophrenias, the personality disorders, the mood disorders, and anxiety disorders are more commonly diagnosed in adulthood. However, the distinction is not an absolute, and a single set of criteria is followed regardless of whether the diagnosis is made in childhood or adulthood. In addition, some of these early diagnoses may only come to clinical attention later in life, while diagnoses associated with later life may already be made in preadolescence. Several reasons may account for disorders not being diagnosed until later in life. Foremost among these may be that the signs and symptoms exhibited by the individual were not severe enough in the early stages to receive attention. Attention may only focus on symptoms when the problem is significant enough to interfere with school performance, employment, or relationships. Thus, a speech–language problem associated with ADHD in the early years may not have been apparent, but may become apparent when a greater demand is placed on abstract language skills in the later school years, and possible compensatory strategies are more difficult. Difficulties with the law because of unacceptable behaviors may also play a role in later diagnoses (Wagner, 1995). However, later diagnoses of childhood and adolescent disorders may also relate to ethnicity or socioeconomic status or lack of readily available services.

While there are few follow-up studies, the age ranges in the earlier review of the literature on language and psychiatric disorders indicate that communication disorders (in particular language disorders) continue to exist through the lifespan. While problems with speech may disappear and problems with grammar may subside, problems with abstract language, auditory language processing, and word finding, as well as social communication, may continue to exist. Furthermore, as some research has shown, children, particularly those with language disorders, have an increasing incidence of psychiatric disorders in adolescence (Cantwell & Baker, 1987b).

CAUSE AND EFFECT RELATIONSHIPS BETWEEN PSYCHIATRIC DISORDERS AND COMMUNICATION DISORDERS

While studies show that linguistic deficits and psychiatric disorders are associated (Baltaxe & Simmons, 1988a, 1990; Beitchman et al., 1986a; Cantwell & Baker, 1991a), the cause and effect relationships between psychiatric disorders and communication difficulties are not at all clear (Baltaxe & Simmons, 1988a, 1990). Cantwell and Baker (1977) and Rutter and Martin (1972) postulated that early language dysfunction may lead to impaired social relations and that these social deficits are etiologically important to the development of later psychopathology. Children with all types of disabilities, especially those involving the brain, are at risk for the development of social and emotional problems. Beitchman (1985a) reported that language-impaired children, at least those with receptive deficits, lack both an effective internalized map of their environment and also the ability to generalize from the individual item to the whole class of items. Because of this lack of generalization, the world is often confusing and unmanageable. Beitchman described those children as showing a wide range of behavior problems. However, even though it has been proposed that communication disturbances may lead to psychiatric disturbances, it is likely that in many instances linguistic impairment in itself may not be sufficient to cause a psychiatric disturbance. A number of unexamined variables may also play a role. These variables include type and severity of any cognitive impairments co-occurring with linguistic problems, psychosocial stressors, socioeconomic status, and other variables (Beitchman, 1985a; Cantwell & Baker, 1991a; Fundudis et al., 1979).

Beitchman (1985a) postulated that neurodevelopmental immaturity may underlie speech language delays. However, most authors agree that it is quite likely that in many cases a poor or impaired neurodevelopmental course may lead to both communication problems and psychiatric disorder (Baltaxe & Simmons, 1988a, 1990). In some instances, it is also plausible that the emergence of a psychiatric disorder may bring about the emergence of a communication problem (Baltaxe & Simmons, 1988a, 1990). This may be the case particularly in the schizophrenias and the psychoses. In addition, there may be a mutual interactive effect between communication impairment and psychiatric disorder as suggested by Prizant et al. (1990).

THE COMMUNICATION SPECIALIST AND PSYCHIATRIC DISORDERS

The fact that 50 percent of speech–language disturbed children have psychiatric disorders means that speech–language pathologists must become attuned to the psychiatric aspects of their patients. This calls for interdisciplinary cooperation between mental health professionals and communication disorders specialists. The speech–language pathologist's contributions are important from both a diagnostic and an intervention perspective. The speech–language pathologist can play an important role on the interdisciplinary team or as a consultant to individual mental health professionals. Such a team generally consists of, but is not limited to, a psychiatrist, psychologist, social worker, education specialist, and nursing professional. The interdisciplinary team may also include a speech–language pathologist as a regular member.

In an **interdisciplinary** team approach, the child or adolescent is seen for a psychiatric complaint by individuals from these disciplines who all work together for the benefit of the patient. Diagnosis and evaluation become a team effort, with input from all team members. Depending on the presenting complaints, the member of each discipline will observe and evaluate the child using the tools and knowledge of the specific discipline. Speech–language pathologists play an important role on such a team. Their input to diagnosis and treatment plan relates to communication behaviors and incorporates information from chart review, parental interview, school observation, informal observation of the patient, and formal testing. Their contributions include the identification of normal speech language behaviors as well as specific deficits, such as deficits in pragmatics, auditory processing and other areas of speech and language function, level of development in relation to chronological age, identification of characteristics of delay and deviance, indications of organicity, as well as strengths and weaknesses seen in the profile of communication behaviors.

The speech–language pathologist's input to the team will also include how well a particular communication profile fits a particular psychiatric diagnosis in the process of differential diagnosis, since specific communication behaviors often corroborate a specific psychiatric diagnosis. For example, the specific pragmatic deficits seen in an adolescent suspected of having schizophrenia may corroborate the presence of a thought disorder. On the other hand, a linguistic profile that includes abnormal prosodic features, comprehension problems, and specific pragmatic deficits, may corroborate the diagnosis of autism. Auditory language processing, slight word-finding difficulties, and specific pragmatic deficits, as well as reading and writing difficulties, may be expected for some children with ADHD.

The information on communication behaviors contributed by the speech–language pathologist on the interdisciplinary team complements and supports that provided by professionals from other disciplines. It may provide the basis for additional referrals, including neurological or audio-logical assessments. The information provided by the speech–language pathologist also assists in determining school placement and services needed. When the speech–language pathologist is a member of the interdisciplinary team, collaboration in the arena of intervention is also provided. The type of medication and/or behavior management may also play a role with respect to speech–language intervention, as may the sequencing of these approaches. The more knowledgeable speech–language pathologists are with respect to psychiatric disorders, the more valuable they can be to others as a member on the interdisciplinary team or as a consultant to other professionals. However, this is also true for non-mental health settings, in which speech–language pathologists can act as knowledgeable sources in further addressing possible emotional, behavior, and mental health problems in the children and adolescents for whom they provide services.

When examining a youngster suspected of having a mental health problem or psychiatric disorder, communication specialists need to take into account the frequency of occurrence of a specific type of psychiatric disorder in the population at large, and the frequency of a particular language disorder associated with psychiatric disorders.

There is a timetable for the emergence of specific psychiatric disorders. Different psychiatric disorders emerge at different times during life. Pervasive developmental disorders are present at birth or close to birth. Mental retardation is present before the age of 18, while ADHD and disruptive behavior disorders emerge in mid-childhood, and personality disorders and schizophrenias generally emerge in adolescence or adulthood, but may also occur in preadolescence.

There may be a diagnostic change in symptoms of the psychiatric disorder over time. Thus, the presenting symptoms for ADHD vary with age of child. In young children, hyperactivity symptoms may include excessive running or climbing, while older children may display extremely restless and fidgety behaviors, particularly in group situations. For autism, the symptom picture may have been autistic by history and later in life change to schizophrenia, or change due to the development of seizure activity.

Consideration must also be given to the possible coexistence of other psychiatric disorders in the same individual. The symptom picture may indicate comorbidity and may impact the communication disorder as well. For example, high comorbidity has been found among ADHD and the disruptive behavior disorders. Also, consideration must be given to the differential diagnosis of related disorders. For example, the category of disorders which has been loosely termed *social communication spectrum disorders* includes autism, pervasive developmental disorder not otherwise specified (PDD NOS), schizotypal personality disorder, schizophrenia, and psychosis. Care must be taken by the psychiatrist or other mental health professional to determine the appropriate diagnosis by taking a careful history and completing the child's mandatory observations, in addition to administering formal tests. A detailed analysis of the child's existing communication problems will aid in the diagnosis.

Knowledge of the frequencies of specific communication problems across psychiatric disorders in general, and/or specific pragmatic disorders, is also desirable. For psychiatric disorders, a high frequency of deficits is expected for the communication areas of pragmatics, abstract language, auditory processing, and the expressive and receptive language areas.

There are age-related variables of communication problems in psychiatric disorders. Speech variables across different psychiatric disorders show an age effect, while pragmatics, receptive and expressive language, and auditory processing remain very significantly impaired across all age groups with psychiatric disorder.

There are gender-related variables in communication problems, in psychiatric disorder, as well as in the co-occurrence of psychiatric and communication disorders. More males than females generally show both communication disorders and psychiatric disorders, but females, when impaired, show more pervasive impairment.

To serve their clients optimally, speech–language pathologists should be aware of and knowledgeable regarding the signs and symptoms of a possible psychiatric disorder in individuals with communication disorders. This is important for the development of a comprehensive treatment plan that may include referral to and consultation with a mental health professional, so that treatment can be extended to ameliorate the psychiatric signs and symptoms as well as the communication deficits.

Major Points of Chapter

- Psychiatric disorders include internalizing or emotional disorders, and externalizing or behavioral disorders.
- Mental disorders with onset in childhood include autism and Asperger's syndrome; those diagnosed in adulthood include schizophrenia, psychoses, and mood and personality disorders.
- Communication and language impairments may be either an integral component of a psychiatric disorder or a related feature of a psychiatric disorder.
- A wide range of psychiatric disorders co-occur with language disorders.

Discussion Guidelines

1. Describe some of the developmental, behavioral, linguistic, social, academic, and family characteristics of a child who may be diagnosed with autism.
2. Contrast the psychiatric and communication problems of a child with emotional problems versus a child with behavioral problems.
3. Provide a case history of a hypothetical 10-year old boy with severe ADHD and a communication problem. Identify the behavioral, cognitive, and language characteristics you might expect to find.

REFERENCES

Affolder, F., Brubaker, R., & Bischofberger, W. (1974). Comparative studies of normal and language dis-turbed children based on performance profiles. *Acta Otolanryngologia, 323* (Suppl.), 1–32.

Alessi, N. E., Eisner, S. J., & Knight, C. (1990). *The association of language disturbances with cognitive and motoric impairments in psychiatrically hospitalized children.* Poster session presented at the meeting of the Society for Research in Child and Adolescent Psychopathology. Costa Mesa, CA.

Alessi, N. E., & Loomis, S. (1988, October). *The frequency and severity of language disturbances in depressed children.* Paper presented at the 35th annual meeting of the American Academy of Child and Adolescent Psychiatry. Seattle, WA.

American Psychiatric Association. (1980). *Diagnostic and statistical manual of mental disorders* (3rd ed.). Washington, DC: Author.

American Psychiatric Association. (1987). *Diagnostic and statistical manual of mental disorders* (3rd ed. revised). Washington, DC: Author.

American Psychiatric Association. (1992). Consumer leaflet on depression in children.

American Psychiatric Association. (1994). *Diagnostic and statistical manual of mental disorders* (4th ed.). Washington, DC: Author.

Anderson, J. C., Williams, S., McGee, R., & Silva, P. A. (1987). DSM-III disorders in preadolescent children. *Archives of General Psychiatry, 44,* 69–76.

Andreason, N. C. (1979a). Thought, language, and communication disorders: I. Definition of terms and their reliability. *Archives of General Psychiatry, 36*(12), 1315–1321.

Andreason, N. C. (1979b). Thought, language, and communication disorders: II. Diagnostic significance. *Archives of General Psychiatry, 36*(12), 1325–1330.

Aram, D. M., & Nation, J. E. (1980). Preschool language disorders and subsequent language and academic difficulties. *Journal of Communication Disorders, 13,* 159–170.

Arboleda, C., & Holzman, P. S. (1985). Thought disorder in children at risk for psychosis. *Archives of General Psychiatry, 42*(10), 1004–1013.

Baker, L., & Cantwell, D. P. (1985). Psychiatric and learning disorders in children with communication disorders: A critical review. In K. D. Gadow (Ed.), *Advances in learning and behavioral disabilities, 4* (pp. 29–47). Greenwich, CT: JAI Press.

Baker, L., & Cantwell, D. P. (1987a). A prospective psychiatric follow-up of children with speech/language disorders. *Journal of American Child and Adolescent Psychiatry, 26,* 546–553.

Baker, L., & Cantwell, D. P. (1987b). Comparison of well, emotionally disordered, and behaviorally disordered children with linguistic problems. *Journal of the American Academy of Child and Adolescent Psychiatry, 26,* 190–196.

Baltaxe, C. (1984). The use of contrastive stress in normal, aphasic, and autistic children. *Journal of Speech and Hearing Research, 27*(1), 97–104.

Baltaxe, C. (1993). Pragmatic language disorders in children with social communication disorders and their treatment. *Publication, American-Speech Language-Hearing Association, Neurophysiology and Neurogenic Speech and Language Disorders, 3*(1), 2–9.

Baltaxe, C. (in press). Prevalence of communication handicaps in 400 children and adolescents with psychiatric disorders: A descriptive study. *Journal of Orthopsychiatry.*

Baltaxe, C., & d'Angiola, N. (1992). Cohesion in the discourse interaction of autistic, specifically language impaired, and normal children. *Journal of Autism and Developmental Disabilities, 22*(1), 1–21.

Baltaxe, C., & d'Angiola, N. (in press). Communication deficits associated with tuberous sclerosis. *Journal of Autism and Developmental Disabilities.*

Baltaxe, C., & d'Angiola, N. (1996). Referencing skills in children with autism and specific language impairment. *European Journal of Disorders of Communication,* 31, 245–258.

Baltaxe, C., & Guthrie, D. (1987). The use of primary sentence stress by normal, aphasic, and autistic children. *Journal of Autism and Developmental Disabilities, 17*(2), 255–271.

Baltaxe, C., Russell, A., d'Angiola, N., & Simmons, J. Q. (1995). Discourse cohesion in the verbal interactions of individuals diagnosed with autistic disorder or schizotypal personality disorder. *Australian and New Zealand Journal of Communication Disorders, 20*(2), 79–96.

Baltaxe, C., & Simmons, J. Q. (1975). Language in childhood psychosis: A review. *Journal of Speech and Hearing Disorders, 40,* 439–458

Baltaxe, C., & Simmons, J. Q. (1977). Language patterns of German and English autistic adolescents. In P. Mittler (Ed.), *Proceedings of the International Association for the Scientific Study of Mental Deficiency* (pp. 267–278). Baltimore, MD: University Park Press.

Baltaxe, C., & Simmons, J. Q. (1981a). Disorders of language in childhood psychosis: Current concepts and approaches. In J. Darby (Ed.),. *Speech evaluation in psychiatry* (pp. 285–328). New York: Grune & Stratton.

Baltaxe, C., & Simmons, J. Q. (1981b). Acoustic characteristics of prosody in autism. In P. Mittler (Ed.), *Frontiers of knowledge in mental retardation, Proceedings Fifth Congress, International Association for the Scientific Study of Mental Deficiency* (pp. 223–233). Baltimore, MD: University Park Press.

Baltaxe, C., & Simmons, J. Q. (1983). Communication deficits in adolescent and adult autistics. *Seminars in Speech and Language, 4*(1), 27–41.

Baltaxe, C., & Simmons, J. Q. (1985). Prosodic development in normal and autistic children. In E. Schopler & G. Mesibov (Eds.), *Communication problems in autism* (pp. 95–125). New York: Plenum Press.

Baltaxe, C., & Simmons, J. Q. (1987). Communication deficits in the adolescent with autism, schizophrenia, and language-learning disabilities. In T. S. Layton (Ed.), *Language and treatment of autistic and developmentally disordered children* (pp. 155–180). New York: Charles C. Thomas.

Baltaxe, C., & Simmons, J. Q. (1988a). Communication deficits in preschool children with psychiatric disorders. *Seminars in Language, 9*(1), 81–91.

Baltaxe, C., & Simmons, J. Q. (1988b). Pragmatic deficits in emotionally disturbed children and adolescents. In J. Schiefelbusch & L. Lloyd (Eds.), *Language perspectives: Acquisition, retardation, and intervention* (pp. 223–253). Austin, TX: Pro-Ed Press.

Baltaxe, C., & Simmons, J. Q. (1990). The differential diagnosis of communication disorders in child and adolescent psychopathology. *Topics in Language Disorders, 10*(4), 17–31.

Baltaxe, C., & Simmons, J. Q. (1991). *Communication disorders in children and adolescents with psychiatric disorders: Age related variables.* Paper presented at the Annual Meeting American Academy of Child and Adolescent Psychiatry, San Francisco, CA.

Baltaxe, C., & Simmons, J. Q. (1992a) Gender-related vulnerability to communication disorders in children and adolescents with psychiatric disorders. *Brain Dysfunction, 5,* 239–252.

Baltaxe, C., & Simmons, J. Q. (1992b). A comparison of language issues in-high-functioning autism and related disorders with onset in childhood and adolescence. In E. Schopler & G. Mesibov (Eds.), *High-functioning individuals with autism* (pp. 201–225). New York: Plenum Press.

Baltaxe, C., & Simmons, J. Q. (1995). Speech and language disorders in children and adolescents with schizophrenia. *Schizophrenia Bulletin, 21*(4), 125–140.

Baltaxe, C., Simmons, J. Q., Russell, A., & Bott, L. (1987). *Thought, language, and communication disorders in prepubertal onset schizophrenia and schizotypal personality disorders.* Paper presented at the Academy of Child and Adolescent Psychiatry, Washington, DC.

Baltaxe, C., Simmons, J. Q., & Zee, E. (1984). Intonation patterns in normal, autistic, and aphasic children. *Proceedings of the Tenth International Congress of Phonetic Sciences* (pp. 713–718). Dortrecht, Holland: Foris Publications.

Baron-Cohen, S. (1988). Social and pragmatic deficits in autism: Cognitive or affective? *Journal of Autism and Developmental Disorders, 18*(3), 379–403.

Baron-Cohen, S. (1989). The autistic child's theory of mind: A case of specific developmental delay. *Journal of Child Psychology and Psychiatry, 30,* 285–297.

Baron-Cohen, S., Leslie, A., & Frith, U. (1985). Does the autistic child have a "theory of mind"? *Cognition, 21,* 37–46.

Bartak, L., & Rutter, M. (1975). Language and cognition in autistic and "dysphasic" children. In N. O'Connor (Ed.), *Language, cognitive deficit and retardation* (pp. 193–202). London: Butterworths.

Baumeister, J. J., Canino, G., & Bird, H. (1994). Epidemiology of disruptive behavior disorders. *Child and adolescent psychiatric clinics of North America, 3*(2), 177–194.

Baumgartner, S. (1980). The social behavior of speech disordered children as viewed by parents. *International Journal of Rehabiliative Research, 3,* 82–84.

Beitchman, J. H. (1985a). Speech and language impairment and psychiatric risk: toward a model of neurodevelopmental immaturity. *Psychiatric Clinics of North America, 8,* 721–735.

Beitchman, J. H. (1985b). Childhood schizophrenia: A review and comparison with adult-onset schizophrenia. *Psychiatric Clinics of North America, 8,* 793–814.

Beitchman, J. H., Hood, J., & Inglis, A. (1990). Psychiatric risk in children with speech and language disorders. *Journal of Abnormal Child Psychology, 18*(3), 283–296.

Beitchman, J. H., Hood, J., Rochon, J., & Peterson, M. (1989a). Empirical classification of speech/language impairment in children I: Identification of speech/language categories. *Journal of American Academy of Child and Adolescent Psychiatry, 28,* 112–117.

Beitchman, J. H., Hood, J., Rochon, J., & Peterson, M. (1989b). Empirical classification of speech/language impairment in children, II: Behavioral characteristics. *Journal of American Academy of Child and Adolescent Psychiatry, 28,* 118–123.

Beitchman, J. H., Nair, R., Clegg, M., Ferguson, B., & Patel, P. (1986a). Prevalence of psychiatric disorders in children with speech and language disorders. *Journal of the American Academy of Child Psychiatry, 25,* 528–535.

Beitchman, J. H., Nair, R., Clegg, M., Ferguson, B., & Patel, P. (1986b). Prevalence of speech and language disorders in 5-year-old kindergarten children in the Ottawa-Carleton region. *Journal of Speech and Hearing Disorders, 51,* 98–110.

Beitchman, J. H., Peterson, M., & Clegg, M. (1988). Speech and language impairment and psychiatric disorder: The relevance of family demographic variables. *Child Psychiatry and Human Development, 18,* 191–207.

Bell-Dolan, D., & Brazeal, T. (1993). Separation anxiety disorder, overanxious disorder, and school refusal. *Child and Adolescent Psychiatric Clinics of North America, 2*(4), 563–580.

Biederman, J., Farraone, S., & Lapey, K. (1992). Comorbidity of diagnosis in attention-deficit hyperactivity disorder. *Child and Adolescent Psychiatric Clinics of North America, 1*(2), 335–360.

Bird, H. R., Gould, M. S., Yagert, T., Staghezza, R., & Canino, R. (1989). Risk factors for maladjustment in Puerto Rican children. *Journal of American Child and Adolescent Psychiatry, 28,* 847–850.

Bleuler, E. (1950). *Dementia praecox or the group of schizophrenias* (J. Zinkin, Trans.). New York: International Universities Press. (Original work published 1911).

Blood, G. W., & Seiden, R. (1981). The concomitant problems of young stutterers. *Journal of Speech and Hearing Disorders, 46,* 31–33.

Bolton, P., & Rutter, M. (1990). Genetic influences in autism. *International Review of Psychiatry, 2,* 67–80.

Brandenburg, N. A., Freidman, R. M., & Silver, S. (1989). *Research on children and adolescents with mental, behavioral, and developmental disorders: Mobilizing a national initiative.* Washington, DC: National Academy Press.

Bubenickova, M. (1977). The stuttering child's relation to school. *Psychologia a Patopsychologia Dietata, 12,* 535–545.

Butler, K. G. (1965). The Bender Gestalt Visual Motor Test as a diagnostic instrument with children exhibiting articulation disorders. *ASHA, 7,* 380–381.

Caceres, V. A. (1971). Retardo del lenguaje verbal [Verbal language delay]. *Revista de Neuropsiquiatria, 34,* 210–226.

Camarata, S., Hughes, C, & Ruhl, K. (1988). Mild/moderate behaviorally disordered students: A population at risk for language disorders. *Language Speech and Hearing Services in the Schools, 19,* 191–200.

Cantwell, D. P., & Baker, L. (1977). Psychiatric disorder in children with speech and language retardation: A critical review. *Archives of General Psychiatry, 34,* 583–591.

Cantwell, D. P., & Baker, L. (1980). Psychiatric and behavioral characteristics of children with communication disorders. *Journal of Pediatric Psychology, 5,* 161–178.

Cantwell, D. P., & Baker, L. (1985). Psychiatric and learning disorders in children with speech and language disorders: A descriptive analysis. *Advances in Learning and Behavioral Disabilities, 4,* 29–47.

Cantwell, D. P., & Baker, L. (1987a). Prevalence and type of psychiatric disorder and developmental disorders in three speech and language groups. *Journal of Communicative Disorders, 20,* 151–160.

Cantwell, D. P., & Baker, L. (1987b). Clinical significance of childhood communication disorders: perspectives from a longitudinal study. *Journal of Child Neurology, 2,* 257–264.

Cantwell, D. P., & Baker, L. (1991a) *Psychiatric and developmental disorders in children with communication disorder.* Washington, DC: American Psychiatric Press.

Cantwell, D. P., & Baker, L. (1991b). Association between attention deficit-hyperactivity disorder and learning disorders. *Journal of Learning Disabilities, 24*(2), 88–95.

Cantwell, D. P., & Baker, L. (1992). Attention deficit disorder with and without hyperactivity: A review and comparison of matched groups. *Journal of the American Academy of Child and Adolescent Psychiatry, 31*(3), 432–438.

Cantwell, D. P., Baker, L., & Mattison I. (1979). The prevalence of psychiatric disorder in children with speech and language disorder: An epidemiological study. *Journal of the American Academy of Child Psychiatry, 18,* 450–461.

Cantwell, D. P., Baker, L., & Mattison I. (1980). Factors associated with the development of psychiatric disorder in children with speech and language retardation. *Archives of General Psychiatry, 37,* 423–426.

Caplan, R. (1994a). Childhood schizophrenia assessment and treatment: A developmental approach. *Child and Adolescent Psychiatric Clinics of North America, 3*(1), 15–50.

Caplan, R. (1994b). Thought disorder in childhood. *Journal of the American Academy of Child Psychiatry, 33,* 605–615.

Caplan, R., Perdue, S., Tanguay, P. E., & Fish, B. (1990). Formal thought disorder in childhood onset schizophrenia and schizotypal personality disorder. *Journal of Child Psychology and Psychiatry, 31*(7), 1103–1114.

Castellanos, F., & Rapoport, J. (1992). Etiology of attention-deficit hyperactivity disorder. *Child and Adolescent Psychiatric Clinics of North America, 1,* 373–384.

Chess, S., & Rosenberg, M. (1974). Clinical differentiation among children with initial language complaints. *Journal of Autism and Childhood Schizophrenia, 4,* 99–109.

Cohen, N.J., Davine, M., Horodesky, N., Lipsett, L., & Isaacson, L. (1993). Unsuspected language impairment in psychiatrically disturbed children: Prevale and language and behavioral characteristics. *Journal of the Amerencican Academy of Child and Adolescent Psychiatry, 33*(3), 595–603.

Costello, E. J., Costello, A. J., & Edelbrock, C. (1988). Psychiatric disorders in pediatric primary care: Prevalence and risk factors. *Archives of General Psychiatry, 45,* 1107–1116.

Cox, A. D., Rutter, M., & Yule, B. (1977). Bias resulting from missing information: Some epidemiological findings. *British Journal of Preventive and Social Medicine, 31,* 131–136.

Crosson, B., & Hughes, C. W. (1987). Role of the thalamus in language: Is it related to schizophrenic thought disorder? *Schizophrenia Bulletin, 13*(4), 605–621.

Crowther, J. H., Bond. L. A., & Rolf, J. E. (1981). The incidence, prevalence, and severity of behavior disorders among preschool-aged children in day care. *Journal of Abnormal Child Psychiatry, 9,* 23–42.

Cutting, J., David, A., & Murphy, D. (1987). The nature of overinclusive thinking in schizophrenia. *Psychopathology, 20*(3–4), 213–219.

Cutting, J., & Murphy, D. (1990). Preference for denotative as opposed to connotative meanings in schizophrenics. *Brain and Language, 39*(3), 459–468.

de Ajuriaguerra, J., Jaeggi, A., Guignard, F., Kocher, F., Marquard, M., Roth, S., & Schmidt, E. (1976). The development and prognosis of dysphasia in children. In D. Morehead & A. Morehead (Eds.), *Normal and deficient child language* (pp. 345–385). Baltimore, MD: University Park Press.

Despert, J. L. (1946). Psychosomatic study of 50 stuttering children. *American Journal of Orthopsychiatry, 16,* 100–113.

Duncan, M. H. (1947). Personality adjustment techniques in voice therapy. *Journal of Speech Disorders, 12,* 161–167.

Earls, F. (1987). Sex differences in psychiatric disorders: origins and developmental influences. *Psychiatric Development, 5,* 1–23.

Erwin, R., Van Lancker, D., Guthrie, D., Schwafel, J., Tanguay, P., & Buchwald, J. (1991). P3 responses to prosodic stimuli in adult autistic subjects. *Electroencephalography and Clinical Neurophysiology, 80*(6), 561–571.

Esser, G., Schmidt, M., & Woerner, W. (1990). Epidemiology and course of psychiatric disorders in school-age children: Results of a longitudinal study. *Journal of Child Psychology and Psychiatry, 31,* 243.

Faraone, S. V., & Biederman, J. (1994). Genetics of attention-deficit hyperactivity disorder. In L. L. Greenhill (Ed.), *Child and adolescent psychiatric clinics of North America, 3*(2), 285–302.

Ferry, P. C., Hall, S. M., & Hicks, J. L. (1975). Dilapidated speech: developmental verbal dyspraxia. *Developmental Medical Child Neurology, 17,* 749–756.

Fitzsimons, R. (1958). Developmental, psychosocial, and educational factors in children with nonorganic articulation problems. *Child Development, 29,* 481–489.

Folstein, S., & Rutter, M. (1977). Infantile autism: A genetic study of 21 twin pairs. *Journal of Child Psychology and Psychiatry, 18,* 297–321.

Fraser, W. I., King, K., & Thomas, P. (1989). Computer-assisted linguistic analysis of two mentally retarded psychotic female's texts. *Journal of Mental Deficiency Research, 33*(5), 429–435.

Fraser, W. I., King, K., Thomas, P., & Kendell, R. (1986). The diagnosis of schizophrenia by language analysis. *British Journal of Psychiatry, 148,* 275–278.

Fundudis, T., Kolvin, I., & Garside, R. (1979). *Speech retarded and deaf children: Their psychological development.* New York: Academic Press.

Gemilli, R. J. (1982). Classification of child stuttering, I: Transient developmental, neurogenic acquired, and persistent child stuttering. *Child Psychiatry and Human Development, 12,* 220–253.

Gillberg, C., Gillberg, I. C., & Steffenburg, S. (1992). Siblings and parents of children with autism: A controlled population-based study. *Developmental Medicine and Child Neurology, 34,* 389–398.

Gillespie S., & Cooper, E. (1973). Prevalence of speech problems in junior and senior high schools. *Journal of Speech and Hearing Research, 16,* 739–743.

Glasner, P. J. (1949). Personality characteristics and emotional problems of stutterers under the age of five. *Journal of Speech and Hearing Disorders, 14,* 135–138.

Goldberg, T. E. Ragland, J. D., Torrey, E. F., Gold, J. M., Bigelow, L. B., & Weinberger, D. R. (1990). Neuropsychological assessment of monozygotic twins discordant for schizophrenia. *Archives of General Psychiatry, 47*(11), 1066–1072.

Goldberg, T. E., Weinberger, D. R. Pliskin, N. H., Berman, K. F., & Podd, M. H. (1989). Recall memory deficit in schizophrenia. A possible manifestation of prefrontal dysfunction. *Schizophrenia Research, 2*(3), 251–257.

Goldfarb, W., Goldfarb, N, Braunstein P., & Lorge (1972). Speech and language faults of schizophrenic children. *Journal of Autism and Childhood Schizophrenia, 2,* 219–233.

Goldson, E., & Hagerman, R. J. (1992). The fragile-X syndrome. *Developmental Medicine and Child Neurology, 34*(9), 826–32.

Gould, M. S., Wunsch-Hitzig, R., & Dohrenwend, B. P. (1980). Formulation of hypotheses about the prevalence, treatment, and prognostic significance of psychiatric disorders in children in the United States. In B. P. Dohrenwend, M. B. Dohrenwend,

M. S., Gould, et al. (Eds.), *Mental illness in the United States: Epidemiological Estimates* (pp. 9–44). New York: Praeger.

Graham, P. (1986). *Child psychiatry: A developmental approach.* Oxford, England: Oxford Medical Publications.

Griffiths, C. P. S. (1969). A follow-up study of children with disorders of speech. *British Journal of Disordered Communication, 4,* 46–56.

Grinnell, S. W., Scott-Hartnett, D., & Larson-Glasier, J. L. (1983). Language disorders [Letter to the editor]. *Journal of the American Academy of Child Psychiatry, 22,* 580–581.

Gualtieri, C. T., Koriath, V., Van Bourgondien, M., & Saleeby, N. (1983). Language disorders in children referred for psychiatric services. *Journal of the American Academy of Child Psychiatry, 22,* 165–171.

Hagerman, R. J., & Falkenstein, A. R. (1987). An association between recurrent otitis media in infancy and later hyperactivity. *Clinical Pediatrics, 26,* 253–257.

Hall, P. K., & Tomblin, J. B. (1978). A follow-up study of children with articulation and language disorders. *Journal of Speech and Hearing Disorders, 43,* 227–241.

Halliday, M., & Hasan, R. (1976). *Cohesion in english.* London: Longman.

Harper, D. C., & Richman, L. C. (1978). Personality profiles of physically impaired adolescents. *Journal of Clinical Psychology, 34,* 636–642.

Harvey, P. S., & Brault, J. (1986). Speech performance in mania and schizophrenia: The association of positive and negative thought disorders and reference failures. *Journal of Communication Disorders, 19*(3), 161–173.

Hechtman, L., & Offord, D. R. (1994). Long-term outcome of disruptive disorders. *Child and Adolescent Psychiatric Clinics of North America, 3*(2) 379–404.

Hier, D. B., & Kaplan, J. (1980). Are sex differences in cerebral organization clinically significant? *Behavioral Brain Science, 3,* 238–239.

Hindley, P. A., Hill, P. D., McGuigan, S., & Kitson, N. (1994). Psychiatric disorder in deaf and hearing impaired children and young people: A prevalence study. *Journal of Child Psychology and Psychiatry and Allied Disciplines, 35*(4), 917–934.

Hinshaw, P. (1992). Intervention for social competence and social skill. *Child and Adolescent Psychiatric Clinics of North America, 1*(2), 539–552.

Hodges, K., & Plow, J. (1990). Intellectual ability and achievement in psychiatrically hospitalized children with conduct, anxiety, and affective disorders. *Journal of Consulting Clinical Psychologist, 58,* 589–595.

Hull, F. M., Mielke, P. W. Jr., Timmons, R. J., & Willeford, P. A. (1971). The national speech and hearing survey: Preliminary results. *ASHA, 13,* 501–509.

Huttenlocher, P., & Huttenlocher, J. (1973). A study of children with hyperlexia. *Neurology, 23,* 1107–1116.

Kanner, L. (1943). Autistic disturbances of affective contact. *Nervous Child, 2,* 217–250.

Kapp, K. (1979). Self concept of the cleft lip and or palate child. *Cleft Palate Journal, 16,* 171–176.

King, K., Fraser, W. I., Thomas, P., & Kendell, R. (1990). Re-examination of the language of psychotic subjects. *British Journal of Psychiatry, 156,* 211–215.

Kraepelin, E. (1971). *Dementia praecox and paraphrenia* (R. M. Barclay, Trans.). New York: Robert E. Krieger Publishing. (Original work published 1919).

Lerner, J. A., Inui, T. S., Trupin, E. W., & Douglas, E. (1985). Preschool behavior can predict future psychiatric disorders. *Journal of the American Academy of Child Psychiatry, 24,* 42–48.

Leslie, A., (1987). Pretense and representation: The origin of "theory of mind." *Psychological Review, 94,* 412–426.

Leslie, A., & Frith, U. (1987). Metarepresentation and autism: How not to lose one's marbles. *Cognition, 27,* 291–294.

Leslie, A., & Frith, U. (1988). Autistic children's understanding of seeing, knowing, and believing. *British Journal of Developmental Psychology, 6,* 315–324.

Loomis, S., & Alessi, N. E. (1988, October). *Speech/language disorders in a group of child psychiatric inpatients.* Paper presented at the 35th annual meeting of the American Academy of Child and Adolescent Psychiatry, Seattle, WA.

Love, A. J., & Thompson, M. G. (1988). Language disorders and attention deficit disorders in young children referred for psychiatric services: Analysis of prevalence and a conceptual synthesis. *American Journal of Orthopsychiatry, 58,* 52–64.

Ludlow, C., & Cooper, J. (1983). *Genetic aspects of speech and language disorders.* New York: Academic Press.

McCauley, E., & Meyers, K. (1992). The longitudinal clinical course of depression in children and adolescents. *Child and Adolescent Clinics of North America, 11*(1), 183–196.

McGee, R., Partridge, F., Williams, S., & Silva (1991). A twelve year follow-up of preschool hyperactive children. *Journal of the American Academy of Child and Adolescent Psychiatry, 30,* 224.

McGee, R., Williams, S., & Feehan, M. (1992). Attention deficit disorder and age of onset of problem behaviors. *Journal of Abnormal Child Psychiatry, 20*(5), 487–502.

McWilliams, B. J., & Musgrave, R. H. (1972). Psychological implications of articulation disorders in cleft palate children. *Cleft Palate Journal, 9,* 294–303.

Menuyk, P., & Quill, K. (1985). Semantic problems in autistic children. In E. Schopler & G. B. Mesibov (Eds.), *Communication Problems in Autism* (pp. 124–144). New York: Plenum Press.

Milisen, R. (1971). The incidence of speech disorders. In L. Travis (Ed.), *Handbook of speech pathology and audiology* (pp. 619–633). Englewood Cliffs, NJ: Prentice-Hall.

Miller, J. (1981). *Assessing language production in children: Experimental procedures.* Baltimore, MD: University Park Press.

Minshew, N. (1995, March). *The autistic spectrum: Clinical aspects.* Paper presented at the Conference on Spectrum of Developmental Disabilities, Johns Hopkin University, Baltimore, MD.

Morice, R., & McNicol, D. (1985). The comprehension and production of complex syntax in schizophrenia. *Cortex, 21*(4), 567–580.

Muma, J. R., Laeder, R. L., & Webb, C. E. (1968). Adolescent voice quality aberrations: Personality and social status. *Journal of Speech and Hearing Research, 11,* 576–582.

Neils, J., & Aram, D. M. (1986). Family history of children with developmental language disorders. *Perceptual Motor Skills, 63,* 655–658.

Nuechterlein, K. H., & Dawson, M. E. (1984). Information processing and attentional functioning in the developmental course of schizophrenic disorders. *Schizophrenia Bulletin, 10*(2), 160–203.

O'Callaghan, E., Larkin, C., & Waddington, J. L. (1990). Obstetric complications in schizophrenia and the validity of maternal recall. *Psychological Medicine, 20*(1), 89–94.

Offord, D. R., Boyle, M. H, Szatmari, P., Rae-Grant, N. I., Links, P. S., Cadman, D. T., Byles, J. A., Crawford, J. W., Byrne, C., Thomas, H., & Wood-

ward, C. A. (1987). Ontario child health study. II: Six-month prevalence of disorder and raters of service utilization. *Archives of General Psychiatry, 44,* 69–76.

Ounsted, M., Moar, V. A., & Scott, A. (1986). Factors affecting development: Similarities and differences among children who were small, average, and large for gestational age at birth. *Acta Paediatrica Scandanavica, 75,* 261–266.

Paul, R., & Cohen, D. J. (1984). Outcomes of severe disorders of language acquisition. *Journal of Autism and Developmental Disorders, 14,* 405–421.

Paul, R., Cohen, D. J., & Caparulo, B. K. (1983). A longitudinal study of patients with severe developmental disorders of language learning. *Journal of the American Academy of Child Psychiatry, 22,* 525–534.

Piacentini, J. (1987). Language dysfunction and childhood behavior disorders. In B. B. Lahey & A. Kazdin (Eds.), *Advances in clinical child psychology* (pp. 259–287), New York: Plenum Press.

Pierce, S., & Bartolucci, G. (1977). A syntactic investigation of verbal autistic, mentally retarded, and normal children. *Journal of Autism and Childhood Schizophrenia, 7*(2), 121–134.

Prizant, B. M. (1983). Language acquisition and communication behavior. Toward an understanding of the 'whole of it.' *Journal of Speech and Hearing Disorders, 48*(3), 296–307.

Prizant, B. M., Audet, L., Burke, G., Hummel, L., Maher, S., & Theodore, G. (1988) *Serving children and adolescents with communication disorders and emotional/behavioral disorders.* Paper presented at the annual convention of the American Speech–Language–Hearing Association, Boston, MA.

Prizant, B., Audet, L., Burke, G., Hummel, L., Maher, S., & Theodore., G. (1990). Communication disorders and emotional/behavioral disorders in children and adolescents. *Journal of Speech and Hearing Disorders, 55,* 179–192.

Richman, N., & Stevenson, J. E. (1977). Language delay in 3-year-olds: Family and social factors. *Acta Paediatrica Belgica, 30,* 213–219.

Ricks, D., & Wing, L. (1975). Language, communication, and the use of symbols in normal and autistic children. *Journal of Autism and Childhood Schizophrenia, 5,* 191–221.

Rochester, S., & Martin, J. (1979). *Crazy talk: A study in the discourse of schizophrenic speakers.* New York: Plenum Press.

Rogeness, G. A. (1994). Biologic findings in conduct disorder. In L. L. Greenhill (Ed.), *Child and Adolescent Psychiatric Clinics of North America, 3*(2), 217–284.

Ross, N. (1979). *Manifestations of hyperlexia in eight autistic boys.* Unpublished master's thesis. University of California.

Rudel, R. G., Denckla, M. B., & Browman, M. (1981). The effect of varying stimulus context on word-finding ability: Dyslexia further differentiated from other learning disabilities. *Brain and Language, 13,* 130–144.

Ruess, A. L. (1965). A comparative study of cleft palate children and their siblings. *Journal of Clinical Psychology, 21,* 354–360.

Rumsey, J., Andreason, N., & Rapoport, J. (1986). Thought, language, communication, and affective flattening in autistic adults. *Archives of General Psychiatry, 48,* 771–777.

Rutter, M. (1971). Psychiatry. In J. Wortis (Ed.), *Mental retardation: An annual review,* (Vol. 3, pp. 186–221). New York: Grune & Stratton.

Rutter, M. (1974a). The development of infantile autism. *Psychological Medicine, 4,* 147–163.

Rutter, M. (1974b). Emotional disorder and educational underachievement. *Archives of Disease in Childhood, 49*(4), 249–256.

Rutter, M. (1987). The role of cognition in child development and disorder. *British Journal of Medical Psychology, 60,* 1–6.

Rutter, M., Cox, A., Tupling, C., Berger, & Yule. (1975). Attainment and adjustment in two geographical areas, I: The prevalence of psychiatric disorder. *British Journal of Psychiatry, 126,* 493–509.

Rutter, M., & Lockyer, (1967). A five to fifteen year follow-up study of infantile psychosis. I: Description of sample. *British Journal of Psychiatry, 113,* 1169–1182.

Rutter, M., & Martin, J. (Eds.). (1972). *The child with delayed speech.* London: Heinemann.

Rutter, M., & Schopler, E. (1987). Autism and pervasive developmental disorders: Concepts and diagnostic issues. *Journal of Autism and Developmental Disorders, 17*(2), 159–187.

Rutter, M., Tizard, J., & Whitmore, K. (1970). *Education, health, and behavior.* London: Longman.

Schuler, A., & Prizant, B. (1985). Echolalia. In E. Schopler and G. B. Mesibov (Eds.), *Communication problems in autism* (pp. 163–182). New York: Plenum Press.

Schweckendiek, W., & Danzer, C. (1970). Psychological studies in patients with clefts. *Cleft Palate Journal, 7,* 533–539.

Shaffer, D. (1986). Brain damage. In M. Rutter & L. Hersov (Eds.), *Child and adolescent psychiatry: Modern approaches* (pp. 129–151). Oxford, England: Blackwell Scientific Publications.

Sheridan, M. D., & Peckham, C. S. (1973). Hearing and speech at seven. *Special Education, 62,* 16–20.

Shriberg, L., Kwiatkowski, J., Best, S., Hengst, J., & Terselic-Weber, B. (1986). Characteristics of children with phonologic disorders of unknown origin. *Journal of Speech and Hearing Disorders, 51,* 140–161.

Silva, P. A., Justin, C., McGee, R., & WIlliams, S. M.. (1984). Some developmental and behavioral characteristics of seven year old children with delayed speech development. *British Journal of Disorders of Communication, 19,* 147–154.

Silverstein, M. L., McDonald, C., & Meltzer, H. Y. (1988). Differential patterns of neuropsychological deficit in psychiatric disorders. *Journal of Clinical Psychology, 44*(3), 412–415.

Simmons, J. Q., & Baltaxe, C. (1975). Language patterns of adolescent autistics. *Journal of Autism and Childhood Schizophrenia, 5,* 333–351.

Simonds, J. F., & Heimburger, R. E. (1978). Psychiatric evaluation of youth with cleft lip-palate matched with a control group. *Cleft Palate Journal, 15,* 193–201.

Slater, E., Beard, A. W., & Clithero, E. (1963). The schizophrenia-like psychoses of epilepsy. *British Journal of Psychiatry, 109,* 95–105.

Solomon, A. I. (1961). Personality and behavior patterns of children with functional defects of articulation. *Child Development, 32,* 731–737.

Spriesterbach, D.C., (1973). *Psychosocial aspects of "the cleft palate problem"* (Vol. 1). Iowa City: University of Iowa Press.

Steffenburg, S., Hellgren. L., Andersson, L., Gillberg, I. C., Jakobsson, G., & Bohman, M. (1989). A twin study of autism in Denmark, Finland, Iceland, Norway and Sweden. *Journal of Child Psychology and Psychiatry, 30,* 405–416.

Steinberg, D. (1985). Psychotic and other disorders in adolescence. In M. Rutter & L. Hersov (Eds.), *Children and adolescent psychiatry: Modern approaches* (pp. 567–583). Oxford, England: Blackwell Scientific Publications.

Stevenson, J. E., & Richman, N. (1976). The prevalence of language delay in a population of three-year-old children and its association with general retardation. *Developmental Medical Child Neurology, 18,* 431–441.

Stevenson, J. E., & Richman, N. (1978). Behavior, language and development in three-year-old children. *Journal of Autism and Childhood Schizophrenia, 8,* 299–313.

Stewart, J. M. (1981). Multidimensional scaling analysis of communicative disorders by race and sex in a mid-south public school system. *Journal of Communicative Disorders, 14,* 467–483.

Stewart, J. M., & Spells, V. R. (1983). Learning disabilities with communicative disorders as related handicaps: A two year study. *Journal of Communicative Disorders, 16,* 345–355.

Swisher, L., & Demetras, M. (1985). The expressive language characteristics of autistic children compared with mentally retarded or specific language impaired children. In E. Schopler & G. B. Mesibov (Eds.), *Communication problems in autism* (pp. 147–162). New York: Plenum Press.

Szatmari, P. (1992). The epidemiology of attention-deficit hyperactivity disorders. *Child and Adolescent Psychiatric Clinics of North America, 1*(2), 361–372.

Tallal, P., Dukette, D., and Curtiss, S. (1989). Behavioral/emotional profiles of preschool language-impaired children. *Development and Psychopathology, 1,* 51–67.

Tanguay, P. (1990). Infantile autism and social communication spectrum disorders [Editor's Note]. *Journal of the American Academy of Child and Adolescent Psychiatry, 29,* 51.

Tantam, D., Holmes, D, & Cordess, C. (1993). Nonverbal expression in autism of Asperger type. *Journal of Autism and Developmental Disorders, 23*(1), 111–133.

Theodore, G., Maher, S., & Prizant, B. (1990). Early assessment and intervention with emotional and behavioral disorders and communication disorders. *Topics in Language Disorders, 10*(4), 42–56.

Thomas, P., King, K., & Fraser, W. I. (1987). Positive and negative symptoms of schizophrenia and linguistic performance. *Acta Psychiatrica Scandinavica, 76*(2), 144–151.

Thomas, P., King, K., Fraser, W. I., & Kendell, R. E. (1990). Linguistic performance in schizophrenia: A comparison of acute and chronic patients. *British Journal of Psychiatry, 156,* 204–210, 214–215.

Trapp, E. P., & Evan, J. (1960). Functional articulatory defect and performance on a non-verbal task. *Journal of Speech and Hearing Disorders, 25,* 176–180.

Trautman, J., Giddan, J. J., & Jurs, S. (1990). Language risk factors in emotionally disturbed children within a school and day treatment program. *Journal of Child Communication Disorders, 13,* 123–133.

Velez, C. N., Johnson, J., & Cohen P. (1988). The children in the community project: A longitudinal analysis of selected risk factors for childhood psychopathology. *Journal of the American Academy of Child and Adolescent Psychiatry, 28,* 861–864.

Volkmar, F. R., & Cohen, D. (1994). Autism: Current concepts. *Child and Adolescent Psychiatric Clinics of North America, 3*(1), 43–52.

Volkmar, F. R., & Nelson, D. S. (1990). Seizure disorders in autism. *Journal of the American Academy of Child and Adolescent Psychiatry, 29* (1), 127–129.

Wagner, M. (1995). Outcomes for youth with serious emotional disturbance in secondary school and early adulthood. In *The Future of Children (Critical Issues for Children and Youths) 5,*(2) Menlo Park, CA: The David and Lucille Packard Foundation.

Wagner, M., Newman, L., & Shaver, B. (1993) *The national Longitudinal Transition Study of Special Education Students: Sample characteristics and procedures* Menlo Park, CA: SRI International, 90–112.

Watson, L. (1988). Pragmatic abilities and disabilities in autistic children. In T. L. Layton (Ed.), *Language and treatment of autistic and developmentally disordered children* (pp 89–127). Springfield, IL: Charles C. Thomas.

Weber, J. L. (1965). The speech and language abilities of emotionally disturbed children. *Canadian Psychiatry Journal, 10,* 417–420.

Weiss, K. M., Vrtunski, P. B., & Simpson, D. M. (1988). Information overload disrupts digit recall performance in schizophrenics. *Schizophrenia Research, 1*(4), 299–303.

Werry, J. S. (1992). Child and adolescent (early onset) schizophrenia: A review in light of DSM-III-R. *Journal of Autism and Developmental Disorders, 22*(4), 601–624.

Werry, J. S. (1994). Pharmacotherapy of disruptive behavior disorders. *Child and Adolescent Psychiatric Clinics of North America, 3*(2), 321–342.

Whalen, C., & Henker, B. (1992). Social profile of attention-deficit hyperactivity disorder: Five fundamental facets. *Child and Adolescent Psychiatric Clinics of North America, 1*(2), 395–410.

Whalen, C. K., Henker, B., & Granger, D. A. (1990). Social judgment processes in hyperactive boys: Effects of methylphenidate and comparisons with normal peers. *Journal of Abnormal Child Psychology, 18*, 297–316.

Wiig, E., & Semel, E. (1973). Comprehension of linguistic concepts requiring logical operations by learning disabled children. *Journal of Speech and Hearing Research, 16*, 627–636.

Wiig, E., & Semel, E. (1975). Productive language abilities in learning disabled adolescents. *Journal of Learning Disabilities, 8*, 578–586.

Wilcox, J., & Nasrallah, H. (1987). Childhood head trauma and psychosis. *Psychiatry Research, 21*, 303–306.

Wolff, S., Narayan, S., & Moyes, B. (1988). Personality characteristics of parents of autistic children: A controlled study. *Journal of Child Psychology and Psychiatry, 29*, 143–153.

Wyatt, G. L. (1958). Mother-child relationship and stuttering in children. *Dissertation Abstracts, 19*, 881.

APPENDIX A

Mental Disorders First Diagnosed in Infancy, Childhood, and Adolescence

1. *Mental retardation.* The defining characteristics of *mental retardation* are significantly subaverage general intellectual functioning accompanied by significant limitations in adaptive functioning in at least two of the following skill areas: communication, self-care, home living, social/interpersonal skills, use of community resources, self-direction, functional academic skills, work, leisure, health, and safety. The onset must occur before age 18 years. Mental retardation has many different etiologies and may be seen as the final common pathway of various pathological processes that affect the functioning of the central nervous system.

2. *Learning disorders* (reading disorder, mathematics disorder, disorder of written language expression). *Learning disorders* are diagnosed when the individual's achievement on individually administered standardized tests in reading, mathematics, or written expression is substantially below that expected for age, schooling, and level of intelligence. The learning problems significantly interfere with academic achievement or activities of daily living that require reading, mathematical, and writing skills.

3. *Motor skills disorder* (developmental coordination disorder). The essential features of *developmental coordination disorder* are marked impairment in the development of motor coordination and performance on daily activities requiring motor coordination that is substantially below that expected, given the person's chronological age and that measured intelligence, and that is not due to a generalized medical condition.

4. *Communication disorders.* Types of communication disorder included in *DSM-IV* (1994) include expressive language disorder, mixed receptive expressive language disorder, phonological disorder, and stuttering. *Communication disorders* are defined by scores on standardized tests, interference with academic or occupational achievement, or with social communication. Exclusionary criteria relate to mental retardation; speech, motor, or sensory deficits; environmental deprivation, and pervasive developmental disorder.

5. *Pervasive developmental disorders.* *Pervasive developmental disorders* include autism, Rett's disorder, childhood disintegrative disorder, Asperger's disorder, and pervasive developmental disorder not otherwise specified (PDD NOS). This class of disorders is characterized by severe and pervasive impairment in several areas of development, including reciprocal social interaction skills, communication skills, or the presence of stereotyped behavior, interests, and activities. The qualitative impairments that define these conditions are distinctly deviant relative to the individual's developmental level or mental age. In *DSM-III* (APA, 1980) and *DSM-III-R* (APA, 1987), the above five classes of disorders were grouped under the category of Developmental Disorders and often are reported under this rubric in research articles on language and psychiatric disorders.

6. *Attention deficit and disruptive behavior disorders.* This group of disorders includes attention deficit/hyperactivity disorder (ADHD), conduct disorder, and oppositional defiant disorder. The essential feature of *ADHD* is a persistent pattern of inattention and/or hyperactivity-impulsivity that is more frequent and severe than is typically present in individuals at a comparable level of development, observed in more than one environment such as home and school, with some hyperactive-impulsive or inattentive symptoms present by age 7 years. *Oppositional defiant disorder* is characterized by a pattern of hostile and defiant behavior lasting at least six months. The disturbance in behavior causes clinically significant impairment in social, academic, or occupational functioning. The essential feature of *conduct disorder* is a repetitive and persistent pattern of behavior in which the basic rights of others or major age appropriate societal norms or rules are violated and the disturbance in behavior causes clinically significant impairment in social, academic, or occupational functioning. Conduct disorder includes aggression toward people and animals, destruction of property, deceitfulness or theft, and serious violations of rules. In *DSM-III* and *DSM-III-R* this class of disorders was grouped as disruptive behavior disorders. There is significant comorbidity among these disorders and ADHD is likely to occur with conduct disorder or oppositional disorder.

7. *Feeding and eating disorders of infancy and early childhood.* This group of disorders is characterized by persistent feeding and eating disturbances and includes *pica* (the persistent eating of nonnutritive substances), *rumination disorder* (the repeated regurgitation and rechewing of food), and *feeding disorder of infancy and childhood* (the persistent failure to eat adequately as reflected by a significant failure to gain weight).

8. *Tic disorders* (Tourette's disorder, chronic motor or vocal tic disorder, transient tic disorder). A tic is a sudden, rapid recurrent, nonrhythmic, stereotyped motor movement or vocalization. It is experienced as irresistible but can be suppressed for varying lengths of time. All forms of tics may be exacerbated by stress and attenuated during absorbing activities.

9. *Elimination disorders.* This includes enuresis and encopresis. *Encopresis* is characterized by the repeated passage of feces into inappropriate places, whether involuntary or intentional after the age of 4, and not due to a general medical condition. The essential feature of *enuresis* is the repeated voiding of urine during the day or at night into bed or into cloth, generally involuntarily but on occasion intentional, in a child of at least 5 years of chronological age or mental age.

10. *Other disorders of infancy, childhood, and adolescence.* These include separation anxiety disorder, reactive attachment disorder, and selective mutism. In *separation anxiety disorder* there is excessive anxiety concerning separation from the home or from those to whom the person is attached. The essential feature of *selective mutism* is the persistent failure to speak in specific situations (i.e., in school) where speaking is expected, despite speaking in other situations. The essential feature of *reactive attachment disorder* is markedly disturbed and developmentally inappropriate social relatedness in most contexts that begins before age 5 and is associated with grossly pathological care.

APPENDIX B

Adult Psychiatric Disorders Also Identified in Childhood and Adolescence

1. *The schizophrenias and other psychotic disorders.* The essential feature of the schizophrenias and psychoses is a mixture of characteristic signs and symptoms that have been present for a significant portion of time (and for schizophrenia, with some signs of the symptoms persisting over at least six months. These signs and symptoms are associated with marked social or occupational dysfunction and include a range of cognitive and emotional dysfunctions that include perception; inferential thinking; language and communication; behavioral monitoring; affect, fluency, and productivity of thought and speech; hedonic capacity, volition, and drive; and attention.

2. *Personality disorders.* This group of disorders includes schizoid, schizotypal, antisocial, and other personality disorders. The common feature of a *personality disorder* is an enduring pattern of inner experience and behavior that deviates markedly from the expectations of the individual's culture, is pervasive and inflexible, has an onset in adolescence or early adulthood, is stable over time, and leads to distress or impairment. Personality disorders are differentiated from each other by specific characteristics.

3. *Anxiety disorders.* This group of disorders includes panic disorders, phobias, obsessive–compulsive disorder, post-traumatic stress disorder, and generalized anxiety disorder. The different types of anxiety disorders carry different essential features. Thus, *panic disorders* are characterized by the sudden onset of intense apprehension, fearfulness, or terror, often associated with feelings of impending doom. *Phobias* are characterized by clinically significant anxiety provoked by exposure to a specific feared object or (social) situation, often leading to avoidance behavior. *Post-traumatic stress disorder* is characterized by the re-experiencing of an extremely traumatic event accompanied by symptoms of increased arousal and by avoidance of stimuli associated with trauma. *Generalized anxiety disorder* is characterized by persistent anxiety and worry for a period of at least six months.

4. *Adjustment disorders.* The essential feature of an *adjustment disorder* is the development of clinically significant emotional or behavioral symptoms in response to an identifiable psychosocial stressor or stressors.

5. *Mood disorders.* In mood disorders, disturbance in mood is the predominant features. *Mood disorders* include major depressive disorder, bipolar disorder, manic and **hypomanic episode, dysthymic disorder,** and **cyclothymic disorder.**

5

DIFFERENTIATING THE DEMENTIAS

SUSAN DE SANTI

The term *successful aging* is used to characterize older persons who are healthy, have lived a long life, and report being satisfied with their life (Palmore, 1979). Unsuccessful aging results when changes occur that are beyond what one expects during normal aging. *Dementia* is an umbrella term for a group of pathological conditions or syndromes that occur with unsuccessful aging (Fraser, 1987). The dementias are acquired disorders, characterized by progressive deterioration in several cognitive domains (Cummings and Benson, 1982). According to the *Diagnostic and Statistical Manual of Mental Disorders IV (DSM-IV)* (American Psychiatric Association, 1994), in order to be classified as a dementia, memory must be impaired, and at least one of the following must also be impaired: abstract thinking, judgment, higher cortical functions, or personality. There are several types of dementia, each with a different underlying cause, producing different clinical expressions and disease processes.

This chapter will focus on the differentiating characteristics of cortical dementia (e.g., Alzheimer's disease and Pick's disease), subcortical dementia (i.e., Parkinson's disease and Huntington's chorea), dementia resulting from multiple brain infarctions (i.e., multi-infarct dementia), and those resulting from infectious diseases (i.e., Creutzfeldt–Jakob disease). Each dementia will be discussed separately. First, the clinical presentation and description of the neuropathological condition associated with the dementia will be reviewed to introduce each disease and explain how each disorder is a result of a different underlying neuropathology. Next, neuropsychological behaviors associated with dementia including memory, language, motor functioning and visuospatial abilities will be examined. Psychological complications will be discussed in addition to both medical and behavioral treatments. Following this, *in-vivo* brain assessment using scanning technologies that include MRI and PET will be considered. These imaging techniques provide pictures of the brain which may assist in diagnosis. A section discussing the role of the speech-language pathologist in the diagnosis and treatment of the various dementias will be included. Lastly, caregiver intervention programs designed to assist caregivers in managing their family member who has dementia will be presented.

CORTICAL DEMENTIAS

Alzheimer's Disease

Alzheimer's disease (AD) was identified in 1906 by Alois Alzheimer who reported on a patient initially displaying memory changes, disorientation in her own home, jealousy and suspiciousness toward her spouse and paranoid thoughts (i.e., someone was trying to kill her). Her condition deteriorated, showing increased memory changes, perceptual problems, and comprehension problems, but no motor difficulties. At autopsy (four-and-one-half years after initial symptoms), Alzheimer noted that her brain was atrophic (shrunken). When an examination of brain tissue was done under a microscope, changes were seen in **neurons.** Some neurons had a few prominent neurofibrils (a cytoskeletal filamentous structure seen with an electron microscope), others had many neurofibrils bundled together (forming **neurofibrillary tangles**). In some regions there were no neurons, only bundled neurofibrils (known today as "**ghost tangles**"). In addition, throughout the cortex, Alzheimer noted the "deposition of a peculiar substance" (p. 3) known as **senile plaques.**

Clinical Presentation. Alzheimer's disease has a slow, insidious onset and proceeds steadily until death. The duration of the disease varies, with death occurring approximately 10 years after diagnosis. The prevalence of Alzheimer's disease is approximately 6 percent of the population over the age of 65, increasing to over 15 percent in those over 80 years of age (Clark & Witte, 1993).

Alzheimer's disease is a heterogeneous disease (i.e., a disease that shows different behavioral characteristics) in which patients do not follow a definitive clinical course. Three characteristic clinical presentations have been described by Martin (1987), each demonstrating a different primary behavioral impairment of memory, language, or visuo–spatial skills. Although there is no single presentation of the disease, various clinicians and researchers have described progressive stages of Alzheimer's disease following a behavioral paradigm (Reisberg Ferris, de Leon, & Crook, 1982), a linguistic paradigm (Obler & Albert, 1984), and a neuropathological paradigm (Braak & Braak, 1991).

The behavioral schema developed by Reisberg, Ferris, de Leon, and Crook (1982), known as the Global Deterioration Scale (GDS), is a seven-point rating scale that assesses the cognitive and functional capacity of the elderly and provides a staging scale from normal aging to severe Alzheimer's disease. A person at Stage 1 has no subjective memory complaints and upon clinical interview shows no memory impairment. In Stage 2, subjective memory complaints (i.e., forgot where the keys are, forgot someone's name) without objective evidence of memory impairment on clinical interview are noted. Stages 1 and 2 are considered within the limits of normal aging. Patients in Stage 3 are considered to have a mild cognitive impairment. Their behavior is characterized by deficits including getting lost traveling to an unfamiliar location, performance changes at work, word finding difficulties, poor reading retention, decreased memory for names of people, and concentration difficulties during formal testing. It is only upon extensive interviewing that objective evidence for performance problems is seen. Stage 4 is considered to be the first stage of Alzheimer's disease in which problems during a clinical interview are noted. Deficits in knowledge of current and recent events, memory of one's personal history, concentration, ability to travel and handle finances, orientation to time and person, and performing complex tasks, are characteristic of this stage. With progression to Stage 5, the patient needs assistance with activities of daily living. During an interview, patients in Stage 5 typically are unable to recall their address, telephone number, or the names of close family members, although they may remember their own name and their spouse's name. Disorientation to time or place is often noted at this stage.

In Stage 6, there is a lack of awareness of recent events and experiences, although some knowledge of the patient's past life may be retained. Due to this lack of awareness of their surroundings, the year, the season of the year, and so on, patients usually require some assistance for survival (e.g., for traveling, dressing). Sleep patterns are frequently disturbed. Personality and emotional changes occur, including delusional behavior (e.g., talk to self in mirror), obsessive behavior (e.g., repeat a simple task over and over), anxiety symptoms (e.g., fear of someone hurting them), agitation, and violent behavior.

At Stage 7, all verbal ability may be lost, with only grunts being produced. Patients usually need assistance with feeding and bathroom activities. A loss of psychomotor skills which effects the ability to walk may be noted. Frequently these patients are bedridden with their extremities in contracted positions. Generalized and cortical neurologic signs and symptoms such as primitive reflexes (e.g., sucking reflex, plantar reflex) are frequently present.

Neuropathology. The neuropathological changes noted by Alzheimer (1987) can only be seen with a microscope and tissue staining. Gross brain changes, however, can be seen without the aid of a microscope. These include gyral atrophy and ventricular enlargement. The brain of an Alzheimer's disease patient shows diffuse atrophy resulting in a weight reduction of approximately 20 percent (Koo & Price, 1993) compared to normal controls. Kemper (1984), on the other hand, noted great individual variability in brain weight with much overlap between Alzheimer's disease cases and normal elderly control subjects. The change in brain weight attributed to atrophy of brain tissue appears most pronounced in the temporal, frontal, and parietal lobes (Kemper, 1984). Additionally, the **ventricles** become larger, a change more prominent when compared to age-matched controls (Tomlinson, Blessed, & Roth, 1970). It appears that the brain atrophy and ventricular enlargement are related to underlying neuropathologic change (Tomlinson, Blessed, & Roth, 1970) such as the deposit of senile plaques and the formation of neurofibrillary tangles.

Alzheimer's disease has been termed "a hippocampal dementia" (Ball, et al., 1985) because of the extensive damage to the cells of the **hippocampus** and the **entorhinal cortex** (the cortical area adjacent to the hippocampus, located in the **parahippocampal** gyrus), affecting the connections between these two areas, the **amygdala** (a nucleus in the temporal lobe), and the **neocortex**

(Braak, et al., 1991). Regions of the neocortex that are particularly vulnerable to cell loss in Alzheimer's disease include the temporo-parietal association areas, premotor frontal regions, and cortex of the frontal pole (Kemper, 1984). While cellular loss is seen in the brains of normal-aged individuals, neuropathologic changes occur in the hippocampus of nondemented persons as well (de la Monte, 1989), suggesting that this region may be an early site of pathologic change prior to the alterations of cortical regions.

Senile plaques, seen in gray matter, are round in shape, found outside the neuron, and contain a center core composed of **amyloid peptides** (known as beta/A4), which are surrounded by dystrophic neurites (abnormal dendrites and axons). It is important to note that there are other components inside this center core (e.g., **apolipoprotein E**), the relevance of which are unknown at this time. The amyloid peptide (an **amino acid**) is derived from the **amyloid precursor protein** (APP) which is cleaved (separated) at specific sites along the protein chain. The abnormal processing of the precursor protein can give rise to abnormal amounts of amyloid or abnormal structures of amyloid (Selkoe, 1994) suggesting a plausible mechanism for Alzheimer's disease. The function of the amyloid precursor protein in normal cells is not yet known.

In order to better understand why abnormal processing of the precursor protein can be a plausible mechanism, we must look at Familial Alzheimer's Disease (FAD), a group of genetically transmitted forms of Alzheimer's disease. FAD has an onset before the age of 65, resulting from a chromosomal mutation. One type of FAD is caused by a mutation on chromosome 21 (Citron, et al., 1992). This mutated gene is associated with changes in the amyloid precursor protein and accounts for Alzheimer's disease in these familial cases. While nonfamilial cases of Alzheimer's disease do not possess this gene, they do have abnormal processing of the amyloid precursor protein. Therefore, it may be possible that abnormal processing of the amyloid precursor protein can account for Alzheimer's disease in nonfamilial cases as well (Selkoe, 1994). However, there are several other mechanisms that may be involved in the formation of plaques or in the pathological impact of plaques on the brain. For example, a variety of different cell types around the plaques such as **microglia,** or **astrocytes,** may be involved in the formation of the plaques.

The other classical neuropathological finding in Alzheimer's disease is neurofibrillary tangles (NFT) which are composed of bundles of helically twisted filaments called paired helical filaments (PHF) (Terry, 1963). Tangles are found inside the neuron and are formed largely from abnormally phosphorylated (decomposed) **tau protein.** Tau is a **microtubule**-associated protein, which is an important intracellular system assisting in the movement of cell components (chemicals) from the cell body down to the axon (Trojanowski, Schmidt, Shin, Bramblett, Rao, & Lee, 1993). When tau becomes abnormally phosphorylated, the transportation of cell components is impeded and the axon does not get what it needs for healthy functioning.

Other neuropathologic changes such as neuronal loss and synaptic loss are noted in Alzheimer's disease and are correlated with the degree of cognitive impairment (Terry, et al., 1991). That is, more advanced stages of Alzheimer's disease are correlated with greater neuronal and synaptic loss. Changes such as reduced amounts of neurotransmitters, the chemicals that allow transmission of a signal from one neuron to the next, have also been reported, affecting **acetylcholine,** serotonin, norepinephrine, and other neuro chemicals. (Hedera & Whitehouse, 1995). These neurotransmitter changes have directed much of the drug treatment protocols in the past few decades.

Neuropsychological Changes

Memory. Memory problems appear to be the most obvious behavioral change associated with Alzheimer's disease. Specifically, memory deficits affecting information acquired in the recent past are seen early in Alzheimer's disease and are manifested by difficulty learning new material such as word lists, paired word associates, stories,

and visuo–spatial information. Retention of newly learned material is difficult and performance on delayed word (Martin, Bowers, Cox, & Fedio, 1985) and story recall (Convit, et al., 1995b) and delayed visual recall (Flicker, Bartus, Crook, & Ferris, 1984) is poor. Remote memory (knowledge about personal and public events that occurred in the past) is less impaired initially but deteriorates with disease progression. Procedural memory (knowledge of how to carry out a task) seems maintained until late in the disease.

Language. Language may or may not be affected early in the disease. General language changes associated with mild cognitive impairment as well as with stages of Alzheimer's disease will be presented next. The staging system described earlier, the Global Deterioration Scale (GDS) (Reisberg et al., 1982), is the framework within which language changes will be discussed.

1. **Mild cognitive impairment (GDS 3),** as was stated previously, is not a stage of Alzheimer's disease, but one in which some cognitive change has occurred. Language problems are noted on naming tasks, and the patient will actively search for words when this occurs. During conversation, subtle word-finding problems and delayed word responses are found. Circumlocuting can often result in producing the correct word. During discourse the patient might initially drift from the topic, but will be able to return to it. A variety of syntactic structures are used during production. Comprehension of complex syntactic sentences (e.g., passives) is difficult due to memory and attention deficits as well as the rate at which language is processed. Difficulties repeating complex or long sentences are also related to memory and attention problems. Reading and writing are intact.

2. **Moderate cognitive impairment (GDS 4),** the first stage of Alzheimer's disease, is characterized by naming problems. Semantic paraphasias (a word-substitution error in which the meaning of the substituted word is related to the target word) are produced and are particularly evident on low frequency items. Self-corrections, nevertheless, often result in the appropriate response.

Syntactic variety continues to be present during verbal production. However, word finding problems, characterized by delayed word responses, are noted. At the earlier stage (GDS 3), circumlocutions were helpful, but at this stage (GDS 4), they no longer lead to finding the correct word. Comprehension of complex syntactic sentences continues to be problematic due to overt memory, attention, and rate of processing deficits. Additionally, comprehension diminishes as material increases in length and complexity. The patient may ask for information to be repeated as a strategy to improve comprehension, but this is not usually successful. There is much difficulty making inferences and extrapolating the meaning.

Repetition of high frequency words and sentences is unremarkable but low frequency words or long sentences are problematic. Patients may produce a more frequent word for a low frequency word, and only fragments of a long sentence may be repeated. Those at Stage 4 can initiate automatic series, but may run on at the end or omit several items. Both reading and writing are compromised in many cases. During conversational discourse, the patient may digress from the topic and is not likely to return to it.

3. Moderate/severe cognitive decline (GDS 5) is characterized by naming errors that may reflect language as well as perceptual problems. Production of semantic paraphasias may be more distant from target. There are less self-corrections due to less awareness. Vocabulary is reduced, negatively affecting the variety of words used. While complex sentences continue to be produced during verbal output, there is a reduction in their amount. Pronoun confusion is prominent and the listener often becomes confused. Some patients become withdrawn and say less while others talk excessively. During conversation, a complete digression from the topic is likely without the ability to recognize this switch, or the ability to return back to the topic. Regarding comprehension, there is a failure to understand less familiar lexical items. Syntactic structure is often used to help comprehend sentences. This strategy fails, however, with idiomatic language. The patient's ability to follow commands that contain more than two bits of information is compromised.

Repetition of familiar/overlearned sentences is adequate if the sentences are not too long. However, unfamiliar sentences, regardless of their length, are problematic. When producing automatic sequences (e.g., numbers, days of the week) the patient experiences difficulty starting the sequence, omits a portion of the sequence, or abandons the task. While other skills such as writing or reading are possible to perform, they are characterized by errors. Writing single words and simple sentences is possible, but errors are noted. The grammatical structure of the sentence may be impaired, but the patient does not realize these errors. When reading, substitution errors are seen. It may be impossible for the patient to read a paragraph or answer questions about it.

4. Severe cognitive decline (GDS 6) is characterized by an exacerbation of naming error without awareness by the patient. Conversations may be filled with vague generic words rather than specific ones. Jargon is often heard at this stage and vocabulary is severely reduced. Syntactic impairments are noted and an increase in automatic sequences/language is produced.

There is minimal comprehension of simple familiar phrases with a tendency to comprehend intonation patterns rather than words. During the repetition of phrases, the intonation pattern may be reproduced although the words are not available to the patient. Automatic sequences require assistance in order for the patient to initiate them and only a few items in the sequence may be produced. Writing and reading of some simple words may be possible but longer sequences are not possible.

5. Marked cognitive decline (GDS 7) is characterized by severe communication problems. Echolalia and mutism are often noted at this stage. While some patients may still be verbal, their output is limited to overusing the words that remain in their repertoire. Comprehension, reading, and writing are severely impaired.

TABLE 5.1   Language Changes Associated with Alzheimer's Disease

GDS	LANGUAGE
3	*Mild Cognitive Impairment*
	a. word problems noted on naming tasks
	b. word finding problems and delayed word responses
	c. circumlocuting often results in finding of correct word
	d. memory, attention deficits, and rate at which language is processed affects ability to understand and repeat complex sentences (e.g., passives)
	e. reading and writing intact
4	*Moderate Cognitive Impairment*
	a. characterized by naming problems
	b. self-corrections may often result in appropriate response
	c. word finding problems and delayed word responses
	d. circumlocuting no longer leads to finding of correct word
	e. continued difficulty with comprehending and repeating complex sentences
	f. reading and writing compromised
5	*Moderate/Severe Cognitive Decline*
	a. naming errors reflect language and perceptual problems
	b. less self-corrections (related to reduced self-awareness)
	c. reduced vocabulary and increased pronoun confusion
	d. during conversation topic digression is likely (patient unaware of digressing)
	e. ability to repeat short familiar sentences
	f. reading and writing skills characterized by errors unrecognized by patient
6	*Severe Cognitive Decline*
	a. exacerbation of naming errors with continued lack of awareness by patient
	b. severely reduced vocabulary
	c. conversations filled with vague generic words
	d. minimal comprehension of simple familiar phrases
	e. reading and writing of only simple phrases may be possible
7	*Marked Cognitive Impairment*
	a. characterized by severe communication problems
	b. echolalia and mutism often noted
	c. verbal output extremely limited
	d. comprehension, reading, and writing severely impaired

Visuo-spatial Abilities. Visuo-spatial problems have been noted in some patients early in Alzheimer's disease. Patients may lose their way while traveling and become disoriented while driving. While this may not be a problem early in the disease for some patients, it usually becomes problematic with disease progression.

Motor Abilities. Motor abilities are remarkably intact in the early stages of Alzheimer's disease. With moderate change, however, motor restlessness is noted and is expressed through idle pacing. In the late stages, especially when patients are bedridden, limbs may be rigid and contracted. The fact that motor abilities are relatively spared may reflect the relatively small accumulation of neuropathological changes in motor brain areas such as the primary motor strip (precentral gyrus) (Kemper, 1984).

Medical Treatments.   At this time there are no effective treatments to change the course of the disease, halt the degenerative process, or reverse the disease process in AD. Several types of drug treatment strategies have been attempted including modulating neurotransmitters (a method to improve cognitive performance and therefore the quality of life), administering nerve growth factors, and administrating anti-inflammatory agents (e.g., prednisone), to name a few. Neuroleptics have been used to treat behavioral symptoms such as agitation, paranoia, anxiety, and so on.

Memory enhancing drugs such as tacrine show inconsistent effectiveness. Tacrine is a **cholinesterase** inhibitor. Cholinesterase, a chemical excreted into the synaptic space, assists in the breakdown of acetylcholine (a neurotransmitter) allowing it to be reabsorbed into the presynaptic terminal for later use. Tacrine prevents this acetylcholine breakdown from occurring, enabling its prolonged availability in the synapse. It theoretically affects the cognitive system, improving delayed recall and selective reminding skills (Becker & Giacobini, 1988). Tacrine, approved by the Food and Drug Administration (FDA) in 1994, has adverse affects, the most serious of which is liver toxicity, causing many patients to be withdrawn from treatment (Knapp, Gracon, Davis, Solomon, Pendlebury, Knopman, 1994). It should be noted, however, that patients can be reintroduced to the drug after a period of time with improved tolerance (Knapp et al., 1994), the reasons for which are not clearly known.

An experimental drug trial using tacrine (Knapp et al., 1994) demonstrated that mild–moderately severe Alzheimer's disease patients who completed the study showed significant improvement over baseline performance as compared to the group receiving a placebo. Treatment effectiveness has been measured using objective cognitive tests (the Alzheimer's Disease Assessment Scale–cognitive subscale [ADAS–cog]), clinician-based assessments, caregiver-based assessments, and assessment of activities of daily living.

Pick's Disease

Pick's disease is a cortical dementia characterized by focal behavioral symptoms (e.g., language problems) and circumscribed lobar cortical atrophy. In 1892, Arnold Pick described a patient experiencing progressive cognitive deterioration and severe aphasia. Upon autopsy, left temporal lobe cortical atrophy was noted suggesting that specific lobar atrophy could account for the focal behavioral symptoms (Hodgers, 1994). Pick described several other cases presenting with severe aphasia, and showing temporal as well as frontal lobe atrophy. It was Alzheimer (Hodgers, 1994), however, who characterized the neuronal cell changes associated with Pick's disease, called **Pick bodies** and **Pick cells** (to be described below).

Although familial cases have been found, Pick's disease, which is rare, occurs sporadically in the general population (less than 1 percent). The onset of Pick's disease occurs in midlife, usually when patients are in their mid 40s with the most prominent feature of the disease being lobar cortical atrophy, affecting the frontal and/or temporal lobes. The cortical changes may show further hemispheric asymmetry, manifesting greater atrophy in one of the two hemispheres. The cause of Pick's disease is unknown.

Clinical Presentation.   According to *DSM-IV* (APA, 1994) Pick's disease is "characterized clinically by changes in personality early in the course, deterioration of social skills, emotional blunting, behavioral disinhibition and prominent language abnormalities" (p. 150). Additionally impairments in insight and judgment have been noted (Cummings et al., 1982). Language changes, such as naming problems, empty speech (speech conveying little meaning) and circumlocutions are also noted early and become exacerbated as the disease progresses. Memory and visuo–spatial skills remain intact until later in the disease when they also progressively deteriorate. Motor problems such as tremor and rigidity are noted as the disease nears the end.

Neuropathology. Two disease presentations associated with Pick's disease have been reported, one showing changes associated predominantly with frontal lobe pathology, and the other showing changes associated predominantly with temporal lobe pathology. Upon gross visual inspection of the brain, atrophy of the frontal and/or temporal lobes affecting one or both hemispheres has been noted (Hodgers, 1994; Roth & Meuers, 1975). Specific gyri within a lobe may show more or less change than other gyri. For example, it is the orbital and medial portions of the frontal lobe that are most atrophic. The pole is most affected in the temporal lobe, followed by the inferior and medial temporal gyri (Hodgers, 1994). Further, the anterior portion of the superior temporal gyri tend to be atrophic, whereas the posterior portions remain spared (Hodgers, 1994).

Microscopically, severe neuronal loss and gliosis (increased amount of glial cells) are observed (Civil, Whitehouse, Lanska, & Mayeux, 1993). Pick bodies (dense structures the size of the nucleus) found inside the cytoplasm of cortical cells, occur in approximately one-fourth of the cases (Hodgers, 1994). Pick bodies are characteristic of Pick's disease; they do not occur in normal aging brains and rarely are found in other diseases (Cummings et al., 1982). These bodies displace the nucleus and push it toward the cell edge. The second characteristic, inflated or enlarged neurons (Pick cells), can be seen in about half of the cases with Pick's disease. In Pick cells the nucleus shifts to one side. There is no cell structure that causes this shift.

Neuropsychological Changes

Memory. Memory change is not prominent in the early phase of the disease. Changes emerge at the later stages.

Language. Language changes are an early and prominent feature of Pick's disease. Reports of naming problems, circumlocutions, and empty speech are seen (Cummings et al., 1982). Aphasia and mutism (Holland, McBurney, Moosey, & Rernmirth, 1985) are reported in the middle and late stages of Pick's disease.

Visuo-spatial Abilities. Visual-spatial abilities are preserved until later in the disease.

Motor Abilities. The motor system is not affected early in Pick's disease. Rather, in the late stage in the disease, extrapyramidal signs (e.g., tremor, rigidity, slowness of movement) are noted and pyramidal changes (e.g., muscle weakness) may be evidenced (Cummings et al., 1982). (See Chapter 8.). Mutism, immobility, and incontinence have been reported at the end of the disease (Cummings et al., 1982).

Medical Treatments. There is no treatment for the progressive deterioration of Pick's disease. Personality changes which tend to be noted early can be treated medically with major tranquilizers. Training of the caregiver may allow the patient to remain at home for as long as possible.

SUBCORTICAL DEMENTIA

Parkinson's Disease

Parkinson's disease is a degenerative disorder that affects the extrapyramidal system. Describing six patients in 1817, James Parkinson noted a condition that included rigidity, tremor, postural and balance problems, with intact personality and normal intellectual functioning (Parkinson, 1817). As Parkinson's disease became better understood, both intellectual (e.g., dementia) and personality changes (e.g., depression) further characterized this disorder.

Parkinson's disease generally affects the aged population with occasional reports of juvenile onset (Rajput, 1994). The characteristic neuropathological changes of neuronal loss in the substantia nigra and **Lewy body** inclusions within a cell has been called Idiopathic Parkinson's Disease. This disease manifests itself through bradykinesia (slowness of movement), rigidity, tremor, disturbances in gait and balance, and a masked-like face. For a description on the motor outcome of the disease, see Chapter 8.

Clinical Presentation. Cummings and Benson (1992) reported that bradykinesia is the primary symptom of Parkinson's disease. Further, rigidity is often associated with slowness of movements. There are problems spontaneously initiating activity, difficulties in problem–solving, reductions in the ability to generate word lists, slowness in memory abilities, problems in concept formation, and difficulties changing set (e.g., on a sorting task, the patient cannot change the sorting strategy from color to number). Some of these difficulties (poor concept formation, word generation, and problems with changing set) are indicative of frontal lobe dysfunction. Dementia is not an initial symptom, but gradually appears with usually mild to moderate severity (Cummings et al., 1982). Additionally, depression is associated with Parkinson's disease and may be an early presenting sign of the disease.

Neuropathology. Changes to the substantia nigra, a nucleus located in the midbrain, are the hallmark of Parkinson's disease. The pars compacta, a portion of the substantia nigra, contains pigmented cells. These pigmented cells, providing **dopamine** (an inhibitory neurotransmitter) for the brain, become depleted in Parkinson's disease. As a result nuclei that are linked or connected to the substantia nigra such as those of the basal ganglia system (an extra-pyramidal system linked to the motor system) show reduced inhibition and excessive excitatory input, producing excessive movement.

Lewy body inclusions are round in shape and are found primarily in the cell of the substantia nigra nuclei and to a lesser extent in other midbrain and diencephalic nuclei (e.g., nucleus basalis, locus ceruleus). Lewy bodies consist of an outer region of loosely packed neurofilaments and an inner region of tightly packed neurofilaments. These structures are deleterious to neurons but the exact reason for this is unknown.

Neuropsychological Changes
Memory. Procedural memory (knowledge of how to carry out a task) and memory during spontaneous recall tasks and temporal ordering tasks become impaired.

Language. Aphasic-like language changes are not associated with Parkinson's disease, although difficulty comprehending syntactically complex sentences has been reported (Grossman, Cavell, Stern, Gollomp, & Hurtig, 1992).

The most frequently occurring speech problem associated with Parkinson's disease is hypokinetic dysarthria. It is characterized by bradykinesia (slow initiation of motor movement, motor responses, and motor planning), muscle rigidity (a resistance to passive movement), reduced range of muscle movements, and variable speed of repetitive movements (Rosenbek, & LaPointe, 1978). These deficits affect respiration, phonation, articulation, and resonance. Speech impairments include reduced loudness (may be inaudible at late stages), slow speech rate, monopitched or limited pitch range, breathy and harsh voice quality, imprecise articulation, and palilalia (repeating a word or phrase with increased rapid speed). For further discussion, see Chapter 8.

Visuo-spatial Abilities. Impaired spatial orientation, gestural representation, and copying complex figures perception are seen with Parkinson's disease (Cronin-Golomb, Corkin, & Rosen, 1993).

Motor Abilities. Rigidity and bradykinesia affect the general neuromuscular system. Passively moving a limb can produce a rhythmically jerky movement that has been called "cogwheeling." Included within the scope of bradykinesia is the loss of arm swing during walking, loss of voluntary smile, speech hesitations, and false starts (Prater, & Swift, 1984). Fingers and toes show a resting tremor which disappears during intentional movement or during sleep. Disease progression produces an intention tremor (tremors during intended movements). Postural and balancing problems are noted and can interfere with the ability to change from a standing position to a sitting position. A shuffling gait (small steps, rapid pace) is also characteristic of Parkinson's disease.

Medical Treatments. Drug treatments for Parkinson's disease include several different strategies that attempt to affect the dopaminergic system. One way to address the problem of too little inhibition (from reduced dopamine) resulting in too much motor excitement is to reduce the amount of excitatory neurotransmitters. The administration of anticholinergic drugs (usually given to newly diagnosed patients), which has little effectiveness in controlling the disease and has several side effects (e.g., dry mouth, memory impairment), has been used as a strategy.

Another strategy in the treatment of Parkinson's disease is to administer a drug that increases dopamine levels in the brain. Levodopa, a precursor of dopamine, has been used as an effective treatment. The drug is incorporated into neurons in the substantia nigra where it is changed into dopamine. There are problems and side effects associated with this drug. Levodopa is metabolized in the stomach; therefore, an additional drug must be administered to reduce this effect, producing greater availability of levodopa to the brain. Nausea and vomiting may be an early side effect, and psychiatric side effects may occur with high doses. Over time, the effectiveness of the drug fluctuates and symptoms gradually reappear.

Huntington's Disease

Huntington's disease was first described by George Huntington in 1872. Huntington observed patients displaying intellectual deterioration with signs of insanity. Another profile of this disease includes both intellectual decline and physical deterioration, progressing steadily until death.

Huntington's disease is an inherited progressive disease, resulting from a genetic defect on the short arm of chromosome 4 (APA, 1994). It is associated with changes in personality, intellectual functioning, motor functioning, and memory. There are prominent psychological features including depression, mania, delusional thoughts,

and paranoia (Greenamyre, & Shoulson, 1994). A child (regardless of gender) of a parent with Huntington's disease has a 50 percent chance of developing the disorder. The disease typically manifests itself in adulthood (usually in the late 30s). However, juvenile onset (age 4) as well as late onset (age 85) have been identified. The disease duration is approximately 14 years (Cummings et al., 1982).

Clinical Presentation. Initial symptoms of Huntington's disease are involuntary choreatic movements and behavioral changes. Chorea movements are irregular and abrupt, or rapid, and can move a body part. (For a more detailed discussion of chorea, see Chapter 8.) When the disease first begins, these movements may appear deliberate; however, as the disease progresses, these movements obviously are involuntary, and affect facial, trunk, and limb muscles. Other involuntary movement disorders seen with Huntington's disease include dystonia (distorted static posture resulting from excess muscle tone), athetosis (slow, irregular, writhing movements), and myoclonus (abrupt, brief contraction of a muscle). With disease progression, voluntary movements show change characterized by rigidity, bradykinesia (reduced speed of movement of a muscle through its range), and difficulty performing and sustaining complex movement patterns.

Personality changes have been noted and include mood disorders (resembling a manic–depressive condition with a higher likelihood of depression), delusions with paranoia (resembling schizophrenia), and a tendency toward suicide. Progressive changes in cognition and memory characterize the intellectual decline that is noted following the presence of chorea. Aphasia or agnosia do not appear to be associated with this disease.

Neuropathology. Multiple pathological changes occur in patient's with Huntington's disease. The hallmark of the disease is a loss of neurons in the caudate nucleus, specifically medium-sized projection neurons that project to the **globus pallidus**

and substantia nigra. The projection neurons of the putamen are also depleted. (See Chapter 8 for further description of these basal ganglia nuclei.) Changes in the substantia nigra have been the subject of much controversy. The debate is whether the changes are primary, or secondary—a result of the severe pathology in the caudate nucleus and the putamen (both these structures project to the substantia nigra). As the disease progresses, cortical atrophy, specifically in the frontal lobe, is noted. The relationship between the genetic abnormality on the short arm of chromosome 4 and the loss of neurons is not known at this time.

Gamma aminobutyric acid (GABA), an inhibitory neurotransmitter within the extra-pyramidal system is reduced, resulting in an overabundance of dopamine, producing a hyperkinetic state (Fraser, 1987). Further, glutamic acid decarboxylase, an enzyme responsible for GABA synthesis, is also reduced. Other neurotransmitters and synthesizing enzymes are reduced but to a lesser degree.

Neuropsychological Changes

Memory.   The co-occurrence of recent and remote memory problems is characteristic of Huntington's dementia (Albert, Butters, & Brandt, 1981). While initial registration of information is only mildly impaired, problems with effective encoding of information occur, as do severe retrieval difficulties (Butters, Wolfe, Cranholm, & Martone, 1986). With disease progression, memory problems become exacerbated.

Language.   Language problems such as aphasia, apraxia, or agnosia are not associated with Huntington's dementia. However, language may be disorganized with psychotic features present (American Psychiatric Association, 1994). (See Chapter 4 for a detailed discussion of the disruption in language function with mental problems.) Verbal fluency (as tested by giving exemplars of a semantic or phonological category) is reduced and is related to frontal lobe pathology. Gordon and Illes (1987) reported word-finding difficulties, some paraphasic errors, reduced word production, and increases in pauses in verbal production. A

hyperkinetic dysarthria, characterized by movements that are quick, jerky, irregular, and involuntary, affecting the lips, tongue, diaphragm, and laryngeal muscles is present (Prater, & Swift, 1984). Speech shows abnormal prosody, imprecise articulation, and intermittent pauses. Dysphagia is noted and aspiration pneumonia is common. Chapter 10 presents an in-depth description of types of swallowing problems.

Visuo–spatial Abilities.   Visuo–spatial problems characterized by performance difficulties on the block design subtest of the Wechsler Adult Intelligence Scale (WAIS) (Wechsler, 1955) as well as right–left discrimination difficulties (Fedio, Cox, Neophytides, Canal-Frederick, & Chase, 1979) are associated with Huntington's disease.

Motor Abilities.   There are motor problems both with voluntary and involuntary muscles. Initially, involuntary movements are noted, including chorea, dystonia, athetosis, motor restlessness, and myoclonus. A hyperkinetic dysarthria (as described above) is also present.

Medical Treatments.   As with the other dementia conditions discussed thus far, there is no successful treatment for Huntington's disease. Drugs that replace the chemical abnormalities (reduced GABA, reduced glutamate) have been attempted, but are unsuccessful at changing the course of the disease or altering the disease process.

Genetic testing and counseling are available. Gene carriers can be identified presymptomatically, as the gene for Huntington's disease has been isolated and cloned (Huntington's Disease Collaborative Research Group, 1993). Counseling should be made available to family members of Huntington's patients.

AIDS Dementia Complex

AIDS dementia complex (ADC) is a primary neurological disorder of the AIDS **retrovirus.** Neuropathologically, it is characterized by changes in white matter and subcortical structures of the brain, and behaviorally, by problems in attention, learning new information, and performing speeded information processing tasks. Ataxia, coordination problems, and motor slowing also occur. ADC, also known as HIV cognitive motor complex, HIV dementia, and HIV-1 associated dementia (HAD), is found in the late stage of **HIV-1 infection** (the cause of acquired immunodeficiency syndrome [AIDS]). When this infection invades the central nervous system, dementia may result.

Acquired immunodeficiency syndrome (AIDS), the result of HIV-1 infection, was first identified in 1981. It is a syndrome resulting from a breakdown in the immune system. This malfunction is specifically related to **cell-mediated immunity** which protects the body from viruses and cancers. **T-cells** (a type of immune cell) responsible for cell-mediated immunity, become depleted by the HIV-1 infection, making the body vulnerable to viruses and opportunistic infections.

AIDS was first detected in homosexual men and soon after was recognized in intravenous drug users, sexual partners of infected persons, hemophiliacs, recipients of blood transfusions, and children (infected mothers transmit the disease in utero). It is a transmissible disease—through blood, semen, breast milk, cerebrospinal fluid, and vaginal secretions. Although the virus is not virulent, it is highly pathological.

HIV-1 infection is a pathological process involving a virus that affects various biological systems (for our purposes we will only consider the central nervous system). The infection is complicated and has a variable course. There are multiple pathological processes that result from HIV-1 infection. Only dementia, with its behavioral and neuropathological manifestations, will be considered here. AIDS dementia complex is a clinical syndrome identified by symptoms or signs which are thought to reflect the HIV-1 infection in the central nervous system. Several groups have reported on the prevalence of ADC, with estimates ranging from 7 to 67 percent. A group studying AIDS in San Diego reported a yearly incidence of ADC to be 14 percent (Day, et al., 1992), while the Multi-Center AIDS Cohort study showed the rate to be 7 percent. The differences in the numbers may reflect factors such as which patients get referred, the criteria used for diagnosis, and the stage when examination occurs (McArthur, Selnes, Glass, Hoover, & Bacellar, 1994).

Clinical Presentation.   Criteria have been developed that define the existence of ADC (Janssen, Cornblath, Epstein, McArthur, & Price, 1989). A "probable" dementia exists if there is an abnormality in at least two of the following cognitive domains: attention, information processing speed, abstraction/reasoning skills, visuo–spatial abilities, memory, learning, speech and language. The cognitive problems must affect work or activities of daily living (ADL). Further, one of the following behaviors must also exist (but cannot be responsible for the cognitive impairment): abnormality in motor function, change in social behavior or emotional control, alterations in consciousness affecting cognition, coexistence of CNS opportunistic infection or malignancy, or a psychiatric disorder. A "possible" dementia exists if the etiology of the cognitive impairments cannot be determined, or if other potential etiologies for the cognitive impairment are present.

Six stages of ADC have been identified (Price, & Brew, 1988), ranging from Stage 0 to Stage 4. At Stage 0 there is normal cognitive and motor functioning. Stage 0.5 is a subclinical stage of dementia. Cognitive change is minimal or questionable but some subtle neurological signs (e.g., snout response) may be noted. Neither work nor ADL are affected at this stage. At Stage 1, mild dementia is present. Challenging and demanding aspects of work and ADL may be affected and neuropsychological testing reveals cognitive or motor impairment. Moderate dementia (Stage 2) is accompanied by an inability to work and a need for ambulatory assistance (e.g., cane). Basic ADL skills remain intact. Stage 3 indicates severe dementia, accompanied by cognitive impairment affecting complex conversation as well as other skills and motor involvement. The last stage of dementia (Stage 4) is the end stage. Patients may be mute, paraplegic, and incontinent. Intellectual and social functioning is minimal.

Neuropathology. Neuropathological analysis of the brain of a person with ADC shows cerebral atrophy occurring in the frontal, parietal, and temporal regions. The ventricles are enlarged, specifically in the frontal and temporal regions (Gelman, & Guinto, 1992).

Multinucleated giant cells (MNGC) are a microscopic feature of ADC (Rhodes, 1987). Additionally, many small inflammatory nodules (containing microglia, macrophages, and lymphocytes) are found in the white matter and subcortical nuclei, such as the thalamus and basal ganglia. The tissue surrounding the veins in the brain also become inflamed (McArthur, 1994) and the white matter looks pale.

Neuropsychological Changes

Memory. There are inconsistent findings regarding memory functioning in ADC. Some researchers have reported learning and memory deficits in early stages of dementia (Wilkie, Eisdorfer, Morgan, Lowenstein, & Szapocznik, 1990), while others do not support this finding (Miller, et al., 1990). In a study examining several cognitive abilities, delayed memory for stories and reproducing geometric figures was not impaired in ADC, but delayed recall of a word list and recognition performance was problematic (Martin, et al., 1992). Maruff, Currie, Malone, McArthur-Jackson, Mulhall & Benson (1994) reported deficits in a selective reminding task, a long-term recall task, and in digit span backwards. Performance on the recognition of the selective reminding task and digit span forward were not impaired.

Working memory performance (Martin 1994), and other frontal lobe tasks such as Wisconsin Card Sort (Grant et al., 1948) or the Tower of London (Shallice, 1982) are not problematic. However, reaction time was remarkably slow for the ADC group.

Language. Language problems do not appear to be an early feature of ADC. Verbal fluency, naming, and writing were not significantly impaired in early-staged patients (Maruff et al., 1994). Motor speech disorders (ataxic dysarthria) have been reported in HIV-1 infection patients but this reflects cerebellar dysfunction rather than dementia (Lopez, Becker, Dew, Banks, Dorst, & McNeil, 1994). (Refer to Chapter 8 for a discussion of ataxic dysarthria.)

Visuo–spatial Abilities. Visuo-spatial abilities are not impaired early in the course of ADC.

Motor Abilities. Simple and complex reaction time tasks were impaired early in ADC, moreover, motor skill learning was problematic for some early cases (Martin, 1994).

Medical Treatments. Patients with ADC are treated with drugs designed to counteract the proliferation of the virus. For example, azidothymidine (AZT) has been widely used and has shown some improvements in cognitive functioning (Yarchoan et al., 1987) but it does not reverse the dementia. Currently there are several drugs [zidovudine (AZT); didanosinc (ddi); dideoxycytidine (ddc)] approved by the FDA for the treatment of HIV. There is considerable research being done using these drugs at early stages of HIV-1 infection with patients who exhibit mild cognitive changes but who do not have dementia. The hope is that treatment will diminish and prevent dementia in AIDS patients.

VASCULAR DEMENTIA

Multi-infarct Dementia

Multi-infarct dementia, a term introduced by Hachinski and colleagues (1974), describes a disease state characterized by dementia resulting from multiple small infarctions in persons with hypertension. While individuals with hypertension usually have occlusion of their arteries, it is not the amount of blood that reaches the brain, but rather, the loss of brain tissue at many sites, that accounts for the dementing condition (Cummings et al., 1982).

Clinical Presentation. Multi-infarct dementia (MID) has several features that distinguish it from

Alzheimer's disease. Unlike AD (which has a gradual onset), MID occurs abruptly and shows stepwise deterioration. Hachinski, Larson, & Marshall (1975) developed the Modified Ischemic Scale that identifies features likely to occur with MID. The higher the score on the scale (above 4), the greater the likelihood that the patient has MID rather than Alzheimer's disease. Conversely, a score of 4 or below may indicate Alzheimer's disease. In addition to the abrupt onset and stepwise deterioration, the course of MID fluctuates, showing alternating improvement and deterioration. The patient exhibits somatic complaints, as well as difficulties expressing emotions. Generally there is a history of hypertension and/or stroke. Upon examination, evidence of focal neurological signs and symptoms such as muscle weakness may be noted. (For further discussion, see Chapter 7.) The personality of the patient is usually preserved, although depression may be present.

Since MID is a result of repeated infarctions, the clinical presentation will reflect the damaged brain regions. Marshall (1993) described several presenting features that prompt patients to seek treatment. These include confusional state (e.g., disorientation to time or place), gait disturbances, transient aphasic episode, apraxia, extrapyramidal symptoms, pseudobulbar palsy, and urinary problems (e.g., incontinence).

Neuropathology. The underlying pathology in MID is usually infarcts located in both cortical and subcortical areas (white matter). Subcortical lesions in white matter, fed by striate arteries (medial striate artery), cause insignificant problems until several of these lesions coexist or unless the lesion affects nuclei such as the caudate, putamen, or thalamus. Cortical brain regions lying between two arterial regions (e.g., the posterior watershed area that lies between the middle and posterior cerebral arteries) are vulnerable to small infarcts due to both the small size of the branches and their location as furthest away from the main artery. It is the combination of the distribution and the amount of lesions that produces the variety and severity of MID symptoms.

Neuropsychological Changes
Memory. Memory problems appear early, affecting recent memory while sparing long-term memory abilities (Marshall, 1993). The patient is aware when memory difficulties arise, and does not attempt to deny they exist.

Language. If lesions exist in important language areas, language deficits will be noted. If the lesion is small, language problems may be transient producing some comprehension or word finding problems that seem to resolve after a short period of time. Subcortical lesions produce problems affecting speech production.

Visuo–spatial Abilities. Visuo–spatial problems may be noted if parietal lobe lesions exist.

Motor Abilities. Regarding motor functioning, extrapyramidal symptoms (e.g., tremor) will be noted with subcortical lesions. Additionally, slowing of movements, rigidity, and problems walking have been noted (Marshall, 1993).

Medical Treatments. There is no cure for MID, although the underlying pathologies that cause the lesions can be treated. For example, if the patient is hypertensive, then treatments (administration of appropriate drugs) that alter the hypertensive state of the patient should be administered. If the patient is aphasic, then speech–language therapy is appropriate. (See Chapter 7.) When motor problems exist, physical therapy should be recommended.

INFECTIOUS DEMENTIAS

Creutzfeldt–Jakob's Disease

Creutzfeldt–Jakob's disease is a transmissible spongiform encephalopathy (brain looks like a sponge) characterized by progressive vacuolation (empty spaces) in the gray matter, as well as the death of neurons (Brown, 1994). The disease has historically been called Jakob–Creutzfeldt's disease. The current name for the disease, Creutzfeldt–Jakob's disease, will be used in the chapter.

Creutzfeldt–Jakob's disease is an uncommon disease with onset usually occurring in the sixth decade of life, but cases have been noted as early as age 16 (Creutzfeldt's case) and as late as age 82. It is caused by infectious agents (i.e., virus) that are not easily detectable since patients do not show overt signs such as fever (McArthur, Roos, & Johnson, 1993) or immune responses (a reaction such as a rash, antibodies in the blood, inflammation and so on). The virus is said to be unconventional, having small proteinaceous infectious particles without nucleic acid (Prusiner, 1987) which make it resistent to traditional treatments.

This is a transmissible disease, although the mode and spread of the disease is not clearly understood. Transmission between humans has been documented in patients who received a corneal transplant, in individuals who received growth hormone injections, and in situations where electrodes were reused (from a patient who had the disease) without being sterilized. Since there are few accounts of health care workers or partners of infected patients contracting the disease (Brown, Cathala & Gajdusek, 1979), it appears to be not easily transmissible. The disease has been transmitted to other species including monkeys, sheep, goats, mice, and cats. It has been genetically transmitted in about 100 families worldwide (Brown, 1994). In genetic cases, the disease shows an autosomal dominant pattern (non sex-linked gene where only one parent needs to carry the gene). Creutzfeldt–Jakob's disease is unique in that it is both transmissible to humans as well as other species and also may be genetically transmitted. As the disease is transgenic (transmitted to other species), it is hoped that the exact cause can be determined and an effective treatment discovered.

Clinical Presentation. Before the onset of clear symptoms, patients report an awareness of changes affecting eating and sleeping habits. They note weight loss and a feeling of anxiety (Cummings et al., 1982). There are three initial presentations of neurological symptoms. Mental deterioration (e.g., memory loss), confusion, and changes in behavior are the initial symptoms of about one-third of the cases; cerebellar changes (e.g., ataxia) and extrapyramidal symptoms (e.g.,

tremor) occur in another third of the cases, and a combination of the two occurs in the remaining third (Cummings et al., 1982). Aphasia, agnosia, apraxia, and dysarthria (combination of cerebellar and extrapyramidal types) (Maxim et al., 1994) as well as a full dementia (Cummings et al., 1982) have been reported after the appearance of the initial neurological symptoms. The patient deteriorates over a relatively short period of time (approximately 9 months to a year) and eventually dies.

Neuropathology. Neuropathological analysis of the brain typically results in a definite diagnosis of Creutzfeldt–Jakob's disease. Upon gross examination, the brain may appear normal or show varying degrees of diffuse or focal atrophy which may reflect the underlying pathology. Ventricular enlargement may also be present.

The neuronal changes associated with Creutzfeldt–Jakob's disease include neuron degeneration and death, gliosis (increase in number of glial cells within the gray matter), and spongiform changes (holes in the gray matter). Neuronal loss is not consistent throughout the brain, but affects portions of the cortex, caudate and putamen, thalamus, brainstem, and spinal cord (Cummings et al., 1982). The spongiform changes occur in the neocortex, caudate nucleus and putamen, thalamus, cerebellar cortex, and dentate nucleus of the cerebellum (Brown, 1994). McArthur, Roos, and Johnson (1993) reported white matter changes whereas Brown did not (Cummings et al., 1982). Brown suggested that neuronal degeneration and death account for the myelin loss (myelin is found in white matter) rather than a primary white matter change.

Neuropsychological Changes. As with other forms of dementia, Creutzfeldt–Jakob disease presents in a heterogeneous fashion. The behaviors discussed below may be present in some cases and not other cases.

Memory. Memory loss is a hallmark of this form of dementia. Initially, recent memory may be affected but with disease progression, long-term memory becomes compromised. Thirteen cases of Creutzfeldt–Jakob disease, among Jewish persons of Libyan descent, presented with a prime cognitive impairment in memory (Chapman, Brown, Goldfarb, Arlazoroff, Gajdusek, & Korczyn, 1993). Short-term memory problems were reported initially in a case of Creutzfeldt–Jakob disease that presented as a Wernicke–Korsakoff syndrome (Pietrini, 1992) and one presenting as a regressive confusional syndrome (Azorin, Donnet, Dassa, Gambarelli, 1993).

Language. A case was reported by Kirk and Ang (1994) where a rapid and progressive Broca's aphasia was the primary symptom. The language was characterized initially by word-finding difficulties which progressed to one-word conversational speech, severe comprehension problems, and inability to repeat, read, or write. Paraphasic errors were noted in another case where cortical deafness was the primary presenting problem (Tobais, Mann, Bone, Silva, & Ironside,1994). Additionally, verbal fluency has been reported to be decreased in some forms of this dementia (Mendez, Selwood, & Frey, 1994). Akinetic mutism occurs late in the disorder and appears to be a consistent phenomenon (Heye & Cervos–Navarro, 1992; Otto, Patzold, Donhuijsen, & Walter, 1995). Of interest is the loss of the use of French by a bilingual speaker whose primary language remained intact (Azorin, et al., 1993).

Visuo-spatial Abilities. Visuo-spatial problems are noted (Mendez, et al., 1994) but are not as prominent as primary visual disturbances (Chapman et al., 1993).

Motor Abilities. Motor speech problems were noted at the initial stage of the disease in several cases described by Heye and Cervos–Navarro (1992). Nine cases were described by Chapman, et al. (1993) where dysphagia, dysphonia, and dysarthria were present. Abnormalities of gait have been reported (Pietrini, 1992; Heye & Cervos–Navarro, 1992; Chapman, et al., 1993), as well as intention tremor of the hand (Pietrini, 1992), and

extrapyramidal signs (e.g., cogwheel rigidity and bradykinesia) (Chapman, et al., 1993).

Medical Treatments. There is no effective treatment for this disease.

NEUROIMAGING TECHNIQUES

Neuroimaging is becoming widely available and these techniques provide important information about disease states. As speech–language pathologists working in medical settings, one is likely to be exposed to neuroimaging reports or actual scans. This section will provide a brief overview of some imaging techniques and findings in some dementia diseases. There are several neuroimaging techniques available including computed axial tomography (CAT), magnetic resonance imaging (MRI), positron emission tomography (PET), and single photon emission tomography (SPECT). MRI and CAT techniques provide scans that show the anatomy, whereas PET and SPECT scans provide information about the way the brain works. Each scanning technique uses different energy sources (e.g., x rays, magnetic fields) from which images are derived. For example, CAT scanners use x rays to acquire their images, whereas MRI scanners use magnetic fields. MRI and PET, representing techniques to examine anatomy (MRI) and physiology (PET) will be described.

Magnetic Resonance Imaging (MRI)

Magnetic Resonance Imaging (MRI) has developed over the past 20 years into potentially the most powerful diagnostic tool available to medicine. The technique involves noninvasive irradiation by harmless radio waves directed to subjects located within a powerful magnetic field. The technique is capable of providing images of static tissue with a high degree of natural contrast between normal and abnormal tissue, between gray matter and white matter, and between gray matter and cerebral spinal fluid. It is capable of quantitatively measuring blood flow, producing angiograms (visualizations of blood vessels) that are beginning to rival x-rays. Most recently, it has been used to look at the activation of specific regions of the brain during various tasks (e.g., visual stimulation, auditory stimulation), a technique known as functional MRI (fMRI).

MRI and the Dementias. Alzheimer's disease produces atrophy that is measurable on an MRI scan. Ventricles become enlarged and gyri become atrophic. One area of the brain that has been studied extensively in patients with Alzheimer's disease using MRI techniques is the hippocampus (Jobst, et al., 1992; Kesslak, Nalcioglu, & Cotman, 1991; Timo, et al., 1993). As stated earlier, this region is important in memory functioning. Using MRI scans and measuring the volume of regions within the temporal lobe, volume loss was found in the hippocampus in over 90 percent of Alzheimer's disease patients relative to normal-aged individuals (de Leon, George, Golomb, Tarshish, Convit, Kluger, et al., in press). Reduction in lateral temporal lobe areas were also noted in Alzheimer's disease. Further, hippocampal volume loss (approximately 14 percent) but not lateral temporal lobe volume loss was noted in cases at risk for developing Alzheimer's disease (Convit et al., 1995a). It has been shown that the size of the hippocampus is related to qualitative and quantitative aspects of memory performance (Deweer et al., 1995). While hippocampal change suggests the possibility of Alzheimer's dementia, it is not a definitive marker of the disease even in cases with possible/or probable Alzheimer's disease. Hippocampal atrophy is also noted in normally aging individuals and the incidence of hippocampal change increases with advanced age (Golomb, et al., 1993).

MRI studies of MID show lesions in the white matter. However, white matter changes are not unique to MID. There is a high prevalence of hyperintensities (bright regions on an MRI scan) found around the ventricles in normal aging individuals over the age of 60 (Fazekas, Niederkorn, Schmidt, Offenbacher, Horner, Bertha, & Lechner, 1988). Further, patients with Alzheimer's disease show these hyperintensities and they do not distinguish Alzheimer's disease patients from normal-aged individuals (Erkinjuntti, Gao, Lee, Eliasziw, Merskey, & Hachinski, 1994). Patients with Creutzfeldt–Jakob's disease also exhibit hyperintensities on MRI. Since hyperintensities occur in normal aging and in many dementia diseases there is no specificity for this finding. Persons with MID may have lesions in the cortex or in the nuclei (e.g., thalamus, caudate) that are indicative of a stroke. When these lesions occur in an individual with dementia, one can be confident that this is not Alzheimer's disease but MID.

MRI changes in Huntington's disease are specific in that there is atrophy of the head of the caudate nucleus, giving the anterior horns of the lateral ventricles an enlarged and flattened appearance. In fact, when one looks at an MRI in the coronal plane (slices of the brain from front to back), the caudate nucleus may not be visible at all. Such an appearance supports the existence of Huntington's disease.

Positron Emission Tomography (PET)

Positron emission tomography (PET) is an imaging technique that allows one to view brain metabolism (i.e., the brain at work). A PET scanner looks for gamma rays that are emitted from the brain. In order for these gamma rays to be produced, a radioactive substance is injected into the patient. The radioactive substance or isotope to be discussed here is [18]F-2flouro-2-deoxy-D-glucose, commonly known as FDG (radioactive glucose or sugar). Glucose, the major substrate for brain metabolism, is useful in examining brain activity. The isotope is injected into the blood and passes through the blood-brain barrier. An enzyme called hexokinase acts upon the radioactive glucose and enables its absorption into neurons (called phosphorylation of FDG). It is the accumulation of FDG in brain tissue that is visualized on a PET scan. FDG releases positrons (positively charged electrons) that collide with electrons and are annihilated, releasing two gamma rays. These gamma rays are detected by the machine to identify the quantity and location of the isotope.

PET and the Dementias. In Alzheimer's disease (AD), the greatest changes in regional cerebral glucose metabolism relative to normal individuals is in the temporal lobes and the parieto-temporal association areas (Cutler, et al., 1985; Haxby, et al., 1986; de Leon, et al., 1983; Smith, et al., 1992). Haxby, et al. (1986) reported glucose metabolic change in parieto-temporal brain areas of mild and moderately severe AD patients as compared to normal elderly controls. They also tested memory, language, and visuo–spatial abilities and correlated these measures with metabolism. The moderately severe Alzheimer's disease patients performed significantly worse than normals on all neuropsychological measures. Their performance was strongly related to the amount of metabolic change in neocortical areas. It was interesting to note that this was not the case with the mild Alzheimer's disease patients. Performance of mild Alzheimer's disease patients on these neuropsychological measures was not related to metabolism, indicating that brain metabolic alterations existed prior to observable changes in behavior.

Patients at risk for AD show glucose metabolic change using PET techniques. In a study by Kennedy, et al. (1995), 24 cases at risk for familial Alzheimer's disease (FAD), and 19 affected FAD cases were examined. Parieto-temporal hypometabolism was noted in the at-risk cases for FAD. These metabolic rates were similar to those with affected FAD cases, indicating that there are neocortical metabolic brain changes prior to the outward expression of the disease process. Glucose metabolic change was also noted in the medial temporal lobe (the hippocampus is located here) in patients at risk for Alzheimer's disease (De Santi, et al., 1995). Cerebral glucose metabolism was measured in several areas of the brain and the medial temporal lobe differentiated patients at risk for Alzheimer's disease from normal individuals but not from patients with probable AD. This is further evidence that cerebral glucose metabolic change can occur prior to observable AD.

While MRI and PET studies have provided information about brain changes in dementia diseases, there is much overlap between these conditions, as well as between dementia and normal aging. Therefore, one must use caution when interpreting information from neuroimaging. It is only with information from many sources (i.e., medical, neurological, neuropsychological, and imaging) that a possible/or probable diagnosis of the dementia condition can be made.

THE ROLE OF THE SPEECH–LANGUAGE PATHOLOGIST

There is considerable discussion about the role of the speech–language pathologist in treatment and diagnosis of dementia illnesses. Diagnosing communication problems is one of the primary functions of the speech–language pathologist. However, there are several issues that arise due to the progressive nature of dementia. One issue, the continual deterioration of function in dementia, is inconsistent with successful long-term treatment effectiveness, and presents an ethical dilemma to speech–language pathologists regarding intervention—should treatment be provided if progressive deterioration will occur? Progressive deterioration, however, does not preclude short-term successes producing effective communication. The American Speech-Language-Hearing Association (ASHA) advocates for the active involvement of speech–language pathologists in assessing communication skill, providing treatment programs to facilitate and maintain functional communication, and helping caregivers understand the communication problems associated with dementia.

Assessment

Assessment of speech and language abilities is important in providing differential diagnosis between dementias, as well as differentiating dementia from aphasia. This knowledge is essential for prognosis and management. Additionally, understanding the communicative strengths and weaknesses of patients can provide important information to family members and caregivers about strategies useful for successful communication (Causino Lamar, Obler, Knoeful, & Albert, 1994).

A diagnostic workup should include a complete case history, as this information is crucial in assisting accurate diagnosis. Unlike other disease processes, dementias, such as Alzheimer's disease and Pick's disease, do not have identifying pathological *in-vivo* markers. A thorough history will permit the possible identification of other diseases that might mimic dementia (e.g., depression). Further, Alzheimer's disease is a diagnosis of exclusion in which one rejects all other possible diseases before the diagnosis of probable/or possible Alzheimer's disease is given. For example, a patient may exhibit language problems consistent with anomia and the underlying cause (dementia or stroke) may not be clear. The speech–language pathologist can contribute to the diagnostic process by evaluating the patient, describing the language functioning, and providing evidence that the language behavior is consistent with one of the two conditions.

Historically, standardized aphasia batteries have been used to assess language abilities of demented populations. These batteries, such as the Boston Diagnostic Aphasia Battery (Goodglass, & Kaplan, 1983) and the Western Aphasia Battery (Kertesz, 1982) provide information about linguistic functioning, including both expressive and receptive language skills. Aphasia tests were developed to reveal language patterns of aphasic disorders. Language changes in AD or other dementing illnesses (with the exception of multi-infarct dementia) are not aphasias. Therefore, it is necessary to supplement aphasia tests with other types of tests (e.g., functional communication tests such as the Communicative Abilities in Daily Living [CADL] [Holland, 1980]) to obtain a complete picture of the patient's communication abilities. Standardized aphasia batteries were not designed to differentiate dementia from aphasia and must be interpreted with this limitation in mind. Further, these tests provide some information about language abilities of dementia but do not reveal the whole language picture of these patients. A recent test, The Arizona Battery for Communication Disorders of Dementia (ABCD) (Bayles, & Tomoeda, 1993), was developed spe-

cifically to examine the communication problems of dementia. Areas assessed include orientation and memory, receptive and expressive language, and perception.

Diseases which affect the motor system, such as Parkinson's disease and Huntington's disease, produce dysarthrias that need to be assessed. Respiration, phonation, articulation, resonance, and timing are the processes that can be affected. A thorough examination of each process should be part of assessment, and can provide information about the type of communication difficulties that arise, and what might be done to prevent complications or minimize their effects. (See Chapter 8 for further information on assessment.)

Behavioral Treatment Programs

Since dementia produces progressive deterioration, treatment strategies and approaches must reflect this change. Maintaining communication strengths is possible using direct treatment approaches, especially in the early stages of dementia. Using strategies such as asking the patient to circumlocute to self cue, or to use semantically related words, may assist when word finding problems interfere with communication. Oftentimes the clinician knows exactly what the patient wants to say and phonologic cueing (providing the first sound of a target word) is helpful. Furthermore, patients have unique communication styles and strategies that they naturally will attempt when difficulties arise. It is important to find out what these individual styles and strategies are and to assist the patient in utilizing them when experiencing communication failure.

A rehabilitation technique resource called "Techniques for Aphasia Rehabilitation: Generating Effective Treatment" (TARGET) (Santo Pietro, & Goldfarb, 1995) brings together treatment technique prototypes from existing literature, providing information about the development of the technique and its usefulness. Techniques for remediating oral expression, auditory comprehension, reading comprehension, and writing are included. The authors suggest which language behaviors and techniques might be successful with patients suffering from dementia.

Another treatment program (Glickstein, 1988) that focuses on activities of daily living provides therapeutic techniques and materials for clinicians working with AD patients and their caregivers. This workbook provides lessons and incorporates the caregiver into the treatment process. Training the caregiver can facilitate follow-up of treatment strategies and techniques and practice, may improve communication.

Direct therapy for remediation of language problems associated with multi-infarct dementia is more straightforward than treatment for AD patients, reflecting principles associated with the remediation of aphasia. (See Chapter 7.) Speech production problems associated with Parkinson's disease and Huntington's disease also follow more traditional treatment methods (Prater, & Swift, 1984). (See Chapter 8.) The association of dysphagia with dementia is becoming widely appreciated. (See Chapter 10 for a discussion of therapeutic principles.) Both assessment and treatment of these problems are the responsibility of the speech–language pathologist. Some forms of dysphagia are due to physical causes and respond to traditional treatment methods. Other forms (associated with advanced stages of AD) require more creative treatment approaches. Successful treatment of these different areas of function provides the opportunity for patients to remain at home and independent for longer periods of time, improving their quality of life. In addition to traditional direct treatment programs, group communication programs have developed over the years for demented populations, providing socialization, the opportunity to participate in structured therapy programs, a relaxed atmosphere in which to practice communication strategies, and an environment in which to experience communicative success.

Caregiver Programs

Since the dementias discussed in this chapter have no known cures, the most effective management of these cases occurs with the assistance of care-givers. Several caregiver programs have been developed over the years to assist in the behavioral management and communication of patients with dementia. These programs educate family members and caregivers as to the expected course of the dementia, including the expected stages and changes (both functional and behavioral) that patients will experience. For example, at a certain point in Alzheimer's disease the patient becomes incontinent. Incontinence makes the patient feel uncomfortable and makes travel difficult, reducing the amount of time the patient can be away from the home. It increases the workload for the caregiver (larger amounts of laundry), and increases caregiver stress. A program developed to assist caregivers (Shulman, Steinberg, Mittelman, Ambinder, Mackell, & Hertz, 1993) provides a step-by-step treatment/behavioral regimen to reduce the incidence of incontinence and to assist the caregiver with strategies to effectively deal with the new situation.

Therapy programs for caregivers and family members also provide an opportunity to share feelings, frustrations, successes, fears, and so on regarding the disease and the effect it has on families. Dealing with a patient with dementia is time consuming and emotionally and financially stressful. These therapy sessions provide an outlet for these stresses, a discussion of possible solutions to problems, information about what do to next, or suggestions of how another member has dealt with their problems.

Communication problems of individuals with dementia also contribute to caregiver stress (Kinney, & Stephens, 1989; Stephens, Kinney, & Ogrocki, 1991). The loss of the ability to effectively communicate and to maintain social interaction through successful communication is overwhelming. Many caregivers do not fully understand the communication problems associated with dementia (Clarke, & Witte, 1990) and this adds to their stress. They may have either too low or too high an expectation of the patient's communication skills (Ripich, 1994). Furthermore, they may not know what to do when communication breaks down. FOCUSED, a communication program developed by Ripich (1994), assesses the caregiver's knowledge of the patient's communication abilities, provides information that will assist the caregiver in obtaining realistic communication expectations, and furnishes management strategies to increase successful communication. There are six training modules in this program, which begins by describing communication and language problems associated with Alzheimer's disease and then examines normal forgetting versus depression and dementia. The next two modules address general communication issues and ethical issues in Alzheimer's disease. The fifth module discusses language and communication changes in various stages of Alzheimer's disease. The last module teaches seven strategies and techniques for promoting communication success at three stages of Alzheimer's disease.

Another approach to working with caregivers and Alzheimer's disease patients directly assesses caregivers' communication skills. Ostuni and Santo Pietro (1991) developed questionnaires for caregivers that examine their communication style, feelings, and sense of burden. Helpful hints are provided to assist in successful communication.

SUMMARY

Dementia is a devastating disease that continues to affect a large portion of our aging population. By the year 2030, 17 to 20 percent of the population (approximately 51 million people) will be over the age of 65 (Schoenberg, 1986), with 1 to 6 percent of those of 65 years and 10 to 20 percent of those over 80 years being affected by Alzheimer's disease (Clark, & Goate, 1993). Continued research and greater understanding will hopefully lead to the effective treatment of these disorders. The job of the speech–language pathologist is to understand the nature of the communication problems associated with each type of dementing, to assess and maximize the current level of communication of the patient, and to provide education, understanding, and support to family members and caregivers who are dealing with these patients every day of their lives.

Major Points of the Chapter

- Dementias may result from cortical, subcortical, vascular, or infectious disease processes.
- Dementias may be distinguished by different neuropsychological and language changes and their progression over time.
- Neuroimaging techniques are increasingly used to characterize different types of dementias.
- Treatment programs are directed at maintaining a patient's communication strengths, as well as providing information and assistance for caregivers.

Discussion Guidelines

1. Describe the differences between a cortical dementia and a subcortical dementia.
2. Contrast the communication problems of Alzheimer's disease with those of Huntington's disease. Provide strategies for improving communication in these patients and their caregivers.
3. Prepare an questionnaire for a caregiver of a patient with dementia. Include questions about past and present communication abilities, as well as cognitive and memory function.

REFERENCES

Albert, M. S., Butters, N., & Brandt, J. (1981). Patterns of remote memory in amnestic and demented patients. *Archives of Neurology, 38,* 495–500.
Alzheimer, A. (1907). A characteristic disease of the cerebral cortex (Original title: Uber eine eigenartige Erkrankung der Hirnrinde). *Allgemeinne Zeitschrift fur Psychiatrie und Psychisch-Gerichtliche Medizin, 64,* 146–148.
Alzheimer, A. (1987). A characteristic disease of the cerebral cortex. In K. Bick, L. Amaducci, & G. Pepeu (Eds.), *The early story of Alzheimer's disease.* (pp. 1–3). Padova: Liviana Press.
American Psychiatric Association. (1994). *Diagnostic and Statistical Manual of Mental Disorders.* (4th ed.). Washington, D.C., American Psychiatric Association.

Azorin, J. M., Donnet, A., Dassa, D., & Gambarelli, D. (1993). Creutzfeldt-Jakob disease misdiagnosed as depressive psuedodementia. *Comprehensive Psychiatry, 34*, 42–44.

Ball, M. J., Hachinski, V., Fox, A., Kirshen, A. J., Fisman, M., Blume, W., Kral, V. A., & Fox, H. (1985). A new definition of Alzheimer's disease: A hippocampal dementia. *Lancet, 5 January 1985*, 14–16.

Bayles, K., & Tomoeda, C. L. (1993). *The Arizona Battery for Communication Disorders (ABCD)*. Phoenix: Canyonland Publishing.

Becker, R. E., & Giacobini, E. (1988). Mechanisms of cholinesterase inhibition in senile dementia of the Alzheimer type: Clinical, pharmacological, and therapeutic aspects. *Drug Development Research, 12*(163), 195.

Braak, H., & Braak, E. (1991). Neuropathological staging of Alzheimer related changes. *Acta Neuropathologica (Berlin), 82*, 239–259.

Brown, P. (1994). Transmissible human spongiform encephalopathy (infectious cerebral amyloidosis): Creutzfeldt–Jakob disease, Gerstmann–Straussler–Scheinker syndrome, and kuru. In D. B. Calne (Ed.), *Neurodegenerative diseases*. (pp. 839–876). Philadelphia: W.B. Saunders Co.

Brown, P., Cathala, F., & Gajdusek, D. (1979). Creutzfeldt–Jakob disease in France. III. Epidemiological study of 170 patients dying during the decade. *Annals of Neurology*, 38–46.

Butters, N., Wolfe, J., Granholm, E., & Martone, M. (1986). An assessment of verbal recall, recognition and fluency abilities in patients with Huntington's disease. *Cortex, 22*, 11–32.

Causino Lamar, M. A., Obler, L. K., Knoefel, J. E., & Albert, M. L. (1994). Communication patterns in end-stage Alzheimer's disease: Pragmatic analysis. In R. L. Bloom, L. K. Obler, S. De Santi, & J. L. Ehrlich (Eds.), *Discourse analysis and applications: Studies in adult clinical populations*. (pp. 217–235). Hillsdale, N.J.: Lawrence Erlbaum Associates.

Chapman, J., Brown, P., Goldfarb, L. G., Arlazoroff, A., Gajdusek, D. C., & Korczyn, A. D. (1993). Clinical heterogeneity and unusual presentations of Creutzfeldt-Jakob disease in Jewish patients with the PRNP codon 200 mutation. *Journal of Neurology, Neurosurgery & Psychiatry, 56*, 1109–1112.

Citron, M., Oltersdorf, T., Haass, C., McConlogue, L., Hung, A. Y., Seubert, P., Vigo-Pelfrey, C., Lieberburg, I., & Selkoe, D. (1992). Mutation of the B-amyloid precursor protein in familial Alzheimer's disease increases B-protein production. *Nature, 360*, 672–674.

Civil, R., Whitehouse, P., Lanska, D., & Mayeux, R. (1993). Degenerative dementias. In P. Whitehouse (Ed.), *Dementia*. (pp. 167–214). Philadelphia: F.A. Davis Co.

Clark, R. F., & Goate, A. M. (1993). Molecular genetics of Alzheimer's disease. *Archives of Neurology, 50*, 1164–1172.

Clarke, L., & Witte, K. (1990). Nature and efficacy of communication management in Alzheimer's disease. In R. Lubinski (Ed.), *Dementia and Communication*. (pp. 238–256). Philadelphia: B.C. Decker.

Convit, A., de Leon, M. J., Tarshish, C., De Santi, S., Kluger, A., Rusinek, H., & George, A. (1995a). Hippocampal volume losses in minimally impaired elderly. *The Lancet, 345*, 266.

Convit, A., de Leon, M. J., Tarshish, C., De Santi, S., Tsui, W., Rusinek, H., & George, A. (1995b). Hippocampal volume in pre-clinical and early Alzheimer's dementia: Relationship to cognitive function. Submitted for publication.

Cronin-Golomb, A., Corkin, S., & Rosen, T. J. (1993). Neuropsychological assessment of dementia. In P. Whitehouse (Ed.), *Dementia*. (pp. 130–164). Philadelphia: F.A. Davis Co.

Cummings, J. L., & Benson, D. E. (1982). *Dementia: A clinical approach*. Boston: Butterworth-Heinemann.

Cutler, N. R., Haxby, J. V., Duara, R., Grady, C. L., Kay, A. D., Kessler, R. M., Sundaram, M., & Rapoport, S. I. (1985). Clinical history, brain metabolism, and neuropsychological function in Alzheimer's disease. *Annals of Neurology, 18*, 298–309.

Day, J., Grant, I., Atkinson, J. H., Brysk, L., McCutchan, A., Hesselink, J., Spector, S., & Richman, D. (1992). Incidence of AIDS dementia in a two year follow-up of AIDS and ARC patients on an initial phase II AZT placebo-controlled study: San Diego cohort. *Journal of Neuropsychiatry and Clinical Neurosciences, 4*, 15–20.

de Leon, M. J., Ferris, S. H., George, A. E., Christman, D. R., Fowler, J. S., Gentes, C., Reisberg, B., Gee, B., Emmerich, M., Yonekura, Y., Brodie, J., Kricheff, I. I., & Wolf, A. P. (1983). Positron emission tomography studies of aging and Alzheimer's disease. *American Journal of Neuroradiology, 4*, 568–571.

de Leon, M. J., George, A. E., Golomb, J., Tarshish, C., Convit, A., Kluger, A., De Santi, S., McRae, T., Ferris, S. H., Reisberg, B., Ince, C., & Rusinek, H.

(in press). Frequency of hippocampus atrophy in 405 normal elderly and Alzheimer's Disease patients. *Neurobiology of Aging.*

de la Monte, S. M. (1989). Quantitation of cerebral atrophy in preclinical and end-stage Alzheimer's disease. *Annals of Neurology, 25,* 450–459.

De Santi, S., de Leon, M. J., Rusinek, H., Golomb, J., Convit, A., Tarshish, C., McRae, T., Kluger, A., Fowler, J., Volkow, N., & Wolf, A. P. (1995). Selective medial temporal lobe pathology in cases at-risk for AD: Diagnostic role of PET. In K. Iqbal, J. Mortimer, B. Winbald, & H. Wisniewski (Eds.), *Research Advances in Alzheimer's Disease and Related Disorders.* Sussex, England: John Wiley & Sons.

Deweer, B., Lehericy, S., Pillon, B., Baulac, M., Chiras, J., Marsault, C., Agid, Y., & Dubois, B. (1995). Memory disorders in probable Alzheimer's disease: The role of hippocampal atrophy as shown with MRI. *Journal of Neurology, Neurosurgery and Psychiatry.*

Erkinjuntti, T., Gao, F., Lee, D. H., Eliasziw, M., Merskey, H., & Hachinski, V. C. (1994). Lack of difference in brain hyperintensities between patients with early Alzheimer's disease and control subjects. *Archives of Neurology, 51,* 260–268.

Fazekas, F., Niederkorn, K., Schmidt, R., Offenbacher, H., Horner, S., Bertha, G., & Lechner, H. (1988). White matter signal abnormalities in normal individuals: Correlation with carotid ultrasonography, cerebral blood flow measurements, and cerebrovascular risk factors. *Stroke, 19,* 1285–1288.

Fedio, P., Cox, C., Neophytides, A., Canal-Frederick, G., & Chase, T. N. (1979). Neuropsychological profile of Huntington's disease: Patients and those at risk. *Advances in Neurology, 23,* 239–255.

Flicker, C., Bartus, R. T., Crook, T., & Ferris, S. H. (1984). Effects of aging and dementia upon recent visuospatial memory. *Neurobiology of Aging, 5,* 275–283.

Fraser, M. (1987). *Dementia: Its nature and management.* Chichester: John Wiley & Sons.

Gelman, B. B., & Guinto, F. C. (1992). Morphometry, histopathology and tomography of cerebral atrophy in the acquired immunodeficiency syndrome. *Annals of Neurology, 32,* 31–40.

Glickstein, J. K. (1988). *Therapeutic intervention in Alzheimer's disease: A program of functional communication skills for activities of daily living.* Rockville, MD: Aspen Publishers.

Golomb, J., de Leon, M. J., George, A. E., Convit, A., Kluger, A., de Santi, S., Litt, A., & Foo, S. H. (1993). Hippocampal atrophy in normal pressure hydrocephalus is associated with severity of cognitive impairment [Abstract]. *Neurology, 43,* A211-A212.

Goodglass, H., & Kaplan, E. (1983). *The assessment of aphasia and related disorders* (2nd ed.). Philadelphia: Lea and Febiger.

Gordon, W. P., & Illes, J. (1987). Neurolinguistic characteristics of language production in Huntington's disease: A preliminary report. *Brain and Language, 31*(1), 10.

Grant, D. A., & Berg, E. A. (1948). A behavioral analysis of degree of reinforcement and ease of shifting to new responses in a Weigl-type card sorting problem. *Journal of Experimental Psychology: Learning, Memory and Cognition, 34,* 404–411.

Greenamyre, J. T., & Shoulson, I. (1994). Huntington's disease. In D. Calne (Ed.), *Neurodegenerative diseases.* (pp. 685–704). Philadelphia: W.B. Saunders Co.

Grossman, M., Carvell, S., Stern, M. B., Gollomp, S., & Hurtig, H. (1992). Sentence comprehension in Parkinson's disease: The role of attention and memory. *Brain and Language, 42,* 347–384.

Hachinski, V. C., Lassen, N. A., & Marshall, J. (1974). Multi-infarct dementia, a cause of mental deterioration in the elderly. *Lancet, ii,* 207–209.

Haxby, J. V., Grady, C. L., Duara, R., Schlageter, N., Berg, G., & Rapoport, S. I. (1986b). Neocortical metabolic abnormalities precede nonmemory cognitive defects in early Alzheimer's-type dementia. *Archives of Neurology, 43,* 882–885.

Hedera, P., & Whitehouse, P. (1995). Neurotransmitters in neurodegeneration. In D. Calne (Ed.), *Neurodegenerative diseases.* (pp. 97–117). Philadelphia: W.B. Saunders.

Heye, N., & Cervos-Navarro, J. (1992). Focal involvement and lateralization in Creutzfeldt-Jakob disease: Correlation of clinical, electroencephalographic and neuropathological findings. *European Neurology, 32,* 289–292.

Hodgers, J. R. (1994). Pick's disease. In A. Burns & R. Levy (Eds.), *Dementia.* (pp. 739–752). London: Chapman & Hall.

Holland, A. (1980). *Communicative abilities in daily living.* Baltimore, MD: University Park Press.

Holland, A., McBurney, D., Moossy, J., & Rernmirth, O. (1985). The dissolution of language in Pick's disease with neurofibrillary tangles: A case study. *Brain and Language, 24,* 36–58.

Huntington, G. (1872). On chorea. *Medical Surgical Reporter, 26,* 317–321.

Huntington's Disease Collaborative Research Group. (1993). A novel gene containing a trinucleotide repeat that is expanded and unstable on Huntington's disease chromosome. *Cell, 72,* 971–983.

Janssen, R. S., Cornblath, D. R., Epstein, L. G., McArthur, J., & Price, R. W. (1989). Human immunodeficiency virus (HIV) infection and the nervous system: Report from the American Academy of Neurology AIDS Task Force. *Neurology, 39,* 119–122.

Jobst, K. A., Smith, A. D., Szatmari, M., Molyneux, A., Esiri, M. E., King, E., Smith, A., Jaskowski, A., McDonald, B., & Wald, N. (1992). Detection in life of confirmed Alzheimer's disease using a simple measurement of medial temporal lobe atrophy by computed tomography. *The Lancet, 340,* 1179–1184.

Kemper, T. (1984). Neuroanatomical and neuropathological changes in normal aging and in dementia. In M. L. Albert (Ed.), *Clinical neurology of aging.* New York: Oxford University Press.

Kennedy, A. M., Frackowiak, R. S., Newman, S. K., Bloomfield, P. M., Seaward, J., Roques, P., Lewington, G., Cunningham, V. L., & Rossor, M. N. (1995). Deficits in cerebral glucose metabolism demonstrated by position emission tomography in individuals at risk of familial Alzheimer's disease. *Neuroscience Letters, 186,* 17–20.

Kertesz, A. (1982). *The Western Aphasia Battery.* New York: Grune & Stratton.

Kesslak, J. P., Nalcioglu, O., & Cotman, C. W. (1991). Quantification of magnetic resonance scans for hippocampal and parahippocampal atrophy in Alzheimer's disease. *Neurology, 41,* 51–54.

Kinney, J. M., & Stephens, M. A. P. (1989). Hassles and uplifts of giving care to a family member with dementia. *Psychology and Aging, 4,* 402–408.

Kirk, A., & Ang, L. C. (1994). Unilateral Creutzfeldt-Jakob disease presenting as rapidly progressive aphasia. *Canadian Journal of Neurological Sciences, 21,* 350–352.

Knapp, M. J., Gracon, S. I., Davis, C. S., Solomon, P. R., Pendlebury, W. W., & Knopman, D. S. (1994). Efficacy and safety of high-dose tacrine: A 30-week evaluation. *Alzheimer Disease and Associated Disorders, 8*(2), 22–31.

Koo, E., & Price, D. (1993). The neurobiology of dementia. In P. Whitehouse (Ed.), *Dementia.* (pp. 55–91). Philadelphia: F.A. Davis Co.

Lopez, O. L., Becker, J. T., Dew, M. A., Banks, G., Dorst, S. K., & McNeil, M. (1994). Speech motor control disorder after HIV infection. *Neurology, 44,* 2187–2189.

Marshall, J. (1993). Vascular dementias. In P. Whitehouse (Ed.), *Dementia.* (pp. 215–236). Philadelphia: F.A. Davis Co.

Martin, A. (1987). Representation of semantic and spatial knowledge in Alzheimer's patients: Implications for models of preserved learning in Amnesia. *Journal of Clinical and Experimental Neuropsychology, 9*(2), 191–224.

Martin, A. (1994). HIV, cognition, and the basal ganglia. In I. Grant & A. Martin (Eds.), *Neuropsychology of HIV infection.* (pp. 234–259). New York: Oxford University Press.

Martin, A., Brouwers, P., Cox, C., & Fedio, P. (1985). On the nature of the verbal memory deficit in Alzheimer's disease. *Brain and Language, 25,* 323–341.

Martin, A., Heyes, M. P., Salazar, A. M., Kampen, D. L., Williams, J., Law, W. A., Coats, M. E., & Markey, S. P. (1992). Progressive slowing of reaction time and increasing cerebrospinal fluid concentrations of quinolinic acid in HIV-infected individuals. *Journal of Neuropsychiatry and Clinical Neuroscience, 4,* 270–279.

Maruff, P., Currie, J., Malone, V., McArthur-Jackson, C., Mulhall, B., & Benson, E. (1994). Neuropsychological characterization of the AIDS dementia complex and rationalization of a test battery. *Archives of Neurology, 51,* 689–695.

Maxim, J., & Bryan, K. (1994). *Language of the elderly: A clinical perspective.* San Diego: Singular Publishing Group.

McArthur, J. (1994). Neurological and neuropathological manifestations of HIV infection. In I. Grant & A. Martin (Eds.), *Neuropsychology of HIV infection.* (pp. 56–107). New York: Oxford University Press.

McArthur, J., Roos, R., & Johnson, R. (1993). Viral dementias. In P. Whitehouse (Ed.), *Dementia.* (pp. 237–275). Philadelphia: F.A. Davis Co.

McArthur, J. C., Selnes, O. A., Glass, J. D., Hoover, D. R., & Bacellar, H. (1994). HIV dementia: Incidence and risk factors. In R. W. Price & S. W. I. Perry (Eds.), *HIV, AIDS, and the brain.* (pp. 251–272). New York: Raven Press.

Mendez, M. F., & Selwood, A., Frey II, W. H. (1994) Clinical characteristics of chronic Creutzfeldt–Jakob disease. *Journal of Geriatric Psychiatry and Neurology, 7,* 206–208.

Miller, E. N., Selnes, O. A., McArthur, J. C., Satz, P., Becker, J. T., Cohen, B. A., Sheridan, K., Machado, A. M., Van Gorp, W. G., & Visscher, B. (1990). Neuropsychological performance in HIV-1-infected homosexual men: The Multicenter AIDS Cohort Study (MACS). *Neurology, 40,* 197–203.

Obler, L. K., & Albert, M. L. (1984). Language in aging. In M. L. Albert (Ed.), *Clinical neurology of aging.* (pp. 245–253). New York: Oxford University Press.

Ostuni, E., & Santo Pietro, M. J. (1991). *Getting through: Communicating when someone you care for has Alzheimer's disease.* Vero Beach, FL: The Speech Bin.

Otto, V., Patzold, U., Donhuijsen, K., &Walter, G. F. (1995). Severe cerebellar atrophy in the panencephalopathic type of Creutzfeldt–Jakob disease: A case report. *Journal of Neurology, 242,* 348–353.

Palmore, E. (1979). Predictors of successful aging. *Gerontologist, 19,* 427–431.

Parkinson, J. (1817). *An essay on the shaking palsy.* London: Sherwood, Neely & Jones.

Pietrini, V. (1992). Creutzfeldt-Jakob disease presenting as Wernicke-Korsakoff syndrome. *Journal of the Neurological Sciences, 108,* 149–153.

Prater, R., & Swift, R. (1984). *Manual of voice therapy.* (1st ed.). Boston: Little, Brown and Company.

Price, R. W., & Brew, B. J. (1988). The AIDS dementia complex. *Journal of Infectious Diseases, 158,* 1079–1083.

Prusiner, S. (1987). Prions and neurodegenerative diseases. New England *Journal of Medicine, 317,* 1571–1581.

Rajput, A. H. (1994). Clinical features and natural history of Parkinson's disease (special consideration of aging). In D. Calne (Ed.), *Neurodegenerative diseases.* (pp. 555–582). Philadelphia: W.B. Saunders Co.

Reisberg, B., Ferris, S. H., de Leon, M. J., & Crook, T. (1982). The global deterioration scale for assessment of primary degenerative dementia. *American Journal of Psychiatry, 139,* 1136–1139.

Rhodes, R. H. (1987). Histopathology of the central nervous system in the acquired immunodeficiency syndrome. *Human Pathology, 18,* 636–643.

Ripich, D. (1994). Functional communication with AD patients: A caregiver training program. *Alzheimer Disease and Associated Disorders, 8*(95), 109.

Rosenbek, J., & LaPointe, L. (1978). The dysarthrias: Description, diagnosis, and treatment. In D. Johns (Ed.), *Clinical management of neurogenic communicative disorders.* (pp. 251–310). Boston: Little, Brown and Company.

Roth, M., & Meuers, D. H. (1975). *British Journal of Psychiatry, 9,* 87.

Santo Pietro, M. J., & Goldfarb, R. (1995). *Techniques for aphasia rehabilitation: Generating effective treatment (TARGET).* Vero Beach, FL: The Speech Bin.

Schoenberg, B. S. (1986). Epidemiology of Alzheimer's disease and other dementing disorders. *Journal of Chronic Disease, 39,* 1095–1104.

Selkoe, D. (1994). Alzheimer's disease: A central role for amyloid. *Journal of Neuropathology & Experimental Neurology, 53*(4), 438–447.

Shallice, T. (1982). Specific impairment of planning. *Philosophical Transactions of the Royal Society of London B, 298,* 199–209.

Shulman, E., Steinberg, G., Mittelman, M. S., Ambinder, A., Mackell, J., & Hertz, S. (1993). Incontinence in AD: Home management and delay of institutionalization [Abstract]. *The Gerontologist, 33,* 231.

Smith, G. S., de Leon, M. J., George, A. E., Kluger, A., Volkow, N. D., McRae, T., Golomb, J., Ferris, S. H., Reisberg, B., Ciaravino, J., & La Regina, M. A. (1992). Topography of cross-sectional and longitudinal glucose metabolic deficits in Alzheimer's disease: Pathophysiologic implications. *Archives of Neurology, 49,* 1142–1150.

Stephens, M. A. P., Kinney, J. M., & Ogrocki, P. K. (1991). Stressors and well-being among caregivers to older adults with dementia: The in-home versus nursing home experience. *The Gerontologist, 31,* 217–223.

Terry, R. D. (1963). The fine structure of neurofibrillary tangles in Alzheimer's disease. *Journal of Neuropathology and Experimental Neurology, 22*(629), 642.

Terry, R. D., Masliah, E., Salmon, D. P., Butters, N., DeTeresa, R., Hill, R., Hansen, A., & Katzman, R. (1991). Physical basis of cognitive alterations in Alzheimer's disease: Synapse loss is the major correlate of cognitive impairment. *Annals of Neurology, 30,* 572–580.

Timo, E., Lee, D. H., Gao, F., Steenhuis, R., Eliasziw, M., Fry, R., Merskey, H., & Hachinski, V. C. (1993). Temporal lobe atrophy on magnetic resonance imaging in the diagnosis of early Alzheimer's disease. *Archives of Neurology, 50,* 305–310.

Tobais, E., Mann C., Bone I., de Silva, R., & Ironside, J. (1994). A case of Creutzfeldt-Jakob disease presenting with cortical deafness. *Journal of Neurology, Neurosurgery and Psychiatry, 57,* 872–873.

Tomlinson, B. E., Blessed, G., & Roth, M. (1970). Observations on the brains of demented old people. *Journal of Neurological Sciences, 11,* 205–242.

Trojanowski, J. Q., Schmidt, M. L., Shin, R., Bramblett, G. T., Rao, D., & Lee, V. M.-Y. (1993). Altered tau and neurofilament proteins in neuro-degenerative diseases: Diagnostic implication for Alzheimer's disease and Lewy body dementias. *Brain Pathology, 3,* 45–54.

Wechsler, D. (1955). *Wechsler Adult Intelligence Scale.* New York: Psychological Corporation.

Wilkie, F. L., Eisdorfer, C., Morgan, R., Loewenstein, D. A., & Szapocznik, J. (1990). Cognition in early human immunodeficiency virus infection. *Archives of Neurology, 47,* 433–440.

Yarchoan, R., Berg, G., Brouwers, P., Fischl, M. A., Spitzer, A. R., Wichman, A., Grafman, J., Thomas, R. V., Safai, B., Brunetti, A., Perno, C. F., Schmidt, R. J., Larson, S. M., Meyers, C. E., & Broder, S. (1987). Response of human immunodeficiency-virus-associated neurological disease to 3'-azido-3'-deoxythymidine. *Lancet, 1,* 132–135.

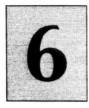

6

COGNITIVE-COMMUNICATIVE DISORDERS FOLLOWING TRAUMATIC BRAIN INJURY

CARL A. COELHO

ommunication is a process of interaction by which two or more individuals strive to exchange information (Davis, 1993). The ability to communicate requires a complex interaction between cognition and language (Adamovich, 1991). Cognitive skills important for communication include such processes as attention, memory, reasoning, problem-solving, and executive functioning (i.e., self-awareness and goal setting, planning, self-directing/initiating, self-inhibiting, self-monitoring, self-evaluation, flexible thinking). Language skills involve transmission of spoken, written, or nonverbal (e.g., gestures, facial expression) messages and reception of auditory, printed, or nonverbal messages. Difficulty or failure at any point along this expressive–receptive continuum, or with critical aspects of cognition, may result in a breakdown in communication and thus the inefficient exchange of information. A variety of brain injuries may result in impairments of cognitive and language skills. The most common are strokes and traumatic brain injuries (TBI), each of which yields distinctive patterns of deficits and recovery.

This chapter provides a general overview of TBI. The chapter begins with a comparison of TBI and stroke because both conditions may result in

permanent brain damage and therefore need to be distinguished from one another. Next, a discussion of the nature of TBI is presented including the incidence and effects of the disorder. The cognitive–communicative deficits that result from TBI are reviewed, as are language, speech, and swallowing impairments. Next, the role of the speech–language pathologist in the management of the individual with TBI is presented. This is followed by a discussion of assessment and treatment approaches for TBI individuals. Finally, the stages of recovery following TBI are presented along with future research needs.

STROKE VERSUS TRAUMATIC BRAIN INJURY

Two primary features that distinguish TBI from stroke are the survivor's age and the mechanism of injury. Strokes typically occur in individuals who are middle-aged or older, consistent with the observation that strokes are often associated with the arteriosclerotic processes of aging (degenerative changes in arteries resulting in thickening of the walls, loss of elasticity, and occasionally calcium deposits). By contrast, the vast majority of TBIs occur in individuals who are under the age of 35 years. Therefore, TBI survivors are, as a group, younger than the stroke population.

With regard to mechanism of brain injury, strokes typically result in focal lesions to either hemisphere, leading to fairly specific deficit patterns, depending on the region of the brain involved. For example, aphasia may result from a lesion or lesions to the left hemisphere in the region of the posterior frontal lobe, anterior temporal lobe, and/or inferior parietal lobe (i.e., anywhere along the distribution of the middle cerebral artery). (See Chapter 7.) Traumatic brain injuries result from a variety of causes including motor vehicle accidents, falls, gunshot wounds, or other trauma involving a blow to the head. The extent of the brain damage following traumatic head injury is the result of a combination of the primary and secondary damage, as well as the concomitant physiologic changes affecting brain function (North, 1984). **Primary damage,** caused by impact to the head, ranges from large brain lesions to microscopic brain lesions. **Secondary damage** results from such factors as infection, hypoxia (oxygen deprivation resulting from injuries to the chest or airway that limit the ability of the lungs to oxygenate the blood), edema (brain swelling due to an increase in fluid content following the trauma), elevated intracranial pressure (due to increased brain mass in the case of swelling or accumulation of fluid as in hematomas, decreasing the protective capacity of the cerebrospinal fluid within the finite intracranial space which if left unchecked may lead to brain herniation), infarction (death of brain tissue in a focal area which has been deprived of the blood supply for that region), and hematomas (focal areas of bleeding within the skull due to tearing of blood vessels) (Sohlberg & Mateer, 1989). Physiologic changes may result from a variety of metabolic disturbances such as hyperthermia (excessive fever), electrolyte imbalances (salt and water retention), damage to the hypothalamus (which exerts neural control over the pituitary gland) or pituitary gland (which releases hormones involved in many bodily functions). In

summary, strokes result in damage to fairly specific areas within the brain while TBIs may result in both focal and diffuse brain damage.

THE NATURE OF TRAUMATIC BRAIN INJURY

Traumatic brain injuries are classified as *open* (also referred to as penetrating) or *closed* head injuries depending on whether or not the meninges (the three layers of tissue that cover the brain) remain intact. Open head injuries result when the scalp and skull are penetrated. Materials commonly involved in open head injuries are bullets, stones, shell fragments, knives, and blunt instruments (Mierowsky, 1984). Primary brain damage in open head injuries is typically localized along the path of the penetrating object. Primary damage may also result from bone fragments when the skull fractures. In many instances the remainder of the brain is spared any damage. However, wartime injuries involving high-velocity missiles may produce damage remote from the point of entry and subsequent path because of displacement forces. In the case of low-velocity projectiles such as bullets that do not exit, further damage is caused as the bullet ricochets off the inner surfaces of the skull (Levin, Benton, & Grossman, 1982).

Open head injuries also produce an array of secondary damage resulting from the effects of increased intracranial pressure, swelling, bleeding, and infections. Open head injuries rarely lead to coma as in closed head injuries but the risk of epilepsy (a disorder characterized by a recurring excessive neuronal discharge related to scarred brain tissue, manifested in varying degrees of seizure activity) is greater (Sohlberg & Mateer, 1989).

Primary damage associated with closed head injuries is the result of mechanical forces including the effects of both direct contact and inertia (Alexander, 1984). Damage results from the inward compression of the skull at the point of impact and the subsequent rebound effects. The point of impact is referred to as **coup;** while the damage to the side of the brain opposite from the side which receives the blow is **contra coup.** The force of such blows literally causes the brain, which is somewhat gelatinous, to forcefully bounce around the rough, somewhat jagged inner surfaces of the skull, resulting in contusions and bruising. These lesions occur most often on the lateral and undersurfaces of the frontal and temporal lobes of the brain (Alexander, 1984). These contusions result in decreased capacities to regulate behavior, affect, emotions, and a host of cognitive abilities such as attention and memory (Sohlberg & Mateer, 1989).

The inertial forces involved in closed head injuries occur in incidents involving high levels of acceleration and deceleration as in whiplash injuries in motor vehicle accidents. Twisting movements result in rapid rotation of the brain within the skull, which in turn strains delicate blood vessels and nerve fibers, causing stretching, shearing, and tearing of microscopic structures (Langfitt & Gennarelli, 1982). This type of injury is referred to as **diffuse axonal injury** and almost always results in widespread brain dysfunction and frequently coma (Alexander, 1984). **Coma** (prolonged period of unconsciousness) results from a disruption of the **reticular activating system** within the brainstem. The reticular activating system is responsible, to a large extent, for the initiation, maintenance, and degree of wakefulness on which higher nervous functions depend. Unless these specific brain structures are damaged in an open head injury, coma typically does not occur. Diffuse axonal injury (stretching, tearing, and shearing of nerve fibers), is also associated with deficits of attention and reduced speed of information processing.

Closed head injury may result in focal lesions to specific regions of the brain, diffuse axonal injury, or a combination of both. Consequently, TBI survivors are a far less homogeneous population than individuals with stroke and are difficult to group for comparison purposes. Although each type of injury may occur in any region of the brain and result in very different patterns of deficits, certain regions of the brain are highly vulnerable in closed head injury. For example, the prefrontal region (the front of the brain just behind the forehead) and the limbic system (located deep within the center of the brain) may be affected, as well as the connections between the limbic system and the prefrontal region (Levin & Kraus, 1994).

INCIDENCE OF TRAUMATIC BRAIN INJURY

The National Head Injury Foundation (1983) defines head injury (i.e., TBI) as a traumatic insult to the brain capable of producing physical, intellectual, emotional, social, and vocational changes. An estimated 500,000 individuals sustain TBI each year (200 per 100,000 population). Of this number, 200,000 will die, 50,000 to 100,000 survive with significant impairment preventing independent living, and more than 200,000 suffer continuing sequelae that interfere with daily living skills (Jennett, Snoek, Bond, & Brooks, 1981; Kalsbeek, McLauren, Harris, & Miller, 1981; Kraus, 1978, 1993). Of the individuals who sustain TBI, nearly twice as many males as females are injured. The risk of TBI is higher for children 4 to 5 years of age, males 15 to 24 years of age, and the elderly (over 75 years). In the United States, trauma is the third leading cause of death among individuals under the age of 35 (National Head Injury Foundation, 1983).

The yearly incidence of new cases of penetrating head wounds that survive account for less than 10 percent of all head injuries (Grafman & Salazar, 1987). More than two-thirds of all head injuries are classified as mild, defined by a loss of consciousness, if any, of less than 30 minutes or a score of 13 to 15 on the Glasgow Coma Scale (Kraus & Nourjah, 1989). Symptoms following mild brain injury are quite variable, but include difficulty concentrating under distracting conditions (e.g., reading with the television on) or problems managing tasks involving multiple demands (e.g., typing and answering the telephone). Three additional areas commonly disrupted are aspects of attention, memory, and executive functioning. Mild brain injuries may also result in word-finding difficulties, decreased motivation, anxiety, depression, and irritability (Levin, Eisenberg, & Benton, 1989; Sohlberg & Mateer, 1989).

THE CONSEQUENCES OF TRAUMATIC BRAIN INJURY

The effects of TBI on the survivor and family are dependent in large measure on the nature and severity of the injury. As stated earlier, no two injuries are the same; each injury yields a diverse constellation of cognitive–communicative, physical, and psychosocial deficits. The degree to which these deficits impede the performance of everyday activities depends on the nature of the activities a particular individual was engaged in premorbidly. Generally, the most devastating impact of TBI is a reduced capacity to pursue premorbid interests and daily activities at the same functional level. Such disability exists along a broad continuum that can range from requiring additional time to complete tasks to near total dependence on others for all basic needs.

Jacobs (1988) surveyed the families of 142 survivors of severe TBI to determine the extent of independence in a variety of behavioral skills. The skill areas included a range of abilities (e.g., reading, writing, telling time, concentration, remembering, and orienting) and a range of complexity (e.g., for reading: from reads and recognizes directional signs to reads books; or, for writing: from writes own name to writes paper or reports). Results indicated that TBI had a significant impact on the survivor's ability to independently perform a variety of daily living skills. The impact of TBI on the family may be equally devastating. Jacobs (1988) noted that many survivors of severe TBI lived with their families, did not work or attend school, and were dependent upon others for skills, finances, and services outside the home.

Overview of Cognitive and Communicative Deficits Secondary to Traumatic Brain Injury

Coma.   **Coma** is a condition in which a patient displays minimal, if any, purposeful response to

the external environment. Coma is relatively common and believed to result from damage to the central portions of the brain stem. In **deep coma** a patient demonstrates no discernable behavioral responses to touch, pain, sound, or movement, although autonomic physiologic responses (those not under voluntary control) such as blood pressure or heart rate sometimes change with various sensory stimuli. In lighter stages of coma the patient may respond to external stimuli, but responses may be generalized—for example, whole body movements or nonspecific motor responses. An intense level of stimulation may be required to elicit such responses. Duration of coma has some prognostic implications in determining long-term recovery. However, the predictive capability is not perfect, since some individuals who undergo lengthy comas may demonstrate good recovery, and other individuals who experience no loss of consciousness may be left with extensive physical and cognitive deficits.

Cognitive Disturbances.   The hallmark of TBI is the resulting cognitive disturbances that are most often present. Sohlberg and Mateer (1989) have described several areas of **cognition** that may be disrupted following TBI, including orientation, attention, memory, reasoning/problem solving, and executive function. Although each of these processes is discussed separately, it is important to emphasize that this is an artificial approach, because these processes are inextricably related components of cognition, each dependent on the others for maximal functioning.

Orientation.   **Orientation** refers to a person's awareness of four spheres: person, place, time, and circumstance. Orientation to person pertains to autobiographic memory, that is, information that was acquired and stored prior to the onset of the injury. This information does not need to be relearned or acquired but simply retrieved. Typically, this aspect of orientation returns rapidly during recovery. Orientation to time, place, and circumstances requires the capacity to take in, store, and recall new information presented after injury. Of these three aspects of orientation, recalling circumstances returns first, followed by place and time (High, Levin, & Gary, 1990). Time (year, month, season, time of day) constantly changes, and therefore information must be continually updated, requiring an increased level of awareness and the ability to sequence and order ongoing events. The frontal lobes, which are commonly damaged in TBI, have been implicated in this process of time tagging.

Attention.   Deficits of attention and concentration often go unrecognized or are misdiagnosed following TBI. Attentional problems may be mild or severe and often resolve; however, they may also be present years after the injury. Concentration problems are a common post-TBI complaint of long-term survivors. There are numerous definitions of attention that have contributed to the confusion and in some instances to the oversight of deficits of attention. Sohlberg and Mateer (1989) have outlined five dimensions of attention: (1) **focused attention,** pertaining to the ability to respond discretely to specific visual, auditory, or tactile stimuli, for example, visually tracking an object; (2) **sustained attention** or vigilance, the ability to maintain a consistent behavioral response during continuous repetitive activities for more than a few minutes or seconds, for example, sorting shapes correctly; (3) **selective attention,** the ability to maintain a behavioral set in the presence of distracting extraneous stimuli, for example, reading the newspaper with a television or music playing in the background; (4) **alternating attention,** the ability to shift the focus of attention and move between tasks with different behavioral requirements, for instance, a waitress serving tables and also working the cash register; and (5) **divided attention,** the ability to respond simultaneously to multiple task demands, such as driving while talking on a car phone. Obviously, problems at any level of attention can lead to significant deficits in communicative function, either with the receptive processing of auditory or printed messages, or expressively, with the ability to sustain the content or focus of what is being said or written.

Memory.   Just as there are many definitions of attention, there are many definitions of memory. Most definitions or models of memory include the dimensions of attention, **encoding** (or coding of information to facilitate later recall), storage, and **consolidation** (integrating new memories with old). Although memory deficits may occur in isolation, they are typically accompanied by deficits in other cognitive abilities such as orientation, attention, and language. Using this generic model of memory, various deficits can be classified by stage of memory implicated (for example, memory problems secondary to attention deficits). Difficulty with any level of attention prohibits complete processing of information for subsequent recall. Memory problems that are secondary to encoding deficits may result from impaired language or perceptual ability; in other words, if the individual does not understand or perceive what was presented, memory of that information is reduced. Memory problems related to storage may be the result of a decreased ability to put or keep information in memory. Such individuals may have normal immediate and short-term memory, but long-term memory is reduced owing to a progressive deterioration of retained information over time.

Problem-Solving and Reasoning.   Both problem-solving and reasoning are considered to be aspects of high-level thought processes (Adamovich, Henderson, & Auerbach, 1985; Hagan, 1984; Sohlberg & Mateer, 1989). There is general consensus that **problem-solving** involves at least three components: strategy selection, application of the strategy for resolution of the problem, and evaluation of the outcome. Difficulty in this process may result from being unable to analyze all aspects of the problem or to anticipate potential outcomes, formulation of incomplete solutions, or acting on the problem impulsively. Reasoning concerns the drawing of inferences or conclusions from known or assumed facts, in other words, determining what follows from what. Various types of reasoning have been described, including **deductive reasoning,** which pertains to the drawing of conclusions based on premises or general principles in a step-by-step manner; **inductive reasoning,** which involves the formulation of solutions given information that leads to but does not necessarily support a general conclusion; and convergent thinking, which involves the recognition and analysis of information relevant to a central theme or main point.

Executive Function. Damage to the frontal lobes results in behavioral and emotional deficits as well as cognitive deficits, particularly decreased **executive function.** The frontal lobes coordinate input from all other regions of the brain and therefore are important for coordinating and actualizing activities involved in cognitive processing. Executive function, more than any other cognitive dimension, determines the extent of social and vocational recovery. Executive function is not a discrete process but rather an umbrella function that comes into play with all realms of cognitive processing. When executive function is impaired, all other cognitive systems have the potential to be affected even though individually they may remain intact. Executive functioning may be considered a composite of activities related to achievement/completion of a goal, including anticipation, goal formulation, planning, implementing, self-monitoring, and the use of feedback. Individuals with deficits in the area of executive function may be able to perform single-step operations but may be unable to plan, sequence, and monitor multistep activities (for example, they may be able to answer the phone in an office but be unable to function as an office manager).

Language Disturbances

Aphasia. McKinley (1981) has noted that language is disturbed in 75 percent or more of individuals with TBI. The nature of this language disturbance in TBI—that is, whether it is aphasic, aphasic-like, or nonaphasic—is not clear-cut. **Aphasia** is an acquired impairment of language processes underlying receptive and expressive modalities caused by damage to areas of the brain that are primarily responsible for language function (Davis, 1993). Aphasia is manifested in grammatical disturbances, deficits of word retrieval, auditory comprehension, reading, and writing, in the presence of relatively intact cognitive abilities (e.g., orientation, attention, memory). (For a more complete discussion of aphasia see chapter on Communication Disorders Following Focal Brain Damage). It has been estimated that nearly 80 percent of aphasic individuals receiving speech and language therapy in hospital settings suffered strokes (Davis & Holland, 1981). Aphasia may also result from TBI, but the incidence reported in the literature varies greatly. Reports range from approximately 2 percent of 750 (Heilman, Safran, & Geschwind, 1971) and 2 percent of 614 (Schwartz-Cowley & Stepanik, 1989) consecutive admissions to two city hospitals, to nearly 50 percent (Levin, Grossman, & Kelly, 1976; Thomsen, 1975). Sarno, Buonaguro, and Levita (1986) reported on a group of 125 closed head injured patients admitted to a rehabilitation center. The population studied fell into three groups: those with classic aphasia (30 percent), those with dysarthria accompanied by subclinical aphasia (34 percent), and those with subclinical aphasia (36 percent). The authors classified patients as aphasic if their use of speech for expression and/or reception was impaired. Subclinical aphasia referred to evidence of linguistic processing deficits on formal testing in the absence of clinical manifestations of linguistic impairment. The apparent discrepancies regarding the incidence of aphasia following TBI are difficult to resolve owing to the lack of consistency in the descriptions of the head-injured patients studied, the different measures employed to document the presence of aphasia, as well as the varied definitions of aphasia applied.

An examination of specific linguistic deficits following TBI that are reported in the literature indicates that anomia, difficulty retrieving words, (Heilman et al., 1971; Levin et al., 1976, 1979; 1981; Sarno 1980; Sarno et al., 1986; Thomsen, 1976) and impaired auditory comprehension (Levin et al., 1976; Sarno et al., 1986) are the most commonly observed symptoms. Holland (1982) noted that there is overlap in these deficit areas between aphasic and TBI patients as well as in the associated reading and writing deficits that both groups often demonstrate. However, it is the qualitative differences in the naming errors between the two groups that may be most useful in distinguishing between aphasic and nonaphasic responses. Both aphasic and TBI individuals produce circumlocutions and various paraphasias and have reduced fluency in the generation of category-specific words; TBI individuals, however, demonstrate additional naming errors. For example, TBI individuals may also produce naming errors related to their personal situations or make errors of confabulation (bizarre responses related to the patient's disorientation). Milton, Turnstall, and Wertz (1983) have described a system for qualitatively evaluating naming behavior for TBI individuals. The system permits descriptions of correct responses, and, when responses are incorrect, descriptions of their semantic, phonemic, and other relationships to the target. For example, for the target stimulus "apple," semantically related responses might include such responses as *fruit, Granny Smith,* or *pear.* Phonemically related responses might include: *able* or *ubel.* Other responses might include such things as *saw* or *We grew them in our backyard.* Use of such a system provides the speech–language pathologist with far more information than can be used for treatment planning than a basic plus/minus scoring system.

Confused Language.   In addition to specific linguistic deficits, individuals with TBI may also demonstrate significant problems in the area of what has been termed confused language (Groher, 1977; Halperin, Darley, & Brown, 1973; Levin, Grossman, & Rose, 1979; Prigatano, 1986). Confused language is described as receptive/expressive language that may be phonologically, syntactically, and semantically intact, yet lacks meaning because responses are irrelevant, confabulatory, circumlocutory, or tangential in relation to a specific topic; confused language also lacks a logical sequential relationship between thoughts (Hagan, 1984). Such language dysfunction may be mistaken for a fluent aphasia, but is more appropriately considered cognitively based as opposed to

linguistically based (that is, as a symptom of cognitive rather than linguistic deficits).

Pragmatics.   Up to this point in the discussion of language disorders subsequent to TBI, it has been noted that the incidence of aphasia reported in the literature varies considerably. The discrepancies are probably the result of the approach the investigators have taken to evaluate language abilities in TBI patients, as well as their definition of aphasia. Confused language has been described as a possible sequela of TBI. A variety of cognitive deficits commonly seen after TBI may interfere with communication. Although some TBI patients exhibit language disorders most consistent with aphasia, and many, particularly in the acute stages of recovery from TBI, demonstrate language behavior consistent with confused language, the primary basis of language dysfunction in the majority of TBI survivors pertains to disordered language use (this term is used synonymously with the term pragmatics). Pragmatics refers to a system of rules that structures the use of language in terms of situational and social context. Sohlberg and Mateer (1989) observed that whereas aphasic individuals may communicate better than they talk, individuals with TBI appear to talk better than they communicate.

Pragmatic deficits are probably most prevalent in those patients with injuries to the frontal lobes. Although the frontal lobes are not thought to be responsible for primary cognitive functions, it appears they are involved in coordinating and actualizing many functions involved in cognitive processing, such as attention, motivation, regulation, and self-monitoring (Stuss & Benson, 1986). Alexander, Benson, and Stuss (1989) noted that individuals with prefrontal injury frequently demonstrate problems with disorganized discourse, inappropriate social interactions (e.g., difficulty interpreting social cues), and abstract forms of language (e.g., irony or sarcasm) among other things.

Speech and Swallowing Disturbances.   In addition to the disorders of communication described above that deal with the form and content of language, TBI may also affect motor control systems. Included in this section are brief reviews of dysarthria, mutism, and dysphagia, which are relatively common sequelae of TBI. (For detailed descriptions, see Chapters 8 and 10.)

Dysarthria.   *Dysarthria* is a speech disorder resulting from weakness or incoordination of the muscles that control respiration, phonation, resonation or articulation. Yorkston, Beukelman, and Bell (1988) noted that the incidence of dysarthria following TBI is not well documented. Additionally, the characteristics of the dysarthria are poorly described due to the limited number of studies that have been undertaken. Rusk, Block and Lowmann (1969) observed dysarthria in approximately 30 percent of 96 head-injured patients they studied. This is consistent with the findings of Sarno, Buonaguro, and Levita (1986), who noted that 34 percent of the 125 TBI patients in their study demonstrated dysarthria. Thomsen (1976) observed that in the group of head-injured individuals that she monitored longitudinally, those with dysarthria showed little improvement up to 15 years after onset. Rusk et al. (1969) reported that of their dysarthric head-injured patients, half had improved and half had not improved 5 to 15 years after injury.

Although there are no reports in the literature regarding the incidence of specific types of dysarthria following TBI, a few studies suggest a variety of characteristics that depend on the nature and locale, as well as the severity, of the brain injury. Ataxic dysarthria has been the predominant dysarthria reported among TBI survivors in a few recent studies (Simmons, 1983; Yorkston & Beukelman, 1981; Yorkston, Beukelman, Minifie, & Sapir, 1984). Ataxic dysarthria results from damage to the cerebellum. The cerebellum regulates the force, speed, range, timing, and direction of movements originating in the other motor systems of the brain. Primary characteristics of ataxic dysarthria are marked breakdown in the articulation of consonants and vowels, abnormalities in the prosody of speech, dysrhythmia, slow rate, and harsh vocal quality.

Flaccid dysarthria as well as mixed dysarthrias (flaccid-spastic, spastic-ataxic) have also been described in TBI survivors (Netsell & Daniel, 1979; Yorkston & Beukelman, 1981). Flaccid dysarthria results from damage to motor units required for speech, resulting in weakness, loss of muscle tone, reduced reflexes, and paralysis. Primary characteristics of flaccid dyarthria are hypernasality, nasal emission, and breathiness. Spastic dysarthria results from damage to the upper motor neurons and impairs movements necessary for efficient speech production. Spastic muscles are stiff, move sluggishly, and tend to be weak. The resulting speech is slow and is produced effortfully with imprecise articulation, low pitch, and harsh vocal quality.

Mutism.   Levin and colleagues (1983) have defined a condition called **mutism,** secondary to severe TBI but not attributable to cranial nerve injury, in which the patient is speechless in the presence of an ability to comprehend simple commands and to communicate nonverbally. These investigators observed the incidence of mutism in a group of 350 TBI patients to be approximately 3 percent. Two types of mutism were identified— one associated with lesions to the left basal nuclei (subcortical structures deep within the brain) believed to have a better prognosis, and the other associated with severe diffuse brain injury, considered to be a permanent condition.

Dysphagia.   *Dysphagia* is a condition in which the action of swallowing is difficult or painful to perform. The incidence of dysphagia following TBI has been carefully studied. Winstein (1983) reported an incidence of 27 percent for consecutive TBI patient admissions to a rehabilitation center, and Cherney and Halper (1989) noted a nearly identical incidence of 26 percent in the 189 TBI patients they studied. Lazarus and Logemann (1987) reported that of a group of 53 dysphagic patients with TBI referred for videofluoroscopic evaluation, 39 percent demonstrated severe dysphagia, 33 percent moderate dysphagia, and 27 percent mild dysphagia. The most frequently occurring dysfunctions were delayed triggering of the swallow response (81 percent), reduced tongue control (53 percent), and reduced pharyngeal transit (32 percent). (See chapter on Swallowing Disorders.) Relatively few of these patients demonstrated difficulties related to laryngeal function (14 percent) (for example, reduced layngeal closure, elevation, or spasm). Of the 53 TBI patients studied, 20 (38 percent) aspirated (swallowed materials entering the airway below the level of the vocal folds) during the videofluoroscopic examination.

THE ROLE OF THE SPEECH–LANGUAGE PATHOLOGIST

The speech-language pathologist is a member of the team of rehabilitation professionals that collaboratively assesses and treats individuals who have sustained TBI (see Ylvisaker, 1994 for a discussion of collaboration in TBI rehabilitation). Speech–language pathologists assume primary responsibility for the assessment of all aspects of communication: hearing (screening with referral to an audiologist for comprehensive audiologic assessment); spoken language (comprehension and production); written language (reading and writing); cognitive communication (i.e., exploring the communicative implications of impairments in such areas as orientation, attention, memory, reasoning, problem solving, and executive functions); speech production (articulation, fluency, voice, and resonance); augmentative and alternative communication; as well as swallowing. Upon completion of this assessment the findings are interpreted, and a prognosis and treatment recommendations formulated. Treatment planning includes collaboration with educational and vocational specialists to enable the TBI individual to succeed educationally and/or vocationally.

Speech–language pathologists are responsible for the establishment of treatment programs aimed at decreasing the effects of impairments in all aspects of speech, language, cognitive-communicative functioning, and swallowing. The treatment plan includes long- and short-term objectives (re-

viewed on a regular basis) and information regarding frequency, estimated duration, type of service, and follow-up or referral to other professionals as necessary. In addition, speech–language pathologists help to identify effective supports to enable cognitively disabled individuals to be as independent and successful as possible. Such supports may include cognitive prosthetic devices (e.g., memory log such as an appointment book); adjustment of work expectations by employer; changes in classroom/work environment (e.g., allowing individual to work where distractions are minimal); and modification of teaching procedures to be consistent with individual's cognitive strengths and weaknesses (e.g., untimed exams). Treatment programs vary depending on the stage of recovery of the TBI individual (Adamovich, Henderson, & Auerbach, 1985).

MANAGEMENT OF COGNITIVE-COMMUNICATIVE DEFICITS IN TRAUMATIC BRAIN INJURY

Just as stage of recovery after TBI guides the management approach of the speech–language pathologist, the assessment and treatment approaches to TBI patients need to be discussed with regard to stage of recovery.

Scaling of Behaviors

Historically, TBI patients have been classified according to such categories as coma, stupor, delirium, and confusion (Hagan, 1984). The Glasgow Coma Scale (GCS) (Jennett & Teasdale, 1981; Teasdale & Jennett, 1974) has been widely used for several years. This scale (Table 6.1), designed to characterize the continuum of coma in a practical and reliable fashion, evaluates three components of wakefulness independent of each other: the stimulus required to induce eye opening, the best motor response, and the best verbal response. Each behavior is described along a gradient of responses indicative of degree of increasing dysfunction. Coma is defined as absence of eye opening, inability to obey commands, and failure to produce intelligible utterances, corresponding to a GCS score of 8 or less. Although the major function of the GCS is for early prediction of mortality and morbidity, the scale is useful for describing categories of patient responses during the early phases of treatment. The GCS has been criticized because the scale has no means of rating TBI patients who are on ventilators and who are thus unable to produce intelligible utterances.

A second scale, the Levels of Cognitive Functioning (LOCF) (Hagan et al., 1979) is useful in identifying a patient's most intact level of cognitive functioning over the entire course of rehabilitation (Table 6.2). While the GCS is used for prognosis, the LOCF is used to identify the patient's best level of functioning and therefore is in-

dicative of the best way to approach the patient throughout the continuum of treatment. The LOCF represents a progression of recovery of cognitive abilities in the TBI population as manifested through behavioral change. Advantages of the LOCF include: it is an assessment that does not require the patient's cooperation; it provides behavioral descriptions of cognitive recovery along a severity continuum; it enables professionals, from a variety of disciplines, to discuss TBI patients using common and descriptive terminology; and it provides baseline information for the development of team treatment goals.

Early Stages of Recovery. For the purposes of our discussion the early stage of recovery will be

TABLE 6.1 The Glascow Coma Scale

		Eye Opening
None	1	Not attributable to ocular swelling
To Pain	2	Pain stimulus is applied to chest or limbs
To Speech	3	Nonspecific response to speech or shout, does not imply the patient obeys command to open eyes
Spontaneous	4	Eyes are open, but does not imply intact awareness
		Motor Response
No Response	1	Flaccid
Extension	2	"Decerebrate." Adduction, internal rotation of shoulder, and pronation of the forearm
Abnormal Flexion	3	"Decorticate." Abnormal flexion, adduction of the shoulder
Withdrawal	4	Normal flexor response; withdraws from pain stimulus with abduction of the shoulder
Localizes Pain	5	Pain stimulus applied to supraocular region or fingertip causes limb to move so as to attempt to remove it
Obeys Commands	6	Follows simple commands
		Verbal Response
No Response	1	(Self-explanatory)
Incomprehensible	2	Moaning and groaning, but no recognizable words
Inappropriate	3	Intelligible speech (e.g., shouting or swearing), but no sustained or coherent conversation
Confused	4	Patient responds to questions in a conversational manner, but the responses indicate varying degrees of disorientation and confusion
Oriented	5	Normal orientation to time, place, and person
		Summed Glascow Coma Scale Score = E + M + V (3 to 15)

Source: Reprinted with permission from Hagan, C. (1984). Language disorders in head trauma. In A. Holland (Ed.), *Language disorders in adults* (pp. 245–281). San Diego, CA: College-Hill Press.

TABLE 6.2 Levels of Cognitive Functioning and Associated Language Behaviors

GENERAL BEHAVIORS	LANGUAGE BEHAVIORS
I. No Response	
Patient appears to be in a deep sleep and is completely unresponsive to any stimuli.	Receptive and expressive: No evidence of processing or verbal or gestural expression.
II. Generalized Response	
Patient reacts inconsistently and nonpurposefully to stimuli in a nonspecific manner. Responses are limited and often the same, regardless of stimulus presented. Responses may be physiologic changes, gross body movements, or vocalization.	Receptive and expressive: No evidence of processing or verbal or gestural expression.
III. Localized Response	
Patient reacts specifically, but inconsistently, to stimuli. Responses are directly related to the type of stimulus presented. May follow simple commands such as "close your eyes" or "squeeze my hand" in an inconsistent, delayed manner.	Language begins to emerge.
	Receptive: Patient progresses from localizing to processing and following simple commands that elicit automatic responses in a delayed and inconsistent manner. Limited reading emerges.
	Expressive: Automatic verbal and gestural responses emerge in response to direct elicitation. Negative head nods emerge before positive head nods. Utterances are single words serving as "holophrastic" responses.
IV. Confused–Agitated	
Behavior is bizarre and nonpurposeful relative to immediate environment. Does not discriminate among persons or objects; is unable to cooperate directly with treatment efforts; verbalizations are frequently incoherent or inappropriate to the environment; confabulation may be present. Gross attention to environment is very short, and selective attention is often nonexistent. Patient lacks short-term recall.	Severe disruption of frontal–temporal lobes, with resultant confusion apparent.
	Receptive: Marked disruption in auditory and visual processing, including inability to order phonemic events, monitor rate, and attend to, retain, categorize and associate stimuli. Disinhibition interferes with comprehension and ability to inhibit responses to self-generated mental activity.
	Expressive: Marked disruption of phonologic, semantic, syntactic, and suprasegmental features. Output is bizarre, unrelated to environment, and incoherent. Literal, verbal, and neologistic paraphasias appear with disturbance of logico-sequential features and incompleteness of thought. Monitoring of pitch, rate, intensity, and suprasegmentals is severely impaired.
V. Confused, Inappropriate, Nonagitated	
Patient is able to respond to simple commands fairly consistently. However, with increased complexity of commands or lack of any external structure, responses are nonpurposeful, random, or fragmented.	Linguistic fluctuations are in accordance with the degree of external structure and familiarity-predictability of linguistic events.

TABLE 6.2 Continued

GENERAL BEHAVIORS	LANGUAGE BEHAVIORS

V. Confused, Inappropriate, Nonagitated (continued)

Has gross attention to the environment but is highly distractible and lacks. ability to focus attention on a specific task; with structure, may be able to converse on a social-automatic level for short periods; verbalization is often inappropriate and confabulatory; memory is severely impaired, often shows inappropriate use of subjects; individual may perform previously learned tasks with structure but is unable to learn new information.

Receptive: Processing has improved, with increased ability to retain temporal order of phonemic events, but semantic and syntactic confusions persist. Only phrases or short sentences are retained. Rate, accuracy, and quality remain significantly reduced.

Expressive: Persistence of phonologic, semantic, syntactic, and prosodic processes. Disturbances in logico-sequential features result in irrelevancies, incompleteness, tangent, circumlocutions, and confabulations. Literal paraphasias subside, while neologisms and verbal paraphasias continue. Utterances may be expansive or telegraphic, depending on inhibition-disinhibition factors. Responses are stimulus bound. Word retrieval deficits are characterized by delays, generalizations, descriptions, semantic associations, or circumlocutions. Disruptions in syntactic features are present beyond concrete levels of expression or with increased length of output. Written output is severely limited. Gestures are incomplete.

VI. Confused–Appropriate

Patient shows goal-directed behavior but depends on external input for direction; follows simple directions consistently and shows carryover for relearned tasks with little or no carryover for new tasks; responses may be incorrect due to memory problems but appropriate to the situation; past memories show more depth and detail than recent memories.

Receptive: Processing remains delayed, with difficulty in retaining, analyzing, and synthesizing. Auditory processing is present for compound sentences, while reading comprehension is present for simple sentences. Self-monitoring capacity emerges.

Expressive: Internal confusion-disorganization is reflected in expressions, but appropriateness is maintained. Language is confused relative to impaired new learning and displaced temporal and situational contexts, but confabulation is no longer present. Social-automatic conversation is intact but remains stimulus bound. Tangential and irrelevant responses are present only in open-ended situations requiring referential language. Neologisms are extinguished, with literal paraphasias present only in conjunction with an apraxia. Word retrieval errors occur in conversation but seldom in confrontation naming. Length of utterance reflects inhibitory-initiation mechanisms. Written and gestural expression increases. Prosodic features reflect the "voice of confusion," characterized by monopitch, monostress, and monoloudness.

continued

TABLE 6.2 Continued

VII. Automatic–Appropriate

Patient appears appropriate and oriented within hospital and home settings, goes through daily routine automatically, but is frequently robotlike with minimal-to-absent confusion; has shallow recall of activities; shows carryover for new learning but at a decreased rate; with structure, is able to initiate social or recreational activities; judgment remains impaired.

Linguistic behaviors appear "normal" within familiar, predictable, structured settings, but deficits emerge in open-ended communication and less structured settings.

Receptive: Reductions persist in auditory processing and reading comprehension relative to length, complexity, and presence of competing stimuli. Retention has improved to short paragraphs but without the ability to identify salient features, organize, integrate input, order, and retain detail.

Expressive: Automatic level of language is apparent in referential communication. Reasoning is concrete and self-oriented. Expression becomes tangential and irrelevant when abstract linguistic concepts are attempted. Word retrieval errors are minimal. Length of utterance and gestures approximate normal. Writing is disorganized and simple at a paragraph level. Prosodic features may remain aberrant. Pragmatic features of ritualizing and referencing are present, while other components remain disrupted.

VIII. Purposeful and Appropriate

Patient is able to recall and integrate past and recent events and is aware of and responsive to the environment, shows carryover for new learning, and needs no supervision once activities are learned; may continue to show a decreased ability relative to premorbid abilities in language, abstract reasoning, tolerance for stress, and judgment in emergencies or unusual circumstances.

Language capacities may fall within normal limits. Otherwise, problems persist in competitive situations and in response to fatigue, stress, and emotionality, characterized in reduced effectiveness, efficiency, and quality of performance.

Receptive: Rate of processing remains reduced but unremarkable on testing. Retention span remains limited at paragraph level but improve with use of retrieval-organization strategies. Analysis, organization, and integration are reduced in rate and quality.

Expressive: Syntactic and semantic features fall within normal limits, while reasoning and abstraction remain reduced. Written expression may fall below premorbid level. Prosidic features are essentially normal. Pragmatic features of referencing, presuppositions, topic maintenance, turn taking, and use of paralinguistic features in context remain impaired.

defined as LOCF II (Generalized Response) and III (Localized Response). During this phase of recovery communicative functioning is dependent on arousal and alertness mechanisms. Kennedy and DeRuyter (1991) noted that there are two types of variables that need to be considered in the assessment of brain-injured patients: task and performance variables. Task variables are within the clinician's control and include such things as: (1) stimulus intensity; (2) rate of presentation; (3) type of stimulus presented and type of response required (receptive versus expressive); (4) duration of task and length of testing sessions; (5) familiarity of task to patient; (6) level of task complexity; and (7) context in which stimulus is presented. Performance variables are aspects of the response the clinician observes while task variables remain constant or change. These include such factors as: (1) response duration; (2) response delay; (3) ability of the patient to shift response sets from one task to the next; (4) number of times a response needs to be repeated for the response to be elicited; (5) type of response; and (6) pattern of responses, or response consistency.

With regard to assessment of cognitive/communicative skills in the early stages of recovery, the speech–language pathologist must rely primarily on observational skills as TBI patients at LOCF II and III are typically unable to participate in standardized testing. Attempts should be made to "standardize" the observations by presenting comparable stimulation across input modalities (e.g., auditory, visual, tactile) and consistent stimulation activities (i.e., with regard to rate, complexity, duration, intensity, etc.) across sessions. By using replicable stimulation, responses observed in one session under a specific pattern of stimulation, can be attempted to be re-elicited under the same conditions during another session as a measure of the consistency of the response. The Western Neuro Sensory Stimulation Profile (Ansell & Keenan, 1989), which was designed to assess TBI patients' arousal/attention, expressive communication, and response to auditory, visual, tactile, and olfactory stimulation, is one approach to standardizing observations of lower functioning patients.

Table 6.3 provides examples of common stimuli used in the evaluation of TBI patients at LOCF II and III. Table 6.4 lists several abilities that should be addressed during the evaluation of such patients.

TABLE 6.3 Commonly Used Stimuli for Evaluating Individuals at LOCF II and III

Tactile
Shapes (cubes, balls)
Surfaces (cloth, Velcro, cotton ball)
Fur
Brushes and combs
Firm touch

Kinesthesia
Range of motion
Positioning (extremities and body)

Auditory
Bells
Chimes
Clapping
Music
Voice (familiar and unfamiliar)
Snapping fingers

Olfactory
Extracts
Perfumes and colognes
Spices
Soap
Vinegar

Visual
Objects from home
Pictures of family and individual
Mirror
Colorful items
ADL items

Gustatory
Extracts
Lemon
Vinegar

Source: Reprinted with permission from Kennedy, M. R. T. & DeRuyter, F. (1991). Cognitive and language bases for communication disorders. In D. R. Beukelman & K. M. Yorkston (Eds.), *Communication disorders following traumatic brain injury* (pp. 123–190). Austin, TX: Pro-Ed.

TABLE 6.4   Assessment of Individuals at LOCF II and III

ABILITIES	METHODS
Alertness: amount, frequency timing, activities, body positions	Team evaluation
Arousability: types of stimulation and responses	Systematic presentation of hierarchical tasks
Sensory modalities: tactile, kinesthetic, olfactory, gustatory, auditory, visual	Observe at various times and during various tasks
Communication: following commands, type of response, communication system, basic reading	Interview family members Observe individual with family, note responses
Presence of reflexes: oral chewing, defensiveness, whole body reflexes	Use familiar items: music, pictures
Balance: posture, head control, limb alignment, sitting, standing	Record frequency, rate, duration, variety, and quality of responses
Arm and hand function: reaching, grasping, gestures	Observe responses with cuing (manual, verbal, gestural, nonverbal
Tone: overall, at rest, in motion, various positions	

Adapted from Reimer, T. J. and Donoghue, K. (1987). The speech pathologist's role in the stimulation of the low level brain injured patient. Presented at the California Speech-Language-Hearing Association Convention, San Diego, CA.

Once a TBI patient is responding in a more consistent fashion, that individual's best input modality and best response mode need to be identified for the purposes of establishing a system for communicative interactions. Such information should be communicated immediately to the other treatment team members and the patient's family to facilitate their interactions with the patient. DeRuyter and Becker (1988) observed that for nonspeaking individuals functioning at LOCF III (localized response), the success of yes-no response systems depended on the most natural and automatic body movement. The most successful yes-no systems were head nods, with decreasing success for systems requiring less automatic movement and the use of other cognitive and/or motor processes (e.g., visual tracking and reading for using yes-no cards).

The ability to follow verbal commands in individuals who have been unresponsive is a significant turning point in patients progressing out of coma (Bricolo, Turazzi, & Feriotti, 1980). Ansell and Keenan (1989) have reported on patterns of communication recovery in "slow to recover pa-

tients" (at LOCF II and III for extended periods of time). They observed that if responses to auditory information (following commands) began to improve, the patient had a 50 percent chance of progressing to LOCF V. If responses to auditory and visual information returned simultaneously, the probability of improving to LOCF V were considerably better. If however, responses to visual or tactile stimulation were the only responses to emerge, the likelihood for cognitive improvement was minimal. These results are consistent with previous research which has indicated retardation of development and diminished recovery of central nervous system function in the presence of environmental and sensory deprivation (Finger & Stein, 1982). It also emphasizes the importance of the cognitive-language system to recovery after TBI.

Intermediate Stages of Recovery.   At LOCF IV (confused, agitated) and V (confused, inappropriate, nonagitated), TBI patients' alertness improves and they are bombarded with a multitude of stimuli from their environment. Because they are unable to focus and sustain attention for more than a few seconds, the stimuli may be meaningless or at best confusing. Consequently, these patients may demonstrate marked agitation. Their arms, legs, trunk, and head may be in constant motion and their speech is often completely irrelevant beyond a few automatic social responses. The term *confusion* is usually applied to such pervasive attentional deficits. This period is almost always reversible in TBI patients; however, in some severely injured patients confusional states may become chronic (Sohlberg & Mateer, 1989).

With time less agitation is noted, but TBI patients may still be unable to maintain a coherent line of thought or to maintain concentration. Severe disruption of language function at this stage is common, even in the absence of aphasia. Confused language, described previously, is the best characterization of the cognitive-communicative impairments. Impaired attentional processes, including initiation, maintenance, shifting, and inhibiting (i.e., the ability to ignore distractions), affect both language comprehension and expression. Poor topic maintenance, topic shifting in conversation, and stimulus bound responses result from ideational perseveration (i.e., becoming fixated on certain ideas or thoughts), verbal disinhibition (i.e., saying whatever comes to mind), and

impaired impulse control (Hagan, 1984; Adamovich, Henderson, & Auerbach, 1985). In the presence of damage to the frontal lobes (a relatively common consequence of TBI), although the structural components of language remain intact, the intent and use of language may be significantly impaired (Alexander, Benton, & Stuss, 1989; Lezak, 1976; Stuss & Benson, 1984; Stuss, 1987). Language behaviors associated with frontal lobe injuries include confabulation, impaired word fluency, perseveration of thought, inappropriate turn-taking, inattentiveness to listener's needs, repetitive and/or disorganized messages, and social inappropriateness due to poor self-monitoring.

Kennedy and DeRuyter (1991) noted that because individuals functioning at LOCF IV and V are frequently unable to focus and sustain their attention to specific tasks, to discriminate, and to sequence and organize their responses, nonstandardized procedures must be employed during the assessment. Adamovich et al. (1985) presented several activities arranged in a hierarchy from low-level (arousal and alertness) to high-level (reasoning and abstraction) cognitive tasks. Table 6.5 summarizes important considerations for the assessment of TBI patients at this level of recovery. Although the use of standardized materials is not always practical, baseline data gathered as early

TABLE 6.5 Assessment of Individuals at LOCF IV and V

ABILITIES	METHODS
Hyper-attentiveness and hypo-attentiveness	Team evaluation
Selectivity, attention span	Systematic presentation of hierarchical tasks
Orientation or confusion: time, place, persons, objects	Use standardized tests if able
Sequencing: in expression, thought activity	Present simple, motor, functional activities
Inhibition or disinhibition	Evaluate in sessions 15 to 30 minutes long
Organization: associating, categorizing	Vary tasks to allow for attention and disinhibition
Agitation: causes, frequency, duration, what reduces it	Include behavioral reinforcements to reduce agitation
Communication: modalities, content, generalized vs. focal, comprehension, use of social skills	Include familiar persons to elicit best response

Adapted from Becker, M. (1986). Cognitive-linguistic assessment protocol: Revised. Presented at the Ninth Annual Conference, "Coma to Community." Santa Clara Valley Medical Center, San Jose, CA.

as possible can document the pattern of recovery and provide prognostic information. Standardized procedures should be incorporated into the evaluation process as soon as possible.

Later Stages of Recovery. For TBI patients in the later stages of recovery, that is, LOCF VI (confused-appropriate), VII (automatic-appropriate), and VIII (purposeful and appropriate), the interdisciplinary approach to cognitive-communicative-behavioral evaluation is critical. Subtle deficits of attention and speed of performance are delineated by neuropsychological assessment, while the occupational therapist analyzes the TBI patient's behavior during activities of daily living. The speech–language pathologist often assumes the role of analyzing the effects that impaired processes have on performance in daily activities and communication (Kennedy & DeRuyter, 1991).

Evaluation of patients at LOCF VI-VIII must be tailored to the individual's specific injury, severity level, and overall communicative needs. With individuals who are confused and disoriented and have difficulty with learning (LOCF V), assessment should focus on impaired processes (e.g., attention and memory) as well as on the impact of the deficits on everyday tasks. With regard to the direct measurement of such deficits, Levin, O'Donnell, and Grossman (1979) developed the Galveston Orientation and Amnesia Test (GOAT), a brief schedule of questions to measure post-traumatic amnesia (the period following coma characterized by an inability to store or recall information on a day-to-day or even minute-to-minute basis) and disorientation following TBI (see Table 6.6). The GOAT asks for the patient's name, address, and birthdate (question 1) because patients recovering from severe TBI are often confused about basic biographic data and this information can usually be verified. Asking the patient to state the city or town and to identify the building as a hospital (question 2) probes for possible geographic disorientation. Recall of the date of hospital admission (question 3) is included because it is assumed that most patients are inclined to obtain this information, which is verifiable. Questions 4

TABLE 6.6 Questions from the Galveston Orientation and Amnesia Test (GOAT)

1. What is your name?
   When were you born?
   Where do you live?
2. Where are you now?
   City?
   Hospital?
3. On what date were you admitted to this hospital?
   How did you get here?
4. What is the first event you can remember *after* the injury?
   Can you describe in detail (e.g., date, time, companions) the first event you can recall *after* injury?
5. Can you describe the last event you recall *before* the accident?
   Can you describe in detail (e.g., date, time, companions) the first event you can recall *before* the injury?
6. What time is it now?
7. What day of the week is it?
8. What day of the month is it?
9. What is the month?
10. What is the year?

and 5 probe events after and prior to the injury, respectively. The GOAT has been standardized on the TBI population and validated for serial testing. It is a useful measure that may be presented on a daily basis, and when graphed, serial GOAT scores provide a clear record of recovery.

Assessment of individuals at LOCF VII and VIII who display impairment in higher thought processes (e.g., reasoning, problem-solving, executive functions) along with mild cognitive deficits will require a more detailed task-specific evaluation to determine the extent of impairment within underlying processes. The use of standardized tests are most appropriate for TBI patients in the later stages of recovery.

There are numerous standardized batteries available that were either designed for or are appropriate for use with the TBI population. Table 6.7 lists and describes several useful measures for

TABLE 6.7 Standardized Tests Applicable to the Traumatic Brain Injured Population

BATTERIES	DESCRIPTION
Minnesota Test for Differential Diagnosis of Aphasia (Schuell, 1972)	Screening test of categorical areas, hierarchical tasks for complexity and predictability
Boston Diagnostic Aphasia Exam (Goodglass & Kaplan, 1983a)	Provides a range of language tasks for comprehension, expression in multimodalities
Boston Naming Test (Goodglass & Kaplan, 1983b)	Assesses confrontation naming, word retrieval with or without cuing
Clinical Evaluation of Language Functions (Semel & Wiig, 1980)	Visual and verbal subtests test word fluency, verbal retention, associations, reasoning
Detroit Tests of Learning Aptitude-2 (Hammill, 1985)	Specific subtests evaluate verbal–visual sequencing, visual analysis, conceptual thinking
Discourse Comprehension Test (Brookshire & Nicholas, 1993)	Assesses comprehension of paragraph length materials with regard to main ideas, stated and implied details
Woodcock-Johnson Psychoeducational Battery (Woodcock & Johnson, 1977)	Specific subtests evaluate visual analysis, problem-solving, reasoning, concept formation
Illinois Test of Psycholinguistic Abilities (Kirk & colleagues, 1968)	Visual and auditory subtests test closure, differentiation, memory, analysis-synthesis
Wechsler Adult Intelligence Scale (Wechsler, 1955)	Verbal subtests assess attention, recall, (immediate and remote), knowledge, abstract comprehension, reasoning, fluency; performance subtests assess visual attention, speed of response, organization, scanning, eye–hand coordination
Wide Range Achievement Test (Jastak & Jastak, 1978)	Reading section is useful for measuring reading rate and single word recognition
Word Test (Jorgenson & colleagues, 1981)	Tests word retrieval, association/categorization, similarities/differences
Revised Visual Retention Test (4th Ed.) (Benton, 1974)	Sensitive to visual attention, recall span, visuo-spatial organization
Raven's Coloured Progressive Matrices (Raven, 1965	Nonlinguistic test measures visual reasoning and visuo-spatial analysis
Reporter's Test (DeRenzi & Ferrari, 1978)	Assessment of verbal formulation and organization (verbal counterpart to the Token Test)
Scales of Cognitive Ability for Traumatic Brain Injury (Adamovich & Henderson, 1992)	Assesses a range of cognitive skills: perception/discrimination, orientation, organization, recall, reasoning along a continuum of difficulty
Test of Problem Solving (Zachman & colleagues, 1984)	Assesses visual attention and synthesis, reasoning, deductive and inferential processing
Ross Test of Higher Cognitive Processes (Ross & Ross, 1979)	Assesses complex abstract reasoning and problem-solving
Fullerton Language Test for Adolescents (Thorum, 1979)	Subtests assess retention, verbal, formulation, association, retrieval, abstract reasoning

continued

TABLE 6.7   Continued

BATTERIES	DESCRIPTION
Goldman-Fristoe-Woodcock Auditory Skills Test Battery (Goldman & colleagues, 1974)	Assesses auditory processing including discrimination, attention, figure–ground
Wechsler Memory Scale-Revised (Wechsler, 1985)	Assesses visual and auditory retention for verbal and nonverbal input at varying levels of complexity; useful for testing processes of attention, organization, analysis-synthesis, learning with repetition
Revised Token Test (McNeil & Prescott, 1978)	Assesses auditory comprehension for increasingly complex and lengthy instructions; tests auditory attention and retention
Rivermead Behavioral Memory Test (Wilson & colleagues, 1985)	Functional memory test for immediate and delayed recall for stories, faces, objects, and multistep procedures
Reading Battery for Aphasia (LaPointe & Horner, 1979)	Subtests range from word to picture matching to functional reading at sentence level
Nelson Reading Skills Test (Hanna, Schell, & Schreiner, 1977)	Assesses vocabulary and literal and inferential comprehension at varied levels of difficulty
Peabody Picture Vocabulary Test (Dunn & Dunn, 1981)	Receptive vocabulary test that evaluates visual attention, scanning, and knowledge base

Source: Reprinted with permission from Kennedy, M. R. T. & DeRuyter, F. (1991). Cognitive and language bases for communication disorders. In D. R. Beukelman & K. M. Yorkston (Eds.), *Communication disorders following traumatic brain injury* (pp. 123–190). Austin, TX: Pro-Ed.

the assessment of such individuals. The information collected from such tests (1) provides baseline information to measure improvement; (2) helps to differentiate deficits attributable to diffuse cognitive-communicative disorganization versus focal-specific symptoms; (3) facilitates the identification of primary and secondary processes responsible for communicative breakdown; and (4) identifies the point at which remediation should begin (Kennedy & DeRuyter, 1991). Assessment tasks will logically involve many cognitive processes, making it difficult to isolate the role of a single process. However, formal assessment should attempt to estimate degree of impairment in single critical processes such as attention (alertness, arousal, processing speed, attention span, selective attention); discrimination; sequencing; organization (association and categorization); memory processes (e.g., retention span,

retrieval mechanisms, recent versus remote, episodic, procedural, semantic); reasoning; integration; and ability to sustain goal-directed activities over time (Hagan, 1984; Adamovich, Henderson, & Auerbach, 1985; Kennedy & DeRuyter, 1991).

Assessment of Functional Activities and Pragmatics

As previously mentioned, an important aspect of the assessment process with TBI patients at both the intermediate and later stages of recovery is not only to assess performance in traditional testing environments, but also to observe performance during functional activities and/or in more natural environments. This aspect of the assessment is important because there are often significant differences in a TBI patient's performances across the two settings. Deficits that are not evident during formal testing are often apparent in unstructured everyday environments (Starch & Falltrick, 1990). For example, a TBI patient may demonstrate concentration abilities that are adequate for functional reading comprehension when distractions are at a minimum. However, when this same individual attempts to read in a noisy/busy environment, concentration abilities may be significantly limited, thus leaving reading comprehension nonfunctional. Such a finding is important for the planning of treatment programs. Examples of functional activities include banking skills, using the telephone, grocery shopping, planning trips, note taking, preparing for an exam, and so on. Milton (1988) described an approach to assessment in which higher level patients (LOCF VII and VIII) preparing for return to school or work are assessed in the environment and on the tasks they will be expected to perform. Treatment is then focused on very specific impairments and the types of compensations that will be necessary for the TBI individual to function independently.

Sohlberg and Mateer (1989) have noted that pragmatic deficits may be the most pervasive communication problem in adults with TBI. Traditionally, assessment of communication skills in TBI patients has involved the administration of a language battery, most of which were designed to diagnose aphasia, and focusing on the assessment of vocabulary and grammatical abilities at the single word and sentence levels. Hagan (1984) has observed that individuals with TBI often appear to have minimal language impairments based on the results of such language batteries, yet demonstrate significant functional communication difficulties in natural environments. Therefore, several investigators have advocated assessing communication skills at the level of discourse (Coelho, Liles, & Duffy, 1991a, 1991b, 1991c, 1993, 1994; Ehrlich, 1985, 1988; Hartley & Jensen, 1991; Liles, Coelho, Duffy, & Zalagens, 1989, 1989; Mentis & Prutting, 1987, 1991). *Discourse* is a series of related linguistic units that convey a message. The length of a given discourse is determined by the communicative function of the message. There are various types of discourse and

each type has different cognitive and linguistic demands. Types of discourse include descriptions (listing static attributes or relations); narratives (convey actions and events that unfold in time); procedures (provide instructions or directions in a specific order); persuasion (giving reasons or facts to support an opinion); and conversation (interaction with others).

Discourse Analysis.   It has been suggested that **discourse** is the most natural and basic unit of normal verbal communication (Haliday & Hasan, 1976). Furthermore, accurate production or comprehension of a narrative requires a complex interaction of linguistic, cognitive, and social abilities (i.e., language use) that are sensitive to the particular disruption following TBI.

Discourse analyses typically begin with the elicitation of a spoken narrative, ideally at least five sentences in length. A variety of types of narrative discourse may be studied including procedural (e.g., describing how to change a tire), descriptive (e.g., describing a favorite activity), story narratives, and conversation. The discourse narratives are audiotaped and transcribed verbatim. Once transcribed, the narratives are divided into basic units for analysis, such as T-units (independent clause plus any dependent clauses associated with it). Depending on the type of discourse and the focus of the analysis, the actual discourse analysis may be done at a variety of levels. For example, in a narrative story, at the sentence level the number of T-units may be tallied as a measure of narrative length, or the number of subordinate clauses may be counted as a measure of grammatical complexity. Across-sentence analyses may involve examining how speakers link meaning units across several sentences (complete or incomplete ties), referred to as intersentential cohesion. In story narrative analysis, episodes are examined. Episode components are defined as information units pertaining to stated goals, attempts at solutions, and consequences of these attempts. The ability to generate episodes requires a variety of cognitive abilities that may be susceptible to disruption in brain injuries (Liles, Coelho, Duffy, &

Zalagens, 1989). Additional analyses include productivity measures such as total words produced or total speaking time, content measures such as accurate content units, and measures of conversational speech, for example, appropriateness of an utterance or topic maintenance.

Numerous recent investigations have illustrated the clinical utility of discourse analyses with the TBI Population (Coelho, et al., 1991a, 1991b, 1991c, 1993, 1994; Ehrlich, 1985, 1988; Hartley & Jensen, 1991; Liles, et al., 1989; Mentis & Prutting, 1987, 1991). Cohesion has been noted to be an area of inconsistent impairment. For example, the cohesive adequacy of TBI subjects was found to be comparable to that of normal speakers in story retelling, but was impaired for story generation. Similarly, the proportion of types of cohesive ties used by the TBI subjects changed from story retelling to story generation, which was not the case for the normal speakers. Overall, analysis of cohesion is useful for detecting subtle discourse organization deficits in TBI individuals. However, performance may vary considerably depending on the discourse elicitation task presented (Liles et al., 1989; Mentis & Prutting, 1987).

In a similar manner, TBI subjects' ability to generate complete episodes is frequently affected by the nature of the task, with story retelling being easier than story generation. Story generation requires a complex interaction of language and various cognitive abilities that has been shown to be difficult for even mildly impaired TBI subjects (Liles et al., 1989). Analysis of story structure (i.e., episodes) in conjunction with cohesion enables discourse samples to be examined at multiple levels (i.e., individual sentences, cohesion, episodes) allowing for the delineation of distinct discourse patterns.

The applicability of findings on discourse productivity and content analysis of TBI subjects has also been limited by the inclusion of individuals with aphasia and dysarthria in the groups studied. In very general terms, it has been observed that TBI individuals demonstrate decreased discourse efficiency, generating information at a slower rate in lengthier utterances than normal individuals.

Results from various pragmatic rating scales and analyses of response appropriateness and topic management all suggest that TBI individuals experience difficulty when called upon to function as a discourse partner, whether in conversation or referential communication (i.e., a structured exchange of information on a specific topic, requiring extensive listener feedback). These individuals demonstrate problems initiating and sustaining topics in conversation and frequently rely on their discourse partner to assume a greater proportion of the communicative burden to ensure a successful interchange of information. Finally, TBI individuals appear to make attempts at implementing a variety of compensatory strategies for their discourse deficits with varying success.

TREATMENT OF COGNITIVE-COMMUNICATIVE DEFICITS FOLLOWING TRAUMATIC BRAIN INJURY

Cognitive Rehabilitation

The treatment of cognitive-communicative deficits that result from TBI is referred to as **cognitive rehabilitation.** This term implies a treatment regimen aimed at increasing functional abilities in everyday life by improving an individual's capacity to process and interpret incoming information (Sohlberg & Mateer, 1989). There are essentially two approaches to cognitive rehabilitation: restorative and compensatory (Ben-Yishay & Diller, 1993). The rationales for these approaches are very different. The restorative approach is based on the notion that neuronal growth (the neuron, or nerve cell, is the basic anatomic and functional unit of the nervous system), and thus improvement in function, is associated with repetitive exercise of neuronal circuits. The restorative approach is sometimes referred to as the "muscle-building approach" and involves repetitive exercises and drilling. In contrast, the compensatory approach concedes that certain functions cannot be recovered, and the development of strategies to circumvent the impaired functions is the primary goal (Benedict, 1989). This view of cognitive rehabilitation implies that "restoration" and "compensation" are distinct phases of rehabilitation. In other words, compensatory strategies are not implemented until restorative exercises have failed. It has been observed that helping TBI individuals to become increasingly aware of their cognitive needs and to be strategic in approaching cognitively demanding tasks (typically associated with a compensatory approach to cognitive rehabilitation) is actually restorative—that is, it restores the strategic, deliberate aspect of cognitive processing—which may be more important after the injury than before. Therefore, it is a mistake to contrast "restorative" and "compensatory" as though they were not overlapping approaches. Rather, these approaches should occur simultaneously in rehabilitation (M. Ylvisaker, personal communication, April, 1995).

Planning for Cognitive Rehabilitation. In planning for cognitive rehabilitation it is necessary to consider the TBI individual's ultimate needs. The individual's needs will focus the answers to the following questions: (1) Are the treatment goals realistic? and (2) What is the individual's capacity to benefit from treatment? According to Lezak (1987), the identification of realistic treatment goals requires the evaluation of two aspects of the TBI individual's cognitive behaviors: (1) the capacity for taking an abstract attitude; and (2) the status of executive functions. Abstract attitude refers to such capacities as appreciating the point of view of others, being aware that there is a world beyond one's own personal perspective, and being free of concrete or literal interpretations of daily experience. As discussed previously, executive functions are those capacities necessary to have an intention and thus formulate goals, to plan and organize goal-directed behavior, to carry out goal-directed behavior effectively, and to monitor and self-correct one's behavior as needed (Lezak, 1982, 1983). Unfortunately, unlike some cognitive deficits that improve with rehabilitation, an impaired capacity to take an abstract attitude and impaired executive functions may often be chronic problems resistant to treatment. Retraining these

capacities requires the individual to have in mind what no longer comes to mind or what that individual no longer appreciates as missing. Generally speaking, the major limitations to an individual's ability to profit from rehabilitation are (1) impaired executive functions; (2) loss of abstract attitude; (3) chronic attentional and/or memory disorders; and (4) learning deficits (Lezak, 1987).

Stages of Recovery

The usual course of recovery following onset of TBI involves a period of unconsciousness followed by some duration of confusion with gradual return of functions. The time frame for these phases as well as extent of recovery varies greatly among individuals and therefore, it is impossible to outline a common course of recovery among the TBI population (Sohlberg & Mateer, 1989). A more practical approach is to consider cognitive-communicative treatment with regard to stage of recovery.

Early Stages of Recovery. In the early stages of recovery, LOCF II (Generalized Response) and III (Localized Response), the speech–language pathologist directs efforts at eliciting and sustaining responses from the patient. All sensory modalities (auditory, visual, tactile, taste, olfaction) may be used and the clinician must identify the best techniques for interacting with the patient. Treatment at this stage is essentially diagnostic in nature and directed toward the elicitation of consistent responses to increasingly more complex stimuli. As the patient becomes more responsive to verbal stimuli, the establishment of a communication system becomes a priority, so that family, medical, and rehabilitation staff can initiate interactions with the patient. Augmentative and alternative communication systems may be introduced at this stage; however, high technology or very complicated systems typically are not appropriate at this time. The consistent and reliable signaling of yes/no responses enables the patient to interact with nearly everyone in the medical setting and will greatly facilitate overall care. With time, certain patients may be able to respond verbally, provided assisted ventilation is not required.

The benefits of early aggressive rehabilitation that includes speech–language pathology services during acute hospitalization following TBI has been documented (MacKay, Bernstein, Chapman, Morgan, & Milazzo, 1992). Comparison of outcome data for a group of 38 TBI patients/clients who were involved in an early intervention program with a second group who were not, indicated that the early intervention group had significantly shorter lengths of coma and rehabilitation stays. Further, the early intervention group was discharged at higher levels of cognitive functioning and had a significantly higher percentage of discharges to home versus extended care facilities.

Intermediate Stages of Recovery. In the intermediate stage of recovery, LOCF IV (Confused-Agitated) and V (Confused-Inappropriate-Nonagitated) traditional cognitive rehabilitation and speech–language management may be initiated as needed. In the beginning, such individuals may only be able to participate meaningfully in individual sessions as group sessions may be too distracting and may overstimulate the patient. As the patient becomes more oriented and less confused, the individual sessions may be supplemented by group therapy. Group intervention is useful for assessing generalization of targeted behaviors in a more natural setting (i.e., a setting full of competing stimuli that is less structured and controlled). Group intervention is very useful for social skills training. Social skills include a variety of abilities (e.g., conversing, sharing, cooperating, greeting others) that enable an individual to interact effectively with peers and others at home, in school, on the job, and in other environments (Ylvisaker, Szekeres, Haarbauer-Krupa, Urbanczyk, & Feeney, 1992). These abilities are vulnerable to disruption following TBI.

Individual and/or group treatment may also be supplemented by computer-assisted treatment. Computers are useful for the presentation of repetitive drills and can be programmed to provide varying levels of reinforcement. Computers can also record precise facets of the patient's response such as accuracy and delays. Family or significant other training/counseling, as well as interdisciplinary consultation and dismissal/discharge planning, is also ongoing during this stage.

Later Stages of Recovery. For individuals in the later stages of recovery, LOCF VI (Confused-Appropriate), VII (Automatic-Appropriate), and VIII (Purposeful and Appropriate), the final phase of intervention should be directed toward carryover of treatment objectives in home or community environments. Consultations with teachers, employers, and fellow workers take place in the later stages of recovery. This is not to imply that programming for carryover begins during the final stages of treatment. Rather, to facilitate carryover of treatment objectives to nonclinical environments, contextualization of treatment (i.e., working on skills the TBI individual needs, in the environment where they are needed) should take place as soon as it is feasible.

Sustained community reentry at the highest level of productivity, independence, and social adaptation an individual is capable of is the desired goal of TBI rehabilitation (Malkmus, 1989). Concerns have been expressed about the generalization of treatment gains demonstrated in clinical settings. Such concerns have arisen from the research indicating that individuals with TBI often demonstrate chronic memory problems and/or frontal lobe injuries. It has been suggested that functional gains are most easily achieved when cognitive remediation is carried out in the patient's home and community involving activities of high interest to the individual (Kneipp, 1991). Recently, numerous case reports of treatment intended to enhance daily living, educational, and vocational activities provided by professionals who travel to the TBI individual's home, school, or job have cited positive results with regard to return to school (Blosser & DePompei, 1989; DePompei & Blosser, 1987) or gainful employment (Kneipp, 1991; Story, 1991; Wehman, 1991).

Individual Differences. When the effectiveness of cognitive rehabilitation is evaluated, individual differences among TBI patients/clients must be considered. For example, Ryan and Ruff (1988) noted that attention and memory training were effective for a group of 20 mildly to moderately impaired TBI individuals, but not for a severely impaired group. At the very least, the cognitive rehabilitation programs for more severely involved patients need to be structured differently, with perhaps greater intensity, more cuing and reinforcement, and longer duration. In addition, without awareness of deficits and motivation, it is difficult to engage an individual with TBI in sustained and effective treatment (Ben-Yishay & Diller, 1993; Haarbauer-Krupa, Szekeres, & Ylvisaker, 1985). Finally, individuals with TBI benefit from programs of cognitive rehabilitation as long as four (Cicerone & Wood, 1987) to six (Benedict, 1989) years post-onset. Time post-onset should not preclude an individual's participation in such a program, on at least a trial basis.

Research Needs for the Future

Without question, the most important research needs related to the management of cognitive-communicative deficits secondary to TBI is that of treatment efficacy. **Treatment efficacy** is a broad term that addresses several questions related to treatment effectiveness (does treatment work?), treatment efficiency (does one treatment work better than another?), and treatment effects (in what ways does treatment alter behavior?) (Olswang, 1990). Treatment efficacy studies conducted to date have utilized both group (e.g., see Prigatano, Fordyce, Zeiner, Roueche, Pepping, & Wood, 1984; or Ruff, Mahaffey, Engel, Farrow, Cox, & Karzmark, 1994) and single-subject (Sohlberg & Mateer, 1987; or Sohlberg, Sprunk, & Metzelaar, 1988) experimental designs to address these questions. Ongoing research is needed to identify the most effective and efficient interventions for the cognitive-communicative impairments that result from TBI (see Coelho, DeRuyter, & Stein, 1996

for a review of this topic). Speech–language pathologists are essential members of the team of professionals that collaboratively manage the rehabilitation of individuals with TBI.

Major Points of Chapter

- Traumatic brain injury produces a cognitive and linguistic disorder that is distinct from aphasia.
- Open and closed head injury have different mechanisms of damage, and different consequences.
- The hallmark of traumatic brain injury is cognitive deficits in orientation, attention, memory, reasoning, and executive function.
- Language deficits following traumatic brain injury may include aphasia, confused language, and pragmatic difficulty.
- Oral motor deficits may include dysarthria and/or dysphagia.
- Treatment of cognitive-communicative function is related to the patient's level of recovery.

Discussion Guidelines

1. Present an inservice to your classmates about the effects of traumatic brain injury on the survivor and their family.
2. Describe what is meant by "mechanisms of damage." Identify several of these mechanisms and explain their cognitive-communicative consequences.
3. Discuss the restorative, compensatory, and environmental approaches to cognitive rehabilitation.

REFERENCES

Adamovich, B. L. B. (1991). Cognition, language, attention, and information processing following closed head injury. In J. S. Kreutzer & P. H. Wehman (Eds.) *Cognitive rehabilitation for persons with traumatic brain injury.* Baltimore, MD: Brookes Publishing.

Adamovich, B. L. B., & Henderson, J. A. (1992). *Scales of cognitive ability for traumatic brain injury.* New York: Riverside Publishers.

Adamovich, B. L. B., Henderson, J. A., & Auerbach, S. (1985). *Cognitive rehabilitation of closed head injured patients.* San Diego, CA: College-Hill Press.

Alexander, M. P. (1984). Neurobehavioral consequences of closed head injury. *Neurology and Neurosurgery, 20,* 1–8.

Alexander, M. P., Benson, D. F., & Stuss, D. T. (1989). Frontal lobes and language. *Brain and Language, 37,* 656–691.

Ansell, B. J., & Keenan, J. E. (1989). The Western neuro sensory stimulation profile: A tool for assessing slow-to-recover head-injured patients. *Archives of Physical Medicine and Rehabilitation, 70,* 104–108.

Benedict, R. H. B. (1989). The effectiveness of cognitive remediation strategies for victims of traumatic brain injury: A review of the literature. *Clinical Psychology Review, 9,* 605–626.

Benton, A. L. (1974). *Revised visual retention test* (ed. 4). New York: Psychological Corp.

Ben-Yishay, Y., & Diller, L. (1993). Cognitive remediation in traumatic brain injury: Update and issues. *Archives of Physical Medicine and Rehabilitation, 74,* 204–213.

Beukelman, D. R., & Yorkston, K. M. (1991). Traumatic brain injury changes the way we live. In D. R. Beukelman & K. M. Yorkston (Eds.), *Communication disorders following traumatic brain injury: Management of cognitive, language, and motor impairments.* Austin, TX: Pro-Ed.

Blosser, J. L., & DePompei, R. (1989). The head injured student returns to school: Recognizing and treating deficits. *Topics in Language Disorders, 9.*

Bricolo, A., Turazzi, S., and Feriotti, G. (1980). Prolonged posttraumatic unconsciousness. *Journal of Neurosurgery, 52,* 625–634.

Brookshire, R. H., & Nicholas, M. A. (1993). *Discourse comprehension test.* Tucson, AZ: Communication Skills Builders.

Cherney, L. R., & Halper, A. S. (1989). Recovery of oral nutrition after head injury in adults. Journal of head trauma rehabilitation, *4,* 42.

Cicerone, K. D. & Wood, J. C. (1987). Planning disorder after closed head-injury: A case study. *Archives of Physical Medicine and Rehabilitation, 68,* 11–115.

Coelho, C. A., DeRuyter, F., & Stein, M. (1996). Treatment efficacy for cognitive-communicative disorders resulting from traumatic brain injury in adults. *Journal of Speech and Hearing Research, 39,* S5–S17.

Coelho, C. A., Liles, B. Z., & Duffy, R. J. (1991a). The use of discourse analyses for the evaluation of higher level traumatically brain-injured adults. *Brain Injury, 5,* 381.

Coelho, C. A., Liles, B. Z., & Duffy, R. J. (1991b). Discourse analyses in closed head injured adults: Evidence for differing patterns of deficits. *Archives of Physical Medicine and Rehabilitation, 72,* 465.

Coelho, C. A., Liles, B. Z., & Duffy, R. J. (1991c). Analysis of conversational discourse in head injured adults. *Journal of Head Trauma Rehabilitation, 6,* 92.

Coelho, C. A., Liles, B. Z., Duffy, R. J., Clarkson, J. V., & Elia, D. (1993). Conversational patterns of aphasic, closed head injured, and normal speakers. *Clinical Aphasiology, 12,* 145–155.

Coelho, C. A., Liles B. Z., & Duffy R. J. (1995). Impairments of discourse abilities and executive functions in traumatically brain injured adults. *Brain Injury, 9,* 471–477.

Davis, A. (1983). *A survey of adult aphasia.* Englewood Cliffs, NJ: Prentice-Hall.

Davis, A. (1993). *A survey of adult aphasia and related language disorders.* Englewood Cliffs, NJ: Prentice-Hall.

DePompei, R., & Blosser, J. (1987). Strategies for helping head-injured children successfully return to school. *Language, Speech, and Hearing Services in Schools, 18,* 292–300.

DeRenzi, E., & Ferrari, C. (1978). The Reporter's Test: A sensitive test to detect expressive disturbances in aphasia. *Cortex, 14,* 279–293.

DeRuyter, F., & Becker, M. R. (1988). Augmentative communication: Assessment, system selection, and usage. *Journal of Head Trauma Rehabilitation, 3,* 35–44.

Dunn, L. M., & Dunn, L. (1981). *Peabody Picture Vocabulary Test-Revised.* Circle Pines, MN: American Guidance Service.

Ehrlich, J. S. (1988). Selective characteristics of narrative discourse in head injured and normal adults. *Journal of Communication Disorders, 21,* 1.

Ehrlich, J. S., & Sipes, A. (1985). Group treatment of communication skills for head trauma patients. *Cognitive Rehabilitation, 3,* 32.

Finger, S. & Stein, D. G. (1982). *Brain damage and recovery.* New York: Academic Press.

Goldman, R., Fristoe, M., & Woodcock, R. (1974). *Goldman-Fristoe-Woodcock Auditory Skills Test Battery.* Circle Pines, Minnesota: American Guidance Service.

Goodglass, H., & Kaplan, E. (1983a). *Boston Diagnostic Aphasia Exam.* Philadelphia: Lea & Febiger.

Goodglass, H., & Kaplan, E. (1983b). *Boston Naming Test.* Philadelphia: Lea & Febiger.

Grafman, J., & Salazar, A. (1987). Methodological considerations relevant to the comparison of recovery from penetrating and closed head injuries. In H. S. Levin, J. Grafman, & H. M. Eisenberg (Eds.). *Neurobehavioral recovery from head injury.* New York: Oxford University Press.

Groher, M. (1977). Language and memory disorders following closed head trauma. *Journal of Speech and Hearing Research, 20,* 212–223.

Haarbauer-Krupa, J., Szekeres, S. F., & Ylvisaker, M. (1985). Cognitive rehabilitation therapy: Late stages of recovery. In M. Ylvisaker (Ed.). *Head injury rehabilitation: Children and adolescents.* San Diego, CA: College-Hill Press.

Hagan, C. (1984). Language disorders in head trauma. In A. Holland (Ed.), *Language disorders in adults: Recent advances.* (pp. 245–282). San Diego, CA: College-Hill Press.

Hagan, C., Malkmus, D., & Burditt, G. (1979) Levels of cognitive functioning. In *Rehabilitation of the head injured adult: Comprehensive physical management.* Downey, CA: Professional Staff Association of Rancho Los Amigos Hospital.

Haliday, M. A. K., & Hasan, R. (1976). *Cohesion in english.* London: Longman Group.

Halpern, H., Darley, F., & Brown, J. R. (1973). Differential language and neurologic characteristics in cerebral involvement. *Journal of Speech and Hearing Disorders, 38,* 162–173.

Hammill, D. D. (1985). *Detroit Tests of Learning Aptitude-2.* Austin, TX: Pro-Ed.

Hanna, G., Schell, L. M., & Schreiner, R. (1977). *The Nelson Reading Skills Test.* Chicago: Riverside Publishing Co.

Hartley, L., & Jensen, T. (1991). Narrative and procedural discourse after closed head injury. *Brain Injury, 5,* 267–285.

Heilman, K. M., Safran, A., & Geschwind, N. (1971). Closed head trauma and aphasia. *Journal of Neurology, Neurosurgery, and Psychiatry, 34,* 265.

High, W. M., Levin, H. S., & Gary, H. E. (1990). Recovery of orientation following closed-head injury.

Journal of Clinical and Experimental Neuropsychology, 12, 703.

Holland, A. L. (1982). When is aphasia aphasia? The problem of closed head injury. In R. H. Brookshire (Ed.) *Clinical aphasiology conference proceedings 12,* 345.

Jacobs, H. E. (1988). The Los Angeles head injury survey: Procedures and initial findings. *Archives of Physical Medicine and Rehabilitation, 69,* 425–431.

Jastak, J., & Jastak, S. (1965). *The Wide Range Achievement Test manual* (rev. ed.). Wilmington, DE: Jastack Association.

Jennett, B., Snoek, J., Bond, M., & Brooks, N. (1981). Disability after severe head injury: observations on use of the Glasgow Coma Scale. *Journal of Neurology, Neurosurgery, and Psychiatry, 44,* 285–293.

Jennett, B., & Teasdale, G. (1981). *Management of head injuries.* Philadelphia: Davis.

Jorgenson, C., Barrett, M., Huisingh, R., & Zachman, L. (1981). *The Word Test.* Moline, IL: Lingui Systems.

Kalsbeek, W., McLauren, R., Harris, B., & Miller, J. (1981). The national head and spinal cord injury survey: Major findings. *Journal of Neurosurgery, 53,* 519–531.

Kennedy, M. R. T., & DeRuyter, F. Cognitive and language bases for communication disorders (1991). In D. R. Beukelman & K. M. Yorkston (Eds.), *Communication disorders following traumatic brain injury: Management of cognitive, language, and motor impairments* (pp. 123–190). Austin, TX: Pro-Ed.

Kirk, S. A., McCarthy, J. J., & Kirk, W. D. (1968). *Illinois Test of Psycholinguistic Abilities.* Urbana, IL: University of Illinois Press.

Kneipp, S. (1991). Cognitive remediation within the context of a community re-entry program. In J. S. Kreutzer & P. H. Wehman (Eds.), *Cognitive rehabilitation for persons with traumatic brain injury.* Baltimore, MD: Brookes Publishing.

Kraus, J. (1978). Epidemiologic features of head and spinal cord injury. *Advances in Neurology, 19,* 261–279.

Kraus, J. F. (1993). Epidemiology of head injury. In P. R. Cooper (Ed.), *Head Injury* (3rd ed.). Baltimore, MD: Williams & Wilkins.

Kraus, J. F., & Nourjah, P. (1989). The epidemiology of mild head injury. In H. S. Levin, H. M. Eisenberg, & A. L. Benton (Eds.), *Mild head injury.* New York: Oxford University Press.

Kreutzer, J., Wehman, P., Conder, R., & Morrison, C. (1989). Compensatory strategies for enhancing independent living and vocational outcome following traumatic brain injury. *Cognitive Rehabilitation,* 30–35.

Langfitt, T. W., & Gennarelli, J. A. (1982). Can the outcome for head injury be improved? *Journal of Neurosurgery, 56,* 19–25.

LaPointe, L., & Horner, J. (1979). *Reading Comprehension Battery for Aphasia.* Tigard, OR: C.C. Publications.

Lazarus, C., & Logemann, J. (1987). Swallowing disorders in closed head trauma patients. *Archives of Physical medicine and Rehabilitation, 68,* 79.

Levin, H. S., Benton, A. L., & Grossman, R. G. (1982). *Neurobehavioral consequences of closed head injury.* New York: Oxford University Press.

Levin, H. S., Eisenberg, H. M., & Benton, H. L. (1989). *Mild head injury.* New York: Oxford University Press.

Levin, H. S., Grossman, R. G., & Kelly, P. J. (1976) Aphasic disorders in patients with closed head injury. *Journal of Neurology, Neurosurgery, and Psychiatry, 39,* 119–130.

Levin, H. S., Grossman, R. G., Rose, J. E., & Teasdale, G. (1979). Long-term neuropsychological outcome of closed head injury. *Journal of Neurosurgery, 50,* 412–422.

Levin, H. S., Grossman, R. G., Sarwar, M., & Meyers, C. A. (1981). Linguistic recovery after closed head injury. *Brain and Language, 12,* 360–374.

Levin, H. S., & Kraus, M. F. (1994). The frontal lobes in traumatic brain injury. *Journal of Neuropsychiatry, 6,* 443–454.

Levin, H. S., Madison, D. F., Bailey, C. B., Meyer, C., Eisenberg, H., & Gunito, F. (1983). Mutism after closed head injury. *Archives of Neurology, 40,* 601.

Levin, H. S., O'Donnell, V. M., & Grossman, R. G. (1979). The Galveston Orientation and Amnesia Test: A practical scale to assess cognition after head injury. *Journal of Nervous and Mental Disease, 167,* 675–684.

Lezak, M. D. (1976). *Mechanisms of neurological disease.* Boston: Little, Brown and Company.

Lezak, M. D. (1982). The problem of assessing executive functions. *Internation Journal of Psychology, 17,* 281–297.

Lezak, M. D. (1983). *Neuropsychological assessment,* (2nd ed.). New York: Oxford University Press.

Lezak, M. D. (1987). Assessment for rehabilitation planning. In M. Meier, A. Benton, & L. Diller (Eds.): *Neuropsychological rehabilitation.* New York: Guilford Press.

Liles, B. Z., Coelho, C. A., Duffy, R. J., & Zalagens, M. H. (1989). Effects of elicitation procedures on the narratives of normal and closed head injured adults. *Journal of Speech and Hearing Disorders, 54,* 356.

Mackay, L. E., Berstein, B. A., Chapman, P. E., Morgan, A. S., & Milazzo, L. S. (1992). Early intervention in severe head injury: Long-term benefits of a formalized program. *Archives of Physical Medicine and Rehabilitation, 73,* 635–641.

Malkmus, D. D. (1989). Community reentry: Cognitive-communicative intervention within a social skill context. *Topics in Language Disorders, 9,* 50–66.

McKinlay, W. W., Brooks, D. N., Bond, M. R., Martinage, D. P., & Marshall, M. M. (1981). The short-term outcome of severe blunt head injury as reported by the relatives of the injured person. *Journal of Neurology, Neurosurgery, and Psychiatry, 44,* 527–533.

McNeil, M. R., & Prescott, T. E. (1978). *Revised Token Test.* Baltimore, MD: University Park Press.

Meirowsky, A. M. (1984). *Penetrating cranicerebral trauma.* Springfield, IL: Charles C. Thomas.

Mentis, M., & Prutting, C. A. (1987). Cohesion in the discourse of normal and head-injured adults. *Journal of Speech and Hearing Research, 30,* 88.

Mentis, M., & Prutting, C. A. (1991). Analysis of topic as illustrated in a head-injured and normal adult. *Journal of Speech and Hearing Research, 34,* 583.

Milton, S. B. (1988). Management of subtle cognitive communication deficits. *Journal of Head Trauma Rehabilitation, 3,* 1–12.

Milton, S. B., Turnstall, C., & Wertz, R. T. (1983). Dysnomia: A rose by any other name may require elaborate description. In R. H. Brookshire (Ed.), *Clinical Aphasiology Conference Proceedings, 14,* 114.

National Head Injury Foundation (1983). *The silent epidemic.* Framingham, MA.

Netsell, R., & Daniel, B. (1979). Dysarthria in adults: Physiologic approach to rehabilitation. *Archives of Physical Medicine and Rehabilitation, 60,* 502.

North, B. (1984). *Jamieson's first notebook of head injury* (3rd ed.). London: Bitterworth's.

Olswang, L. B. (1990). Treatment efficacy: The breadth of research. In L. B. Olswang, C. K. Thompsen, S. F. Warren, & N.J. Minghetti (Eds.), *Treatment efficacy research in communication disorders.*

Rockville, MD: American Speech-Language-Hearing Foundation.

Prigatano, G. (1986). *Neuropsychological rehabilitation after brain injury.* Baltimore, MD: Johns Hopkins Press.

Prigatano, G. P., Fordyce, C. J., Zeiner, H. K., Roueche, J. R., Pepping, M., & Wood, M. C. (1984). Neuropsychological rehabilitation after closed head injury in young adults. *Journal of Neurology, Neurosurgery and Psychiatry, 47,* 505–513.

Raven, J. C. (1965). *Guide to using the coloured progressive matrices.* London: H. K. Lewis.

Ross, J. P., & Ross, C. M. (1979). *Ross Test of Higher Cognitive Processes.* Novato, CA: Academic Therapy Publications.

Ruff, R., Mahaffey, R., Engel, J., Farrow, C., Cox, D., & Karzmark, P. (1994). Efficacy study of THINKable in the attention and memory training of traumatically head-injured patients. *Brain Injury, 8,* 3–14.

Rusk, H., Block, J., & Lowmann, E. (1969). Rehabilitation of the brain injured patient: A Report of 157 cases with longterm follow-up of 118. In E. Walker, W. Caveness, and M. Critchley (Eds.), *The late effects of head injury.* Springfield, IL: Charles C. Thomas.

Ryan, T. V., & Ruff, R. M. (1988). The efficacy of structured memory retraining in a group comparison of head trauma patients. *Archives of Clinical Neuropsychology, 3,* 165–179.

Sarno, M. T. (1980). The nature of verbal impairment after closed head injury. *Journal of Nervous and Mental Disease, 168,* 685.

Sarno, M. T., Buonaguro, A., & Levita, E. (1986). Characteristics of verbal impairment in closed head injury. *Archives of Physical Medicine and Rehabilitation, 67,* 400.

Schuell, H. (1972). *Minnesota Test for Differential Diagnosis of Aphasia; Revised.* Minneapolis, MN: University of Minnesota Press.

Schwartz-Cowley, R., & Stepanik, M. J. (1989). Communication disorders and treatment in the acute trauma center setting. *Topics in Language Disorders, 9,* 1.

Semel, E. M., & Wiig, E. (1980). *Clinical evaluation of language functions.* Columbus, OH: Charles Merrill Publications.

Simmons, N. (1983). Acoustic analysis of ataxic dysarthria: An approach to monitoring treatment. In W. R. Berry (Ed.), *Clinical dysarthria.* San Diego, CA: College-Hill Press.

Sohlberg, M. M., & Mateer, C. A. (1987). Effectiveness of an attention training program. *Journal of Clinical and Experimental Neuropsychology, 9,* 117–130.

Sohlberg, M. M., & Mateer, C. A. (1989). *Introduction to cognitive rehabilitation theory and practice.* New York: Guilford Press.

Sohlberg, M. M., & Sprunk, H., & Metzelaar, K. (1988). Efficacy of an external cuing system in an individual with severe frontal lobe damage. *Cognitive Rehabilitation, 6,* 36–41.

Starch, S., & Falltrick, E. (1990). The importance of a home evaluation for brain-injured clients: A team approach. *Cognitive Rehabilitation, 8,* 28–32.

Story, T. B. (1991). Cognitive rehabilitation services in home and community settings. In J. S. Kreutzer & P. H. Wehman (Eds.), *Cognitive rehabilitation for persons with traumatic brain injury.* Baltimore, MD: Brookes Publishing.

Stuss, D. T. (1987). Contribution of frontal lobe injury to cognitive impairment after closed head injury: Methods of assessment and recent findings. In H. S. Levin, J. Grafman, & H. M. Eisenberg (Eds.), *Neurobehavioral recovery from head injury* (pp. 166–176). New York: Oxford University Press.

Stuss, D. T., & Benson, D. F. (1984). Neuropsychological studies of the frontal lobes. *Psychological Bulletin, 95,* 3–28.

Stuss, D., & Benson, F. (1986). *The frontal lobes.* New York: Raven Press.

Teasdale, G., & Jennett, B. (1974). Assessment of coma and impaired consciousness: A practical scale. *Acta Neurochirugie, 34,* 45–55.

Thomsen, I. V. (1975) Evaluation and outcome of aphasia in patients with severe closed head trauma. *Journal of Neurology, Neurosurgery, and Psychiatry, 38,* 713.

Thomsen, I. V. (1976) Evaluation and outcome of traumatic aphasia in patients with severe verified lesions. *Folia Phoniatrica, 28,* 362.

Thorum, A. (1978). *Fullerton Language Test for Adolescents.* Palo Alto, CA: Consulting Psychologists Press.

Wechsler, D. (1955). *Manual for the Wechsler Adult Intelligence Scale.* New York: Psychological Corp.

Wechsler, D. (1985). *Wechsler Memory Scale - Revised.* San Diego, CA: Psychological Corp./Harcourt Brace Jovanovich.

Wehman, P. H. (1991). Cognitive rehabilitation in the workplace. In J. S. Kreutzer & P. H. Wehman

(Eds.), *Cognitive rehabilitation for persons with traumatic brain injury.* Baltimore, MD: Brookes Publishing.

Wilson, B., Cockburn, J., & Baddeley, A. D. (1985). *The Rivermead Behavioral Memory Test.* Reading, England: Thames Valley Test Company.

Winstein, C. J. (1983). Neurogenic dysphagia: Frequency, progression and outcome in adults following head injury. *Physical Therapy, 12,* 1992.

Woodcock, W., & Johnson, M. B. (1977). *Woodcock-Johnson Psychoeducational Battery: Tests of cognitive ability.* Allen, TX: DLM Teaching Resources.

Ylvisaker, M. (1994). Collaboration in assessment and intervention after TBI. *Topics in Language Disorders, 15,* 1–81.

Ylvisaker, M., Szekeres, S., Haarbauer-Krupa, J., Urbanczyk, B., & Feeney, T. (1992). Speech and language intervention. In G. Wolcott & R. Savage (Eds.), *Educational programming for children and young adults with acquired brain injury.* Austin, TX: Pro-Ed.

Yorkston, K. M., & Beukelman, D. R. (1981). Ataxic dysarthria: Treatment sequences based on ineligibility and prosodic considerations. *Journal of Speech and Hearing Disorders, 46,* 398.

Yorkston, K. M., Beukelman, D. R., & Bell, K. R. (1988). *Clinical management of dysarthric speakers.* San Diego, CA: College-Hill Press.

Yorkston, K. M., Beukelman, D. R., Minifie, F., & Sapir, S. (1984). Assessment of stress patterning in dysarthric speakers. In M. McNeil, A. Aronson, & J. Rosenbek (Eds.), *The Dysarthrias: Physiology, acoustics, perception, management.* Boston: College-Hill Press.

Zachman, L., Jorgenson, C., & Huisingh, R. (1984). *Test of Problem Solving.* Moline, IL: Lingui Systems.

7 COMMUNICATION DISORDERS FOLLOWING FOCAL BRAIN DAMAGE

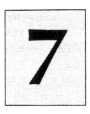

RONALD L. BLOOM

D amage to the brain may be described as **focal** or **diffuse.** Focal damage involves a distinct, circumscribed area of the brain or a single anatomic structure within the brain. Damage that is diffuse relates to neurologic disease that is more widespread or localized to more than one region of the brain. Brain damage that is diffuse may be caused by multiple strokes or by a degenerative process (see Chapter 5) that results in dementia. In patients with closed head injury (see Chapter 6) the effects of both focal damage and diffuse damage are often apparent. Focal damage to the brain is often related to vascular disease, but **neoplastic** and **inflammatory** diseases can produce similar symptoms. Focal brain damage and diffuse brain damage produce different symptoms. Neurologic symptoms most typically reflect the localization of brain damage rather than its specific cause.

Vascular disease is the most common cause of focal damage to the brain. **Cerebrovascular accident (CVA)** is the medical term for a sudden onset of a neurologic deficit due to an interruption of blood supplied to the brain. The term specifically refers to a blockage or a break in the blood vessels of the brain resulting in a long-term neurological disorder. **Stroke** is a more popular term. The terms *CVA* and *stroke* are often used synonymously.

At the onset, stroke is a medical problem. Knowledge of the causes and effects of vascular disease on the nervous system is necessary for all those involved in the treatment of the stroke patient. Efforts in rehabilitation rest upon state of the art medical information, current scientific knowledge, and the ability to clearly communicate this information to all those involved in treatment.

This chapter focuses on the communication disorders that result from focal brain damage. The communication disorders that result from CVA will be emphasized because they are the most common. Following a review of the population at risk for CVA, the physiologic and neuroanatomic basis of stroke will be described. The nature of vascular damage, and the effect it has on different parts of the brain will be presented. Other pathologic conditions that may produce focal brain damage and have an effect on communication are also described. What is known about the relationship between brain structure and language is then considered. This research will provide the background necessary to examine the communication disorders that result from left brain damage (i.e., aphasia) and right brain damage. Finally, some basic principles that guide communication assessment and rehabilitation for these two groups of brain-damaged patients will be introduced.

PATIENT POPULATION AND RISK FACTORS FOR STROKE

Stroke ranks as the third leading cause of death in the United States, behind coronary heart disease and cancer. Stroke affects over 500,000 Americans every year, with people over age 65 accounting for about 70 percent of the total incidence (Bonita, 1992). African Americans have over a 60 percent greater chance of death from stroke than do their Caucasian counterparts. This may be because African Americans are at greater risk for **hypertension** (high blood pressure), a major factor for stroke (Otten, Teutsch, Williamson, & Marks, 1990). It is estimated that in the United States today there are over three million people who have survived stroke, many living with a permanent physical disability or language disorder (Thorngren & Westling,1990). In the 1980s the Asian American population in the United States increased by 65 percent (Keough, 1990), and the number of Hispanic Americans rose from 15 to 23 million (Current Population Reports, 1990). Increasingly, patients with **aphasia** will come from communities in the United States where English may not be the primary or only language spoken.

Although CVA can happen to anybody, a striking number of patients have had a prior history of **cardiovascular** (heart) disease, hypertension (high blood pressure), **atherosclerosis** (hardening of the arteries) and **obesity** (severely overweight). These conditions can influence the long-term medical prognosis of a stroke patient. Many of these patients are clearly at risk for a heart attack that may be fatal. **Diabetic** patients are especially at risk since diabetes speeds up the process of atherosclerosis. As smoking can narrow the blood vessels, it is believed to be a significant contributor to heart disease and stroke.

In comparison to adults, the occurrence of CVA in children is rare. When stroke does occur during childhood it is usually during the first two years of life, and in conjunction with other diseases. Cardiac disease, **sickle-cell disease, hemorrhage,** and **vascular occlusions** or malformations are among the most typical causes of stroke in children (Milliken, McDowell, & Easton, 1987). Recovery from stroke differs in children and adults. In adults, recovery is primarily related to age, as well as to the extent and site of brain damage (Sarno, 1981). By comparison, recovery from CVA in children is usually faster, more complete, and appears to be independent of age, extent, and size of brain injury (Satz & Bullard-Bates, 1981). The relatively robust recovery pattern in childhood may be related to the plasticity (i.e., the capacity to transfer functions from damaged nerve tissue to another brain region) of the immature central nervous system (Geschwind, 1974). Beyond early childhood the brain's capacity for functional reorganization may slow down or be lost (Lenneberg, 1967).

PHYSIOLOGIC AND NEUROANATOMIC BASES OF FOCAL BRAIN DAMAGE

This section provides an overview of the physiologic and anatomic systems that are chiefly compromised following focal damage to the brain. The vascular system and other sources of focal neurologic injury will be discussed. An overview of the organization of the nervous system will be presented. The interaction of the neurologic system with diseases that produce changes in communication behavior is extremely complex. For example, multiple strokes can cause damage to several parts of the brain, obscuring the localization of function. Only a brief outline of the major components are presented here.

The Vascular System

The vascular system includes the **arteries** that carry blood away from the heart, the **veins** that carry blood toward the heart, and the **capillaries** that connect the arteries to the veins. The *cerebrovascular system* refers specifically to the network of blood vessels within the brain. The blood nourishes the brain with life sustaining properties, such as **glucose** and **oxygen.** Loss of blood supply to the brain results in the rapid destruction of brain tissue.

The **aorta** is the main artery of the heart. It transports blood from the left ventricle to all parts of the body except the lungs. There are four branches of the aorta, two **common carotid arteries,** and two **vertebral arteries,** which directly ascend to the brain. The common carotid arteries continue to branch out into the **internal carotid arteries** as they enter the brain through the base of the skull. The internal carotid extends anteriorly where it branches into several smaller divisions that serve the areas of the brain most connected with language processing. Specifically, these divisions include the **anterior cerebral artery** (supplies blood to the area extending from the midfrontal cortex to the parieto-temporal-occipital sulcus) and the largest branch, the **middle cerebral artery** (supplies the lateral surface of cortex including regions of the frontal lobe). The left and right vertebral arteries arise from the two subclavian arteries that extend from the heart. As the vertebral arteries enter the skull they branch out to supply blood to adjoining regions that include the brainstem. The two vertebral arteries unite to form the **basilar artery** at the lower level of the pons. At the upper portion of the pons, the basilar artery divides into numerous small branches that supply blood to the spinal cord, medulla, pons, midbrain, and cerebellum.

The carotid and vertebral arteries form a circular passage at the base of the brain called the **circle of Willis.** In case one of the arteries is unable to transport blood, the circle of Willis provides an alternate channel for blood to reach the brain. When an artery becomes compromised below the circle of Willis, an adequate supply of blood is maintained and damage to the brain is minimized. If an artery above the circle is compromised, alternate circulation routes are limited and brain damage may occur. Although the cerebrovascular system intertwines to produce alternate and redundant routes of blood to the brain, a blockage or break in the blood vessels above the circle of Willis can cause a CVA.

There are two basic types of cerebrovascular accident: **ischemic** and **hemorrhagic.** Ischemic strokes are caused by a complete or partial occlusion of the arteries that transport blood to the brain. Ischemic strokes are commonly related to a condition of aging called atherosclerosis or hardening of the arteries. **Atherosclerosis** causes lipids (fats) and fibrous material to thicken the arterial wall, eventually producing an occlusion or blockage of a blood vessel. This progressive narrowing of a blood vessel may produce a **thrombosis,** which can result in an **ischemia** (a reduction of oxygen) or an **infarction** (death of brain tissue due to lack of oxygen). The ischemia may be temporary, as in a **transient ischemic attack (TIA),** or it may cause permanent damage due to an infarction. Additionally, the thrombosis may break up and be released into the blood stream. Such a traveling mass is called an **embolism.** An embolism may be formed from a thrombosis, or from a blood clot that breaks off from a blood vessel in one part of the arterial system (e.g., heart), and lodges in a narrower part. An embolic stroke results when an artery in the brain becomes occluded.

Hemorrhagic strokes result from an arterial bleed where the blood forces its way into brain tissue. This causes destruction of tissue at the site of the bleed. In addition, inflammation may increase pressure on other areas of the brain due to displacement of tissue at the original site of the bleed. Hemorrhages may occur in two different areas: within the cerebral cortex (intracerebral) and outside the cortex (extracerebral). Intracerebral hemorrhages refer to a rupture within the brain or brainstem. These hemorrhages are typically associated with chronic high blood pressure and arterial walls that have weakened with age. Extracerebral hemorrhages refer to a bleed within the meninges, the layered membranes covering the brain and spinal cord. Extracerebral hemorrhages are often caused by the bursting of an

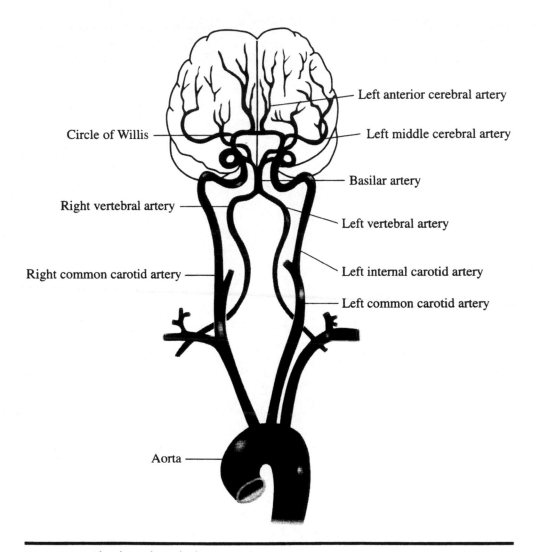

FIGURE 7.1 Blood supply to the brain.

aneurysm, a swelling or bulging of a weakened vessel wall.

Different patterns of recovery result from ischemic and hemorrhagic strokes. This is due to the distinct kind of neuronal damage inflicted by the different types of stroke. With an ischemic stroke, there is often noticeable improvement within the first few weeks. Maximum recovery is usually reached within three months, and then the level of recovery slows somewhat. By contrast, hemorrhagic strokes are often medically severe in the initial stage. If the patient does survive, a period of rapid recovery often occurs after the first or second month. Following a hemorrhagic stroke, the swelling lessens and neurons that were temporarily disabled slowly regain function. In an ischemic stroke neurons are completely and permanently destroyed. Despite the initial severity of the medical condition, a patient who had a hemorrhagic stroke may demonstrate a favorable long-term prognosis for recovery from aphasia.

Other Sources of Focal Brain Damage

Focal brain lesions caused by **neoplastic** disease, and **inflammatory** disease may produce changes in communication that mirror those caused by a single cerebrovascular accident. Neoplastic lesions are spontaneously growing, space occupying tumors that increase intracranial pressure. Benign (i.e., noncancerous) tumors exert mild pressure on adjacent brain regions. Malignant (i.e., cancerous) tumors continue to grow, causing displacement and destruction of surrounding brain tissue. Increased intracranial pressure may also produce swelling and interfere with blood flow to the brain. Such lesions may arise from the brain itself, or from other anatomic regions (such as the lungs) that may spread cancer cells to the brain. Symptoms of aphasia will appear in patterns that depend on the type of tumor, its rate of growth, and its location in the brain.

Inflammation of brain tissue may occur as a reaction to toxic substances, microorganisms, and certain immunologic reactions (Duffy, 1995). In response to the disease, an **abscess** of white blood cells and other anti-inflammatory cells may form to limit the spread of infection. This **abscess** can create a cavity that displaces brain tissue and may produce symptoms of focal brain damage.

The Nervous Systems

The consequences of neurologic insult depend on the extent and site of the damage to the nervous system. The basic building blocks of the nervous system are nerve cells called **neurons** that receive and send electrochemical impulses. Networks of connected neurons create transmission pathways (or fiber tracts) that send and receive information throughout the nervous system. The human nervous system is subdivided into central and peripheral components. The **Central Nervous System (CNS)** is composed of the brain and spinal cord

and is housed in the bony protective encasing of the skull and vertebral column. The **Peripheral Nervous System (PNS)** includes the cranial nerves and the spinal nerves that aid in a variety of sensorimotor behaviors. Because of the importance of the PNS in speech motor control it will be discussed in the chapter on neuromotor speech disorders. (See Chapter 8.)

Knowledge of the CNS is important in understanding neurologically based language disorders. The **spinal cord** carries neural information from the brain to the periphery (where actual motor activity takes place), and from the periphery to the brain. The **brainstem** is an extension of the spinal cord. Cranial nerves originate in the brainstem and many of them are crucial in speech production. The anatomical segments of the brain stem include the **medulla oblongata** (or medulla), the **pons,** and the **midbrain.** Cranial nerves responsible for tongue, laryngeal, and diaphragmatic movement originate in the medulla. The pons and midbrain contain cranial nerves responsible for eye and facial movements and hearing. Damage to the brainstem often results in **dysphagia.** (See Chapter 10 for more information on dysphagia.)

On top of the midbrain sit the two hemispheres of the **cerebellum.** The two cerebellar hemispheres are separated by a midline portion called the **vermis.** Damage to the cerebellum produces disorders in the coordination of movements and related motor speech disorders such as dysarthria and ataxia. (See Chapter 8.) The **transverse fissure** divides the cerebellum from the cerebrum.

The **cerebrum,** the largest part of the brain, is composed of two cerebral hemispheres. The covering of the cerebrum is called the cerebral cortex. The cerebral cortex contains many prominent ridges (called gyri) and grooves (called fissures or sulci). Consciousness, personality, and our ability to think are located in the cerebral cortex. The majority of the cerebral cortex is **neocortex.** The cellular structure of the neocortex is unique to mammals. Deep within the cerebral hemispheres lies the **subcortical gray matter,** which participates in a variety of sensory, motor, and integrative neural functions. The **thalamus** and **basal**

nuclei are two subcortical structures that may be relevant to language processing and communication disorders. Most information that reaches the cerebrum is first processed by the thalamus. The thalamus is believed to play a critical role in regulating attention and memory. Left hemispheric thalamic lesions have been linked to certain aphasia syndromes (Alexander & Loverme, 1980). The basal nuclei is interconnected to many components of the motor system. It is thought to participate heavily in movement control. Damage to the basal nuclei (e.g., Parkinson's disease) results in abnormalities in involuntary motor control (dyskinesia) and in hyperkinetic dysarthria (Darley, Aronson, & Brown, 1975). At the present time,

subcortical participation in language processing is not completely understood (Murdoch, 1990).

Groups of neurons that are similar in structure and function are often organized together. Those arranged in layers on the brain's surface are called cortices (singular, **cortex**) and those arranged in clusters are called **nuclei** (singular, nucleus). Together, nuclei and cortices comprise the gray matter of the brain. Sheets of **white matter** lie directly beneath the cerebral cortex. This white matter is composed of fiber tracts that provide information pathways that connect the cerebral hemispheres, and link the cerebral cortex with other parts of the CNS. **Gray matter** structures of the brain and spinal cord are connected by these

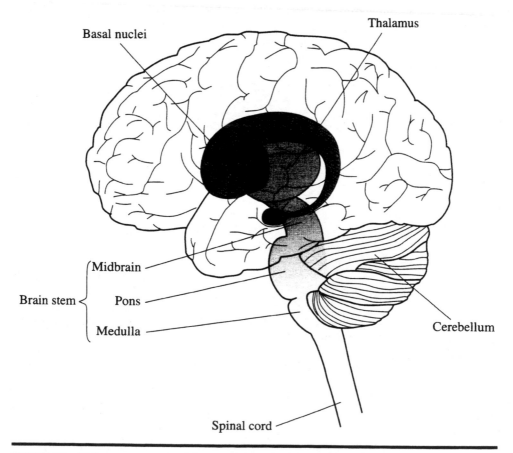

FIGURE 7.2 Major components of the central nervous system.

white matter pathways or fiber tracts. Together the gray matter structures and white matter pathways form complex neural networks involved in cognition, language, and movement.

Neurotransmission across these widely distributed neural networks in the brain gives rise to complex, integrative thought and behavior. A major transmission pathway is the **corpus callosum,** a broad band of fibers at the base of the brain that connects the two cerebral hemispheres. Another important transmission pathway is the **arcuate fasciculus** which interconnects various regions on the same side of the brain. In the left hemisphere, the arcuate fasciculus arches backward from the motor speech area (i.e., Broca's area) to the audi-

tory cortex (i.e., Wernicke's area). Within the last decade sophisticated brain imaging techniques have suggested that white matter pathways that project from the cortex to subcortical structures play an important role in language processing (Naeser, Gaddie, Palumbo, & Shassny-Edner, 1990) and recovery from aphasia (Naeser, Helm-Estabrooks, Hass, Auerbach, & Shrinvasan, 1987).

The left and right hemispheres of the cerebrum are separated by a groove that runs from the front to the back of the brain (**longitudinal cerebral fissure**). Two additional landmarks serve to divide the brain into general regions. The **central sulcus** roughly divides the brain into anterior and

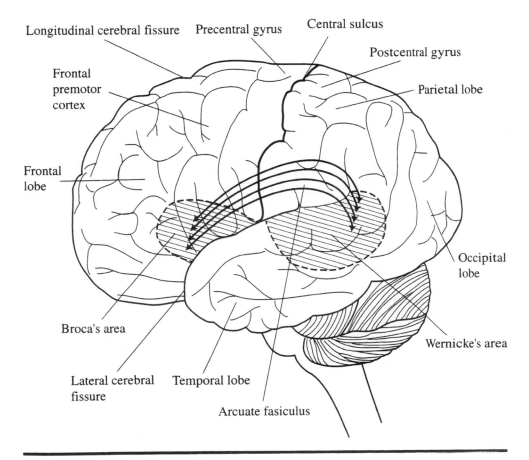

FIGURE 7.3   Major regions of the cortex.

posterior portions. The **lateral cerebral fissure** starts at the base of the brain and runs laterally and upward. Together, the central sulcus and the longitudinal cerebral fissure roughly divide each hemisphere into four general regions or lobes: **frontal, parietal, occipital,** and **temporal.** The lobes of the brain are usually thought of as having a primary or major function and a secondary or supplementary function.

The **frontal lobe** includes the area in front of the central sulcus and comprises about one-third of the neocortex. The area just in front of the central sulcus, called the **precentral gyrus,** contains the primary motor cortex, or motor strip. This cortical area controls voluntary muscle movement on the opposite side of the body. The left, lower portion of the motor strip contains **Broca's area,** a cortical region consistently associated with the execution of speech movements. The **frontal premotor** or supplementary motor cortex has been associated with integrating sensory stimulation from the periphery and in planning and executing speech movements.

The **parietal lobe** is located on the other side of the central sulcus and contains the **postcentral gyrus** or the primary sensory cortex. The primary sensory cortex is also called the somesthetic cortex. Somesthetic refers to sensation for proprioception, touch, pressure, pain, and temperature. Arranged in the mirror image of the motor strip, this region of the brain is believed to be responsible for many aspects of body awareness and sensation. The secondary sensory cortex, located posteriorly in the parietal lobe, has been associated with analysis and integration of the sensations of touch, pressure, and bodily awareness.

The central function of the **temporal lobe** is auditory processing. The primary auditory cortex is concerned with hearing. Posterior to the primary auditory cortex is **Wernicke's area,** located on the superior temporal gyrus, near to where the temporal, parietal, and occipital lobes join. Wernicke's area is believed to be important in comprehension of spoken and written language.

Visual processing is the major function of the **occipital lobe.** The primary visual cortex perceives visual information as patterns of light. Higher order analysis (e.g., recognition, interpretation) to change these patterns into meaningful symbols takes place in the visual association cortex.

APPROACHES TO UNDERSTANDING BRAIN AND LANGUAGE

Historic Perspectives

Inquiry into the nature of language and its relationship to the brain has an ancient history. Theories that have attempted to explain the relationship between brain and language seem to reflect the prevailing technology of the time. Early philosophers passionately argued whether it was the heart or the brain that served as the location of thought. On the basis of the post–mortem observations of nineteenth-century neurologists like Dr. Paul Broca and Dr. Karl Wernicke, the idea that the left cerebral hemisphere played a special role in speech production became prominent. This kind of work led to the widely held belief that the two hemispheres of the brain are asymmetrical in function, with the left side containing the area chiefly responsible for processing words and sentences. This account of the central language mechanism is often referred to as the classical explanation. Contemporary theories of brain organization are an elaboration of this early idea.

The theory that one hemisphere is dominant for a particular function is called **laterality.** Most contemporary theories of brain function lateralize language to left side. The theory that emotion can be lateralized to the right brain is more controversial (Borod, 1993). **Localization** is a complementary theory that suggests that a function can be isolated to a specific part of the brain within a hemisphere. For example, Broca's area, roughly located in the lower, posterior portion of the left frontal lobe, is believed to be responsible for speech production. Wernicke's area, which generally refers to the posterior left superior temporal gyrus, is believed to be responsible for auditory comprehension. In the classical view, the left hemisphere contains all of the cortical centers that support specific language functions. Damage to these centers or the connections between them will produce a predictable form of aphasia. Many current theories of brain and language are based upon the principle that the brain is organized into discrete components that subserve different language functions. A major criticism of the classical explanation is that it does not fully account for the complexity of language in social contexts since it focuses on word and sentence level processing. Another criticism is that it derives an explanation of normal function from patients with brain damage. As early as 1879, neurologist John Hughlings-Jackson cautioned that locating speech and locating brain damage were two separate things. That is, it is not possible to fully describe how the normal brain operates during language processing on the basis of the disorders that result from brain damage.

Data illuminating the relationship of language and the brain has come from sources other than post–mortem examinations of brain-damaged patients. In the 1950s, neurosurgeon W. Penfield and colleagues examined cortical function by directly applying electrodes to the cortices of patients with epilepsy during open brain surgery (Penfield & Roberts, 1959). This work localized right-sided motor and sensory control to the surface of the left cerebral cortex, and left-sided motor and sensory control to the surface of the right cerebral cortex. Penfield and Roberts (1959) pointed out that a relatively large area of the motor strip in the frontal lobe was devoted to control of the vocal tract. Historically, the cortical electrical stimulation technique provided additional evidence that specific functions could be mapped onto certain cortical locations.

Modern technology continues to inform what is known about the brain. By the late 1970s, **computerized axial tomography scans (CT scans)** were widely used to study the location and extent of brain damage more precisely. CT scans have been used to visualize the internal structure of the brain and to study the effects of certain neuropathologies. For example, CT studies have demonstrated that many types of aphasia are linked to damage to specific brain sites (Damasio, 1991). More recently, images of brain tissue have been obtained with **Magnetic Resonance Imaging (MRI).** In the study of the brain, MRI has the advantage over CT scanning because it provides a clearer view of the extent and location of brain damage. MRI studies have been useful in examining the relationship between certain cortical and subcortical areas and language deficits. Both these technologies picture the brain at a single moment in time. However, recent evidence suggests that the brain's activity levels vary from moment to moment. **Positron Emission Tomography (PET)** is the most recent neuroimaging technology. PET measures glucose and oxygen metabolism of cells in a manner that reflects the amount of physiologic functioning. Different processing tasks produce differential neuronal activity patterns. PET may be used to study metabolic activity patterns in neurologically healthy and brain-damaged subjects and has great potential for advancing knowledge about how the brain functions. A study of cellular glucose metabolism in patients with aphasia demonstrated that focal brain pathologies affect the function of distant brain regions (Metter, 1987). This provides evidence that parts of the brain do not work in isolation, challenging a strict localizationist view of brain function.

Functional Asymmetry of the Cerebral Hemispheres

Experimental studies strongly suggest that the left side of the brain and the right side of the brain function quite differently. Although the two sides of the brain are roughly comparable in structure, they seem to process information in different ways. Several explanations have been advanced to explain the functional differences between the two sides of the brain.

The most widely held view is that each side of the brain is specialized to control particular types of behavior. In most people the left hemisphere is the verbal half of the brain, specialized for language, and the right hemisphere the nonverbal half, specialized for processing visuo-spatial perceptual information (Davis, 1983). This dichotomy must be viewed cautiously, as an oversimplified explanation of a complex and interconnected process, because the right hemisphere has been shown to have some linguistic abilities and the left some nonverbal abilities (Searlman,1977; Perecman, 1983).

Each cerebral hemisphere may employ a different cognitive processing style to operate on information (West,1983). Specifically, the left hemisphere may use an analytic and sequential processing style that is equipped to break information down into logical and rational pieces. By contrast, the right brain may employ an intuitive or holistic processing style and may be better equipped to perceive relationships and simultaneously integrate information (Galin, 1976).

Following brain damage, the distinct processing capacities of the two hemispheres may be most apparent. Studying the brain in this manner helps to illustrate the concepts of cerebral lateralization, localization, and asymmetry. Knowledge of how the sides of the brain are different provides a context for examining the consequences of left brain damage and right brain damage.

While the two hemispheres are functionally asymmetrical, all complex cognitive skills, including language, arise from the interaction of overlapping, interconnected neural networks distributed across both sides of the brain. Although many people do sustain a single unilateral lesion confined to one area of the brain, many patients also have brain damage that is diffuse or bilateral. This may give rise to cognitive deficits or disorders such as dysarthria or dysphagia that should be carefully distinguished from the language disorder.

The Neurosciences

Neuroscience, the multidisciplinary study of the structure and function of the nervous system, is a relatively new division of science. The field of neuroscience is comprised of scientists from many branches of medicine, biochemistry, pharmacology, psychology, and speech–language and hear-

ing. Prior to the middle of the 1960s, there was little communication between the numerous disciplines that investigated the brain and the neurobiology of behavior (Webster, 1995). The goal of neuroscience today is to obtain a transdisciplinary picture of how humans perceive information, think, feel, make decisions, control action and movement, and communicate.

Of particular importance to speech–language pathologists are the branches of neuroscience that focus on language and communication. There are several general approaches to interpreting information about language and the brain. **Psycholinguistics** and **neurolinguistics** are two major disciplines that investigate the neurology of language behavior. The ultimate goal of both approaches is to construct models of the psychological processes that make it possible for humans to produce and use language. In the psycholinguistic approach, the focus is on the cognitive processes that underlie language production and comprehension. For example, psycholinguistic studies may examine the role of short-term memory in language processing. Psycholinguistic models are generally constructed by studying language in normal populations. (For a good introduction to psycholinguistics, see Berko-Gleason & Ratner, 1993.) The neurolinguistic approach seeks to explain the anatomic and physiologic correlates of language behavior. Neurolinguists construct models of language processing by studying brain-damaged patients to describe how linguistic breakdown reflects impairment to different parts of the brain. (For a good introduction to neurolinguistics see Caplan, 1987.)

Psycholinguistics and neurolinguistics both have their roots in the discipline of linguistics. **Linguistics** is primarily concerned with describing rules governing the formation of acceptable utterances within a language or across languages. Language is described in terms of the regularities in its sound system (phonology), structure (morphosyntax), vocabulary (lexicon), semantics (meaning or message content), and use (pragmatics). (For a good introduction to linguistics see Ackmajian, Demers, & Harnish,1984.) The basic tenet of contemporary neurolinguistic theory is that discrete areas of the brain are linked to specific aspects of linguistic processing. Familiarity with the basic elements of linguistic structure is crucial for detailing the language impairment that results from brain damage. Research in psycholinguistics and neurolingustics will continue to inform our understanding of how the brain works and how it may recover when it has been damaged. Concepts in psycholinguistics and neurolinguistics form the basis of most current assessment and treatment practices.

LEFT BRAIN DAMAGE: APHASIA

In the 90 percent of the population who are left hemisphere dominant for language (Ojemann, 1979), damage to the left side of the brain causes aphasia. In the broadest sense, aphasia refers to an acquired loss of language or a reduction in the ability to name. The term aphasia does not specify the cause of the language deficit. Vascular disease, abnormal growth of brain tissue (i.e., neoplasm), or head trauma produce damage that can selectively interfere with language processing. The aphasia acquired following a CVA has an abrupt onset. However, aphasic-like symptoms may also appear with a gradual onset. **Primary progressive aphasia** (PPA) is a term given for aphasic-like language symptoms with an insidious onset and slow, gradual progression. Cases of PPA demonstrate that focal symptoms may appear along the course of certain degenerative diseases (Caselli & Jack, 1991). The aphasia considered here is most specifically related to focal damage in the left side of the brain.

Defining and Classifying Aphasia

It is generally agreed that aphasia is a language disorder caused by damage to the brain. However, there is considerable controversy concerning exactly how aphasic language disorders should be conceptualized. Some researchers assert that **aphasia** is a homogenous disorder characterized by an underlying deficit in verbal behavior. In contrast, others believe that there are several types of aphasia that can be classified into distinctly different syndromes. Taking the single disorder view, Scheull and colleagues (1964) defined aphasia as a general deficit in language that enters into a patient's listening, speaking, reading, and writing. Scheull et al. believed that aphasia may vary in terms of severity, but not in kind. Underlying Scheull's definition of aphasia is the view that language is an integrative function that results from the dynamic interaction of complex cortical and subcortical activity.

Goodglass and Kaplan (1983) provided a different view of aphasia. They asserted that there are various types of aphasia and have proposed a classification systems that takes a localizationist approach. That is, they attempt to classify aphasia into syndromes based on the premise that different brain areas control different language functions. Consistent with this view, aphasic patients may be broadly divided into two separate groups characterized by either fluent or nonfluent patterns in oral expression. Nonfluent aphasia results from damage to anterior cortical regions (i.e., frontal lobe lesions) and fluent aphasia results from damage to the posterior regions of the cortex (i.e., temporal or temporal-parietal lesions). Patients with nonfluent aphasia typically produce sparse, perseverative language characterized by disturbed prosody, misarticulations, errors in syntax, and a reduction in phrase length. Because anterior lesions may include a portion of the motor cortex, these patients often are paralyzed on the right side of the body. Patients with fluent aphasia produce a great deal of language with few pauses, normal articulation, and generally intact syntactical skills (Goodglass, 1981). Clinical evidence supports the view that patients with cortical damage can be classified reliably into these two symptom types in a manner that generally localizes the lesion within the left hemisphere.

The Boston aphasia classification system developed by Goodglass and Kaplan (1983a) is widely used to designate different types of aphasia syndromes. In addition to examining verbal expression for fluency, the Boston system considers naming, repetition, and auditory comprehension abilities. On the basis of these behaviors, the Boston system further differentiates three nonfluent and four fluent cortical aphasia syndromes. The nonfluent types include Broca's aphasia, transcortical motor aphasia, and global aphasia. The fluent types of aphasia include Wernicke's aphasia, anomic aphasia, conduction aphasia, and transcortical sensory aphasia. The Boston approach assumes that each type of aphasia may be correlated with a particular site of brain damage. This classification system is a direct outgrowth of the classical view of how language is organized in the brain. The following section a brief summary of each aphasia syndrome and its neuroanatomical basis.

Broca's Aphasia. Broca's aphasia is a nonfluent aphasia usually associated with damage to cortical and subcortical tissue of the lower left frontal lobe, including the precentral gyrus (Goodglass, 1981). Speech is characterized by awkward articulation and restricted prosody. Agrammatism is frequently associated with Broca's aphasia. **Agrammatism** is a loss in the use of grammatical morphemes (e.g., articles, prepositions, inflectional endings) resulting in short utterances that contain content words (e.g., nouns, main verbs). Agrammatic speech is apparent in the conversation of patients with Broca's aphasia as well as during sentence repetition. The ability to name words varies in Broca's aphasia, but most patients are mildly impaired. Word retrieval is often helped by providing an initial sound cue. Auditory comprehension is a relative strength for these patients, but mild-to-moderate difficulties may be displayed. Oral reading and writing reveal deficits that tend to parallel speech production. It has been suggested that patients diagnosed with Broca's aphasia actually demonstrate a language disorder that is complicated by the coexistence of **apraxia of speech** (Darley, 1982). (See Chapter 8.)

Transcortical Motor Aphasia. Another nonfluent variety of aphasia is transcortical motor aphasia. A frontally located lesion that interrupts the connection between Broca's area and the supplementary motor cortex, sparing Broca's area, will produce this kind of aphasia (Helm-Estabrooks & Albert, 1991). Because Broca's area is preserved, articulation remains unimpaired. Sentences produced during conversation frequently contain errors in syntax. The most distinguishable characteristic of transcortical motor aphasia is preserved repetition ability. That is, during the repetition of complex sentences, these patients do not produce errors in syntax or morphology. Auditory comprehension is a relative strength. Reading and writing skills are comparable to patients with Broca's Aphasia.

Global Aphasia. Patients with global aphasia are completely nonfluent. A large lesion involving portions of the frontal, temporal, and parietal regions (from Broca's area to Wernicke's area) and extending deep into the nearby white matter, produces global aphasia. Speech output is severely limited, and is often characterized by meaningless word and syllable repetitions or interjections. Naming and repetition are virtually impossible. Some emotional (e.g., cursing) and automatic speech (e.g., counting) may be preserved. Auditory comprehension is severely impaired, blurring the distinction between what the patient can understand and what the patient can produce. Some patients can answer concrete "yes" and "no" questions and respond to basic commands (e.g., raise your hand). There is usually no functional reading. Writing skills are often limited to copying words or sentences. Some patients with global aphasia retain the ability to write their name.

Wernicke's Aphasia. Wernicke's aphasia is a fluent syndrome associated with lesions in the posterior third of the superior temporal gyrus (also called Wernicke's area). Articulation and intonation remain essentially normal but rate of speech becomes noticeably rapid. Basically, the sentences produced are intact syntactically. However, the patient often uses words that are not recognizable, making language sound empty or vague. For instance, the patient may produce neologistic jargon (meaningless invented words) or words that are semantically unrelated to the context. Wernicke's aphasia is often associated with paragrammatism (subtle mistakes in the use of small grammatical elements). For example, the patient may substitute an adjective for a noun, or place the past tense marker on a noun. Auditory comprehension is usually severely impaired in Wernicke's aphasia. Naming and repetition skills are severely impaired. Reading is usually impaired and written performance is variable. Some patients are not able to write at all while others write in a manner that parallels their oral production.

Anomic Aphasia.   When anomic aphasia results from a focal lesion, it is usually in the angular gyrus or second temporal gyrus. Anomic symptoms are often reported when the brain damage is not focal, as in closed head injury or dementia. Usually a mild or moderate deficit in auditory comprehension is present in anomic aphasia. Speech is characterized by syntactically intact utterances with no impairments in articulation and prosody. A pervasive deficit in word finding often makes conversation sound empty or devoid of content. Failures in word finding are often compensated for by circumlocution, or talking around the word. Reading and writing abilities seem to be tied to the specific site of the lesion. Typicallly, patients with a lesion to the angular gyrus are severely impaired in reading and writing. Patients with damage to the second temporal gyrus may demonstrate mild reading and writing problems that parallel deficits in speech production.

Conduction Aphasia.   Conduction aphasia is associated with lesions in the arcuate fasciculus, the white matter pathway connecting Wernicke's area to Broca's area. Oral motor abilities, prosody, and basic syntax remain intact. Word finding problems are often met with false starts and attempts at self-correction. Auditory comprehension is only mildly affected. The most distinguishable characteristic of conduction aphasia is the selective deficit in repetition; that is, the poor repetition abilities that characterize this syndrome stand in

contrast to the mild impairments in other areas. Reading usually remains intact and writing is marked by spelling errors and problems in syntax.

Transcortical Sensory Aphasia.   Transcortical sensory aphasia is another fluent syndrome. Lesions producing this aphasia are associated with posterior parietal-temporal damage, sparing Wernicke's area. Similar to patients with Wernicke's aphasia, these patients demonstrate intact articulation, a preservation of basic syntax, and deficits in auditory comprehension that are usually severe. Naming is also severely affected. Unlike patients with Wernicke's aphasia, those with transcortical sensory aphasia maintain their ability to repeat sentences that contain complex syntactic constructions. Although these patients are often good at oral reading, comprehension is usually poor. Writing is most often severely impaired.

The Boston system and the formal diagnostic protocol (i.e., the Boston Diagnostic Aphasia Examination) (Goodglass & Kaplan, 1983b) that emerged from it, are not without critics (Caramazza, 1984). Because the Boston classification system is based primarily on unilateral damage to the cortex, findings may not be easily generalized to patients with subcortical and diffuse cortical damage, those patients with atypical medical histories, psychiatric disorders, or bilateral cerebral dominance for language. Proponents of this popular system argue that it is worthwhile from a clinical perspective to get a general description of patients' language strengths and weaknesses. Alternative clinical tools are likely to be developed over the next few years. These approaches will be informed by research in functional communication (e.g., Aten, 1994), pragmatics (e.g., Lubinski, 1994), and discourse processes (e.g., Bloom, Obler, DeSanti, & Ehrlich, 1994).

Other important findings about the nature of aphasia have been obtained by comparing left-brain-damaged patients to neurologically healthy subjects. Generally, on experimental tasks, aphasic individuals perform at a slower rate and produce and comprehend less language than persons

TABLE 7.1   Production Characteristics and the Boston Classification System for Cortical Aphasias (Goodglass and Kaplan, 1983b)

PRODUCTION CHARACTERISTICS	BOSTON DIAGNOSTIC APHASIA CLASSIFICATION	DESCRIPTION
NONFLUENT—sparse perseverative language, disturbed prosody, misarticulations, incomplete syntax, reduced phrase length	BROCA	awkward articulation, agrammatism, relatively intact auditory comprehension, poor repetition
	TRANSCORTICAL MOTOR	unimpaired articulation, errors in syntax, relatively intact auditory comprehension, good repetition
	GLOBAL	severely limited production, some preserved syllables and automatic speech, very poor naming and repetition, severely impaired auditory abilities
FLUENT—word finding problems, normal-lengthy sentences, few pauses, normal articulation, basically intact syntax	WERNICKE	normal articulation and prosody, produces meaningless invented word, intact syntax, poor auditory comprehension
	ANOMIA	pervasive word finding deficit, intact syntax, good articulation and prosody, mild-moderate auditory comprehension deficit, good repetition skills
	CONDUCTION	normal articulation and prosody, basic syntax is spared, frequent self-corrections, mildly impaired auditory comprehension abilities, poor repetition
	TRANSCORTICAL SENSORY	good articulation, preserved syntax, some auditory comprehension deficits, good repetition skills

without aphasia. Interestingly, the kinds of errors people with aphasia produce are apparent, but to a lesser degree, in the speech of normal individuals. Similarities between subjects with aphasia and those without neurological damage have been revealed in terms of the structure and organization of **discourse** (Berko-Gleason, Goodglass, Obler, Green, Hyde, & Weintraub, 1981; Ulatowska, Freedman-Stern, Doyel, Macaluso-Haynes, & North, 1983). Studies that have examined discourse in patients with left brain damage have revealed a preservation of the global organization (i.e., essential elements) of a story despite obvious problems in phonology, morphology, syntax, and semantics (Ulatowska, North, &

Macaluso-Haynes, 1981). It appears that in aphasia, the underlying framework around which discourse is structured essentially remains intact. Additionally, adults with aphasia demonstrate variability in performance as a function of elicitation condition (Hough, Pierce, & Cannito,1989; Glosser, Weiner, & Kaplan, 1986) and linguistic system (Zurif & Caramazza, 1976). For example, a patient may demonstrate deficits in semantics but still have a relatively intact phonological system. Taken together, these findings support the view that aphasia is an interference in the ability to perform linguistic operations, not a loss of **communicative competence** (McNeil, 1982; Holland, 1982). That is, the basic ability to formulate ideas, as well as the knowledge of the words and rules that govern one's language, are not entirely lost in patients with aphasia. Rather, the deficit is in the ability to retrieve words and the linguistic rules that express ideas.

Aphasia cannot be described solely on the basis of its linguistic impairments. Some conceptualizations of aphasia are based on the idea that cognition is central to all aspects of language processing. Cognition includes perception, attention, memory, and conceptualization abilities. Wepman (1976) viewed aphasia as a cognitive–linguistic impairment in which the disturbance may be in language or in the thought processes that underlie linguistic expression. McNeil (1982) conceptualizes aphasia as an inefficiency in verbal symbolic manipulations (e.g., lexical storage, retrieval, and rule generation) stemming from neurophysiological and cognitive inactivity. According to the cognitive view, aphasia includes impairments in memory for language and in strategies for planning, constructing, and retrieving linguistic information.

Psychosocial Considerations

Loss of language has dramatic psychosocial consequences. Adjustment to a disability acquired in adulthood presents many challenges for the patient and the family. For instance, when aphasia occurs after retirement in older persons, it may impede their ability to live without assistance. When aphasia occurs before retirement, it may have devastating financial implications for the entire family. Many people with aphasia become socially isolated. People without aphasia may become intolerant and uncomfortable around an adult with a communication disorder, even if they knew the person before the stroke.

Adjustment to life with aphasia varies greatly from patient to patient. Although many patients go through a process of mourning that may ultimately lead to the realistic acceptance of their functional differences, many patients remain in denial of their limitations (Tanner, 1980). Coping with the effects of stroke is undoubtedly tied to premorbid personality. For example, a patient who values literacy may react differently than a patient who values mobility. Some adults with aphasia may reject being dependent on anyone for help, others may respond wholeheartedly to clinical treatment.

Families may not fully understand the nature of the patient's acquired language disorder and often have unrealistic expectations for recovery. Some families may become burdened by sadness and anxiety. A spouse may become angry, overprotective, or depressed. Persons with aphasia are often perceived by their spouse to be demanding, temperamental, and dependent (Zraich & Boone, 1991). Children must adjust to the new roles of the disabled and nondisabled parent. The entire family may need to make major modifications to accommodate the reality of having a person with a disability living in the home. Changes in managing the details of daily life can overpower the patient and family. The patient and the family must learn to adjust to the short-term effects (e.g., work-related adjustment) and the long-term consequences (e.g., paralysis) of the stroke.

Some psychological changes experienced by the patient are neurological in origin. Many brain-damaged patients experience extreme fatigue and emotional lability (i.e., uncontrolled tears or laughter) following a stroke. Studies have consistently demonstrated an association between emotional disorders and the site of the lesion following stroke (Borod, Bloom, & Santschi-Haywood, 1996). In one study, patients with left brain damage generally demonstrated strong, catastrophic reactions to their condition, and patients with right brain damage appeared to be relatively indifferent (Gainotti,1972). Pathological crying in aphasic patients and pathological laughing in patients with right brain damage has been reported (Sackeim, Greenberg, Weiman, Gur, & Hungerbuhler, 1982). Denial and depression are associated with frontal left brain damage and Broca's aphasia, whereas temporal damage and Wernicke's aphasia may be associated with agitation and lack of awareness (Swindell & Hammons, 1991). Emotional functioning may recover differently in patients with left brain damage and patients with right brain damage. For example, Nelson, Cicchetti, Satz, Sowa, and Mitrushina (1994) reported that at six months post onset emotional functioning stabilized in patients with left brain damage but worsened in patients with right brain damage.

The neurobehavioral and psychosocial aspects of aphasia are intimately tied to a patient's potential for recovery (Hammons & Swindell, 1987). Speech–language pathologists are often in a good position to comment on a patient's adjustment to their acquired deficits. Following stroke reactive depression, catastrophic reaction and severe anxiety may be present to the degree that it hinders the recovery process (Nelson, Cicchetti, Satz, Stern, Sowa, & Cohen, 1993). Although such emotional reactions are not apparent in all individuals with aphasia, some patients should be referred to a physician who may then elect to treat these behaviors pharmacologically.

RIGHT BRAIN DAMAGE

Communication Disorders

Even in patients who are left hemisphere dominant for language, damage to the right side of the brain can result in communication deficits. Except in the rare cases of crossed language dominance (left-handed and right brain dominant for language), the communication disorders from right hemisphere damage are clearly distinct from the aphasia syndromes (Myers, 1984). On experimental tasks, patients with right brain damage have displayed mild deficits in naming (Joanette, LeCours, Lepage, & Lamoureux, 1983), verbal fluency (Diggs & Basili, 1987), and auditory comprehension (Adamovich & Brooks, 1981). If linguistic deficits in these patients are present, they are most often mild and may go undetected on experimental tasks. Many patients with right brain damage demonstrate intact sentence level processing, with language abilities that become compromised in challenging communication situations.

Deficits in selective attention (Bud, Audet, & LeCours, 1990) and unilateral neglect of the left hemispace (Mesulam, 1985) have also been documented in patients with right brain damage. A patient with unilateral left hemispace neglect, for example, may not notice utensils presented on the left side of the table. These kinds of visuospatial perceptual problems have been offered as an explanation for some of the reading and writing problems these patients often experience. According to Myers (1994), patients with right brain damage may have visuo-perceptual disorders that effect communication on a variety of levels. At low levels of visuo-spatial processing, patients with right brain damage demonstrate problems on figure–ground tests (Heir & Kaplan, 1980) and problems identifying fragmented, incomplete figure drawings (Myers, Linebaugh, & Mackisack, 1985). At higher levels of visuo-perceptual processing, these patients may not attend to visual detail or successfully organize visuospatial information into a narrative (Benowitz, Moya, & Levine, 1990).

A wide variety of experimental tasks have suggested that many patients with right brain damage approach language with a concrete orientation. For instance, some patients with right brain damage have demonstrated deficits in fully appreciating the humor in jokes (Brownell, Michell, Powelson, & Gardner, 1983). Other studies have noted that patients with right brain damage respond to language literally, and often fail to interpret the intended meaning of **idioms** (Winner & Gardner, 1977) and **metaphor** (Myers & Linebaugh, 1981).

It is not clear if right hemisphere communication disorders reflect an underlying deficit in language processing, or if problems arise because of perceptual problems, deficits in emotion, or more general cognitive processing disorders. Analytic discourse techniques have been useful in examining the factors that enter into language processing (Bloom, Obler, DeSanti, & Ehrlich, 1994). Because discourse techniques focuses on language beyond the sentence level, these studies have been particularly useful in identifying subtle communication deficits. Such studies have suggested that patients with right brain damage produce poorly structured discourse that contains incomplete and ambiguous information (Bloom, Borod, Obler, & Gerstman, 1992; Myers & Brookshire, 1994). In a comparison to normal control subjects, deficits in integrating contextual information into a narrative and interpreting complex concepts have been described in patients with right brain damage. Patients with right brain damage will often list information, rather than interpret relationships between characters and events in a story (Brownell, Potter, Bihrle, & Gardner, 1986; Hough, 1990). Despite their ability to process sentences on experimental tasks, these studies suggest that the communication abilities of right-brain-damaged patients may be compromised in daily living. Thus, some of these patients may be unable to return to work if their job demands extensive paper work or detailed message taking, for example.

Emotional Processing and Communication

Several studies have suggested that there are major changes in emotional functioning following right hemisphere stroke (Nelson, Cicchetti, Satz, Stern, Sowa, & Cohen, 1993; Robinson & Starkstein, 1990). Clinical reports frequently note that patients with right brain damage speak in a monotone and appear emotionally flat, indifferent, or unaware of their deficits (Myers, 1994). Such observations have led researchers to investigate the role of the right hemisphere in processing emotion, using unilateral brain damaged patients as subjects (Borod, Bloom, & Santschi-Haywood, 1996). Deficits in interpreting emotion in facial expressions (Borod, Koff, Lorch, & Nicholas, 1986; Cicone, Wapner, & Gardner, 1980) and in spontaneously producing facial expressions in response to emotional picture stimuli (Borod, et al., 1986; Buck & Duffy, 1981) have been demonstrated in these subjects. Right-brain-damaged subjects also have demonstrated impairments in identifying and discriminating prosodic information in sentences (i.e., alterations in pitch, volume, and duration) (Heilman, Bowers, Speedie,

& Coslett, 1984; Lalande, Braun, Carlebois, & Whitaker, 1992). Some studies have suggested that right-brain-damaged patients have a selective deficit in the production (Ross & Mesulam, 1979) and comprehension (Tompkins, 1991) of prosody when it conveys emotional information. Deficits in identifying emotion on the face or in interpreting prosodic cues significantly can interfere with conversational skills.

Many patients with right brain damage seem to have a special problem with language that is emotional. In a discourse production task, patients with right brain damage demonstrated a reduction of emotional content, but not neutral content, when their narratives were compared to aphasic patients and normal controls (Bloom, Borod, Obler, & Gerstman, 1992). When the verbal pragmatic aspects of discourse were examined, emotional content interfered with the performance of patients with right brain damage. Interestingly, emotional content seemed to help pragmatic appropriateness in patients with aphasia (Bloom, Borod, Obler, & Gerstman, 1993). Recently, impairments in the perception of emotional words have been noted in subjects with right brain damage, relative to left-brain-damaged and normal subjects (Blonder, Bowers, & Heilman, 1991; Borod, 1993). These studies seem to indicate that cortical structures of the right hemisphere play a dominant role in the facial, prosodic, and verbal aspects of emotional communication. Additional research is needed to examine how emotion is organized in the brain. Emotional processing deficits should be considered during assessment and treatment of communication disorders. Because cognition, emotional processing, language, and social skills are so intermixed, consultation with a neuropsychologist is often necessary to adequately diagnose the nature of the problem.

CLINICAL APHASIOLOGY AND THE SPEECH–LANGUAGE PATHOLOGIST

Clinical aphasiology focuses on the rehabilitation of communication in patients with brain damage.

Clinical aphasiologists are speech–language pathologists who typically work with a team of health care providers in diagnosing and treating individuals with acquired neurogenic disorders (Chapey, 1994). Research in clinical aphasiology has explored issues such as prognosis for language recovery, treatment efficacy, and the social consequences of brain damage. In practice the speech–language pathologist may work in a medical center, community hospital, rehabilitation center, or nursing facility. A major charge of the speech–language pathologist is to assess a patient's communication abilities, identify and describe the disorder, and, if warranted, plan a program of clinical management.

Communication Assessment

Communication assessment is a systematic process of gathering information in order to identify the factors that contribute significantly to the clinical picture. Assessment is geared at differentiating the language component of the disorder from speech problems (e.g., apraxia, dysarthria), and distinguishing aphasia from related disorders (e.g., dementia, right brain damage, and head injury). The initial assessment culminates in a written summary or detailed report that documents the findings and provides baseline data on patient performance. Assessment is really an ongoing process that continues throughout treatment and serves as a basis for treatment planning.

Assessment begins with gathering a patient's case history. The patient, spouse, or relative and the medical records are good sources of information. The case history includes personal data such as age, education, occupation, hobbies, and family structure or support systems. It is important to get a good sense of the patient's personality prior to the stroke. This often provides clues as to how the patient may approach treatment and adjust to the disability. Medical information can often be obtained by reviewing the hospital or referral records. Previous hospitalizations and medical conditions that could complicate recovery should

be noted. Results of the neurological examination, including any neurobehavioral signs (e.g., paralysis) should be summarized along with any neuroradiological information. Type of neurological disorder, etiology, and the size and site of the lesion should be concisely summarized in the report. These factors, taken together with formal testing results and observations, help the speech–language pathologist form an impression of prognosis, the maximum amount of recovery predicted for the patient, and whether the patient is a good candidate for treatment.

Formal Testing for Aphasia

There are many commercially available assessment tools that formally examine aphasia. In addition to determining the presence of a disorder, many of these batteries help characterize the aphasia and purport to estimate how much recovery the patient will experience. As mentioned above, The Minnesota Test for the Differential Diagnosis of Aphasia (MTDDA)(Scheull et al., 1965) and The Boston Diagnostic Aphasia Examination (BDAE) (Goodglass & Kaplan, 1983) are two widely used assessment tools that differ in the conceptual approach to aphasia. The MTDDA views aphasia as a single disorder, whereas the BDAE identifies different aphasic syndromes.

The MTDDA consists of five major sections that examine for disturbances in auditory comprehension, speech and language, reading, writing, numerical relations, and arithmetic. Testing places patients in general categories that describe the degree of language breakdown and suggest the amount of recovery the patient might experience. Speech–language pathologists have used the MTDDA to pinpoint a patient's strengths and weaknesses across different modalities and at different levels of linguistic complexity.

The Boston Diagnostic Aphasia Examination (BDAE) is another widely used assessment tool. The BDAE seeks to identify the presence of aphasia and categorize it in a way that leads to inferences about the site of brain damage. It is estimated that 80 percent of patients with aphasia can reliably be classified in a distinct category (Helm-Estabrooks & Albert, 1991). The BDAE begins with conversational speech, elicited through an interview and picture description task respectively. A profile of speech characteristics, based on dimensions of oral expression (i.e., melodic line, phrase length, grammatical form, paraphasia, word finding) and auditory comprehension aids in classifying patient communication patterns into aphasia symptom types. Procedures for examining a patient's reading and written language are also included. The test manual provides some normative data, making it possible to roughly compare a patient's subtest performance to a sample of male patients with aphasia from the Veteran's Administration Medical Center in Boston. Speech–language pathologists use this test as a comprehensive measure of performance that adheres to the principle that subtyping aphasia into syndromes leads to inferences concerning lesion localization.

Supplementary Aphasia Assessment Strategies

A frequent observation is that patients with aphasia perform better in real life situations than they do on formal language-oriented test batteries. Several supplementary assessment tools have been developed to assess how people with aphasia communicate in everyday situations. In contrast to the language-oriented approach of the MTDDA and the BDAE, the Communications Abilities in Daily Living (CADL) (Holland, 1980) examines whether or not a message was successfully conveyed, rather than the linguistic form of the utterance. The test was designed to capture a patient's functional communication abilities in naturally occurring situations. The Pragmatic Protocol (Prutting & Kirchner, 1987) has also been employed as a guideline for informally observing a patient's natural conversation and noting if the verbal, nonverbal, and paralinguistic aspects of language were used appropriately or not. Lubinski

(1981) emphasized examining the environment in which communication takes place and assessing a patient's accessibility to that environment. Certain environments may provide limited opportunity for communication. Guidelines with applicability to patients in institutionalized settings or at home are provided to evaluate the physical environment (Lubinski, 1981), family, as well as the sociocultural and economic consequences of the disorder (Lubinski, 1994).

Aphasia and the Bilingual Patient

Many factors should be considered when examining acquired aphasia in an individual who is bilingual. In addition to obtaining a clear picture of the language disorder, it is necessary to determine the language or languages that will be used to promote optimal recovery. One critical factor is the degree of bilingualism. A bilingual individual may have equal or native proficiency in both languages or may have greater proficiency in one language than the other. Factors such as the individual's age at the time each language was acquired, the social uses of each language, and the emotional attachment to a particular language help the speech–language pathologist to establish the preferable language for treatment.

Predictions about language recovery in bilingual patients are difficult as differential improvements in both languages are possible. A variety of possible recovery patterns in aphasic patients who speak more than one language have been reported (Albert & Obler, 1978; Paradis, 1977). Three general patterns of language recovery seem to occur with the most frequency in bilingual patients. Sometimes, it is the first language acquired that is less impaired following aphasia, and sometimes the first language is also the first recover. A second pattern is that the most familiar or most recently used language is the first to recover. In the third recovery pattern, affective factors or the emotional attachment to a language seem to account for the language that recovers first. Given these possible recovery patterns, both of a patient's languages should be examined in order to determine the language most appropriate for intervention. In a clinical situation, alternate use of both languages may facilitate word retrieval in bilingual aphasic patients. However, the language used for intervention should be carefully selected on the basis of a patient's premorbid language history, current linguistic abilities, and environmental needs such as the language used by the patient's communication partners. In addition, the patient's culture, religion, and traditions should be understood because these factors may impact on the patient's approach to treatment and their acceptance of help (Wallace & Freeman, 1991).

Assessment of Patients With Right Brain Damage

The MTDDA and the BDAE often do not capture the subtle language difficulties of patients with right brain damage. Some symptoms of right brain damage may be overt, such as hemispatial neglect or dysarthria, but communication problems may only reveal themselves during challenging social and linguistic situations. Administration of the RIC Evaluation of Communication Problems in Right Hemisphere Dysfunction (RICE) (Burns, Halper, & Mogil, 1985) may uncover some of the language and communication deficits in these patients. The RICE includes behavioral observation of communication in a variety of environments, an examination of narrative discourse, a visual tracking test, and writing analysis to evaluate problems that may underlie reading and writing. Complex language processing is examined through the patient's interpretation of metaphors (e.g., proverbs, idioms).

Myers (1994) presented an informal protocol to evaluate neglect and to determine if the deficit is linguistic or perceptually based. The Pragmatic Protocol (Prutting & Kirchner, 1987) may be used to distinguish inappropriate verbal, nonverbal, and paralinguistic communication. Discourse analysis may also be helpful in examining language coherence (Bloom, Borod, Haywood, Obler, & Peck, 1996), cohesion (Berko-Gleason,

Goodglass, Obler, Green, Hyde, & Weintraub, 1981), and global organization or structure of narratives (Chapman & Ulatowska, 1994) in patients with right brain damage.

Treatment of Communication Disorders

In addition to language disorders, brain damage causes related deficits that may influence the outcome of treatment. Hemiplegia or hemiparesis, perceptual deficits, cognitive disorders, reductions in activities of daily living, problems in psychosocial adjustment, depression, and dysphagia often complicate recovery of language function. The complex interaction of these diverse disorders warrants an interdisciplinary approach to rehabilitation. The exact composition of the team is usually determined by the health care setting (Kimbarow, 1994). In addition to a speech–language pathologist, members of the team may include a physical therapist, occupational therapist, social worker, neuropsychologist, rehabilitation nurse, and vocational rehabilitation counselor. Consultations with an audiologist, rehabilitation engineer, and recreational therapist should be considered to fully address the needs of the patient. The team is often headed by a physiatrist, a medical doctor specializing in rehabilitation medicine. The patient and the patient's family should also be included in treatment planning and thought of as members of the rehabilitation team. Interdisciplinary team members collaborate on defining goals directed at enhancing the patient's functional capacity and achieving the highest quality of life possible (Kimbarow, 1994).

Presented here are several general treatment goals that identify what speech–language pathologists do to help the patient overcome the effects of an acquired language disorder. The treatment goals outlined here neither capture the range of intervention strategies that might be used with an individual, nor do they fully account for the scope of clinical practice in speech–language pathology. Goals for the treatment of dysphagia and neuromotor speech disorders are discussed elsewhere. The goals presented here overlap in that they are all related to enhancing a patient's functional communication. That is, the goals of treatment are directed at improving a patient's ability to interact socially and communicate their physical and psychological needs in everyday situations (Aten, 1994). The importance of each goal will vary with the severity of each patient's deficit and particular living circumstances. Goals presented here are broad enough to be applicable to patients with both aphasia and right brain damage. Four general treatment goals are outlined with a few specific clinical approaches presented to illustrate ways these goals might be implemented.

The first general treatment goal is to educate and provide support for patients and their families or significant others. The speech–language pathologist is typically the team member who will explain the nature and impact of the language disorder to the patient and family. Most people understand very little about aphasia or what the patient's world will be like with a communication breakdown such as the inability to organize information into a story. Support for a patient might include modifying the living environment by removing physical barriers to communication and increasing the opportunity for social interaction (Lubinski, 1981). Some of these factors are particularly relevant when the patient resides in a nursing home. Significantly, Lubinski calls attention to factors such as lighting, room acoustics, and the knowledge base and behavior of the patient's communication partners. Facilitation of a realistic attitude toward the recovery process is a related, ongoing treatment objective that continues throughout rehabilitation. Tanner (1980) discussed stages of grieving with respect to loss of communicative function and notes that the speech–language pathologist should avoid behaviors that interrupt the process. Often, denial of deficits may be overcome by setting clear goals and realistically conveying progress. A patient's independence should be emphasized in the recovery process, and dependency on the therapist for communication minimized. In addition, working directly with family members to establish, accept, and practice alternative modes of communication

with the patient is an essential aspect of clinical management (Lyon, 1992).

The second general goal is to develop compensatory strategies that improve the patient's access to the communicative environment. For example, self-cuing strategies, such as silent rehearsal or initial phoneme placement, are taught and practiced to facilitate word retrieval (La-Pointe, 1985). Adaptive speaking, reading, writing, and listening techniques are taught to improve the ability to function in the world and offset any deficits in language. For example, one adaptive listening strategy might be to teach the patient to gesture as a request for a speaker to slow down. Communication notebooks may serve as another adaptive strategy. These notebooks may be designed to contain essential information that can be utilized to help the patient select foods, give biographical information, or discuss family or current events. For patients with right brain damage who demonstrate deficits in structuring story content, Myers (1994) suggested the use of a four-step process to help the patient analyze the information presented. That is, overt instructions are utilized to compensate for a process that was once automatic. At each step, the patient's conscious awareness of story structure is heightened.

The third general goal is to facilitate neurologic recovery in all modalities of communication, through the application of controlled, carefully selected linguistic and cognitive stimulation. Numerous treatment approaches that fit under this goal have been devised to maximize a patient's abilities in listening, speaking, reading, and writing. Scheull's stimulation therapy (Scheull, Jenkins, & Jimenez-Paron, 1964), designed to facilitate reorganization of language, is an excellent example of this approach. Scheull emphasized the use of repetitive and controlled auditory stimulation to prime or excite the damaged language system. Each stimulus item presented to a patient is designed to elicit a particular response. In this approach, the success of each type of stimulation is assessed. The goal is to elicit a large number of adequate responses in order to encourage neurological compensations. Language-oriented treatment

(LOT) (Shewan & Bandur, 1986) is also designed to stimulate recovery at the level of complexity in which language processing breaks down. LOT materials are presented in five modalities: auditory processing, visual processing, gestural and gestural–verbal communication, oral expression, and graphic expression. This approach is arranged in hierarchies of difficulty, presented at a level and pace that the patient can accommodate. Melodic Intonation Therapy (MIT) (Helm-Estabrooks, Nicholas, & Morgan, 1989), which exploits right hemispheric musical and prosodic abilities, is another example of an approach that helps achieve this general goal. Initially, MIT uses melody, repetition, and hand tapping to improve verbal production. As therapy progresses, responses are shaped to become more natural. Other therapy approaches (e.g., Helm-Estabrooks, Fitzpatrick, & Barresi, 1982; West, 1983) that utilize an aspect of the spared neurologic or language system to mediate communication fit under this general goal.

The fourth general treatment goal is to promote maximum independence in a patient's ability to communicate in a variety of common situations. Problem-solving, role playing common or challenging interactions, and practicing newly acquired communication strategies are emphasized. One approach that was designed to help patients with aphasia to transfer strategies from a therapy session to their daily living environment is Prompting Aphasics' Communicative Effectiveness (PACE) (Davis & Wilcox, 1985). PACE emphasizes the idea to be conveyed, not the linguistic accuracy of the message. Patients are encouraged to use gestures, drawings, or any means possible to get the message across to a listener. For some patients, group therapy sessions may be an ideal setting to reinforce strategies learned in individual treatment and to help patients become comfortable using them in real communication situations.

EFFICACY AND CLINICAL PRACTICE

Consumers and health care insurers in the private and public sectors must see that intervention yields measurable benefits that are worth the cost of ser-

vices. Speech and language services must be able to document successful outcomes and demonstrate efficacy. Few studies have explored treatment efficacy with right-brain-damaged patients. Several aphasia treatment studies have been conducted but they are difficult to interpret. Although most research has demonstrated that treatment for aphasia is efficacious, few studies have shown that treatment produces significantly more improvement than no treatment (Rosenbek, LaPointe, & Wertz, 1989). Aphasia treatment studies seem to suffer from some design flaws that prevent generalizing results to the patients actually enrolled in speech–language management programs. Gains from treatment are usually measured using formal instruments that do not account for functional abilities. Group treatment studies often fail to control for patient variables and the effects of spontaneous recovery. Age of subject, education, neurological status, medical history, and time post–onset are just a few of the factors that can influence treatment outcome and confound group treatment designs. Spontaneous recovery, or language abilities that improve without intervention, also complicate aphasia treatment studies. Spontaneous recovery may continue for three months or longer post onset, making it difficult to discern if improvement in language can be attributed to the effects of therapy alone.

Traditional assessment tools (e.g., BDAE, MTDDA) tend to emphasize linguistic performance and ignore the functional aspects of communication (Frattali, 1992). Funding sources for rehabilitation services are increasingly requiring measures of functional gains achieved directly through treatment. Documenting functional improvements in communication has become a primary focus in speech–language pathology (Blomert, 1990). Present demands of consumers and funding sources will inevitably revolutionize the way patients with brain damage are studied and the way their communication disorders are managed within the health care system. To be sure, flexibility will be an operative word for service delivery in the changing face of health services. The benefits of speech–language pathology services to patients who have acquired communication disorders should not be overlooked. If brain damage is defined as a medical problem, there must be resources in that system to provide treatment for its communicative consequences.

Major Points of Chapter

- Stroke (cerebrovascular accident) is the most common cause of focal damage to the brain.
- Neurological symptoms reflect the location of the brain damage.
- Left brain damage and right brain damage produce very different linguistic and pragmatic problems.
- Theories of brain and language reflect the technology of the time.
- New communicative assessment tools are needed to keep up with current neuroimaging techniques.
- Treatment strategies focus on stimulating brain recovery, educating the patient and family, and improving functional communication.

Discussion Guidelines

1. Focal neurological damage and diffuse damage produce different patterns of language behavior. List three causes of each type of damage and describe the language behaviors that differentiate each type.
2. Locate an article by an author who criticizes the Boston Diagnostic Classification System. Summarize the argument presented, and, in a class discussion, indicate the reasons you agree or disagree with the author.
3. Develop a characterization of a typical patient at risk for stroke. Include a description of the patient's history, health, personality, and demographic and social characteristics. Compare your characterization with your classmates' characterization.

REFERENCES

Ackmajian, A., Demers, R. & Harnish, R. (1984) *Linguistics: An introduction to language and communication* (2nd ed.). Cambridge, MA: MIT Press.

Adamovich, B. L., & Brooks, R. (1981). A diagnostic protocol to assess the communication deficits of patients with right hemisphere damage. In R. H. Brookshire (Ed.), *Clinical aphasiology: Conference proceedings* (pp. 244–253) Minneapolis, MN: BRK.

Albert, M., & Obler, L. (1978). *The bilingual brain.* New York: Academic Press.

Alexander, M., & LoVerme, S. (1980) Aphasia after left hemisphere intracerebral hemorrhage. *Neurology, 3,* 1193–1202.

Aten, J. L. (1994). Functional communication treatment. In R. Chapey (Ed.), *Language intervention strategies in adult aphasia.* Baltimore, MD: Williams & Wilkins.

Benowitz, L., Moya, K., & Levine, D. (1990). Impaired verbal reasoning and constructional apraxia in subjects with right hemisphere damage. *Neuropsychologia, 28,* 231–241.

Berko-Gleason, J. B., Goodglass, H., Obler, L. K., Green, E., Hyde, M., & Weintraub, S. (1981). Narrative strategies of aphasic and normal speaking subjects. *Journal of Speech and Hearing Research, 23,* 370–382.

Berko-Gleason, J., & Ratner, N. B. (Eds.). (1993). *Psycholinguistics.* Ft. Worth, TX: Holt, Rinehart and Winston.

Blomert, L. (1990). What functional assessment can contribute to setting goals for aphasia therapy. *Aphasiology, 4,* 307–320.

Blonder, L., Bowers, D., & Heilman, K. (1991). The role of the right hemisphere in emotional communication, *Brain, 114,* 1115–1127.

Bloom, R. L., Borod, J. C., Haywood, C., Obler, L. K. & Pick, L. (1996). An examination of coherence and cohesion in aphasia. *International Journal of Neuroscience, 88,* 125–140.

Bloom, R. L., Borod, J. C., Obler, L. K., & Gerstman, L. J. (1992). Impact of emotional content on discourse production in patients with unilateral brain damage. *Brain and Language, 42,* 153–164.

Bloom, R. L., Borod, J. C., Obler, L. K., & Gerstman, L. J. (1993). Suppression and facilitation of pragmatic performance: Effects of emotional content on discourse following right and left brain damage. *Journal of Speech and Hearing Research, 36,* 1227–1235.

Bloom, R. L., Obler, L. K., DeSanti, S., & Ehrlich, J. (1994). *Discourse analysis and applications: Studies in adult clinical populations.* Hillsdale, NJ: Lawrence Erlbaum Associates.

Bonita, R. (1992). Epidemiology of stroke. *Lancet, 339*–320.

Borod, J. C. (1993). Cerebral mechanisms underlying facial, prosodic and lexical emotional expression: A review of neuropsychological studies and methodological issues. *Neuropsychology, 7*, 445–463.

Borod, J., Bloom, R., & Santschi-Haywood, C. (1996, in press). Lexical aspects of emotional communication. In Beeman, M. and Chiarello, C. (Eds). *Getting it right: The cognitive neuroscience of right brain damage.* Hillsdale, NJ: Lawrence Erlbaum Associates.

Borod, J. C., Koff, E., Lorch, M. P., & Nicholas, M. (1986). The expression and perception of facial emotion in brain-damaged patients. *Neuropsychologia, 24*, 169–180.

Brownell, H. H., Michel, D., Powelson, J., & Gardner, H. (1983). Surprise but not coherence: Sensitivity to verbal humor in right hemisphere patients. *Brain and Language, 18*, 20–27.

Brownell, H. H., Potter, H. H., Bihrle, A. M., & Gardner, H. (1986). Inference deficits in right brain-damged patients, *Brain and Language, 27*, 310–321.

Buck, R., & Duffy, R. J. (1981). Nonverbal communciation of affect in brain-damaged patients. *Cortex, 6*, 351–362.

Bud, D., Audet, T., & LeCours, A. (1990). Re-evaluating the effect of unilateral brain damage on simple reaction time to auditory stimulation. *Cortex, 26*, 227–237.

Burns, M. S., Halper, A. S., & Mogil, S. I. (1985). *Clinical management of right hemisphere dysfunction.* Rockville, MD: Aspen Publishers.

Caplan, D. (1987). *Neurolinguistics and linguistic aphasiology: An introduction.* New York: Cambridge University Press.

Caplan, D. (1990). Psycholinguistic assessment of language disorders. Paper presented at the annual convention of the American Speech-Language-Hearing Association.

Caramazza, A. (1984). The logic of neuropsychological research and the problem of patient classification in aphasia. *Brain and Language, 21*, 9–20.

Caselli, R., & Jack C. (1992). Asymmetric cortical degenerative syndromes: A proposed clinical classification. *Archives of Neurology, 49*, 770.

Chapey, R. (Ed). (1994). *Language intervention strategies in adult aphasia.* Baltimore, MD: Willams and Wilkins.

Chapman, S. D., & Ulatowska, H. K. (1994). Differential diagnosis in aphasia. In R. Chapey (Ed.), *Language intervention strategies in aphasia.* Baltimore, MD: Williams & Wilkins

Cicone, M., Wapner, W., & Gardner, H. (1980). Sensitivity to emotional expressions and situations in organic patients. *Cortex, 16*, 145–158.

Current Population Reports. (1990). *The Hispanic population in the United States: March 1990.* Washington, D.C.: Bureau of the Census.

Damasio, H. (1991). Cerebral localization of the aphasias. In Sarno, M. T. (Ed.). *Acquired Aphasia.* 2nd ed. New York: Academy.

Darley, F. L., Aronson, A. E., & Brown, J. E. (1975). *Motor speech disorders.* Philadephia: W.B. Saunders.

Davis, G. (1983). *A survey of adult aphasia.* Englewood Cliffs, NJ: Prentice Hall.

Davis, G. A., & Wilcox, M. J. (1985). *Adult aphasia rehabilitation: Applied pragmatics.* San Diego, CA: College Hill Press.

Diggs, C., & Basili, A. G. (1987). Verbal expression of right cerebrovascular accident patients: Convergent and divergent language. *Brain and Language, 30*, 130–146.

Fratteli, C. M. (1992). Functional assessment of communication: Merging public policy with clinical views. *Aphasiology, 6*, 63–83.

Gainotti, G. (1972). Emotional behavior and hemispheric side of lesion. *Cortex, 8*, 41–55.

Galin, D. (1976). The two modes of consciousness and the two halves of the brain. In P. Lee, R. Ornstein, D. Galin, A. Deikman, and C. Tart. (Eds.), *Symposium on consciousness.* New York: Penguin.

Geschwind, N. (1974). The development of the brain and the evolution of language. In N. Geschwind (Ed.), *Selected papers on language and the brain.* Dordrecht, Holland: D. Reidel.

Glosser, G., Weiner, M., & Kaplan, E. (1988). Variations in aphasic language behavior. *Journal of Speech and Hearing Disorders, 53*, 115–124.

Goodglass, H. (1981). The syndromes of aphasia. Similiarities and differences in neurolinguistic features. *Topics in Language Disorders, 1*, 1–14.

Goodglass, H., & Kaplan, E. (1983a). *The assessment of aphasia and related disorders.* Philadelphia: Lea and Febiger.

Goodglass, H., & Kaplan, E. (1983b). *Boston diagnostic aphasia examination.* Philadelphia: Lea and Febiger.

Hammons, J., & Swindell, C. (1987). Poststroke clinical depression: Neurologic, diagnostic and treatment implications. *ASHA, 29,* 115.

Heilman, K. M., Bowers, D., Speedie, L., & Coslett, H. B. (1984). Comprehension of affective and non-affective prosody. *Neurology, 34,* 917–921.

Heir, H., & Kaplan, J. (1980). Verbal comprehension deficits after right hemisphere damage. *Applied Psycholinguistics, 1,* 279–294.

Helm-Estabrooks, N., Fitzpatrick, P., & Barresi, B. (1982). Visual action therapy for global aphasia. *Journal of Speech and Hearing Disorders, 44,* 385–389.

Helm-Estabrooks, N., Nicholas, M., & Morgan, A. (1989). *Melodic intonation therapy program.* San Antonio, TX: Special Press.

Holland, A. (1980). *Communicative abilities of daily living.* Baltimore, MD: University Park Press.

Holland, A. (1982F). Observing functional communication in aphasic adults, *Journal of Speech and Hearing Disorders, 47,* 50–56.

Hough, M. (1990). Narrative comprehension in adults with right and left hemisphere brain-damage: Theme organization. *Brain and Language, 38,* 253–277.

Hough, M. S., Pierce, R. S., & Cannito, M. (1989). Contextual influences in aphasia: Effects of predictives versus nonpredictive narratives. *Brain and Language, 36,* 325–334.

Joanette, X., LeCours, A., LePage, Y., & Lamoureux, M. (1983). Language in right-handers with right hemisphere lesions: A preliminary study. *Brain & Language, 20,* 217–248.

Keough, K. (1990). Emerging issues for the professions in the 1990s. *Asha, 32,* 55–58.

Kimbarow, M. L.(1994). Interdisciplinary team intervention. In R. Chapey (Ed.), *Language intervention strategies in adult aphasia* (pp. 584–588). Baltimore, MD: Williams & Wilkins.

Lalande, S., Braun, C., Carlebois, N., & Whitaker, H. (1992). Effects of right and left cerebrovascular lesions on discrimination of prosodic and semantic aspects of affect in sentences. *Brain and Language, 42,* 165–186.

LaPointe, L. L. (1985). Aphasia therapy: Some principles and strategies for treatment. In D. F. Johns (Ed.), *Clinical management of neurogenic communicative disorders* (2nd ed.). Boston: Little, Brown and Company.

Lemme, M. (Ed.), *Clinical aphasiology* (Vol. 22). Austin, TX: Pro-Ed.

Lenneberg, E. (1967). *Biological foundations of language.* New York: Wiley.

Lubinski, R. (1981). Environmental language intervention. In R. Chapey (Ed.), *Language intervention strategies in adult aphasia.* Baltimore, MD: Williams and Wilkins.

Lyon, J. (1992). Communication use and participation in life for adults with aphasia in natural settings: The scope of the problem. *American Journal of Speech–Language Pathology, 1* (30), 7–14.

McNeil, M. R. (1982). The nature of aphasia inadults. In N. J. Lass, L. V. McReynolds, Northern, J. L., & Yoder, D. E. (Eds.), *Speech, language and hearing: Volume III: Pathologies of speech and language* (pp 692–740). Philadelphia: W. B. Saunders.

Mesulam, M. M. (1985). Attention, confusional states and neglect. In M. M. Mesulam (Ed.), *Principles of behavioral neurology* (pp. 125–168). Philadelphia: F. A. Davis.

Metter, E. J.. (1987). Neuroanatomy and physiology of aphasia: Evidence from positron emission tomography. *Aphasiology, 1,* 3–33.

Miliken, C. H., McDowell, F., & Easton, J. D. (1987). *Stroke.* Philadelphia: Lea and Febiger.

Murdoch, B., Kennedy, M., McCallum, W., & Siddle, K. (1991). Persistent aphasia following a purely subcortical lesion: A magnetic resonance imaging study. *Aphasiology, 5,* 183–197.

Myers, P. S. (1984). Right hemisphere impairment. In A. Holland (Ed.), *Language disorders in adults: Recent advances.* San Diego, CA: College Hill Press.

Myers, P. S. (1994). Communication disorders associated with right hemisphere brain damage. In R. Chapy (Ed.), *Language intervention strategies in adult aphasia* (pp. 513–534). Baltimore, MD: Williams and Wilkins.

Myers, P. S., & Brookshire, R. H. (1994). The effects of visual and inferential complexity on the picture descriptions of non-brain-damaged and right hemisphere-damaged adults. In M. Lemme (Ed.), *Clinical aphisiology* (Vol. 22). Austin, TX: ProEd.

Myers, P. S., & Linebaugh, C. W. (1981). Comprehension of idiomatic expressions by right hemisphere-damaged adults. In R. H. Brookshire (Ed.), *Clincial aphasiology: Conference proceedings* (pp. 254–261). Minneapolis, MN: BRK.

Myers, P. S., Linebaugh, C. W., & Mackisack, E. L. (1985). Extracting implicit meaning: Right versus left hemisphere damage. In R. H. Brookshire (Ed.),

Clincial aphasiology (Vol. 15), (pp. 72–82). Minneapolis, MN: BRK.

Naeser, M. A., Gaddie, A., Palumbo, C. L., & Shassny-Eder, D. (1990). Late recovery of auditory comprehension in global aphasia: Improved recovery with subcortical temporal isthmus lesion versus Wernicke's cortical area lesion. *Archives of Neurology, 47,* 425–432.

Naeser, M. A., Helm-Estabrooks, N., Haas, G., Auerback, S., & Srinivasan, M. (1987). Relationship between lesion extent in "Wernicke's area" on CT scan and predicting recovery of comprehension in Wernicke's Aphasia. *Archives of Neurology, 44,* 73–82.

Nelson, L., Cicchetti, D., Satz, P., Sowa, M., & Mitrushina, M. (1994). Emotional sequelae of stroke: A longitudinal perspective. *Journal of Clinical and Experimental Neuropsychology, 16,* 796–806.

Nelson, L., Cicchetti, D., Satz, P., Stern, S.,Sowa, M., & Cohen, S. (1993). Emotional sequelae of stroke. *Neuropsychology, 7,* 553–563.

Ojemann, G. (1979). Individual variability in cortical localization of language. *Journal of Neurosurgery, 50,* 164–169.

Otten, W., Teutsch, S., Williamson, D., & Marks, J. (1990). The effect of known risk factors on the excess mortality of Black adults in the United States. *Journal of the American Medical Association, 263,* 6, 845–850.

Paradis, M. (1977). Bilingualism and aphasia. In H. Whitaker and H. A. Whitaker (Eds.), *Studies in Neurolinguistics, Volume 3.* New York: Academic Press.

Penfield, W., & Roberts, L. (1959). *Speech and brain mechanisms.* Princeton, NJ: Princeton University Press.

Perecman, E. (Ed.) (1983). *Cognitive processing in the right hemisphere.* New York: Academic Press.

Prutting, C., & Kirchner, D. (1987). A clinical appraisal of the pragmatic aspects of language. *Journal of Speech and Hearing Disorders, 52,* 105–119.

Robinson, R., & Starkstein, S. (1990). Current research in affective disorders following stroke. *Journal of Neuropsychiatry, 2,* 1–14.

Rosenbek, J. C., LaPointe, L. L., & Wertz, R. T. (1989). *Aphasia: A clinical approach.* Austin, TX: Pro-Ed.

Ross, E. D., & Mesulam, M. (1979). Dominant language functions of the right hemisphere: Prosody and emotional gesturing. *Archives of Neurology, 36,* 561–569.

Sackeim, H., Greenberg, M. Weiman, A., Gur, R., & Hungerbuhler, J. (1982). Functional brain asymmetry in the expression of positive and negative emotions: Lateralization of insult in cases of uncontrollable emotional outbursts. *Archives of Neurology, 19,* 210–218.

Sarno, M. T. (1981). Analyzing aphasic behaviour. In Sarno, M. and Hook, O. (Eds.) *Aphasia: Assessment and treatment.* New York: Masson.

Satz, P. and Bullard-Bates, C. (1981). Aquired aphasia. In Sarno, M. (Ed.) *Acquired aphasia.* NY: Academic Press.

Scheull, H. M., Jenkins, J., & Jimenez-Pabor, E. (1964). *Aphasia in adults.* New York: Harper and Row.

Searlman, A. (1977). A review of right hemisphere linguistic capabilities. *Psychological Bulletin, 84,* 503–528.

Shewan, C. M., & Bandur, D. L. (1986). *Treatment of aphasia: A language-oriented approach.* Austin, TX: Pro-Ed.

Tanner, D. C. (1980). Loss and grief: Implications for the speech-language pathologist and audiologist. *ASHA, 22,* 916–928.

Thorngren, M., & Westling, B. (1990). Rehabilitation and achieved health quality after stroke. A population-based study of 258 hospitalized cases followed for one year. *Acta Neurological Scandinavia, 82,* 374–380.

Tompkins, C. A. (1991). Redundancy enhances emotional inferencing by right- and left-hemisphere-damaged adults. *Journal of Speech and Hearing Research. 34,* 1142–1149.

Ulatowska, H., Freedman-Stern, R., Doyel, A., Macaluso-Haynes, S., & North, A. (1983). Production of narrative discourse in aphasia. *Brain and Language, 19,* 317–334.

Ulatowska, H., North, A., & Macaluso-Haynes, S. (1981). Production of narrative and procedural disocurse in aphasia. *Brain and Language, 13,* 345–371.

Wallace, G., & Freeman, S. (1991). Adults with neurological impairment from multicultural populations. *ASHA, 33,* 58–60.

Wepman, J. M. (1976). Aphasia: Language without thought or thought without language. *ASHA, 18,* 131–136.

West, J. F. (1983). Heightening visual imagery: A new approach to aphasia therapy. In E. Perecman (Ed.), *Cognitive processing in the right hemisphere.* New York: Academic Press.

Winner, E., & Gardner, H. (1977). The comprehension of metaphor in brain damaged patients. *Brain, 100,* 719–727.

Yorkston, K. M., & Beukelman, D. R. (1980). An analysis of connected speech samples of aphasic and normal speaker. *Journal of Speech and Hearing Disorders, 45,* 27–36.

Zraich, R., & Boone, D. (1991). Spouse attitude toward the person with aphasia. *Journal of Speech and Hearing Research, 34*:1, 123–128.

Zurif, E. B., & Caramazza, A. (1976). Psycholinguistic structures in aphasia. In H. Whitaker and H. A. Whitaker (Eds.) *Studies in neurolinguistics* (Vol. 1). New York: Academic Press.

NEUROMOTOR SPEECH DISORDERS

RONALD L. BLOOM AND CAROLE T. FERRAND

S peech is both a sensory and a motor process that requires complex neural integration and rapid coordination of several physiological systems. These systems include respiration, phonation, resonation, and articulation. Speech can be considered as the oral–motor correlate of language processing. Whereas language is a symbolic and social process, speech is a neuromotor and sensory process. When any of the underlying structural or physiological components of speech processing are disrupted through injury or disease, there are certain predictable consequences. Thus, diagnosis and treatment of motor speech disorders requires that the basic mechanisms underlying speech processing be understood.

This chapter will focus on current conceptualizations of neuromotor speech disorders (i.e., apraxia and the dysarthrias) in children and adults. A brief review of the neurology of motor speech behavior is presented to provide an understanding of normal speech motor control. A distinction is then drawn between psycholinguistic and neuroanatomical models of speech motor function. An extension of the traditional approach (Darley, Aronson, & Brown, 1975) for classifying motor speech disorders will be presented. Measures of acoustic and physiologic speech function will be used to supplement the traditional classification system.

Acoustic measures are those that characterize aspects of the vocal signal produced by the larynx, such as frequency, intensity, and duration. Physiological methods focus on how the speech structures move in isolation and in relationship to other structures. This work has provided a foundation for an approach to motor speech that examines aspects of the disorders with respect to where in the neurologic system the damage can be localized. Using this approach, the examining speech–language pathologist may determine if a patient's motor speech behavior is consistent with the neurological diagnosis. Subsequently, some of the diseases that accompany motor speech disorders across the lifespan will be introduced, including the etiology and symptomatology for the different speech systems. Lastly, contemporary approaches to assessment and treatment of these problems in children and adults are discussed.

Neuromotor speech disorders may be caused by damage to the motor control centers in either the central or peripheral nervous system, resulting in an inability to regulate the movements of the speech musculature. The two major categories of motor speech disorders are **apraxia** and **dysar-**

thria. Apraxia refers to a problem in the coordination of movements that generate sequences of speech sounds. In apraxia, the neuromuscular structures themselves are intact, and the problem is in higher level, cortical and subcortical areas that are responsible for organizing the muscular events involved in articulating speech. By contrast, dysarthria includes those speech disorders that result from damage to the nerves and/or muscles. These problems can manifest themselves as weakness or incoordination in the respiratory, phonatory, or articulatory systems. The term dysarthria refers to a partial disturbance in motor speech, while the term anarthria designates a complete lack of speech due to severe motor involvement.

THE NEUROLOGY OF SPEECH MOTOR BEHAVIOR

Production of speech requires the complex interaction of cortical, subcortical, and peripheral levels of the nervous system. The **Central Nervous System (CNS)** includes the cerebral cortex, cerebrum, subcortical structures including the basal nuclei, the brainstem (pons, medulla, and midbrain), the cerebellum, and the spinal cord. The **Peripheral Nervous System (PNS)** includes the cranial and spinal nerves.

The Cerebral Cortex

The **cerebral cortex** contains motor and sensory areas that are important in skilled voluntary movement. The cortical motor area in the frontal lobe plans and sequences the organization of motor activity. It functions by continually transmitting and receiving updated information on motor and sensory activity from various other cortical and subcortical areas.

Critical to this process is the area of the cortex known as the **primary motor cortex** (or **motor strip**). This area is located on the **precentral gyrus** of the frontal lobe in both the left and right hemispheres. Neurons in the lower portion of the motor strip control the tongue and larynx on the opposite (contralateral) side of the body. Because the tongue and larynx require an extraordinary degree of fine, rapid motor coordination, they have an enormous amount of cortical area dedicated to their functioning. The **premotor area** lies just in front of the motor strip, and is believed to supplement the functioning of the motor strip by integrating and refining oral motor output. This premotor cortex also participates in reasoning and planning. The **supplementary motor cortex** is located on the middle surface of the frontal lobe. The premotor cortex and supplementary cortex receive input from the occipital, parietal, and temporal lobes and pass this information on to the primary motor cortex. An important area that is located only in one hemisphere (usually the left) is **Broca's area.** This area lies at the lower end of the frontal lobe, slightly in front of the motor strip. Broca's area has long been considered the classic motor programming and planning area for speech. The **insula** is a small section of cortex buried within the cerebral hemispheres. Recently, it has been implicated in certain types of apraxic disorders. Motor pathways of the nervous system descend from these cortical motor areas to connect with subcortical and peripheral levels of the nervous system. These pathways include both the direct and indirect fiber tracts.

The Direct Motor System

The direct system is subdivided into the **corticobulbar** and **corticospinal** tracts. The corticobulbar pathway arises from the motor strip and premotor area and extends to the medulla. It is critical to motor speech activity because it directly affects the cranial nerves that control the oral mechanism. The corticospinal pathway arises from the sensorimotor areas of the cortex and descends directly to the spinal cord. Note that the fibers of this pathway, unlike those of the corticobulbar tract, cross over (decussate) to the opposite side of the body in the medulla. Thus, the left side of the corticospinal tract controls movement on the right side of the body, and vice versa. The corticobulbar and corticospinal tracts are concerned with skilled movement, and together, integrate and transmit

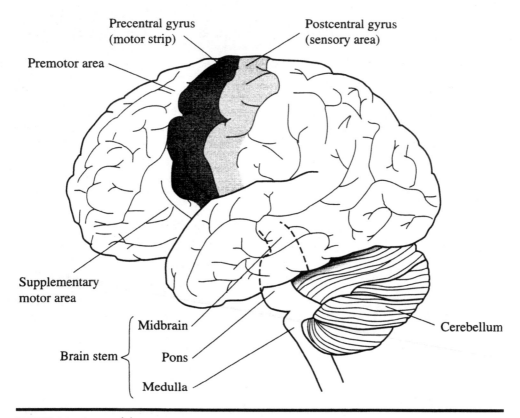

Precentral gyrus
(motor strip)

Postcentral gyrus
(sensory area)

Premotor area

Supplementary
motor area

Brain stem

Midbrain

Pons

Medulla

Cerebellum

FIGURE 8.1   Areas of the cortex.

information from higher brain centers to the brainstem and spinal cord.

The Indirect Motor System

The indirect motor system is made up of the **basal nuclei** and the **cerebellum,** and their many interconnections. This system significantly affects movement by regulating and coordinating the neural impulses of the motor and premotor cortex. The basal nuclei are comprised of collections of nerve cells deep within the white matter of the cerebrum. One important part of the basal nuclei is the **corpus striatum.** This serves as the major receiving area for motor impulses from the cortex and other subcortical structures. Another important section of the basal nuclei is the **globus pallidus.** This serves as a transmitter of motor signals,

and plays a role in coordinating motor activity with the cerebral cortex. Another component, the **substantia nigra,** is thought to be involved in the manufacture of a chemical neurotransmitter called **dopamine,** which is important in maintaining an appropriate degree of muscle tone.

The cerebellum is located directly behind the cerebrum. As Darley, Aronson, and Brown (1975) noted, its primary function is to impose control upon posture and other types of movement that it does not, itself, initiate. The cerebellum functions as an error control device by comparing motor output from the motor cortex with sensory signals from joints and muscles. The cerebellum is furnished with information concerning all levels of motor activity, and thus is an integrating center for coordinated movement, muscle tone and strength, and regulation of posture and position of the body.

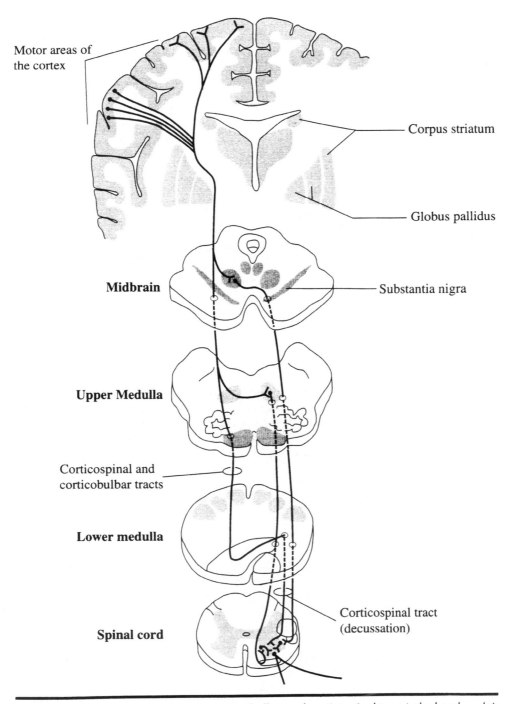

Motor areas of
the cortex

Corpus striatum

Globus pallidus

Midbrain

Substantia nigra

Upper Medulla

Corticospinal and
corticobulbar tracts

Lower medulla

Corticospinal tract
(decussation)

Spinal cord

FIGURE 8.2   The direct motor system (corticolbulbar and corticospinal tracts); the basal nuclei (corpus striatum, globus pallidus, substantia nigra), and adjacent structures.

There is some speculation that speech functions may be more precisely localized in the cerebellum (Gilman, Bloedel, & Lechtenberg, 1981).

The brainstem consists of the pons, medulla, and midbrain. These areas are where the cranial nerves originate, in various nerve cell bodies. The brainstem receives signals from the direct and indirect systems as well as from the spinal cord. It helps to regulate muscle tone and posture, and to control oral motor functions important to speech production. In addition, the brainstem contributes to the control of various respiratory activities.

The spinal cord extends from the base of the skull to the lower back, and is protected by the vertebrae. It is important in regulating many reflexes common in motor activity, including speech. Thirty-one pairs of spinal nerves are attached to the spinal cord at various levels. It is through these nerves that the spinal cord relays sensory information to the cerebrum and transmits motor information from the CNS to the muscles. Similar to the cortex, the spinal cord contains both white and gray matter. The white matter consists of nerve pathways, while the gray matter contains nerve cell bodies.

All neurons of the direct and indirect systems which descend from the cortex via the brainstem to the medulla and spinal cord are known as the **upper motor neuron.**

The Peripheral Nervous System

The peripheral nervous system, consisting of both cranial and spinal nerves, is also known as the **lower motor neuron.** This system can be conceptualized as a summary of the complex integration of the nerve signals from the direct, indirect, and cerebellar pathways and centers. It is known as the final common pathway, because impulses are transmitted by way of the peripheral nerves to activate the muscles of the body so movement may be accomplished.

Cranial Nerves. The nuclei of the cranial nerves receive impulses from the cerebral cortex by way of the corticobulbar tract. Innervation is bilateral for most of the cranial nerve nuclei. In other words, most of the cell bodies of the cranial nerves receive signals from both the right and the left corticobulbar tract. This is an important point because if there is damage to the corticobulbar tract on one side only, the associated cranial nerve (with just three exceptions) will receive impulses from the unaffected corticobulbar tract on the other side. This means that speech production will not be particularly affected. However, if there is unilateral damage to the corticobulbar tract at a point where it is associated with a cranial nerve that receives impulses from only one side, the effects on speech production will be much more severe.

There are 12 pairs of cranial nerves (CNs), of which seven pairs are directly involved in speech production. The cranial nerves provide essential motor and sensory information to the muscles of phonation, articulation, and resonation, and are therefore crucial for speech production. Those cranial nerves important for speech include CN V (trigeminal), which is responsible for mastication and for sensation to the face. This nerve also provides impulses to an important velar muscle, the tensor veli palatini, which is involved in flattening and tensing the soft palate, and opening the auditory tube. Innervation is bilateral. CN VII (facial) is an exceptionally important nerve for speech because it is responsible for all movements of the face (Love & Webb, 1992). The nerve innervates muscles that permit wrinkling of the forehead, closing the mouth, as well as allowing the corners of the mouth to be pulled back and down. The upper part of the face is innervated bilaterally, while the lower part has ipsilateral (same side) innervation. CN VII also innervates the stapedius muscle of the middle ear. CN VIII (vestibuloacoustic) conducts sensory information from the inner ear to the cortex. It is responsible for inner ear structures that control sensitivity to changes in equilibrium. CN IX (glossopharyngeal) contains motor fibers that contribute to the function of the pharyngeal muscles. This nerve is involved in palatal

TABLE 8.1 Cranial Nerves Important in Speech Production

| | | FUNCTIONS | |
NUMBER	NAME	SENSORY	MOTOR
V	Trigeminal	face, jaw, mouth	jaw, soft palate
VII	Facial	taste, mucous membrane of soft palate and pharynx	face, lips
VIII	Acoustic	hearing, balance	
IX	Glossopharyngeal	taste, mucous membrane of pharynx, middle ear, and mouth	pharynx
X	Vagus	mucous membrane of pharynx, larynx, soft palate, tongue, lungs	larynx, pharynx
XI	Spinal-Accessory		soft palate, larynx, pharynx, neck
XII	Hypoglossal	tongue	tongue

movement, swallowing, and salivation. It innervates muscles responsible for elevating the larynx and pharynx, and widening the pharynx to receive food (Love & Webb, 1992). Innervation is bilateral. CN X (vagus) has bilateral innervation, and transmits signals to muscles with many different functions, including the heart, respiratory system, digestive system, palatal muscles, and intrinsic laryngeal muscles. Thus, it is responsible for much of laryngeal function as well as soft palate movement. CN XI (spinal accessory) also receives bilateral information from the corticobulbar tracts. The primary function of this nerve is to innervate muscles involved in moving the head (e.g., sternocleidomastoid muscle). Finally, CN XII (hypoglossal) provides impulses to the muscles that regulate tongue movement, including the intrinsic muscles of the tongue that control shortening, narrowing, elongating, and flattening of the tongue, and the extrinsic muscles that allow the tongue to be protruded, retracted, and depressed. This nerve receives impulses from both corticobulbar pathways, except for those nerve cells sending information to the genioglossus muscle of the tongue, which receives only contralateral fibers (Love & Webb, 1992).

Spinal Nerves. The 31 pairs of spinal nerves project to the muscles of the body excluding the face and neck, which, as discussed, are innervated by the cranial nerves. Innervation from the spinal nerves is contralateral. Corticospinal fibers project mainly to the opposite side of the body. Therefore, damage to one side of the brain will result in paralysis of the opposite side of the body.

The Motor Unit

The concept of the **motor unit** is important to understand, as motor units provide the interface between the nervous system and the peripheral muscles and structures used for speech and other types of movement. A motor unit consists of the nerve cell body located either in the spinal cord (for spinal nerves) or in the brainstem nuclei (for cranial nerves). It also includes the nerve axon or pathway that leads from the neuron to the point where it forms a junction with muscle tissue. This junction is known as a **synapse,** across which nerve impulses must travel to reach the muscle fibers that form the last component of this unit. At the neuromuscular junction, a neurochemical transmitter (e.g., **acetylcholine**) is released in

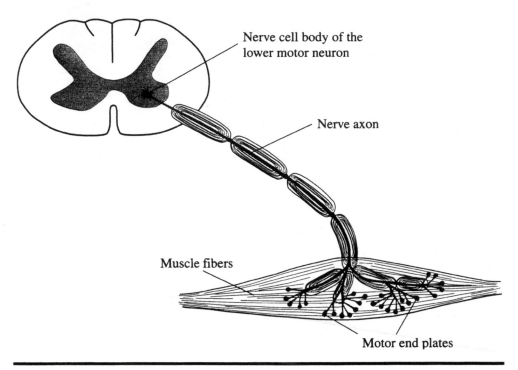

Nerve cell body of the
lower motor neuron

Nerve axon

Muscle fibers

Motor end plates

FIGURE 8.3   Components of the motor unit.

order to facilitate the nerve impulse reaching the muscle from the peripheral nerve.

MODELS OF MOTOR SPEECH DISORDERS

There are two general frameworks for conceptualizing motor speech disorders: neuropsychological and neuroanatomical. These models distinguish types of disorders and describe where the breakdown in processing may have occurred.

Neuropsychological Models

Basically, neuropsychological models look at motor control as a series of processing levels culminating in the execution of the speech movement. The first psychological processing level is an *ideational* one, characterized by the generation of thoughts and feelings, and the desire to express them to a listener. Following is the *language planning* level, during which semantic and syntactic knowledge is used to place utterances into linguistic segments such as syllables and words. The next levels include *motor planning* and *programming* of speech movements. Generally speaking, planning refers to the selection of specific phonemes and their placement into these linguistic segments. Programming describes the stage in which the selected phonemes are transformed into neuromuscular commands. Rate of speech, prosodic patterns, stress, and accent are incorporated into the speech motor signal at this level. Finally, these stages culminate in the actual *execution* of speech. It is important to note that auditory, tactile, and proprioceptive feedback helps to coordinate this process at any of its many levels.

Envisioning the speech production process as a series of levels is useful in differentiating between different kinds of disorders. For instance, when there is widespread neural damage that affects the highest cognitive level, the person may demonstrate a general intellectual impairment, or some form of dementia. (For a thorough description of the dementias, see Chapter 5.) At the language planning level, for example, focal damage to the left hemisphere of the brain may result in aphasia. (For a discussion of aphasia, see Chapter 7.)

Apraxia is thought to be a disturbance at the motor planning stage of speech motor control resulting from damage to various structures in the language dominant hemisphere; for example, Broca's area, the insula, or the supplementary motor cortex. Dysarthria is considered to occur at the later stages of motor programming, in the motor execution level of speech processing. Damage to any of the peripheral or sensory feedback mechanisms may also result in dysarthria.

The Neuroanatomical Model

Neuroanatomical conceptualizations of the motor speech system have been quite useful as a guide to classifying the major types of motor speech disorders. The premise of this classification system is that the speech behaviors of patients with motor speech disorders are consistent with the neurological site of damage. The work of Darley, Aronson, and Brown (1975) at the Mayo Clinic revolutionized the way speech–language pathologists conceptualized motor speech disorders. Darley, et al. outlined an approach to classification that linked damage to a particular area of the nervous system to the resulting speech characteristics. They obtained speech samples of individuals who were diagnosed as having a particular type of neurologic disorder. Based on perceptual ratings of the phonatory, articulatory, and resonatory dimensions of the samples, they determined that each of these diagnostic groups demonstrated a fairly unique pattern of deviant speech characteristics. Following is a description of this sytem, identifying the site of the lesion and the type of disorder associated with the damage. The system of classification used in this chapter has been modified from the original work of Darley et al. (1975).

Apraxia of Speech. Apraxia of speech is a motor speech disorder that is distinct from the dysar-

thrias. Apraxia is a disturbance in planning and programming the sensory and motor commands required for speech sound production. Dysarthria, by contrast, is a weakness in the muscles or an inability to control aspects of the neuromuscular execution of speech. Apraxia of speech is not a loss of the ability to perform the movements of speech, nor is it a deficit in understanding the instructions required to complete such a task. Apraxia of speech is an inability to produce volitional speech, either to command or imitation, despite the fact that automatic speech tasks such as counting or reciting may be performed without error. Apraxia of speech is caused almost exclusively by focal damage to the left side of the brain. It frequently coexists with aphasia, dysarthria, or both. Lesions causing apraxia of speech may be located in the left frontal lobe, the parietal lobe, the basal nuclei, or the insula. Degenerative central nervous system disease, trauma, or tumor, are other possible etiologies. Apraxia of speech may occur with other signs of left brain damage, but it may also appear as an isolated syndrome.

Some patients with apraxia of speech also demonstrate limb apraxia. Limb apraxia refers to deficits in performing volitional movements of nonparalyzed fingers, wrists, elbows, and shoulders. It is critical to examine for limb apraxia, because it may interfere with alternate communication modalities such as writing or gesturing.

Apraxia of speech varies in severity. In severe cases a speaker may produce a limited number of intelligible words or phrases. In moderate cases the speaker may be able to produce words and some sentences but with great effort. Prominent characteristics of apraxia of speech include trial and error searching articulation attempts, speech initiation difficulty, disfluency, and inconsistent speech production errors. Acoustic studies have documented lengthy pause times and increases in vowel and consonant production rates. Further, acoustic studies have shown that individuals with apraxia of speech work toward approximating the correct articulatory position across successive trials (Rosenbek, 1985). This finding has supported the notion that apraxia is a motor disorder, not a linguistic one (McNeil & Kent, 1990). Physiologic measures have consistently demonstrated variable lip, tongue, jaw, and velar movement in apraxic speech (McNeil, Caliguiri, & Rosenbek, 1989).

A distinction needs to be made between apraxia of speech in adults and the childhood form of the disorder, often labeled development apraxia of speech. There is no clear neurologic explanation or cause associated with developmental apraxia of speech as there is for apraxia of speech in adults. Thus, use of developmental apraxia of speech as a diagnostic category has been quite controversial. However, many researchers and clinicians suggest that if a child exhibits difficulty in producing speech gestures when automatic and vegetative movements of the same muscles are unimpaired, a diagnosis of developmental apraxia of speech should be considered. These are children whose speech sound productions vary greatly across tasks, making it difficult to determine which phonological rules they have mastered, and which they have not. Some research suggests that developmental apraxia of speech may be accompanied by deficits in auditory processing, language development, and cognition. Therefore, developmental apraxia of speech appears to be a heterogeneous disorder that may exist by itself or may be accompanied by other neurological signs or language disorders.

The Dysarthrias.   Six major neuroanatomical categories of dysarthrias, which are distinguished from apraxia of speech, are presented. Beginning with the site of the lesion, the discussion then focuses on the perceptual, acoustic, and physiological characteristics of each type of dysarthria. Examples of clinical disorders that exemplify the type of dysarthria are presented.

Lower Motor Neuron Disease: Flaccid Dysarthria.   Lower motor neuron (LMN) diseases refer to those diseases affecting cranial or spinal nerves or the motor unit itself. Recall that the motor unit is composed of a number of components. These include the cell bodies (nuclei) of the cranial and spinal nerves, innervating the structures

involved in motor speech production, the axons of these nerves, the junction between the nerves and the muscle fibers, and the muscle fibers themselves. Damage to any of these components can result in flaccid dysarthria characterized by a weakness in any one or a combination of the speech subsystems, including respiration, phonation, articulation, and resonation. The main symptom is lack of muscle tone resulting in weakness or paralysis of affected muscles. Duffy (1995) has summarized some of the acoustic and physiological observations typically found in flaccid dysarthria. At the respiratory level, the weakness may show itself in reduced vital capacity (the total amount of air one is able to exhale), abnormal movements of the thoracic cavity, and shallow breathing. These respiratory symptoms can reduce the breath support necessary for normal speech. At the laryngeal level, muscle weakness may be evident in weakness or paralysis of the vocal folds, resulting in a breathy voice or even aphonia. Pitch and loudness levels may be reduced, and the person may sound hoarse. The person may also sound monotonous, and be unable to modify loudness appropriately. In terms of resonation, there may be weakness of the soft palate (velum), resulting in hypernasality. Damage to the articulatory structures can lead to lack of tongue and lip strength, causing a lack of precision in forming the sounds of speech.

A disorder in which there is damage to the cell body of a cranial nerve is Moebius syndrome. Moebius syndrome, also called congenital facial diplegia, results from hypoplasia (lack of tissue development) of brainstem nuclei. This problem with the cell bodies causes bilateral paralysis of CN VI (Abducens) and CN VII (Facial). The bilateral damage can cause complete or partial paralysis of the facial muscles, which may often be accompanied by eye muscle weakness. The tongue may or may not be involved. Speech intelligibility ranges from extremely poor to mildly impaired, with many individuals showing good compensatory strategies for improving their articulation. For instance, if the lips are paralyzed so that bilabial sounds are impaired, an individual

TABLE 8.2 The Dysarthrias

TYPE	SITE OF LESION	EXAMPLE OF DISEASE
Flaccid	Lower motor neuron; motor unit	Moebius syndrome, Bell's palsy, Myasthenia gravis
Mild-Moderate Spastic	Unilateral upper motor neuron	Unilateral stroke
Severe Spastic	Bilateral upper motor neuron	Multiple strokes, Degenerative diseases (e.g., primary lateral sclerosis)
Ataxic	Cerebellum	Friedrich's ataxia
Extrapyrmidal: Hyperkinetic	Basal nuclei	Huntington's chorea, Dystonias
Extrapyrmidal: Hypokinetic	Basal nuclei	Parkinson's disease
Mixed	Multiple systems	Amyotrophic lateral sclerosis (ALS), Multiple sclerosis (MS)

with a functioning tongue may substitute lingua alveolar for bilabial sounds (e.g., /n/ for /m/) with good results.

Several diseases can affect the nerve axons themselves. Guillain-Barre syndrome is a disease in which paralysis occurs after the person has suffered some kind of viral infection. Most commonly the facial nerve (CN VII) is involved (Love, 1992), but impairment of CN IX and CN X has also been reported (Love, 1992). In addition, muscles of respiration may be weakened. Approximately 65 percent of individuals with this syndrome recover completely.

Facial palsy (Bell's palsy) is a disorder in which CN VII (Facial) is affected either unilaterally or bilaterally. With severe unilateral paralysis the entire face on the affected side sags. The eye on the affected side stays open and the mouth is drawn toward the normal side. The mouth may also droop on the impaired side, and the person may drool. In a less severe case the person may be able to blink, but slowly and incompletely, and the affected corner of the mouth does not move completely when the person smiles. If other cranial nerves are involved, such as those that provide nerve impulses to the muscles of the eye, the patient may also demonstrate other symptoms such as ptosis (drooping of the upper eyelids).

The neuromuscular junction may be the site of damage resulting in flaccid dysarthria. The most typical example of this kind of problem is

myasthenia gravis (MG). Myasthenia gravis is a relatively common disorder affecting the neuromuscular junction of the motor unit. In this disease there is a rapid weakening of muscles due to difficulty in transmitting the nerve impulse into the muscle itself. The disease may be focal, and affect localized groups of muscles such as the laryngeal muscles, or it may be more generalized. Frequently, the velar muscles are affected. A remarkable characteristic of this disease, and one which is often used diagnostically, is the speed with which the muscles regain their strength after a short rest interval. Thus, an individual with MG affecting the laryngeal and velar muscles will begin an utterance sounding fairly normal, but voice and resonance qualities will deteriorate within a few seconds. The person is likely to become increasingly hoarse and breathy, low-pitched, and hypernasal, during the course of the utterance. However, after a short break, the next utterance will once again start out by being clear and strong, and again will rapidly deteriorate.

Finally, the muscles themselves may be affected by various neurologic diseases. These diseases are the muscular dystrophies (MD), of which the most common is Duchenne MD. This is the most severe type of MD, and affects mostly young boys (Love, 1992). Onset is usually between the ages of 2 to 5, and the disease progresses rapidly, with few affected individuals surviving beyond their early 20s. The disease is characterized by muscle weakness, which typically starts in the muscles of the pelvis and trunk and progresses to all of the skeletal muscles. The weakness is caused by a lack of protein that helps to activate muscle contractions (Love, 1992). Lack of protein eventually leads to the destruction of the muscle cells, with corresponding loss of muscle strength. However, the person looks like they have large muscles, because the muscle fibers are replaced by fat and connective tissue. As the disease progresses, the subsystems of speech (respiration, phonation, and articulation) become increasingly involved, and the person may develop flaccid dysarthria.

Another kind of MD is myotonic dystrophy, which manifests itself in adolescence or adulthood. This disease is characterized by the inability to rapidly relax a contracted muscle. The limbs may be affected, as may the eye, facial, and pharyngeal muscles. An often noted characteristic of a person with this MD is the long, thin, expressionless face, together with drooping eyelids (ptosis), and an open bite. Hypernasality has been reported as a primary dysarthric problem in this disease.

There are many different diseases and conditions associated with damage to the lower motor neuron. A relatively common problem is vocal fold paralysis, due to damage to CN X. (See Chapter 11 for an in-depth discussion of vocal fold paralysis).

Unilateral Upper Motor Neuron Disease: Mild-Moderate Spastic Dysarthria. Recently, a distinction has been made between unilateral (UUMN) and bilateral upper motor neuron (BUMN) disease (Duffy, 1995). The upper motor neurons transmit nerve impulses to the cranial and spinal nerves that supply the speech musculature. Half of the upper motor neuron system originates in the left side of the brain and half originates in the right. Damage to the upper motor neuron system on one side of the brain can produce a distinct form of dysarthria. Stroke is the most common cause of UUMN damage, but focal trauma or a tumor confined to one side of the brain can also cause this type of dysarthria.

UUMN dysarthria is characterized by a mild or moderate articulation disorder that is often temporary. It is often difficult to distinguish this dysarthria from other disorders associated with unilateral brain damage. With left brain damage, UUMN dysarthria may co-occur with aphasia or apraxia. With right brain damage, UUMN dysarthria may accompany cognitive disorders or deficits in prosody.

UUMN dysarthria reflects the effects of weakness of the side of the face and tongue opposite the side of the lesion. In the early stages after onset, drooling, chewing, and swallowing difficulty are frequently reported. Hemiplegia or hemiparesis on the side of the body contralateral to the side of lesion is very common. Speech is characterized by imprecise consonant production, slowed rate, and a reduction in rapid alternating movements of the articulators. Voice quality is frequently reported as harsh (Duffy, 1995).

A limited number of studies have examined the acoustic and physiological characteristics of UUMN dysarthria. An electromyographic (EMG) study confirmed lower facial weakness and unilateral jaw weakness in patients with UUMN dysarthria (Hartman & Abbs, 1992). Acoustic measures matched perceptual ratings and further documented slow and abnormal irregular articulatory movements (Hartman & Abbs, 1992).

Bilateral Upper Motor Neuron Disease: Severe Spastic Dysarthria. The Upper Motor Neuron (UMN) includes the corticobulbar and corticospinal tracts. Together these tracts are known as the direct motor system. The corticobulbar pathway directs nerve impulses from the cortex to the cell bodies of the various cranial nerves; the corticospinal tract relays signals from the cortex to the cell bodies of the spinal nerves. From the cell bodies of the cranial and spinal nerves, the impulses are transmitted via the lower motor neuron to the appropriate muscles. As previously mentioned, the corticobulbar and corticospinal tracts mediate skilled and discrete voluntary movements, including those of speech. Innervation from the tracts to the muscles involved in speech production is bilateral.

The indirect system is also considered part of the UMN. Recall that this system includes the basal nuclei and the cerebellum, as well as the multiple connections between them. This is an inhibitory system, which helps in the fine tuning and regulating of movements initiated in the cortex.

While the UMN is composed of two separate motor systems, each serving a somewhat different function of movement control, damage to the UMN usually is manifested in both systems, due to their proximity in the CNS. Damage to the direct motor system results in weakness and loss of fine motor skills, while damage to the indirect system leads to increased muscle tone, hyperactive reflexes, and spasticity (Duffy, 1995). Affected structures will demonstrate a reduction in range of motion and slowness of movements.

Many different kinds of lesions or injury to the UMN can cause spastic dysarthria, as long as the damage is bilateral. For instance, a single stroke somewhere in the cerebral hemisphere, where the right and left UMN pathways are not close together, will not produce a severe spastic dysarthria. However, a single stroke in the brainstem, where the right and left UMN tracts are close together, can affect both sides and result in spastic dysarthria. Sometimes, an individual suffers from multiple strokes, which, over time, can affect the UMN bilaterally, resulting in spastic dysarthria. Inflammatory diseases such as leukoencephalitis can affect the UMN, as can degenerative diseases such as primary lateral sclerosis. Traumatic brain injury is another cause of spastic dysarthria.

Speech production in an individual with spastic dysarthria tends to be slow, effortful, jerky, and laborious. The voice quality is often harsh and tense, so much so that this kind of quality is called "strained-strangled." A characteristic symptom of this disorder is uncontrollable laughter and crying without any underlying emotion.

Cerebellar Disease: Ataxic Dysarthria. Ataxic dysarthria (AD) is associated with damage to the cerebellar system. Duffy (1995) notes that AD primarily reflects a breakdown in motor organization and control, rather than an impairment at the execution level like the other dysarthria types. AD is an impairment in the coordination of movement that may affect any of the speech subsystems. The most salient speech characteristics of AD are articulatory inaccuracy, prosodic excess characterized by inappropriate loudness modulation, and poor pitch control.

Across the lifespan numerous etiologies have been associated with cerebellar disease and AD. In children, congenital ataxia is a major classification of cerebral palsy, although the incidence of ataxia is substantially lower than it is for spasticity or athetosis (Hardy, 1983). In adults, there are several degenerative diseases that occur more frequently with AD than with other types of dysarthria. AD may appear as the first presenting sign of a neurologic disorder, or it may appear among other changes associated with a particular disease. Degenerative diseases that are largely confined to the cerebellum and nearby structures are likely to cause AD. For instance, Friedrich's ataxia is an inherited fatal disease that typically begins before adolescence and progresses gradually for about 20 years, finally resulting in death. Because it is a metabolic disease, it not only affects the cerebellum, but other brain structures as well. Thus, the speech characteristics of Friedrich's ataxia are associated primarily with AD, but may also include some spastic components (Joanette & Dudley, 1980).

Vascular damage to the cerebellum or cerebellar pathways, such as a cerebellar hemorrhage or occlusion, may also result in AD. Brain tumors within the cerebellum, or which exert a physical pressure upon the cerebellum, may also cause cerebellar signs. In addition, toxic levels of certain prescription drugs such as anticonvulsants or lithium may also produce cerebellar damage (Judd, 1991). Ataxic speech may result from acute alcohol abuse, but permanent dysarthria in chronic alcoholism is not common (Gilman, Bloedel, & Lechtenberg, 1981). Cerebellar signs may appear with malnutrition and vitamin deficiencies.

AD often co-occurs with nonspeech signs of cerebellar disease including decomposition of movement, **dysmetria,** and **dyssynergia.** Decomposition of movement refers to disruptions in producing smooth sequenced and regulated actions, resulting in quick, jerky, and irregular movements. Dysmetria is the inability to gauge the distance and speed of movements. As a result, the person is often unable to estimate the appropriate distance and speed required to carry out a movement, such as reaching for an object. Dyssynergia is characterized by deficits in performing rapid alternating repetitive movements. Prominent characteristics of cerebellar lesions include an irregular stance and a broad-based, high-stepping, awkward gait. Abnormal eye movement (i.e., rapid oscillations or **nystagmus**) often accompanies cerebellar disease.

Acoustic studies have documented elevated and restricted pitch, and unsteady vowel prolongation. For example, Kent and Rosenbek (1982) characterized AD by its scanning quality of equal and excessive stress with little pitch variation across syllables. Physiologic studies of patients with AD have documented a reduction in vital capacity, a decrease in the ability to time respiration with phonation (Murdoch, Chenery, Stokes, & Hardcastle, 1991), and a restricted amount of tongue movement during vowels, which may account for the perception of vowel distortions in AD speech (Kent & Netsell, 1975). Taken together, the acoustic and physiologic data have confirmed the impression that AD is a disturbance of muscular coordination, rather than a loss of muscle strength.

Extrapyramidal Disease. These are a group of disorders resulting from damage to the basal nuclei that involve various types of movement abnormalities. Rosenfield (1991) noted that clinically, extrapyramidal diseases consist of one or a combination of the following: (a) abnormal involuntary movements, (b) altered skeletal muscle tone; (c) decrease or increase in movement; or (d) alteration of automatic associated movements. Rosenfield further stated that the involuntary movements may be patterned or nonpatterned, predictable or unpredictable, and repetitive or nonrepetitive. Extrapyramidal disorders may be classified as hyperkinesia (too much movement) or hypokinesia (too little movement).

Hyperkinesia refers to an excess of movement, ranging in rate from slow to fast, that results when the basal nuclei fail to exert an inhibitory influence on nerve impulses generated by the cortex. Hyperkinesias can also result when the normal equilibrium between excitatory acetylcholine (ACh) and inhibitory dopamine neurotransmittors is disturbed, leading to an increase in ACh excitation (Duffy, 1995). Some hyperkinesias are rapid and unsustained, whereas other movements are slower to develop, and may be sustained for seconds or longer at a time. Some movement disorders include combinations of these quick and slow extraneous movements.

Hyperkinetic Dysarthria. The excessive movements in hyperkinesia include different types of tremors and tics, chorea, and dystonia. Tremor is the nonpurposeful, rhythmic, patterned, to-and-fro oscillation produced by contractions of antagonistic and agonistic muscles (Rosenfield, 1991). Tremor may be classified into different subtypes. Physiologic tremor is a fast tremor that occurs naturally with no damage to the brain. It occurs when a person is under stress or fear, or is fatigued, or holds a posture for a long time. Certain medications, such as steroids, can increase the amplitude of physiologic tremor. Metabolic tremor is a slower tremor seen in metabolic disturbances such as electrolyte imbalance, withdrawal from alcohol or drugs, or in liver, kidney, or lung disease. Intention tremor, on the other hand, is only noticeable when the patient attempts some kind of voluntary movement, but is absent at rest. An intention tremor is often associated with cerebellar disease. Resting tremor is the opposite of intention tremor. Here, the patient's voluntary movements are not affected, but the tremor appears when the patient is at rest. This kind of tremor is very common in Parkinson's disease. Essential tremor is a disorder that usually begins in middle age, although it can occur at any time. Essential tremor consists of involuntary rhythmic movements of the head, face, jaw, tongue, laryngeal muscles, arms, and hands. It is usually treated with medications such as Propranolol or Mysoline.

Tics, according to McDowell and Cedarbaum (1988), are rapid, stereotyped, repetitive, involuntary movements resembling fragments of normal motor acts. Unlike tremors, tics can be voluntarily suppressed for variable amounts of time. Gilles de la Tourette syndrome is a well-known example of a tic disorder. This is a chronic disorder that begins between the ages of 2 and 15 years, and is characterized by multiple motor and vocal tics. Motor tics may be simple; i.e., involving only one movement, or more complex. Some tics involve multiple movements, such as hitting, jumping, skipping, and so on. Vocal tics include barking, grunting, sniffing, snorting, squealing, and such. A majority (but not all persons) afflicted with Gilles de la Tourette syndrome have coprolalia (involuntary swearing). Similar to some kinds of tremors, these tics are worsened with stress and fatigue.

Chorea refers to quick involuntary extraneous movements that are random and unpredictable. Movements last from one-tenth of a second to about one second (Rosenfield, 1991). These movements may occur all over the body, or may be more focal; that is, limited to a particular part of the body. These extraneous movements impair voluntary control by reducing coordination, particularly in those areas that require a rapid succession of movement, such as speech production. Huntington's chorea is such a disease. It is an autosomal dominant disease with complete penetrance, meaning that each child of a person with Huntington's has a 50 percent chance of inheriting the disease. Dysarthria may be an early symptom of the disease, with the individual's speech becoming unintelligible by the interference of the extraneous movements of the tongue, lips, larynx, palate, pharynx, diaphragm, and chest. The person may make continuous facial grimaces, and there may be sucking, grimacing, and lip-smacking movements (Rosenfield, 1991). While there is no cure for Huntington's chorea, the choreic movements can be decreased with various drugs, such as haloperidol.

Chorea can result from long-term usage of psychotropic medications. This is fairly common in young people who may take high doses of drugs to control acute schizophrenia. If these drug-induced choreic movements become permanent, the resulting disorder is known as tardive dyskinesia. Chorea also occurs in many patients with Parkinson's disease, who have been treated with a particular medication called L-Dopa. However, the movements tend to disappear with lower doses of the medication, or if the medication is discontinued. Other causes of chorea include infections, trauma, stroke, and various metabolic and degenerative diseases.

Chorea can affect any or all of the subsystems necessary for motor speech production. According to Duffy (1995), phonation and respiration will be affected by sudden, forced instances of inspiration or expiration, voice stoppages, periods of breathiness, a strained-harsh voice quality, and excessive variations in loudness. In terms of resonance, the individual is likely to have intermittent intervals of hypernasality. Articulation will be impaired, characterized by distortions of speech sounds, and impaired prosody, with the patient demonstrating inappropriate and prolonged pauses.

Dystonia, like chorea, involves random extraneous involuntary movements that interfere with voluntary motor activity. These involuntary movements probably result from dopaminergic and cholinergic overactivity within the basal nuclei (Rosenfield, 1991). However, the movements are slow, sustained, and writhing. As with chorea, the involvement may be generalized, (known as dystonia musculorum deformans), or more restricted (focal dystonia). Dystonia can occur by itself or in conjunction with other complex involuntary movements (Rosenfield, 1991). A variety of CNS disorders can result in dystonias, including trauma, stroke, infections, toxins, and certain medications. Focal dystonias typically begin during adulthood, and include torticollis, writer's cramp, and **blepharospasm** (involuntary eye closure). Spasms of the tongue, mouth, jaw, and pharyngeal muscles are known as oromandibular dystonia.

Drugs and medications that result in chorea can also result in dystonia (tardive dyskinesia). In fact, acute dystonic reactions can occur within minutes after a patient receives an antipsychotic drug. However, tardive dyskinesia usually begins weeks to months after the drug treatment. After discontinuing the drug, 50 percent of patients become asymptomatic within six months.

Speech-related problems commonly found in individuals with dystonia are similar to those associated with chorea. Duffy (1995) listed the following problems in the phonation–respiration domain: strained-harsh voice quality, voice stoppages, audible inspirations, excess loudness variations, and voice tremor. Hypernasality is also commonly found. Articulation is characterized by distorted vowels, and similar to chorea, prosody is affected, with inappropriate intervals of silence and unpredictable stress patterns.

Hypokinetic Dysarthria.   Hypokinesia refers to a lack of appropriate movement. A rigid muscle is one that has too much muscle tone, resulting in an excessive degree of muscle stiffness. Limbs that are rigid cannot move easily; that is, they are restricted in range of motion. Hypokinesia results from damage to the basal nuclei, whose major functions are to regulate muscle tone and control posture. These functions are achieved in part through the action of the neurotransmitter dopamine, which is manufactured in a part of the basal nuclei known as the substantia nigra. In order for appropriate movement to occur, the **dopaminergic** and **cholinergic** (ACh) pathways must be in balance. Many different diseases or other processes can result in hypokinesia; e.g., progressive supranuclear palsy and Shy-Drager syndrome. Antipsychotic medications, which block dopamine receptors, can lead to hypokinetic symptoms, as can exposure to lead and mercury. Repeated head trauma, such as that often sustained by boxers, can damage the substantia nigra and cause hypokinesia. However, the best known disease associated with hypokinetic dysarthria is Parkinson's disease (PD). PD results from a lack of dopamine due to destruction of neurons in the substantia nigra.

PD is associated with some characteristic signs. One of the major signs is bradykinesia. This refers to difficulty and slowness in initiating voluntary movements (often including those necessary for speech). The individual may have long delays, or may be very slow in beginning a movement. Once the movement is begun, it may be slow, and it also may be very difficult to stop. There may also be intermittent "freezing" during the course of the movement (Duffy, 1995, p. 168). Akinesia also is often found. Akinesia includes a reduction in such movements as limb gestures during speech, eye blinking, head movement, and swallowing. Also included in this category is micrographia (excessively small handwriting) and masked facies (patient's face appears blank and devoid of expression, due to reduction in muscle movement). Postural abnormalities also are often present in PD. Patients may sit or walk in a stooped position, or they may have trouble going from sitting to standing. They may have difficulty turning around in bed, and may not be able to adjust their body position to prevent falling. Another very typical characteristic of PD is a resting tremor, often seen as a "pill rolling" movement of the fingers. The tremor may also be present in other body areas, such as the head, jaw, lip, tongue, or in the limbs (Duffy, 1995).

Speech production is often affected in PD. The most common problems are reduced loudness, reduced pitch variability, and imprecisely formed consonants. An extremely fast rate of speech may occur, together with short rushes of speech. Many patients also exhibit a hoarse or breathy voice. Fisher (1978) investigated the speech and voice characteristics of 200 PD patients. They found that 89 percent of these patients had a speech and/or voice problem. Of this 89 percent, 45 percent had a voice problem as the only presenting symptom of the disease.

PD is usually treated with dopaminergic drugs (dopamine agonists) that restore the balance between dopamine and acetylcholine (Duffy, 1995). The best known drug is called Levadopa, which works by increasing the level of dopamine in the substantia nigra. Other drugs used to treat PD are Sinement and Bromocriptine. While these drugs can be very effective in relieving rigidity and in increasing the precision and fluency of speech, they can have unpleasant and serious side effects. Probably the most severe side effect is **tardive dyskinesia** (recall that this is a hyperkinesia resulting in choreic or dystonic movements). Confusion is another side effect. "On-off" effects can also occur as a fluctuation in symptoms during a dosage cycle. For example, symptoms may worsen in severity at the peak, beginning, or end of a medication cycle. This is important for speech–language pathologists to know, because the dysarthria in individuals with PD who are being treated for communication problems may result not only from the disease itself, but also from the effects of medications used to treat it.

Diseases of Multiple Neurologic Systems: Mixed Dysarthria.   Mixed dysarthria, a combination of two or more of the pure types of dysarthria described above, is relatively common. Mixed dysarthria reflects the effects of diffuse neurologic disease that has spread across two or more divisions of the nervous system (Darley, Aronson, & Brown, 1975). Neurologic diseases that can cause mixed dysarthria include degenerative disorders, toxic metabolic conditions, vascular disorders, trauma, tumor, and infectious disease. Amyotrophic lateral sclerosis (ALS) is a degenerative disease characterized by UMN and LMN signs. The cause of ALS has not been determined, but immunologic and viral etiologies are suspected. Males are affected more frequently than females, with the first symptoms of the disease typically appearing between 40 and 70 years of age. Fatigue, muscle atrophy (a wasting of muscle fibers and a loss of muscle bulk), fasciculations (brief visible contractions of the motor unit), and hypotonia (reduced muscle tone) are prominent clinical features of ALS, strongly associated with motor neuron degeneration. Some patients with ALS have dementia, while in others there is no impairment in cognition. Although people have been known to survive the disease for 20 years, the disease typically progresses for 1 to 5 years following initial diagnosis. Death from ALS is usually related to airway obstruction, respiratory failure, or infection (Mulder, 1982).

Anarthria may develop as the disease progresses, and in the chronic stages, communication problems are often one of the most debilitating aspects of the disorder (Yorkston, Strand, Miller, Hillel, & Smith, 1993). Augmentative communication devices may be the only means of communication in the final stages of the disease. Signs of UMN damage (e.g., spasticity), LMN damage (e.g., fasciculation), or both (e.g., dysphagia), may appear as the disease progresses.

Darley, Aronson, and Brown (1975) described ALS patients as having some speech features consistent with spastic dysarthria and some consistent with flaccid dysarthria, and some that may reflect a combination of the two. Thus, the speech of ALS patients generally may be characterized by its labored and slow rate, short phrasing with lengthy silences, severely impaired articulation, and hypernasality (Duffy, 1995). Acoustic examination of ALS speakers has revealed abnormal fundamental frequency, abnormal jitter and shimmer, and reduced harmonic/noise ratios (Kent, et al., 1991). These findings are indicative of slow tongue and laryngeal movement, instability of movement and weakness of movement, during speech.

Multiple sclerosis (MS) is another acquired degenerative disease with no known specific etiology. MS follows a highly unpredictable course that is not always fatal. It is more common in women than men, with onset usually between 20 and 60 years of age (Smith & Scheinberg, 1985). The main characteristic of this disease is diffuse demyelination. Myelin is the covering of fatty tissue that surrounds the axons throughout the nervous system. Demyelination refers to a breakdown in the myelin covering resulting in ineffective neural transmission. Because the demyelination is diffuse in MS, the signs of damage are varied. Problems may include walking difficulties, loss of bladder control, as well as visual or sensory deficits. Memory may be impaired, psychiatric problems may develop, and aphasia and higher-level language processing deficits have also been reported (Lethlean & Murdock, 1993).

Dysarthria frequently emerges in MS, and may change in type and severity as the disease progresses. Specifically, spastic, ataxic, and mixed forms of dysarthria may appear at different times within the course of the disease. Severity of the dysarthria has been linked to the number of impaired neurologic systems (Beukelman, Kraft, & Freal, 1985). Darley, Brown, and Goldstein (1972) noted impaired loudness, harshness, defective articulation, and impaired stress as the most deviant characteristics of patients with MS. Reductions in vital capacity and weakness in the respiratory muscles are often present. Mechanical respiratory support is often provided in the terminal stages of MS to prevent airway obstruction and sleep apnea.

Toxic and metabolic diseases usually produce diffuse neurologic damage. When motor speech disorders are due to toxic or metabolic conditions, the resulting dysarthria is usually mixed. Wilson's disease (WD) is a rare genetic metabolic disorder that usually appears in early adulthood. In WD, there is a build up of dietary copper in the liver, brain, and cornea of the eye. Bizarre arm tremors, slowness of movement, trunk rigidity, drooling, and dysphagia are classic neurologic signs of WD (Adams & Victor, 1991). The dysarthria of WD can be mixed, hypokinetic, ataxic, or spastic (Berry, Aronson, Darley, & Goldstein, 1974). Berry et al. demonstrated significant reductions in impaired speech characteristics when patients' diets were modified to eliminate foods rich in copper.

Multiple strokes, or a single brainstem stroke, may result in mixed dysarthria. Because the direct and indirect nerve pathways and the cranial nerves connect in the brainstem, a single stroke can produce damage to multiple components of the neurologic system. For similar reasons, a tumor within or nearby the brainstem can cause mixed dysarthria. Multiple focal lesions, or diffuse brain injury from closed head injury, can also cause mixed dysarthria.

Cerebral Palsy

Because children with cerebral palsy (CP) demonstrate a high incidence of motor speech disability, this population is considered separately. CP is a nonprogressive disorder of movement and posture due to brain damage generally incurred before the age of three years. CP is a term that has usually been used to describe childhood motor impairments that occur prenatally or perinatally. When motor disability arises from postnatal factors, such as closed head injury or tumor, these are usually described as syndromes separate from CP. The estimated incidence of CP is 2 cases per 1000 live births, with prevalence estimated to be 400,000 living individuals with CP in the United States (Kudyavev, Schoenberg, Kurland, & Groover, 1983). It is estimated that the incidence of dysarthria in CP is 31 to 88 percent (Yorkston, Beukelman, & Bell, 1988). In addition to dysarthria, children with CP frequently have disturbances in cognition, perception, sensation, hearing, language, emotional development, feeding, and seizure control (Love, 1992). There are three major clinical types of CP, named for the predominant pattern of motor involvement: spastic, dyskinetic (or athetoid), and ataxic. Combinations of these three types are often labelled as mixed CP.

The most common types of motor disturbance in CP are the spastic syndromes. Spasticity is often associated with low birth weight, reduced oxygen, and reduced cerebral blood flow in premature infants. There are four classic profiles of spastic CP involvement: spastic hemiplegia, spastic paraplegia, spastic diplegia, and spastic quadriplegia. In cases of congenital spastic hemiplegia, the arm and leg on one side of the body show a spastic weakness. If dysarthria is present, it is often mild. Communication development in children with spastic hemiplegia may be hindered by disturbances in language and cognition. Children with spastic paraplegia are rare. They have CP involving both legs and generally develop normal speech. Cognitive disturbances are not likely. Children with spastic diplegia show involvement of all four extremities, with the lower limbs showing more impairment. In addition to the limb and hand involvement, respiratory muscles may be affected. Classic signs of spastic diplegia include flexion and adduction of the hips, resulting in a crossing of the legs while walking (scissors gait), and toe walking due to tightness in the hamstring muscles of the leg and the tendons of the ankle. Lastly, children with spastic quadriplegia display equal amounts of motor impairment in all four limbs. There may be involvement of respiratory, laryngeal, articulatory, and palatopharyngeal muscles. Drooling and dysphagia may be present. Children with spastic quadriplegia frequently exhibit mental retardation, and demonstrate marked delays in speech and language acquisition.

Spastic dysarthria will occur when the corticobulbar system is bilaterally damaged, as is the case in children with diplegia or quadriplegia. The identifying abnormalities of movement that appear in spastic syndromes are spasticity, weakness, limited range of motion, and slowness of movement. Harsh voice and short phrasing may be related to air waste because the larynx is unable to modify the airstream for voice (Love, 1992). Hypernasality is a major contributor to poor speech intelligibility in this population (Netsell, 1969). Articulatory function is less severely impaired in this population than it is in the other types of CP.

Athetosis is a common syndrome of CP. In the past, athetoid CP was often caused by blood type incompatibility between a mother and her unborn baby. Medical advances to detect and prevent blood incompatibility problems have significantly lowered the current incidence of athetoid CP. Hypotonia and the inability to achieve motor milestones within age expected limits are initial signs of motor disability in the athetoid child. Most athetoid children demonstrate some involvement in all four limbs. The child may present with a long-term history of drooling and dysphagia, and cognitive deficits may or may not be present. Inadequate respiratory patterns may contribute to problems in pitch and loudness. Laryngeal dysfunction is often characterized by difficulty in closing the vocal folds. Insufficient tension in the folds, resulting in weak intensity and breathiness, and hyperadduction of the folds, resulting in aphonia, are possible. In addition, the inability to move the vocal folds may result from generalized

lack of muscle tone (Love, 1992). Poorly regulated vocal fold tension may explain the audible glottal attacks at the initiation of vowels, strained vocal quality, monotone, and inappropriate pitch variation often found in athetoid type CP. Articulation problems appear to be the result of excessive jaw movements, limited tongue shaping, and difficulty in achieving velopharyngeal closure (Kent & Netsell, 1979).

Ataxia is the least frequent type of CP. Clinical evidence suggests that ataxic dysarthria resulting from CP is very similar to the ataxic dysarthria found in adults with cerebellar disease. Ataxic CP is primarily a problem of motor coordination, with a wide-based, lurching, staggering gait as the most prominent feature (Fenicheal, 1988). Ataxic dysarthria is characterized by imprecise consonants and distorted vowels. Mixed ataxic–spastic type dysarthria frequently has been reported as a subtype. Love (1992) noted that in ataxic children, severity of articulation impairment may be related more to intellectual function than to the degree of motor disability. Many children with ataxia present with articulation disorders that are difficult to separate from developmental phonological processing problems (Love, 1992).

TRACHEOSTOMY AND VENTILATOR-DEPENDENT PATIENTS

Patients with neuromotor problems are often at risk for respiratory failure, because many neuromuscular diseases directly affect respiratory function. If breathing becomes compromised to the point at which a person cannot breathe independently, an individual might have to depend, temporarily or permanently, on a tracheostomy and respirator for breathing assistance. Neuromuscular diseases such as ALS, myasthenia gravis, and muscular dystrophy can necessitate external ventilation. It has been estimated that there are close to 12,000 chronic ventilator-dependent patients being treated in hospitals in the United States at any given time (Tippett & Siebens, 1995). While ventilation may be essential to preserve a patient's life, it compromises communication. A respiratory procedure requires that an opening be cut into the trachea (tracheostomy) in order for the breathing apparatus to be hooked up to the patient's lungs. Thus, the patient is unable to phonate naturally. Because air enters and leaves the lungs via the tracheostomy (Mason, 1993), air does not pass through the larynx and the vocal folds are therefore not able to be set into vibration. Alternative methods of communication are essential. Some methods are similar to those used with individuals who have undergone laryngectomy, as discussed in Chapter 12. Other methods are unique to ventilator-dependent patients, and include modifying the attachment tube between the respirator and the patient's lungs so that air is directed to the larynx as well as to the lungs.

ASSESSMENT OF NEUROMOTOR SPEECH DISORDERS

Assessment of neuromotor speech disorders is based on principles of differential diagnosis. Differential diagnosis is the process of describing particular features of the patient's communication in a manner that illuminates all possible explanations for the disorder. Assessment is directed at distinguishing the neuromotor aspects of the impairment from deficits in cognition and language. Further, assessment seeks to differentiate among speech disorders and relate them to the neurologic diagnosis. Information used in the speech diagnosis may be gleaned from the patient's medical, psychological, and, in the case of children, educational records. An interview with the patient and family members may help to develop an understanding of the patient's personality and adjustment to the problem.

Because neuromotor speech disorders so often coexist with other impairments, assessment should account for related language disorders, sensory deficits, and the presence of dysphagia. Differential diagnosis may then progress to drawing a distinction between apraxia and dysarthria. Medical history of the disorder, and performance on a series of oral motor tasks and speech tests help to document the existence or coexistence of

apraxia and dysarthria. Oral motor tasks include voluntary nonspeech movements (e.g., "stick out your tongue"), elicited via command or imitation. When the patient is able, speech tests include spontaneous samples of conversation, as well as samplings of word, phrase, and sentence production during imitation and on tasks of oral reading. Automatic speech (counting, naming days) should also be tested. The patient with dysarthria will show deficits in the strength, tone, range, and steadiness of oral movement on both automatic and volitional tasks. Deficits in dysarthria will be apparent on speech and nonspeech tasks. The patient with apraxia may perform better on automatic tasks, will typically demonstrate some error-free speech, and will exhibit effortful groping attempts at articulation.

Valuable data comes from a complete diagnosis of oral motor structure and function. Symmetry of the face should be observed, with any weakness noted. Inability to close the lips may be indicative of muscle weakness. Tongue position at rest and during voluntary activities such as protrusion and retraction should also be examined. Involuntary twitchings of muscle fibers (fasciculations) in the tongue may suggest peripheral nervous system damage to the hypoglossal nerve. If the tongue deviates to one side when it is at rest, this may reflect damage to the nervous system on the opposite side of the body. Lack of symmetry in the elevation of the soft palate during phonation of a vowel may be indicative of a weakness in its neuromuscular function. Finally, diadochokinesis or measures of rate of articulatory movement may reveal breakdowns in the speed, sequencing, and timing of the speech mechanism.

An important part of differential diagnosis is describing the status of the physiological subsystems involved in speaking. This approach not only helps to distinguish among the different types of dysarthria, but also provides a useful measure of the patient's function prior to treatment. The diagnostic battery should include functional measures of the different speech subsystems. Respiration should be examined to see if there is adequate breath support to drive the vocal tract. Maximum vowel phonation time, number of syllables per breath, and counts of utterance length per inhalation provide some measures of respiratory control. The ability to sustain respiratory driving pressure sufficient for speech may be examined using a waterglass manometer. By blowing into a tube connected to the manometer, it is possible to see if the patient can generate enough subglottal air pressure to drive the vocal folds apart. Water displacement of 5 cm held for five seconds is thought to be sufficient respiratory force for speaking purposes (Hixon, Hawley, & Wilson, 1982). Phonation may be assessed by rating the perceptual quality of vocal tone during vowel prolongation. Laryngeal dysfunction is suspected when there is an apparent reduction in the pitch or loudness range of the vowel, or if the patient's voice wavers or demonstrates voice arrests or pitch breaks. Low pitch may reflect weakness in the longitudinal tension of the vocal folds. Inadequate volume may reflect weakness in medial compression of the vocal folds or a problem with respiratory support. Problems with resonance may reflect velopharyngeal dysfunction, resulting in hypernasality and audible nasal emission. Videofluoroscopic examination of the velopharynx is often used to determine the status of the velopharynx. Articulation testing is a crucial part of the assessment. It is necessary to note sound, syllable, word, sentence, and conversational articulation abilities. A measure of general intelligibility is used to describe how clearly the speaker's message comes across in known and unknown contexts.

Where possible, it is highly desirable to supplement perceptual evaluations with instrumental measures. These types of measures provide a more objective perspective on speech function. For example, perceptual measures of pitch can be confirmed by the use of the Kay Elemetrics Visi-Pitch. This device extracts the voice fundamental frequency (pitch) and intensity (loudness) and provides the specific Hz and dB values. Thus, this kind of instrument is helpful in establishing pitch and prosodic patterns of speech that may require modification. Other acoustic measures include spectrographic analyses that provide visual information about the speech signal in terms of frequency, intensity, and duration. Valuable quantifiable measures of vowel length and stability, voice onset time, and coarticulatory movements may be obtained.

APPROACHES TO NEUROMOTOR SPEECH INTERVENTION

Treatment for Apraxia

There are no widely administered medical or surgical treatments that improve apraxia of speech. Rehabilitative efforts for apraxia of speech must be careful to consider the influence of any coexisting aphasia. Most treatment approaches for apraxia of speech rely on auditory comprehension abilities and self-monitoring of errors. When the aphasia is severe, direct intervention for apraxia is often delayed until language abilities become functional.

Essentially, treatment for apraxia of speech focuses on articulation, because the other subsystems usually remain intact. Intervention programs for apraxia of speech typically introduce strategies to help the patient organize the movement sequences of speech. Intrasystemic reorganization approaches (Rosenbek, 1985) use aspects of the unimpaired speech system to compensate for the articulatory deficits associated with apraxia. Thus, a primitive automatic level of speech function (e.g., singing, social speech) or a higher cortical level of speech control (e.g., imitation, phonetic placement) is exploited to improve performance. Intersystemic reorganization (Rosenbek, 1985) relies upon nonverbal activities; that is, strategies from outside the speech system, to facilitate control of speech. Gestures (Rosenbek, 1985), rhythmic tapping, or a pacing board (Helm, 1979) are used to provide an organizational framework for sequencing speech movements. One such intersystemic approach utilizes prompts to restructure oral muscular phonetic targets (PROMPTS) (Square-Storer & Hayden, 1989). These prompts, provided by the clinician, combine tactile stimulation and specific finger placements placed directly on the patient's articulators. Each prompt helps to cue oral placement and the movement required for speech. Eventually, a sequence of prompts may be joined together to facilitate movement between phonemes, as in connected speech.

Carefully structured speech drills are a major component of apraxia treatment, designed to help the patient regain skill in speech movements. Drills are structured hierarchically to gradually increase the complexity of the stimulus as the patient demonstrates mastery of the target speech gesture. Using such an approach, Rosenbek (1985) provided a general framework for treating apraxia. He presented an eight-step continuum that guides the level of stimulation provided to achieve a targeted response. Initially, auditory and visual cues are combined and production is elicited simultaneously as the clinician models the target production. As the program progresses, stimulus cues are faded, and the patient's response requirements are increased. The last steps of the continuum elicit production in response to a question and in a role playing situation.

Augmentative Alternative Communication systems (AAC) may be appropriate for some patients with apraxia of speech. Because of the reliance on symbol recognition, success with AAC seems to be related to the severity of any accompanying aphasia or cognitive deficit. Electronic or print boards with pictures, letters, and words have successfully been used for patients with apraxia of speech who have relatively good auditory comprehension as well as the ability to remember and use symbolic representations. It is also necessary for the patient to demonstrate sufficient gestural or motor abilities (e.g., the ability to trigger a switch, point, blink) to activate the AAC system.

Treatment of developmental apraxia of speech requires special consideration. The use of the term as a diagnostic label is controversial, and there is little agreement on the behaviors required for such a diagnosis (Guyette & Diedrich, 1981). However, there are many children with a severe articulatory deficit and a restricted phonemic repertoire (Edwards, 1973) whose speech resists modification using traditional means. A predomi-

nance of omission errors, inconsistent performance across trials, and vowel distortions may further distinguish children with developmental apraxia of speech from those with phonological deficits. Treatment focuses on providing cuing strategies to organize speech movements. Rhythmic tapping, stress marking, and movement paired with intonational patterns have been used to facilitate sequences of articulatory movements. Whereas traditional treatment focuses on auditory stimulation and mastery of phonological patterns, Love and Fitzgerald (1984) recommended that for developmental apraxia of speech, the emphasis in treatment should be placed on phonetic placement through the combined use of auditory, visual, and tactile stimulation. Clinical reports also suggest some individual success with finger-spelling cues (Shelton & Graves, 1985) and sign language (Harlan, 1984).

Treatment for Dysarthria

If a patient is to enroll in a clinical management program for dysarthric speech, several factors will affect the selection of treatment goals. Treatment decisions are best made following careful review of an individual's medical records, and for children, following careful review of educational reports. A complete evaluation of linguistic and functional communication abilities is essential. Prognosis, the composition of the individual's communication environment (e.g., settings and partners), and general health status at the time of evaluation should be noted prior to the development of the treatment plan. Some general treatment considerations and approaches are reported here. Appropriate application of a specific therapeutic approach will vary as much as do the individuals with motor speech disorders.

Early Intervention

Early intervention refers to therapeutic programs that begin shortly after identification of the problem. Recently, these programs have targeted children with motor impairments as early as two months of age (Erenberg, 1984). Goals of these programs often focus on feeding, prespeech skills, and stimulating language development. Early intervention, begun once the patient is medically stable, also applies to adults. Providing intensive treatment early on may help the adult dysarthric patient adapt to communication changes and begin to compensate for them. Further, documentation of an individual's initial clinical status serves as baseline data for measuring progress or regression.

Medical Treatment

Pharmacological intervention and surgery are two medical treatments often used to improve motor function and speech. Because of the underlying nervous system pathology, patients with movement disorders are often treated with various types of drugs. It is therefore very important for the speech–language pathologist to be aware of different types of drugs, their effects and side effects, and their impact on speech production. Many speech–language pathologists work in medical settings and communicate on a frequent basis with physicians, neurologists, and other medical personnel, so that familiarity with basic pharmacological issues is crucial. As Rosenfield (1991) pointed out, patients tend to see a speech–language pathologist more often than they do a neurologist. Therefore, a clinician who is knowledgeable about the effects and side effects of different types of drugs may be the first to detect medication-related changes in the patient's speech or other communication behaviors.

In order to understand the effect of drugs on movement disorders, it is necessary to understand the role that chemicals play in the brain and nervous system. Much brain activity relies on certain chemicals that are manufactured by the brain, known as neurotransmittors. These neurotransmittors play a crucial role in the transmission of nerve impulses from the brain to the various muscles and structures of the body. Over 20 different neurotransmittors have been identified to date (Ro-

senfield, 1991). Some of the best known are acetylcholine (ACh), dopamine, and serotonin. ACh is found in the basal nuclei and the neuromuscular junction, between the end of an axon and the actual muscle fiber. ACh helps nerve impulses to crossover synapses and is thus considered to be excitatory. The nerve impulse is transmitted across the neuromuscular junction and into the muscle, which then contracts, resulting in movement. Dopamine occurs in many parts of the brain, and is particularly dense in the basal nuclei. Dopamine is thought to have an inhibiting effect on nerve transmission, and is therefore important in refining and smoothing movement. Serotonin pathways originate in the brainstem (Rosenfield, 1991) and connect with cortical and subcortical areas. This neurotransmitter can cause strong contractions of smooth muscles.

Many medications used to treat movement disorders achieve their effects by actually modifying neurotransmitter characteristics. Rosenfield (1991) noted that pharmacological agents can alter the amount of ACh released by the nerve impulse; alter the response of the muscle to ACh; or act upon the enzymes (chemicals involved in synthesizing and breaking down neurotransmittors) that degrade the ACh after it has been released. Rosenfield (1991) listed five classes of drugs that work by altering ACh characteristics, thereby affecting muscle responses. Choline uptake inhibitors lessen the number of ACh molecules that reach the muscle, resulting in reduced strength of muscle contraction. ACh release blockers halt the process through which a nerve impulse releases ACh into the space between the nerve axon and the muscle, resulting in inadequate ACh to stimulate a muscle contraction. Therefore, a severe muscle weakness ensues. ACh antagonists serve to block muscle activation by ACh, thus producing paralysis. Cholinomimetics mimic the action of ACh. However, rather than increasing the strength of muscle contraction, they work by desensitizing the muscle until paralysis results. Finally, cholinesterase (enzyme) inhibitors decrease the chemical breakdown of ACh after it has been released, and therefore allow the ACh to work for a longer period of time on the muscle, enhancing muscle contraction.

It is important to realize that when a patient is prescribed a drug, the medication affects various sites, both within and outside the brain. Many of the cerebral sites are involved in speech production. As described earlier, vocalization involves the coordination of many bodily systems, including respiration, phonation, and articulation. Lower motor neurons that control respiration are located in various portions of the spinal cord. Motor neurons controlling laryngeal function are situated in the nucleus ambiguus, housed in the brainstem. Cranial nerve neurons responsible for articulatory control, i.e., CN V, VII, and others, are found from the pons to the lower part of the spinal cord. There is also major input from the corticobulbar tracts, the limbic system, the extrapyramidal system, and the cortex itself. Thus, damage to any of these areas can affect speech production. The damage can arise from stroke, trauma, infections, and so on, but importantly, can also arise from medications that affect these areas (Rosenfield, 1991).

Surgery.   Surgery directed at improving speech is sometimes considered a medical option. Pharyngeal flap surgery to decrease hypernasality and increase intelligibility is discussed in Chapter 9. Phonosurgical techniques for voice improvement are presented in Chapter 11. Removal of a tumor or repair of an occluded artery are surgical means aimed at eliminating the neurologic cause of the dysarthria. The speech–language pathologist is often a member of the transdisciplinary team involved in discussions of options with the patient and family.

Prosthetic Considerations

A prosthesis is an artificial device that substitutes for an impaired body part. Two general prosthetic options should be considered in the treatment of dysarthria: the palatal lift, and the use of augmen-

tative alternative communication (AAC) devices. Some dysarthric individuals are able to tolerate placement of an orthodental device into the mouth designed to elevate the soft palate. Gains in intraoral air pressure, increases in utterance length, and improvement in intelligibility have been reported in some cases (Hardy, 1983). AAC devices include a wide range of picture boards and electronic equipment that supplement or substitute as the individual's primary method of expression. Use of such a device should be made in conjunction with the patient, family, and after assessment of the patient's communication environment. For a complete examination of AAC, please refer to Silverman (1993).

Motor Practice and Behavioral Change

Practice is critical to bringing about behavioral changes in speaking. Clinical management is often directed at providing strengthening exercises to directly improve skill in respiration for speech, phonation, resonance, and articulation (Brookshire, 1992). Drill work requiring systematic and repetitive practice may help improve motor performance (Yorkson, Beukelman, & Bell, 1988). Feedback about motor performance may reinforce preferred speech behaviors. Feedback may be verbal, visual, or instrumental, such as biofeedback provided by the Kay Elemetrics Visi-Pitch. Darley, Aronson, and Brown (1975) believed that motor skills could be improved when the patient is given instructions to make the movements of speech as conscious as possible. This method relies heavily on intact language comprehension abilities because self-correction and monitoring are essential to the process.

Physiological Considerations

A subsystems approach to treatment considers each of the physiological components of the speech process and their relationships. Respiratory disturbances are fairly common to UMN and LMN lesions. Dworkin (1991) suggested that the first step in treatment is to position the patient so there is adequate breath support for speech. Training is often provided to prolong breath support and increase control of expiration. Rate control, use of short phrases, and timed inhalations may be used to maximize speech intelligibility. Phonatory problems in the dysarthrias often relate to too much or too little tension in the vocal folds. Inappropriate vocal fold control can result in a voice that is too high, too low, hoarse, breathy, harsh, and so on. (See Chapter 11 for a complete discussion.) Auditory (e.g., tape recorder) and visual biofeedback (e.g., Visi-Pitch, mirror) are useful treatment tools when used to increase the patient's awareness of phonatory control. Resonance has been treated by improving velopharyngeal function through palatal stimulation exercises such as brushing and massage, surgery, and prostheses. Articulation training using a variety of approaches is often administered to teach speech sound placement. Overarticulation (i.e., exaggerated placement of articulators) can be useful in teaching compensatory movements and heightening awareness of correct articulator placement.

Interpersonal Considerations

The psychosocial impact of dysarthria on an individual cannot be overlooked. For some patients a slight imperfection in speech production can cause embarrassment and depression. Lubinski (1991) noted that the family should be considered as a complex factor in the dynamic life of a dysarthric individual, and that family adjustment to the problem is an important part of treatment. In some cases, when the person with dysarthria cannot live independently, or when the person needs daily living assistance, institutionalization may be considered. Regardless of the living situation, Lubinski (1991) recommended careful study of the environment in order to understand the social, physical, and psychological aspects of communication and to propose clinical intervention that yields functional outcomes. A patient's psychosocial adjustment to the problem is best addressed by frequent consultations between medical and rehabilitative personnel.

SUMMARY

Neuromotor speech disorders can have a major impact on an individual's communication abilities. The problems that result can range from mild deficits in speech sound production to totally unintelligible speech. Adjustment to the problem varies from patient to patient. Assessment and treatment of neuromotor speech disorders relies on an understanding of the neurologic and behavioral aspects of speech motor control. When a patient demonstrates dysarthria there is a disturbance of muscular control that is consistent with a neurologic disease or injury. Many diseases associated with dysarthria are progressive, and speech motor control will worsen over time. Some conditions associated with dysarthria remain stable over time, while in other diseases recovery of motor control can be expected. The clinical course of apraxia is not very predictable. The motor programming problems associated with apraxia of speech result in inconsistent speech error patterns. Clinically, the diagnosis of apraxia of speech usually has been linked to deficits in language formulation.

Clinical management of motor speech disorders requires gathering information from a variety of sources to identify any causative factors. Thus, the speech–language diagnosis is intimately related to an understanding of a patient's medical, cognitive, and social status. Inconsistencies between speech behavior and the medical diagnosis may eventually result in more refined neurological information about the anticipated course of the disease. Helping the patient to understand the nature of the communication impairment is a critical component of treatment and a first step in encouraging adjustment to the disability. The goals of treatment may be to improve upon current oral communication abilities or it may be to develop an efficient means of communication using alternative or augmentative means. Speech–language pathology services are an integral part of a team approach designed to give an individual access to the environment. Developing an effective means of communication is the most important aspect of educational programming and a primary goal of rehabilitation services.

Major Points of Chapter

- The two major types of neuromotor speech disorders are apraxia and dysarthria.
- Six categories of dysarthrias are classified according to the site of the lesion and the perceptual and acoustic speech characteristics that result.
- Apraxia in adults has different characteristics than the developmental form of apraxia in children.
- Cerebral palsy is a developmental nonprogressive movement disorder that gives rise to specific types of dysarthrias.
- Patients with tracheostomies who are ventilator-dependent are part of the expanding scope of practice in speech–language pathology.
- Differential diagnosis uses a speech subsystems approach that describes function in respiration, phonation, articulation, and resonance.
- Treatment may include pharmacological, surgical, prosthetic, behavioral, and augmentative approaches.

Discussion Guidelines

1. Compare and contrast the respiratory, phonatory, and articulatory characteristics of a patient with ataxic dysarthria versus a patient with spastic dysarthria.
2. Locate an article by one author who believes in the concept of developmental apraxia of speech and another article by an author who opposes this concept. Summarize their arguments, and discuss whether you agree or disagree with each point raised.
3. Observe a patient who uses an augmentative alternative communication system. Describe how the system works, and indicate the extent

to which the individual is successful in communicating, and the reasons for their success.

REFERENCES

Adams, R., & Victor, M. (1991). *Principles of Neurology.* NY: McGraw-Hill.

Berry W., Aronson, A., Darley, F., & Goldstein, N. (1974). Effects of penicilamine therapy and low copper diet on dysarthria in Wilson's disease. *Mayo Clinic Proceedings, 49,* 405–408.

Beukelman, D., Kraft, G, & Freal, J. (1985). Expressive communication disorders in persons with multiple sclerosis: A survey. *Archives of Physical Medicine and Rehabilitation, 66,* 675–678.

Brookshire, R. (1992). *An introduction to neurogenic communication disorders.* St. Louis: Mosby Year-book.

Darley, F., Aronson, A., & Brown, J. (1975). *Motor speech disorders.* Philadelphia: W. S. Saunders.

Darley, F., Brown, J., & Goldstein, N. (1972). Dysarthria in multiple sclerosis. *Journal of Speech and Hearing Research, 15,* 229–245.

Duffy, J. R. (1995). *Motor speech disorders: Substrates, differential diagnosis, and management.* St. Louis: Mosby Year Book.

Dworkin, J. P. (1991). *Motor speech disorders: a treatment guide.* St. Louis: Mosby Year Book.

Edwards, M. (1973). Developmental verbal dyspraxia. *British Journal of Communication Disorders, 8,* 64–70.

Erenberg, G. (1984). Cerebral palsy. *Postgraduate Medicine, 75,* 87–93.

Fenichel, G. (1988). *Clinical pediatric neurology.* Philadelphia: W. B. Saunders

Fisher, C. (1978). Ataxic hemiparesis. *Archives of Neurology, 35,* 126–129.

Gilman, S., Bloedel, J., & Lechtenberg, R. (1981). *Disorders of the cerebellum.* Philadelphia: F. A. Davis.

Guyette, T., & Diedrich, W. (1981). A critical review of developmental apraxia of speech. In N. Lass (Ed.), *Speech and language: Advances in basic research and practice* (Vol. 1, 1–49). NY: Academic Press.

Hall, P., Jordon, L., & Robin, D. (1993). *Developmental apraxia of speech: theory and clinical practice.* Austin: TX: Pro-Ed.

Hardy (1983). *Cerebral palsy.* Engelwood Cliffs, NJ: Prentice-Hall.

Harlan, L. (1984). Treatment approaches for a young child evidencing developmental verbal apraxia.

Australian Journal of Human Communication Disorders, 12, 121–127.

Hartman, J., & Abbs, J. (1992). Dysarthria associated with focal unilateral upper motor neuron lesion. *European Journal of Disorders of Communication, 27,* 187–195.

Helm, N. (1979). Management of palilalia with a pacingboard. *Journal of Speech and Hearing Disorders, 44,* 350–353.

Hixon, T., Hawley, J., & Wilson, K. (1982). An around-the-house device for clinical determination of respiratory driving pressure: A note on making the simple even simpler. *Journal of Speech and Hearing Disorders, 4,* 13–19.

Joanette, Y., & Dudley, J. (1980). Dysarthric symptomatology of Friedrich's ataxia. *Brain and Language, 10,* 39–45.

Judd, L. (1991). The therapeutic use of psychotropic medications. In K. Wilson et al. (Eds). *Harrison's principles of internal medicine.* NY: McGraw-Hill.

Kent, R. (1976). Anatomical and neuromuscular maturation of the speech mechanism: evidence from acoustic studies. *Journal of Speech and Hearing Research, 19,* 422–447.

Kent, J. F., Kent, R., Rosenbek, J., Weismer, G., Martin, R., Sufit, R., & Brooks, B. (1991). Quantitative description of the dysarthria in women with amyotrophic lateral sclerosis. *Journal of Speech and Hearing Research, 35,* 723–733.

Kent, R., & Netsell, R. (1975). A case study of an ataxic dysarthric: cineradiographic and spectographic. *Journal of Speech and Hearing Disorders, 40,* 115–125.

Kudrjavcev,T., Schoenberg, B., Kurland, L., & Groover, R. (1983). Cerebral palsy-trends in incidence and changes in concurrent mortality: Rochester, MN, 1950–1976. *Neurology, 33,* 1433–1436.

Lethlean, J. B., & Murdock, B. E. (1993). Language problems in multiple sclerosis. *Journal of Medical Speech–Language Pathology, 1,* 47–56.

Love, R. (1992). *Childhood motor speech disability.* New York: Macmillan Publishing Company.

Love, R., & Fitzgerald, M. (1984). Is the diagnosis of developmental apraxia of speech valid? *Australian Journal of Human Communication Disorders, 12,* 170–178.

Love, R. J., & Webb, W. G. (1992). *Neurology for the speech–language pathologist,* 2nd ed. Boston: Butterworth-Heinemann.

Lubinski, R. (1991). Dysarthria: A breakdown in interpersonal communication. In D. Vogel and M. Cannito (Eds.). *Treating disordered speech motor control: By clinicians for clinicians.* Austin, TX: Pro-Ed.

Mason, M. (1993). *Speech pathology for tracheostomized and ventilator dependent patients.* Newport Beach, CA: Voicing.

McDowell, F. H., & Cedarbaum, J. M. (1988). The extrapyramidal system and disorders of movement. In R. J. Joynt (Ed.). *Clinical neurology* (Vol. 3, Chapter 38). Philadelphia: J. B. Lippincott.

McNeil, M. Caliguri, M., & Rosenbek, J. (1989). A comparison of labiomandibular kinematic durations, displacements, velocities and dysmetrias in apraxic and normal adults. In T. Prescott (Ed.), *Clinical aphasiology, 18.* Boston: College-Hill.

McNeil, M., & Kent, R. (1990). Motoric characteristics of adult apraxic and aphasic speakers. In G. Hammond (Ed.). *Cerebral control of speech and limb movements.* New York: North Holland.

Mulder, D. W. (1982). Clinical limits of amyotrophic lateral sclerosis. In L. P. Rowland (Ed.). *Advances in neurology, 36,* Human motor neuron diseases. New York: Raven Press.

Murdoch, B., Chenery, H., Stokes, P., & Hardcastle, W. (1991). Respiratory kinematics in speakers with cerebellar disease. *Journal of Speech and Hearing Research, 34,* 768–778.

Netsell, R. (1969). Evaluation of velopharyngeal function in dysarthria. *Journal of Speech and Hearing Disorders, 34,* 113–122.

Rosenbek, J. (1985). Treating apraxia of speech. In D. Johns (Ed.), *Clinical management of neurogenic communication disorders.* Austin, TX: Pro-Ed.

Rosenfield, D. (1991). Pharmacologic approaches to speech motor disorders. In D. Vogel & M. Cannito (Eds), *Treating disordered speech motor control.* Austin, TX: Pro-Ed.

Shelton, M., & Graves, M. (1985). Use of visual techniques in therapy for developmental apraxia of speech: A case study. *Language Speech and Hearing Services in Schools, 16,* 129–131.

Silverman, F. H. (1993). *Communication for the speechless,* Boston, MA: Allyn and Bacon.

Smith, C. R., & Scheinberg, L. C. (1985). Clinical features of multiple sclerosis. *Seminars in Neurology, 5,* 85–90.

Square-Storer, P., & Hayden, D. (1989). PROMPT treatment. In Square-Storer, P. (Ed.). *Acquired apraxia of speech in aphasic adults.* London: Lawrence Erlbaum.

Tippet, D., & Siebens, A. (1991). Distinguishing psychogenic from neurogenic disfluency when neurologic and psychologic factors coexist. *Journal of Fluency Disorders, 16,* 3–7.

Yorkston, K., Beukelman, D., & Bell, K. (1988). *Clinical management of dysarthric speakers.* San Diego: College Hill.

Yorkston, K., Strand, E., Miller, R., Hillel, A., & Smith, K. (1993). Speech deterioration in amyotrophic lateral sclerosis: Implications for the timing of intervention. *Journal of Medical Speech-Language Pathology, 1,* 35–46.

9

CLEFT LIP AND PALATE, CRANIOFACIAL ANOMALIES, AND VELOPHARYNGEAL INSUFFICIENCY

KAREN J. GOLDING-KUSHNER

The word **cleft** is defined by Webster's College Dictionary as "a space or opening" (1991). Clefts may occur anywhere in the body that structures are meant to fuse during embyronic development but fail to do so. The most common types of clefts are cleft lip and cleft palate, but clefts also occur in other parts of the face and in the spine (spina bifida). A craniofacial **anomaly** is an abnormality of the skull (cranium) and/or face. When the skull, face, or lip are involved, the defect is obvious at the time of birth. However, sometimes anomalies (abnormalities) are not discovered until later on, when difficulties with feeding, speech, or hearing become apparent.

The presence of an oral defect may, at the very least, affect facial and dental development, speech, hearing, and psychological well-being. The purpose of this chapter is to describe oral clefts and some related craniofacial disorders and the way in which they may affect various aspects of development. Relevant normal anatomy and physiology of speech will be reviewed to provide a context for understanding the pathological conditions that may exist in patients with cleft palate. A brief introduction to the embryology and genet-ics of facial development and disorders of clefting is also included.

EMBRYOLOGY

The neural crest theory of development holds that neural crest cells, one type of specialized embryonic cells, give rise to various connective and neural tissues of the skull and face. The cells migrate at different rates to destined locations, where they differentiate into specialized cells with predetermined functions. If this migration fails to occur, or if there is an absence or inadequacy of related cells, clefts and other facial abnormalities may result (Krogman, 1973; Johnston, 1975; Johnston & Sulik, 1984; Stark, 1977). Embryonic development of the lip and palate are illustrated in Figure 9.1. The upper lip and **premaxilla** are formed by the merging of three structures: the frontonasal process and the right and left nasomedial processes of the maxilla. Lip closure occurs during the fifth or sixth week of embryonic development (Krogman, 1979). The palate is formed by the union of the palatal shelves that develop from the maxillary processes and close during the eighth or ninth week of gestation (Krogman, 1979). In embryonic life, the three to four week difference between closure of the lip and closure of the palate is very long. This suggests that cleft lip and palate are embryologically different and explains why one may occur without the other. As seen in Figure 9.1, the mandible first develops relatively high on the face. The embryonic tongue sits above the mandible between the two sides of the palate and fusion of the two lateral sections of the palate can only occur after the mandible and tongue lower out of the

way (Figure 9.2). When this sequence of events (mandible lowering, tongue lowering, palate fusing) is interrupted it results in a condition called Robin sequence, which will be discussed in more detail later.

NORMAL ANATOMY AND PHYSIOLOGY

In order to understand the consequences of a cleft lip, cleft palate, or other craniofacial anomaly, a familiarity with the normal anatomic structures and physiological processes that may be affected

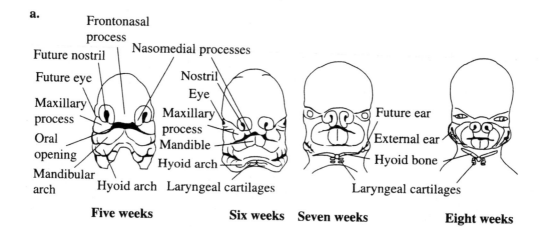

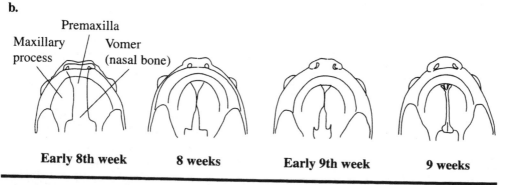

FIGURE 9.1   Embryonic development of the face and lip (a) and palate (b). Lip closure occurs during the fifth and sixth week of gestation. Palatal development follows around the eighth and ninth weeks. Complete fusion of the uvula follows shortly.

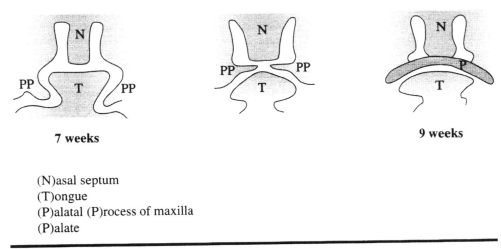

7 weeks   **9 weeks**

(N)asal septum
(T)ongue
(P)alatal (P)rocess of maxilla
(P)alate

FIGURE 9.2   Normal embryonic sequence of palatal development.

is necessary. The hard palate (Figure 9.3) is formed by the palatine processes of the maxilla and the horizontal plates of the palatine bones. Structures of the oral cavity and pharynx are labeled in Figure 9.4. The most important velar (palatal) and pharyngeal muscles for speech (Figure 9.5) are the levator veli palatini (levator), the musculus uvulae (m.u.), and the superior constrictor muscles. Levator is a paired structure with fibers arising from the base of the skull and

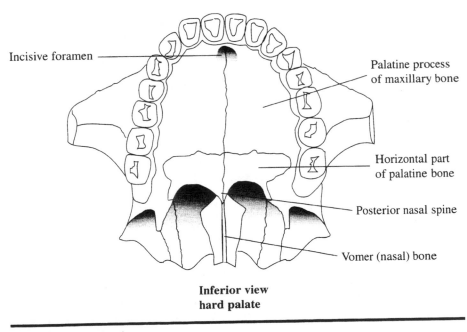

Incisive foramen

Palatine process
of maxillary bone

Horizontal part
of palatine bone

Posterior nasal spine

Vomer (nasal) bone

**Inferior view
hard palate**

FIGURE 9.3   Hard palate.

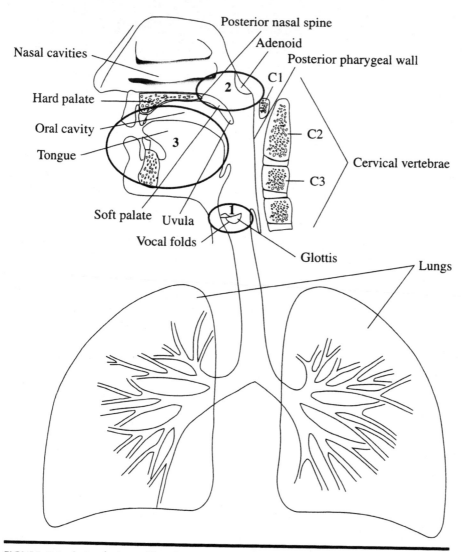

FIGURE 9.4 Lateral view of head and vocal tract showing the nasal cavities, oral cavity, hard palate, posterior nasal spine, velum or soft palate, uvula, tongue, adenoid, posterior pharyngeal wall, upper most cervical vertebrae, vocal folds, and glottis.

cartilage of the eustachian tube. It follows a sling-like course to the midline of the nasal surface of the soft palate, along the palatal aponeurosis. When levator contracts, the palate moves upward and backward toward the posterior pharyngeal wall, and the lateral pharyngeal walls may be pulled inward toward the palate. Cessation of

levator activity allows the palate to return to its rest position.

The musculus uvulae is a short, paired muscle that overlies the junction of the right and left levators. It lies in an anteroposterior direction and, when viewed through the nasal passages, appears as a bulge on the nasal surface of the soft

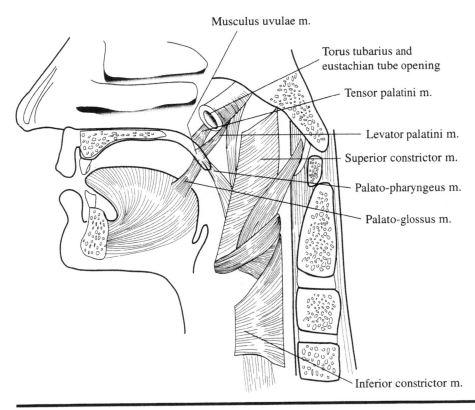

Musculus uvulae m.

Torus tubarius and
eustachian tube opening

Tensor palatini m.

Levator palatini m.

Superior constrictor m.

Palato-pharyngeus m.

Palato-glossus m.

Inferior constrictor m.

FIGURE 9.5 Muscles of the palate and pharynx.

palate (Figure 9.6). The m.u. arises from the posterior nasal spine (bony edge of the hard palate) and terminates in the tip of the uvula. There is disagreement as to whether or not contraction of the m.u. plays a role in velar thickening and elevation during speech. However, there is no question that during speech, the m.u. bulge provides important tissue mass for velopharyngeal closure by contacting the posterior pharyngeal wall and by serving as an area of contact (a target of sorts) for closure of the lateral pharyngeal walls. In a submucous cleft palate, the musculus uvulae bulge is absent, and during speech, the space left vacant by the tissue deficiency is the typical site of **velopharyngeal insufficiency (VPI)** when it occurs (Figure 9.6).

Lateral pharyngeal wall (LPW) motion is an essential component of velopharyngeal closure.

Even when the palate is fully in contact with the posterior pharyngeal wall, absence of LPW motion allows escape of air laterally, around the sides of the palate. However, there is not complete agreement as to what causes this important motion. One view is that the levator influences LPW motion by its action on the torus tubarius, the cartilage that forms the circular border of the opening to the eustachian tube from the pharynx (Dickson & Maue-Dickson, 1972, 1980). This view implies that LPW motion is essentially passive, and that the lateral and posterior pharyngeal walls are simply pulled along by velar movement because of muscular and fibrous connections. A more widely accepted view is that LPW motion is active and is caused by contraction of the superior constrictor muscle (Shprintzen, McCall, Skolnick, & Lencione, 1975; Iglesias, Kuehn, & Morris, 1980). The

Normal

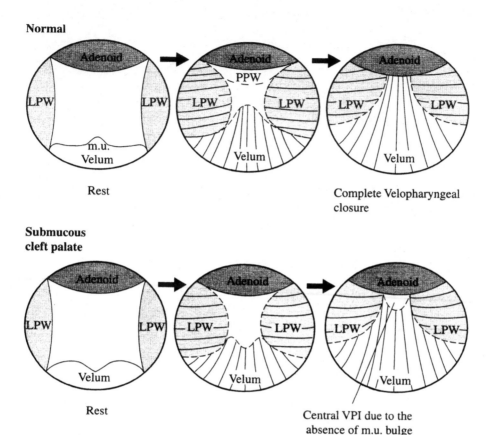

**Submucous
cleft palate**

FIGURE 9.6 Nasal surface of a normal palate (top) and submucous cleft palate (bottom) at rest and during phonation. The solid lines show rest positions and the dotted lines show displacement during speech. Note convexity of the musculus uvulae (m.u.) bulge and complete velopharyngeal closure in the normal palate. In the submucous cleft palate, the m.u. bulge is absent resulting in a central velopharyngeal gap during speech.

superior constrictor muscle forms a circular layer of muscle around the pharynx. Its fibers arise from several sources including the soft palate, the sides of the tongue, the medial pterygoid plate, and the hamulus, and insert into the median pharyngeal raphe. Lower fibers that comprise the middle and inferior constrictor muscles probably have roles in pharyngeal constriction during deglutition but do not appear to play significant roles during normal speech, although the inferior constrictor muscle is thought to be important in

esophageal speech (see Chapter 12). Superior constrictor also forms the posterior pharyngeal wall (PPW) and may be responsible for the localized anterior motion of the PPW, known as **Passavant's ridge,** which is present during phonation in some individuals.

Other muscles in the region important in understanding the interaction between velopharyngeal function and articulation are the palatoglossus and palatopharyngeus muscles. The paired palatopharyngeus muscles form the posterior faucial pillars, extending from the lateral pharyngeal wall to the side of the soft palate. This muscle may contribute to velopharyngeal narrowing, elevation of the larynx, and depression of the pharynx. It may also contribute to the formation of Passavant's ridge. The palatoglossus muscles extend from the oral surface of the velum to the sides of the tongue and these paired muscles form the anterior faucial pillars. They pull the tongue upward and back, and narrow the distance between the pillars. Another muscle in the region is the misnamed tensor veli palatini. It arises from the base of the skull and inserts into the palatine aponeurosis. However, it does not tense the palate or have any other role in velopharyngeal closure. It is active in opening the eustachian tube to equalize middle ear pressure.

PHYSIOLOGY: HOW IS SPEECH PRODUCED?

Speech, which encompasses voice, resonance, and articulation, is produced by the modification of an air stream from the lungs through a series of three basic valves (Figure 9.4). The speech process begins with respiration. Exhaled air passes from the lungs through the larynx. In order to leave the larynx, the air passes through the opening between the vocal folds called the **glottis,** which is the first valve. Rapid opening and closing of the vocal folds causes the outgoing airstream to vibrate, creating a vocal tone (see Chapter 11). Characteristics of the speech signal that are directly related to the respiratory and phonatory activity to this point are referred to as **voice.** Various modifications in respiratory and laryngeal activity result in differences in the frequency, intensity, and quality of vocal fold vibration that are perceived respectively as the pitch, loudness, and clarity of voice. The vocal signal rises through the pharynx, or vocal tract, and is modified by features of the vocal tract's size, shape, and tissue characteristics. The vocal tract may be thought of as a tube that begins at the glottis and extends from the larynx to the mouth. This tube has a branch through the nasal cavities that may be included or excluded during speech

production, as necessary. The process by which the nasal branch is separated from or coupled with the rest of the vocal tract is referred to as **velopharyngeal closure.** The velopharyngeal region is an important vocal tract modifier and is the second valve in the system. Pharyngeal characteristics and activity of the velopharyngeal region impose the feature of **resonance** on the speech signal. When velopharyngeal closure occurs, the nasopharynx and nasal cavities are excluded from the vocal tract, significantly shortening it and eliminating any further modification of the speech signal in the nasal cavities. Normally, velopharyngeal closure occurs during production of all phonemes except /m, n, ŋ/, which are, therefore, referred to as "nasal" sounds. The speech signal with characteristics of phonation and resonance is, in turn, modified by activity of the tongue and lips in the oral cavity that impose on the signal features of place and manner of articulation. Constrictions created by movement of the lips or tongue constitute the third speech valve.

The mechanism of velopharyngeal closure is of great importance in understanding speech disorders in individuals with cleft palate and related disorders, and requires additional elaboration. The velopharyngeal "valve" is formed by the velum, posterior aspect of the pharyngeal wall, and lateral aspects of the pharyngeal walls. Four general patterns of muscle movement to achieve velopharyngeal closure during speech have been observed. These reflect the different relative contributions of velar and pharyngeal motion to closure, and these patterns occur with about equal frequency in individuals with and without cleft palate (Skolnick, McCall, & Barnes, 1973; Croft, Shprintzen, & Rakoff, 1981). The "coronal" pattern, in which the velum moves up and back to contact the posterior pharyngeal wall (the adenoid in children) with just enough lateral wall motion to prevent air escape around the sides of the palate is the most common pattern and occurs in about 40 percent of individuals (Croft, Shprintzen, & Rakoff, 1981). At one time, this was thought to be the only type of normal velopharyngeal closure and was likened to a trap door. The other closure patterns, each of which occur in about 20 percent of speakers, are the *sagittal* pattern, in which the lateral pharyngeal walls move together between the palate and PPW, the *circular* pattern, which results when the velum and lateral pharyngeal walls move equally, and the *circular with Passavant's ridge* pattern in which there is movement of the velum, LPWs and also localized forward motion of the posterior pharyngeal wall (Croft et al., 1981). Velopharyngeal closure occurs during normal swallowing and a small number of individuals with incomplete VP closure (especially adults with acquired velopharyngeal dysfunction and infants) experience nasal regurgitation of fluids when swallowing. However, it is important to understand that the way in which the palate and pharynx move during speech is different from the way in which the very same structures move during blowing, swallowing, gagging, and other nonspeech activities (Shprintzen et al., 1975; Skolnick & Cohn, 1989).

TYPES OF CLEFTS

An individual may be born with a cleft lip, cleft palate, or both, depending on the nature of the interruption in embryologic development. Clefts may affect all or only part of a structure and are described as *complete* or *incomplete*. They may affect one or both sides and are therefore referred to as *unilateral* or *bilateral*. Some of the more common types of clefts may be seen in Figure 9.7.

Cleft Lip

A cleft lip may be so mild that there is only a small notch in the vermillion (red part) on one side of the upper lip. If the cleft does not extend into the floor of the nose, it is incomplete. A cleft lip is complete if the cleft extends into the floor of the nose. Complete cleft lip is usually, although not always, associated with a cleft of the alveolar ridge (gum) on the affected side. A cleft lip is uni-

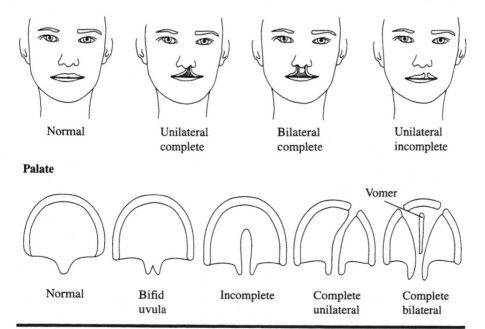

FIGURE 9.7 Common types of cleft lip and palate.

lateral if only one side is affected, and bilateral if both sides are affected. Bilateral cleft lip may or may not be symmetric (the same on both sides). Because complete cleft lip extends into the nasal floor, the appearance of the nose is always affected. A less common anomaly is a submucous cleft lip, in which there is discontinuity of the underlying orbicularis oris muscle but the outer layers of skin are intact. This may appear as an indentation or faint vertical line and often resembles a repaired cleft lip. This is the mildest type of cleft lip, and may require no treatment at all, unless accompanied by a nasal deformity.

Cleft Palate

A cleft palate is an opening in the palate (roof of the mouth) that is present at birth and that results in a total or partial lack of separation between the mouth and nose. Clefts of the palate may be unilateral or bilateral, and complete or incomplete. Overt (open) clefts of the palate are conspicuous and are, therefore, generally noticed at birth. Another type of cleft palate is not readily visible because the overlying mucosa (membrane) is intact. This is called a **submucous cleft palate** (SMCP) and is usually not detected at birth. In many cases, SMCP is never noticed. Other times, a SMCP is found during a careful examination that is conducted because of a problem with feeding, speech, or hearing, or because of sudden onset of hypernasal speech following an adenoidectomy. The three classic features of a SMCP include a bifid (cleft) uvula, zona pellucida, or bluish discoloration along the central part of the palate caused by the separation of underlying muscles (muscular diastasis), and a notch that can be palpated or seen at the posterior edge of the hard palate.

Sometimes all or some of these three anatomic features of SMCP are absent, and the palate looks completely normal when examined orally, even though a submucous cleft palate is present. This is referred to as an **occult submucous cleft palate (OSMCP).** Occult submucous clefts are often misdiagnosed as "short palate," "capacious pharynx," "velopharyngeal disproportion," or "congenital palatal insufficiency." OSMCP is impossible to diagnose by oral examination and cannot consistently be detected using radiographic techniques. OSMCP can only be identified by looking directly at the palatal morphology (structure) from the nasal side of the palate. This is possible using a fiber-optic endoscope which is inserted through the nose during a procedure called nasopharyngoscopy, which will be discussed later in this chapter. The anatomic feature of OSMCP is flattening or grooving of the dorsal (nasal) surface of the velum, reflecting deficiency

TABLE 9.1 Types of Cleft Palate

TYPE OF CLEFT PALATE	AFFECTED REGION
complete	tip of uvula through alveolar ridge including all of soft and hard palate
unilateral	only one side of alveolus cleft
bilateral	both sides of alveolus cleft
incomplete	tip of uvula through soft and/or hard palate but not anterior to the incisive foramen
unilateral	larger palatal segment attached to vomer (nasal bone)
bilateral	(hard and soft palate); neither palatal segment attached to vomer
soft palate only	central; terms unilateral and bilateral do not apply
submucous cleft palate	cleft of palatal muscles and notch in edge of hard palate but with intact mucosa
occult submucous cleft palate	cleft or absence of musculus uvulae without oral manifestations seen in submucous cleft palate

or absence of the musculus uvulae (m.u.) as seen in Figure 9.6.

CLASSIFICATION OF CLEFTS

It is usually adequate to describe a patient's cleft according to the parameters already discussed: lip and/or palate, unilateral/bilateral, complete/incomplete, or overt/submucous. Uniformity and precision in classification are important to facilitate communication among professionals and to group subjects in research. An early system developed by Veau in 1931 included four cleft types (McWilliams, Morris, & Shelton, 1990): (1) cleft of soft palate only; (2) cleft of hard and soft palate extending to the incisive foreman; (3) complete unilateral cleft of the lip, alveolus, hard and soft palate; (4) complete bilateral cleft of the lip, alveolus, hard and soft palate.

The Veau system is still used by some clinicians, but it does not provide a category for submucous clefts, cleft lip without cleft palate, or other possible variations. Many different classification systems have been proposed over the years to classify types of clefts in a descriptive yet succinct way. These include systems by Kernahan and Stark (1958), Olin (1960), and Kriens (1990). However, no one system is accepted universally.

INCIDENCE OF CLEFTS

Reports on the incidence of cleft lip, cleft palate, and other congenital anomalies vary because of differences in how information is ascertained and reported. It is generally agreed that cleft palate and other craniofacial disorders are underreported. For example, most reports are based on birth records, but some reports include all births, while others include only live births. Cleft lip is likely to be seen during an initial examination, but cleft palate without cleft lip is less obvious and may not be noticed until long after a birth has been registered. Submucous cleft palate may not be diagnosed for years, if at all.

A generally accepted estimate of the incidence of overt cleft palate not associated with

TABLE 9.2 Racial Differences in the Incidence of Cleft Lip and/or Cleft Palate (Based on Vanderas, 1987).

GROUP	INCIDENCE PER 1000 LIVE BIRTHS
Native Americans	3.7
Asians	3
Caucasians	1 to 2
African Americans	.2 to 1.7

other malformations is one in 750 live births. Cleft palate without cleft lip occurs more often in females than males (57 percent to 43 percent) (Oka, 1979; Jensen, Kreiborg, Dahl, & Fogh-Anderson, 1988). However, cleft lip with or without cleft palate occurs in twice as many males than females. Gender differences in cleft lip and cleft palate may be related to slight differences in the timing of embryological development. There are no significant racial differences in the incidence of cleft palate without cleft lip, but there are racial differences in the incidence of cleft lip with or without cleft palate. The highest incidence of cleft lip with or without cleft palate is found among Native Americans and the lowest among African Americans.

SYNDROMES

Cleft lip and palate are considered major malformations. The probability of a baby being born with two "unrelated" major malformations, such as a cleft palate and a heart defect, is quite small. However, many children do have other major and minor anomalies in addition to cleft lip and palate. These children used to carry a diagnosis of multiple congenital anomalies. These anomalies often appear, on the surface, to be unrelated. However, they frequently have a common etiology. Recurring patterns of anomalies with a single **etiology** are referred to as **syndromes.** With the rapid growth in recent years of the fields of clinical and molecular genetics, hundreds of patterns of malformations that include clefts as one of many features have been described and are recognized as syndromes. In fact, there are over 342 known syndromes involving orofacial clefting, many of which are genetic (Cohen & Bankier, 1991).

Correct diagnosis of every baby with a cleft lip or palate is very important for several reasons. Some anomalies are easily identified at birth or during infancy. Other problems, such as learning disabilities, may not manifest until later in the developmental process. Knowledge of the natural course of a particular syndrome allows professionals to give reasonably accurate prognostic information to parents. More importantly, it alerts professionals to other medical, developmental, or behavioral disorders that may be associated with a particular syndrome. Medical problems may then be identified and treated promptly, and early intervention may minimize the effects of developmental delays or medical complications. Finally, when a correct diagnosis is established, appropriate genetic counseling can be provided to the parents who may be concerned that future offspring will be similarly affected.

Isolated cleft palate is more likely to be associated with other malformations than other patterns of clefting. An early estimate was that 24 percent of individuals with only cleft palate had other malformations, in contrast to 14 percent of those with cleft lip and palate, and 7 percent of those with cleft lip alone (Greene, Vermillion, Hay, Gibbens, & Kerschbaum, 1964). More recent reports show much higher percentages, probably because of the increased thoroughness of examinations of children with clefts and the addition of clinical geneticists to many cleft palate teams. Shprintzen et al. (1985) found that as many as 63 percent of the patients at one craniofacial center had associated anomalies.

SEQUENCES

A *syndrome* exists when two or more anomalies occur together and both have the same primary etiology. A **sequence** exists when two or more anomalies occur together, but the primary etiology caused the first anomaly and it was the first

anomaly that caused the second one. For example, cleft lip may occur as an isolated finding. However, a wide cleft of the lip during embryological development may prevent subsequent union of the palatal shelves, which do not close until three or four weeks later because of the increased distance between them (Hagerty, 1965). As a result, cleft lip without cleft palate occurs much less frequently than cleft palate without cleft lip. Another example of a sequence that results in cleft palate is **Robin sequence,** formerly called Pierre Robin Syndrome. In this condition, the primary anomaly is mandibular deficiency. The mandible (lower jaw) must descend in order for the palatal shelves to grow horizontally and fuse. In Robin sequence, failure of the mandible to grow properly in utero prevents the tongue from lowering into its normal position. The elevated tongue, in turn, prevents the lateral segments of the palate from growing together, resulting in an incomplete cleft palate which usually is "U" shaped, like the interfering tongue. After birth, infants with Robin sequence may have difficulty breathing because of **glossoptosis,** or collapse of the back of the tongue into the airway related to the small mandible. Glossoptosis sometimes improves without aggressive treatment, but often requires surgery during the first few weeks of life. Robin sequence may occur in isolation, but often is associated with a syndrome. In fact, the failure of the mandible to grow properly in utero (the primary abnormality in Robin sequence), may be caused by chromosomal, genetic, teratogenic, mechanical, or unknown factors.

ETIOLOGY

Four etiologic categories of clefts, syndromes, and sequences have been described (Cohen, 1982). These four categories are: (1) chromosomal abnormalities; (2) genetic abnormalities; (3) teratogenic agents; and (4) mechanical influences. Listing these categories suggests that each is distinct and unrelated, and many instances of cleft palate and syndromes do fall neatly into one category. However, a widely held theory is that clefts result from the interaction of genetic or other factors with environmental influences. This is referred to as *multifactorial inheritance* and helps to explain why two embryos may carry the same genetic predisposition to a disorder but may not exhibit the same anomalies. Conversely, different etiologic factors may result in similar patterns of anomalies. An example is Robin sequence, in which the primary defect of mandibular deficiency may be the result of chromosomal, genetic, teratogenic, or mechanical factors.

Chromosomal Abnormalities

All human cells contain 46 chromosomes arranged in 23 pairs. One member of each pair is inherited from each parent. Each chromosome contains thousands of genes. There are several types of chromosome abnormalities, including deletion of all or part of a chromosome, rearrangement of pieces of a chromosome, or duplication of all or part of a chromosome. Most chromosome abnormalities have devastating effects that may be incompatible with life, and a large percentage of miscarriages are believed to be caused by chromosomal abnormalities. Pregnancies with chromosome abnormalities that come to term often result in the birth of a baby with severe malformations, delays, and mental retardation. A chromosome abnormality with which many people are familiar is Trisomy 21, also called Down syndrome, in which there is an extra (third) chromosome 21. Cleft lip and palate is a commonly associated defect but, in some cases, may be a relatively minor consideration because of the poor long-term medical and developmental prognosis and cognitive limitation of communication skills.

Genetic Abnormalities

Thousands of gene pairs are inherited (one from each parent) and are arranged on the chromosome pairs. Genes may be dominant or recessive. If a gene is dominant, a fetus need inherit only one to display the particular trait for which that gene is responsible. If a gene is recessive, that particular gene must be inherited from both parents to be expressed. An important concept in understanding genetic disorders is variable expression. This means that every individual who has inherited an abnormal version of a gene may not display every symptom or feature, and every feature of the syndrome may not be expressed with the same severity. Examples of genetic syndromes with dominant transmission that are often associated with cleft palate are velo–cardio–facial syndrome, Stickler syndrome, van der Woude syndrome, and Treacher Collins syndrome. Because these syndromes are fairly common in the cleft palate population, they will be described briefly.

Velo–cardio–facial Syndrome. Velo–cardio-facial syndrome (VCF), first described by Shprintzen and colleagues in 1978, is the most common syndrome associated with cleft palate (Shprintzen & Goldberg, 1995). Individuals with VCF usually have incomplete cleft palate or submucous cleft palate (*velo*), cardiac defects (*cardio*), and a characteristic facial appearance (*facial*) (Shprintzen, et al., 1978; Shprintzen & Goldberg, 1995). Infants with VCF may have breathing problems related to Robin sequence and airway obstruction (Shprintzen, 1992), and often appear to have facial asymmetry, especially when crying (Shprintzen, 1995). Laryngeal web has been reported (Lipson, 1995). Speech is almost always characterized by severe compensatory articulation disorders (discussed later in this chapter), severe hypernasality, hoarse voice, and high vocal pitch (Golding-Kushner, 1991). Most children with VCF also have delayed language development and significant learning disabilities that may not be apparent until second or third grade (Golding-Kushner, Weller, & Shprintzen, 1985). The learning disabilities usually involve difficulty with inferential reasoning and abstract thinking that affects mathematics and reading (Golding-Kushner et al., 1985). During the teenage years, psychiatric disorders may appear (Shprintzen, Goldberg, Golding-Kushner & Marion, 1992). VCF is probably caused by a small genetic defect on chromosome 22 (Scambler, et al., 1992).

Stickler Syndrome. Stickler syndrome is a genetic disorder affecting the connective tissue. Features of this syndrome include incomplete cleft palate or submucous cleft palate, severe, progressive myopia (nearsightedness), and early arthritis (Jones, 1988; Gorlin, Cohen, & Levin, 1990). Even young children may be troubled by painful joints. High frequency sensorineural hearing loss and scoliosis are other findings. Infants with Stickler syndrome often have airway obstruction related to Robin sequence and a narrow upper airway. In fact, it has been estimated that one-third of all cases of Robin sequence actually have Stickler syndrome (Shprintzen, 1992). Everyone with Stickler syndrome does not have cleft palate, and many of those who do have normal speech. However, about half of the individuals with cleft palate related to Stickler syndrome are mildly hypernasal and have compensatory articulation disorders (Golding-Kushner, 1991). Language and learning skills are usually normal, especially when hearing is normal and middle ear disease associated with cleft palate is treated vigilantly (Golding-Kushner, 1991).

Van der Woude Syndrome. Van der Woude syndrome (VDW) is characterized by dominantly inherited cleft lip and/or palate with lower lip pits, and congenitally absent premolars (Jones, 1988; Gorlin et al., 1990). In general, it is unusual for different types of clefts to occur within the same family. However, in VDW, expression of clefting is variable (even among siblings), and may range from submucous cleft palate to complete bilateral cleft lip and palate. Language and learning skills are usually normal (Golding-Kushner, 1991). Speech is often normal after palate repair but about 40 percent of individuals have mild- to-moderate hypernasal resonance and compensatory articulation errors (Golding-Kushner, 1991).

Treacher Collins Syndrome. Treacher Collins Syndrome, first described by Berry (1889), involves the face, orbits, and ears bilaterally. Cleft palate and submucous cleft palate are common in this syndrome, and cleft lip may also occur. Max-imum conductive hearing loss secondary to outer and middle ear malformations is common, and is the greatest threat to cognitive, speech, and language development, especially if not detected and treated early. Because of bilateral microtia and/or atresia, use of a bone conduction hearing aid may be necessary. Facial characteristics include defects of the lower eye lids, clefting of the zygomatic arch that gives the eyes a downward-slanting appearance, maxillary hypoplasia, and mandibular deficiency related to Robin sequence (Jones, 1988; Gorlin et al., 1990). The vocal tract is extremely narrow in Treacher Collins syndrome, and airway obstruction is very common in infancy (Shprintzen, Croft, Berkman, & Rakoff, 1979). Following palate repair, nasal resonance is usually normal. When hypernasality occurs it is generally very mild or intermittent and may decrease or even resolve with age because of changes in the nasopharynx and vocal tract that occur as a result of craniofacial growth patterns in this syndrome (Golding-Kushner, 1991). Articulation errors often involve tongue backing, but compensatory errors related to VPI are infrequent (Golding-Kushner, 1991). Oral resonance may be muffled because the oral cavity and vocal tract are small.

Teratogenic Effects

A **teratogen** is an external agent that passes from a pregnant mother to the developing embryo or fetus through the placenta and has the potential to interfere with normal prenatal development. The teratogenic effect of a particular agent in a specific case depends on many factors including the teratogen; the stage of pregnancy; the frequency, duration, and intensity of exposure; exposure to combinations of potential teratogens; the mother's metabolism; and so forth. Well-known teratogens include alcohol, crack/cocaine, many over-the-counter and prescription medications, and viruses such as rubella. Few of these agents are known to cause cleft palate. At the least, these agents may cause intrauterine growth retardation and low birth weight, both of which are risk factors for subsequent language and learning deficits (see Chapter 2). At the worst, they cause severe malformations. Alcohol and cocaine are potent teratogens that do frequently cause cleft lip and palate (Shprintzen, Siegel-Sadewitz, Amato, & Goldberg, 1985; Cohen & Bankier, 1991). Fetal risk is even greater if the mother's substance abuse is chronic because prenatal care may be poor.

Fetal alcohol syndrome (FAS) is characterized by prenatal and postnatal growth deficiency, mental retardation, irritability and hyperactivity, cardiac defects, micrognathia, and cleft lip and/or cleft palate (Jones, 1988; Gorlin, 1990). Language and learning problems are common because of cognitive deficits. Children who have FAS or FAE (fetal alcohol effect, a less severe expression of fetal alcohol syndrome) and who also have cleft palate are at additional risk with regard to speech and language because of chronic ear infections. Compensatory articulation patterns and hypernasality are also common in children with FAS/FAE and cleft palate. Fetal cocaine embryopathy is also often associated with cleft palate. Characteristics of fetal cocaine embryopathy are similar to FAS. The neonatal period is often even more difficult because the baby experiences cocaine withdrawal, making early feeding especially challenging. The most unfortunate thing about this group of disorders is that they are entirely preventable. After the child's birth, parental substance abuse and any associated family dysfunction must be addressed if there is to be any hope for the child to develop to his or her potential.

Mechanical Influences

Mechanical influences are factors that affect a developing embryo which is otherwise normal. Clefts and certain syndromes may be caused by uterine abnormalities or multiple pregnancies that result in intrauterine crowding. Amniotic tears or bands of amniotic tissue may interrupt otherwise normal development and result in severe deformities affecting the face, limbs, and digits. The appearance at birth is shocking because of the severity of the facial, lip, and palatal clefts, and digital amputations that occur in utero. Intrauterine crowding may also cause craniofacial anomalies by depriving the fetus of the necessary room for normal growth. Crowding may be related to the presence of a multiple pregnancy (e.g., twins, triplets) or due to structural abnormalities of the uterus. Robin sequence and hemifacial microsomia (literally "half the face smaller") are two disorders that may sometimes be related to this type of problem.

Acquired Deformities and Neurologic Disease

Maxillofacial deformities resembling cleft palate and related problems may result from trauma (such as a gunshot wound) or ablative surgery (such as for removal of a tumor). Congenital neurologic disorders (such as cerebral palsy and nemaline myopathy) and neurologic diseases of later onset (such as muscular dystrophy, Parkinson's disease, cerebral vascular accidents, and amyotrophic lateral sclerosis) may result in resonance disorders similar to those associated with cleft palate (see Chapters 8 and 14). In these cases, treatment and prognosis may be different, depending on age of onset and stability of the disease process (i.e., if it is stable or progressive).

PSYCHOSOCIAL ISSUES

The birth of a child can be one of the most eagerly anticipated events in a person's life. Throughout the long months of pregnancy, many expectant parents plan for their newborn's homecoming and dream about the future. Therefore, it can be devastating to new parents to learn that there is a problem with their newborn, and especially shocking to see a baby with a facial deformity. When a child is born with an abnormality, especially a highly visible one, parents mourn the loss of the perfect baby they expected. Feeding problems may further complicate acceptance and bonding.

Little is known about the psychological effects of repeated hospitalizations and surgery on a developing child, and different studies have suggested different results. It is clear that there is a significant interaction among many cultural and familial factors that affect the child's ultimate self-image. Communication skills and acceptance by peers are also factors. Fortunately, most parents quickly learn to accept the presence of a defect. Strauss and Broder (1990) summarized a large body of literature on psychological and sociocultural issues related to cleft lip and palate. They found that facial attractiveness appears to affect interactions and expectations for behavior from school age through adulthood. Teachers and parents tend to underestimate the abilities of children with visible clefts and have lower expectations for them, especially if speech intelligibility is also compromised (Richman, 1978; Kapp, 1979). Subjects with facial clefts appear to have lower self-concepts than their noncleft peers and may tend to underachieve relative to their intellectual abilities (Richman & Harper, 1978). Adolescents and adults with clefts report less dating experiences and marry later in life (Peters & Chinsky, 1974). Strauss and Broder concluded that there is no distinctive personality type among cleft subjects, and that relatively low rates of psychopathology are reported in this group. This is not the case among individuals with velo–cardio–facial syndrome, who have been described as having distinctive personality characteristics in childhood and may have a higher than expected risk for psychosis in adolescence (Golding-Kushner et al., 1985; Shprintzen et al., 1992). Some cleft palate teams and independent organizations sponsor support groups for parents, children, and teenagers with cleft palate or specific syndromes. As a result of the excellent coordinated care available in developed nations, most children with cleft lip and/or palate develop into adults who take their place in society and have families of their own. Unfortunately, some non-Western cultures have extremely negative attitudes towards birth defects (Strauss & Broder, 1990). Child neglect and concealment of persons with facial defects keeps some children from receiving surgical and other care in some locations. At the extreme, infanticide has been used as a means of dealing with birth defects.

TEAM CARE

The presence of a cleft lip and palate or other craniofacial anomaly has effects that require treatment at multiple stages of development from birth through adulthood. Treatment should be provided by a variety of medical, dental, and behavioral specialists. Most patients are treated by multidisciplinary teams of specialists who work together to coordinate care. The composition of teams varies, but cleft palate teams almost always include, at the very least, a pediatrician, plastic surgeon, otolaryngologist (ENT), orthodontist, and speech–language pathologist. Teams that treat patients with more complex problems often include professionals from more disciplines, such as oral surgery, audiology, pediatric dentistry, genetics, radiology, nursing, psychology, speech science/physiology, and social work. Other specialties that may participate in the care of patients with cleft palate syndromes are cardiology, ophthalmology, orthopedics, endocrinology, neurology, neuroradiology, neurosurgery, urology, and others.

Team members must be very knowledgeable about their own discipline and about the subspecialty of cleft palate as it relates to their field. In order to work together as a team, each professional must be familiar with the other disciplines, with the vocabulary of the other specialties, and with the treatment goals of the entire team. This challenge can be very exciting and rewarding for speech–language pathologists and audiologists who are integral members of such teams. For example, cleft palate may have a negative effect on dental development and hearing, as well as on early feeding and speech, and certain syndromes may be associated with neurologic and cognitive deficits. Therefore, speech-language pathologists who are part of a craniofacial team have a unique opportunity to work closely with pediatricians, plastic surgeons, dentists, orthodontists, oral surgeons, prosthodontists, otolaryngologists, audiologists, neurologists, and psychologists. Essential but often overlooked members of the team are the parents and the patient. (See Chapter 14.) Cultural and family issues cannot be ignored when recommendations are made for treatment. It is the role of the professional team to examine, diagnose, and propose treatment. However, the family must make the final decision and it is up to them to follow through with the plan. If they are uncomfortable with a particular recommendation, the rationale should be discussed; if possible, other treatment options should be offered.

The Role of the Speech–Language Pathologist

The speech-language pathologist on a cleft palate team has many responsibilities. During the earliest stages of care, the speech-language pathologist may provide the parents with guidance for feeding the newborn. Language and speech evaluations should begin early—no later than the child's first birthday. The speech-language pathologist monitors the child's speech and language development and establishes early intervention programs through home programs and parent training. If needed, the speech-language pathologist may provide therapy, which must usually be intensive. Many children who receive care from cleft palate teams do not live in the community in which the team is located. Therefore, ongoing speech therapy is often provided by a therapist working in a neighborhood hospital, clinic, school, or private practice. In this situation, the speech-language pathologist at the cleft palate center and the treating speech-language pathologist must work as a speech therapy team (Golding-Kushner, Le Blanc, & Tantilb, 1990b; Golding-Kushner, 1995). The speech-language pathologist who is on the cleft palate team acts as a liaison between the team and the treating speech-language pathologist, and is available to offer management suggestions. When the patient is cooperative enough for nasopharyngoscopy and multiview videofluoroscopy (usually at four years of age), the speech-language pathol-

ogist works together with the endoscopist and radiologist in performing the examination and interpreting the results.

Birth and the Newborn Period

The prospect of treatment from such an array of specialists can overwhelm new parents still struggling to cope with the fact that their newborn baby was born with an abnormality of some type. A common practice is for a representative of the cleft palate team to meet with the parents shortly after the birth of a child with a cleft to offer emotional support, provide reassurance that help is at hand, and introduce the parent to the concept of team care. This first meeting also lays the groundwork for providing factual information about cleft palate. Different teams have different practices, and the first specialist with whom the parents have contact may be a pediatrician, speech–language pathologist, social worker, genetic counselor, plastic surgeon, or other specialist. Regardless of who it is, the team representative must, above all else, be a good listener and give the new parents an opportunity to talk. At the same time, enough information should be provided to alleviate concerns without causing more stress.

Pediatric Care

A newborn baby with a cleft is, first and foremost, a baby. The earliest treatment involves routine pediatric care and, if necessary, assistance with feeding. Otologic and surgical care also begin during the first few months of life.

Feeding. After the first cry, the very first task that newborns perform with their mouths is eating, which involves sucking and swallowing. (See Chapter 10 for a complete description of infant sucking behaviors.) Infants who have only a cleft lip usually have no difficulty feeding, and may even be breast-fed. Some mothers have successfully breast-fed infants with cleft palate. However, because of a lack of separation between the mouth and nose, a newborn with a cleft palate cannot create the negative oral pressure needed to extract liquid by sucking on a nipple. Therefore, most infants with cleft palate are bottle fed. This may be an emotional issue, especially for a mother who wanted to breast-feed. Some mothers compromise by expressing breast milk using a pump and feeding their own milk by bottle rather than (or in addition to) formula. Feeding is often the catalyst for bringing together the newborn, the parents, and the cleft palate team for the first time. Feeding instruction is usually provided by the team pediatrician, speech pathologist, or nurse.

The primary goal of the feeding process is to ensure that the infant receives adequate nutrition, but it is also important to maintain maximum normalcy of this early and frequent activity. It is widely accepted that important parent–child (especially mother–child) bonds are formed during feeding. It is a time of close physical and eye contact, and of early and pleasurable communication. If attention is shifted away from this natural exchange and onto the feeding process itself because of awkward feeding devices or methods, much of the pleasure may be lost to both the parent and child, and opportunities for early communication and language stimulation may be missed. Normal feeding also helps to focus the parents' attention on the normalcy of the baby, rather than on the birth defect. If the baby can be fed in the same way as other babies, without special tubes, special bottles, special appliances, and a lot of anxiety, it helps the parents to see their newborn as a child who happens to have a cleft, rather than as a "defective," "handicapped," or "special needs" child. This sets a tone for the way in which the child is perceived by the immediate and extended family, and even by others in the community.

Some professionals advocate the use of feeding appliances. There are various feeding devices and special bottles on the market made especially for infants with cleft palate. However, most infants feed well with a regular bottle and soft nipple, as long as certain minor adjustments are made in position, nipple placement, and the nipple hole. First, when being fed, an infant with a cleft palate

should be held in as upright a position as possible to allow gravity to work with the baby during swallowing, helping the milk reach the stomach and reducing **nasal regurgitation** (food coming out of the nose) and choking. Second, the nipple must be placed against an intact area of the palate, not into the cleft, so the baby can squeeze the nipple between the tongue and side of the palate or cheek to extract liquid. The third adjustment is to make a crosscut (X) in the nipple to replace the small hole so that the formula flows more easily. It is important to allow the infant to use the tongue and intact portion of the palate to take milk from the nipple. Gavage (nasogastric or orogastric), syringe, or other tube feeding essentially bypasses the mouth and deprives the infant of an important prespeech activity. Bypassing the mouth may also increase the development of oral defensiveness and sensitivity, affecting later eating behavior and, possibly, speech. When an infant is fed for several months or even several weeks without using the tongue, lips, cheeks, and palate, it often becomes more difficult to introduce oral feeding.

On occasion, an infant with a cleft palate is unable to feed adequately even when the feeding position, nipple placement, and nipple hole size are optimal. This usually signals the presence of other problems that require medical attention. For example, the pharynx is a common pathway for both eating and breathing, and most infants who present with feeding difficulties actually have a compromised airway (another name for the pharynx or vocal tract), which may be very serious and even life threatening if not treated. When feeding attempts using these procedures are ineffective, the airway must be examined to rule out obstruction or compromise. In most cases, the feeding problem resolves itself once the airway problem is managed. Feeding therapy techniques applied for the treatment of swallowing disorders (dysphagia) are generally inappropriate for babies with cleft palate. In fact, when the underlying cause of a feeding problem is related to structural abnormalities such as airway obstruction, attempts at feeding therapy might delay appropriate medical examination of the airway.

Otologic Care.   It has been said that middle ear disease is "universal" in the cleft palate population (Paradise, Bluestone, & Felder, 1969; Paradise & Bluestone, 1974). While this may be somewhat extreme, there is no question that the prevalence of otitis media in cleft palate is extremely high. Malpositioning of muscles (including levator palatini and tensor palatini) that occurs in the presence of a cleft palate is probably largely responsible for the high prevalence of middle ear disease in this population. The eustachian tube normally ventilates the middle ear cavity and equalizes air pressure. In patients with cleft palate, the pharyngeal opening of the eustachian tube is often elliptical in shape rather than round, and often becomes occluded with muscle tissue during phonation and swallowing, rather than remaining patent as it does in individuals with normal palates (Figure 9.8) (Gereau, et al., 1988). These abnor-

malities may contribute to the prevalence of otitis media in children with cleft palate. It is therefore important that careful otologic examination and routine audiometric testing, including tympanometry, be performed beginning by age three or four months, when otitis tends to begin.

Certain craniofacial syndromes such as Treacher Collins syndrome and hemifacial microsomia are associated with malformations of the outer, middle, or inner ear. Infants with a syndrome associated with high risk for hearing loss should be tested as soon after birth as possible. In patients with cleft palate and otitis media, tympanostomy tubes are often placed at the time of palate repair. Otitis generally decreases with age, especially following palate repair, and most children with cleft palate are free of ear disease by the time they are five years old. However, some individuals continue to have otitis media and second-

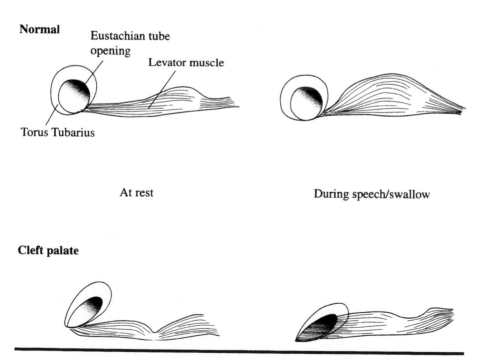

FIGURE 9.8 Eustachian tube orifice and lateral insertion of levator muscle. Note circular shape of normal (top), and patency at rest and during function. In individuals with cleft palate (bottom), the orifice is often elliptical and becomes occluded by the levator veli palatini muscle during speech and swallowing.

ary complications (such as perforated tympanic membranes from repeated tube insertions, cholesteatoma, mastoiditis) into the teen years or adulthood.

SURGICAL MANAGEMENT

Lip Repair

Cleft lip is usually repaired at about three months of age, following the "Rule of 10": the baby should weigh at least 10 pounds, have a hemoglobin of at least 10 grams, a white count no higher than 10,000, and be at least 10 weeks old (Wilhelmsen & Musgrave, 1966). Revisions of the lip and nose are often done at later ages. A few surgeons perform lip repairs or preliminary lip adhesions during the first few days of life. Revolutionary new techniques of fetal surgery have been used in recent years to correct serious defects in fetuses who would otherwise not have survived. Fetal surgery is highly complicated and carries enormous risks to both the fetus and the mother. Cleft lip is sometimes diagnosed prenatally using ultrasound. It has been suggested that fetal surgery could be performed on cleft lip, thus eliminating the life-long scar that is inevitable after traditional surgery (Hallok, 1985; Ortiz-Monasterio & Micolo, 1990; Oberg, Evans, Nguyen, Peckham, Kirsch, & Hardesty, 1995). However, most medical ethicists agree that the risks to the fetus and the mother are far greater than the potential benefit of avoiding a scar. On the other extreme, there are some developing countries in which surgical repair of cleft lip is not readily available, and individuals may never have surgery.

Palate Repair

The purpose of palate repair is to separate the nasal and oral cavities. Whereas the primary purpose of lip repair is aesthetic, the most important reason for repairing the palate is related to speech; other reasons are to facilitate eating and to reduce regurgitation of food and fluid through the nose. Surgical repair between 12 and 18 months of age results

in better speech than later repair because the palate is intact early, before the infant has an opportunity to develop or habituate abnormal compensatory articulation errors that have been referred to as *cleft palate speech* (Lindsay, Le Mesuriers, & Farmer, 1962; Morley, 1973; Hall & Golding-Kushner, 1989; McWilliams, Morris, & Shelton, 1990; Karling, Larson, Leanderson, & Henningsson, 1993).

Children who do not have their palate repaired until after two years of age are at very high risk for severe maladaptive compensatory articulation disorders that can be difficult to treat. Some surgeons delay repair of the hard palate, or even the entire palate, until age five or even 12 years because of concern that repairing the palate at an early age could interfere with subsequent facial growth (Graber, 1954; Schweckendiek, 1978). However, the cleft itself probably signals a tissue deficiency that could result in underdevelopment of the middle third of the face.

The prevalent view among speech–language pathologists, plastic surgeons, oral surgeons, and orthodontists regarding the timing of palate repair may be summarized as follows. Early repair of the palate probably has no effect on subsequent facial growth. Even if it does have a negative effect in a percentage of individuals, mid-facial deficiency is easily corrected with surgery. In contrast, delayed palate repair usually results in the development of deviant articulation patterns that cannot be corrected surgically and will require speech therapy. Because the speech benefit of early palate repair is unquestionable and the detrimental effect on facial growth is doubtful, it is in the best interest of the child to repair the palate between 12 and 18 months of age. Palate repair may be accomplished in a single procedure or in two stages, one for the hard palate and one for the soft palate. The decision is often based on the severity of the cleft, but also depends on each surgeon's philosophy.

Pharyngeal Flap Surgery

Hypernasality due to velopharyngeal insufficiency occurs following palate repair about 16 percent to 20 percent of the time. The purpose of **pharyngeal flap** surgery is to provide the potential for velopharyngeal closure. Most pharyngeal flaps are created by separation of a rectangular flap of tissue from the posterior pharyngeal wall (the top of the flap remains connected), and insertion of the bottom end of the flap into a slit in the soft palate (Figure 9.9). The flap acts as a cork to prevent leakage of air into the nasal cavities and eliminates the need for contact between the velum and posterior pharyngeal wall. Success of the flap is dependent on the ability of the lateral pharyngeal walls to move inward and contact the sides of the flap during speech (Skolnick & McCall, 1972; Argamaso, et al., 1980). The spaces between each side of the flap and the lateral pharyngeal wall on that side are called the lateral ports, and it is through the lateral ports that the postflap patient breathes and drains nasal secretions. The lateral ports also provide nasal coupling for production of nasal phonemes (Figure 9.10). The surgeons with the greatest success in eliminating hyperna-

sality with a pharyngeal flap are those who use diagnostic information based on direct visualization of the amount of lateral pharyngeal motion during speech to plan the general width of the pharyngeal flap (Shprintzen et al., 1979). This can usually be accomplished after the child's fourth birthday using nasopharyngoscopy and multiview videofluoroscopy, which will be discussed later. Construction of a flap that is unnecessarily wide should be avoided because it may increase the risk of airway obstruction, snoring, and hyponasality. When lateral pharyngeal wall motion is asymmetric, the pharyngeal flap can be skewed to one side (Argamaso, Levandoski, Golding, Kushner, & Shprintzen, 1994). Many lay people misunderstand the recommendation for a pharyngeal flap, and think it is needed because it was missing. Therefore, it is important to explain to a potential surgical candidate and the family that infants are not born with a pharyngeal flap, and that "normal" speakers do not have them. A pharyngeal flap is something that is created surgically

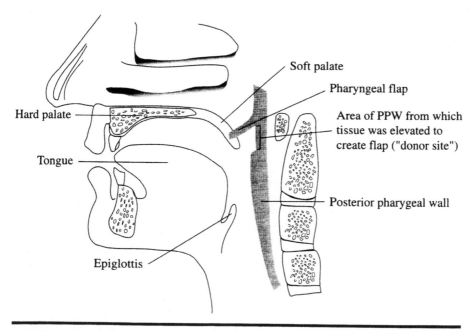

Soft palate

Pharyngeal flap

Hard palate

Area of PPW from which tissue was elevated to create flap ("donor site")

Tongue

Posterior pharygeal wall

Epiglottis

FIGURE 9.9 Lateral sketch of pharyngeal flap. A flap of tissue from the posterior pharyngeal wall is inserted into the velum to create a bridge across the velopharynx.

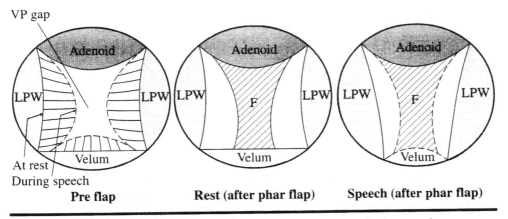

FIGURE 9.10 Superior view of velopharyngeal region showing (a) velopharyngeal insufficiency during speech prior to pharyngeal flap surgery, (b) appearance of the pharyngeal flap and the velopharyngeal port at rest, and (c) closure of the lateral ports during speech achieved due to movement of the lateral pharyngeal walls to the lateral edges of the flap. The solid lines represent rest positions, and the dotted lines represent the position during speech. Velopharyngeal insufficiency has been eliminated.

to enable an otherwise hypernasal speaker to have normal resonance.

Other Surgical Procedures

Fistula Repair.   A palatal **fistula** is an opening that remains or appears after palate repair. Depending on their size and location, fistulae may not affect speech or eating. On the other hand, they may contribute to nasal regurgitation or may be annoying because of food entrapment. They may be detrimental to speech in several ways. First, they may affect articulation, often leading to a pattern of tongue backing errors, which will be discussed later. They may also result in a worsening of velopharyngeal closure (Isberg & Henningsson, 1987), a phenomenon of major surgical consequence.

Alveolar Bone Graft.   Repair of an alveolar cleft is accomplished by grafting bone from the hip to the alveolar ridge. This is done to stabilize the maxillary dental arch and to ensure retention of the secondary teeth in the region. This is usually done between the ages of seven and nine, de-

pending on dental development, and is performed just prior to eruption of the permanent canine tooth. Earlier bone grafting is not recommended by most orthodontists because surgery could damage the permanent tooth buds and interfere with subsequent dental development (Bardach & Salyer, 1995). Also, the bone graft and permanent teeth provide reciprocal stability that may only be achieved by waiting until the canine is about to erupt. However, some oral surgeons, plastic surgeons, and orthodontists do not believe that bone grafting should be performed until 12 years of age, some combine it with the initial lip repair, and some do not advocate the procedure at all.

Craniofacial and Maxillofacial Surgery

Procedures involving the facial skeleton below the orbits are referred to as *maxillofacial surgery.* When at least one orbit is involved, the procedure is referred to as *craniofacial surgery.* Maxillofacial procedures are used to correct abnormalities of the midface, maxilla, or mandible. Craniofacial procedures correct abnormalities of the orbits, forehead, and skull. These types of operations are highly specialized, and are performed by extensively trained plastic or maxillofacial surgeons. Craniofacial surgery is often performed jointly with neurosurgeons and eye surgeons. The most common maxillofacial procedures in patients with cleft palate involve midface advancement in which part or all of the maxilla is detached from the surrounding facial or cranial skeleton and moved forward to a more favorable position. The maxilla may be advanced, rotated, retracted, or tilted. Advancement is commonly needed because of midfacial deficiency, causing a concave profile and a severe Class III malocclusion that affects both the function of the jaws and teeth and appearance. Repositioning may also be used to correct malocclusions when they cannot be corrected adequately with orthodontic therapy alone, or to compensate for facial asymmetry. Craniofacial surgery was pioneered by Tessier, and involves removing segments of the cranium (which exposes the brain), reshaping the segments, repositioning them, and suturing them together. This may be a lifesaving procedure in some patients who have skull deformities that actually cause compression of the brain. Methods of surgical planning for correction of complicated cranial and facial deformities have become very sophisticated over the last five years. "Phantom surgery" may be performed on computerized three-dimensional reconstructed images from CT scans, allowing surgeons to determine the feasibility of their plan, and to rehearse in advance what they will actually do in the operating room. The surgical procedure and anticipated postsurgical appearance can also be shown to the patient and/or parents.

Dental Management.   Children who have undergone surgery in or near the mouth may display oral defensiveness leading to poor oral hygiene. Establishing good dental hygiene at a very young age is especially important for children with clefts so that the primary dentition will not be lost prematurely because of decay or gum disease. Early exfoliation (loss) of the primary teeth could further complicate orthodontic abnormalities of the permanent dentition.

Orthodontic Management.   Orthodontic problems are common among children with cleft lip and/or palate, especially when the alveolus is also cleft. These problems include malocclusions, collapse of the maxillary arches leading to cross bite, and missing, rotated, and/or supernumerary (extra) teeth. The effect of these deviations on speech depends on their severity, but there is not a direct relationship between the presence of a dental abnormality and the presence of a speech problem. Sibilant sounds are most sensitive to malocclusions and abnormal interdental spacing. Sometimes an orthodontic deviation does not affect speech adversely but may, at least temporarily, interfere with tongue placement and lead to multiple sound distortions. An important role of the orthodontist in the care of children with cleft palate is to assess and monitor growth of the facial skeleton using standardized radiographs called *cephalographs*. Standardized measurements can be made and patterns of growth can be predicted in order to guide treatment. Certain skeletal features are also helpful in establishing a syndromic diagnosis.

Prosthodontic Management.   A **prosthodontist** is a dentist or orthodontist with additional special training in the construction of artificial teeth and devices. For example, if permanent teeth are missing they may be replaced prosthetically, or, if there is sufficient underlying alveolar tissue, dental implants may be used. Some cleft palate teams advocate the use of feeding appliances for newborns, which look like orthodontic retainers and may be constructed by dentists, orthodontists, or prosthodonists. Prosthodontists may also treat patients with cleft palate with speech aids known as **obturators**. Obturators are prostheses that are used to cover an unrepaired hard palate in some patients with a primary veloplasty, or to cover large palatal fistulae until they can be repaired.

Another use of obturators is in the management of velopharyngeal insufficiency. Two appliances used for eliminating hypernasality are **speech bulbs** and **palatal lifts**. A speech bulb contains a palatal retainer and pharyngeal extension that terminates in a bulb usually made of

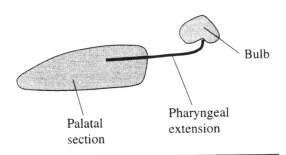

FIGURE 9.11 Speech bulb appliance.

acrylic (Figure 9.11). A speech bulb functions in exactly the same way as a pharyngeal flap, serving as a target in space around which velopharyngeal closure can occur. Another type of speech appliance is a palatal lift. Palatal lifts contain a retainer identical to the anterior portion of a speech bulb, but terminate in a finger-like extension that does not extend beyond the palate. As its name implies, this type of appliance elevates the palate. Speech bulbs are more appropriate than palatal lifts in patients with repaired or submucous cleft palate, especially if the palate appears short. A palatal lift may be better than a speech bulb when there is sufficient palatal tissue to contact the posterior pharyngeal wall when the palate is raised, and enough lateral pharyngeal wall motion to contact the lateral edges of the elevated palate. Palatal lifts are used more commonly in patients with neurologically based velopharyngeal insufficiency than in patients with structurally based velopharyngeal insufficiency. The placement and size of both appliances must be individually designed, and may be guided using multiview videofluoroscopic or nasopharyngoscopic examination (Schechter, Golding, Shprintzen, & Rakoff, 1977; McGrath & Anderson, 1990; Golding-Kushner et al., 1995).

Patient selection must take into account technical issues such as adequacy of dental hygiene and stability of the dentition needed to retain the appliance. More importantly, the use of an appliance demands a very high level of commitment and compliance from the patient and parents (Golding-Kushner et al., 1995). One advantage of a speech appliance over a pharyngeal flap is mod-

ifiability; that is, once surgery is done, it's done. A deficiency can be corrected only with additional surgery. On the other hand, a speech appliance can be elevated, lowered, enlarged, or decreased in size as needed. Speech appliances are removed at night, so the potential for airway obstruction is not an issue. However, speech appliances have many disadvantages. They are constructed over many visits to a dental specialist and demand repeated nasopharyngoscopic examinations to achieve optimum placement and size. They must be maintained and checked by the dental specialist and endoscopist periodically. They must be cleaned on a daily basis, and frequent handling can result in damage. Perhaps most problematic is that when the appliance is not inserted, hypernasality is present. For example, this would occur if the appliance was out for repair, which could take from days to weeks, or if it was lost, which frequently occurs with children.

COGNITIVE DEVELOPMENT

Cleft lip and palate alone are not associated with abnormal cognitive development. Most children with cleft lip and/or palate who do not have any other anomalies enjoy normal development and achieve milestones such as sitting, walking, and talking at the same ages as their peers who do not have cleft palate. Ironically, incomplete cleft palate, which would seem to be the least severe type of overt clefting, is the type of cleft that is most often associated with other anomalies. Individuals with certain syndromes, such as velo–cardio–facial syndrome, are at extremely high risk for developmental, cognitive, and even psychiatric disorders. Therefore, every baby with a cleft palate should undergo thorough medical and developmental examinations to arrive at a proper diagnosis. Only then can intervention be appropriately provided.

LANGUAGE DEVELOPMENT

There have been numerous studies of speech and language development in children with cleft lip and palate. Cleft lip alone has no effect on any aspect of development. The question of whether children with cleft palate are more or less likely than their noncleft peers to experience speech and language problems must be addressed separately for syndromic and nonsyndromic cleft palate. Early studies of language development suggested some delays in children with cleft palate (Spriestersbach, Darley, & Morris, 1958; Morris, 1962). However, patterns of language development are often predictable in specific syndromes. For example, 85 percent of children with velo–cardio–facial syndrome experience delayed language development and the discrepancy between their expected and actual language skills increases with age, as expectations for language performance increase (Golding-Kushner et al., 1985; Golding-Kushner, 1991). In contrast, van der Woude syndrome is associated with average or above average language skills (Golding-Kushner, 1991). Recent investigations that take syndromic diagnoses into account generally suggest that children with isolated cleft palate who have aggressive management of their middle ear disease are essentially no different from their peers who do not have cleft palate (Pecyna, Feeny-Giacoma, & Neiman, 1987; Long & Dalston, 1983). Clearly, the cleft palate population, even including individuals with syndromic cleft palate, is a heterogeneous group with respect to all aspects of development, including language (Shames & Rubin, 1979). Therefore, early language screening for all children with cleft palate and craniofacial disorders is essential (McWilliams et al., 1990).

SPEECH DEVELOPMENT AND DISORDERS

Eighty-four percent of children with nonsyndromic cleft lip and palate or cleft palate alone develop normal resonance and articulation that is free of **compensatory errors** following primary palate repair, without any intervention (Hall & Golding-Kushner, 1989; Peterson-Falzone, 1990). A recent study suggested that children who do not receive optimal team care from infancy may be far less likely to achieve normal speech, even by adulthood (Peterson-Falzone, 1995). When they

occur, the speech disorders associated with cleft palate and velopharyngeal insufficiency are different from other clinical populations and often seem resistant to treatment. Furthermore, certain syndrome groups are at risk for specific types of voice, resonance, and articulation disorders.

Voice

Voice is the result of laryngeal activity. There are some studies that suggest that the prevalence of vocal pathology, such as hoarseness, vocal fold nodules, and vocal hyperfunction is higher in the cleft than in the noncleft population, especially in patients with borderline velopharyngeal closure (McWilliams, Bluestone, & Musgrave, 1969; McWilliams, Lavorato, & Bluestone, 1973). Supporters of that view believe that this is because of the greater effort needed to attain intensity due to the effect of air escape through the velopharyngeal valve. Other studies have found that the incidence of vocal pathology in children with cleft palate is no different than other school age children. Certain vocal characteristics may be associated with certain syndromes. For example, Golding-Kushner (1991) found that 28 percent of patients with velo–cardio–facial syndrome have a higher than normal vocal pitch, and about 20 percent of patients with VCF are hoarse. She observed radiographic evidence of laryngeal immaturity that could account for the perceptual characteristics. Laryngeal web and other structural abnormalities have also been reported in VCF (Lipson, Yuille, Angel, Thompson, Vanderwood, & Beckenham, 1991; Lipson, 1995). Laryngeal examination is critical for all patients with craniofacial disorders, especially those with evidence of abnormal vocal pitch, quality, or loudness. Findings such as underdevelopment of the epiglottis, laryngeal asymmetry, laryngeal web, or even cleft larynx may be of great significance in establishing a syndromic diagnosis.

Resonance

The characteristic acquired by the vocal tone as it passes through the pharynx is called *resonance*. In order to be perceived as normal, a certain balance of oral resonance and nasal resonance must be present.

Hypernasality.   Eighty-four percent of children with nonsyndromic cleft palate obtain normal resonance following palate repair (Hall & Golding-Kushner, 1989; Peterson-Falzone, 1990). The other 16 percent are hypernasal. In most of these cases, hypernasality is consistent. However, it is also possible to have inconsistent hypernasality. Hypernasality is a perceptual phenomenon and can only be diagnosed by the human ear. The presence of hypernasality often suggests the presence of velopharyngeal insufficiency. However, VPI is physiologic, not perceptual, and can only be diagnosed by direct visualization of the region.

Hyponasality.   Hyponasality may occur because of adenoidal obstruction, septal deviation, or other nasal obstruction. It is possible, and not uncommon, for a patient to have both hypernasality and hyponasality. Patients with hyponasality should be examined by an otolaryngologist for diagnosis and to determine if medical or surgical treatment is indicated. Hyponasality is also a frequent sequela of pharyngeal flap surgery. This is usually temporary and resolves over time, except in individuals who have surgery to construct subobstructing pharyngeal flaps as teenagers or adults after growth is complete (Shprintzen, 1988; Hall, Golding-Kushner, Argamaso, & Strauch, 1991; Argamaso et al., 1994; Golding-Kushner, Argamaso, & Mitnick, 1994).

Articulation

Children with cleft palate may exhibit articulation errors related to many sources including delayed development, hearing loss, malocclusion, palatal fistulae, and velopharyngeal insufficiency. Sound errors also may be categorized as functional, **obligatory,** or **compensatory.** It is the task of the speech–language pathologist to determine the source and category of each sound error and the appropriate course of treatment. Judgments about articulation must be based on a comprehen-

sive speech sample that should include administration of a formal test of articulation, repetition of isolated phonemes, words, and phrases, and conversational speech. The speech sample must include nasal-loaded phrases and nasal-free phrases that focus on each class of sounds, such as plosives and fricatives, voiced and voiceless (Shprintzen & Golding-Kushner, 1989; Golding-Kushner, 1990a). Isolated sustained [s, f] should be included because they may reveal the presence of inconsistent velopharyngeal insufficiency.

Developmental Errors.   Children with clefts are subject to the same delays as other children, and they should be managed in the same way, with intervention when appropriate.

Hearing Loss.   The effect of long-term, chronic or intermittent otitis media on speech development is not known. Children with high frequency sensorineural hearing loss, such as may be associated with Stickler syndrome, may evidence difficulty with high frequency phonemes, such as sibilants. When errors are associated with hearing loss, the hearing loss should be treated medically and/or with amplification as early as possible, and speech therapy should be provided as for any other hearing-impaired child.

Malocclusion.   Tongue-tip phonemes [t, d, n, s, z] are the most sensitive to distortion because of malocclusion, endentulous spaces (wider than normal spaces between the teeth), and the presence of an alveolar cleft. Sometimes, speech is acoustically accurate but visually distorted. For example, a severe Class III malocclusion (underbite) may be associated with inversion of labiodental placement for [f, v]; that is, production using the upper lip and lower teeth, which sounds accurate but looks in error. The presence of a dental abnormality does not preclude normal speech. The nature and severity of the speech error, and the proximity in time (months versus years) to resolution of the dental problem must be taken into account when speech therapy is considered. Depending on the degree of accuracy of tongue placement, minor acoustic distortions may resolve without speech therapy when the dental abnormality is corrected.

Palatal Fistulae. Fistulae may be directly responsible for reduced intraoral pressure (IOP), which causes weak pressure consonants, nasal air emission, and nasalization of oral phonemes. Nasal air emission may be audible or inaudible. Because these errors cannot be corrected in the presence of the open fistula, they are considered obligatory. Obligatory errors require orthodontic, prosthetic, or surgical management, and cannot be corrected using speech therapy. Children with unrepaired hard palate clefts or fistulae often develop an articulation pattern of tongue backing, in which the tongue tip is retracted to a position posterior to the fistula during production of alveolar or mid-palatal sounds. For example, instead of lingua-alveolar stops and fricatives, mid-dorsal palatal stops and fricatives, or even pharyngeal stops and fricatives, may be substituted. These are referred to as compensatory errors, and are more commonly heard in the speech of children with cleft palate than any other clinical population. Thus, palatal fistulae may contribute to both obligatory and compensatory articulation errors. The term compensatory is misleading because, as the term is usually used, a compensation is the closest possible approximation in the presence of a defect. For example, following a glossectomy, a patient is taught to compensate by using a remaining tongue segment to produce a sound. Therefore, compensatory errors should be categorized as adaptive, as in the glossectomy example, or maladaptive. Maladaptive compensatory errors require speech therapy.

Velopharyngeal Insufficiency. Velopharyngeal insufficiency (VPI) causes the obligatory errors of reduced intraoral pressure, nasal air escape, and nasalization of oral phonemes. These errors are only treatable by physical management of VPI. Some children with VPI develop otherwise normal articulation. However, some develop a complex pattern of maladaptive compensatory errors often referred to as cleft palate speech. These er-

rors include glottal and pharyngeal stops, pharyngeal and laryngeal fricatives, and nasal snorting (sometimes called a velar or nasal fricative), among others (Trost, 1981). A **glottal stop** is produced by abrupt adduction of the vocal folds, usually used as a substitution for stop consonants. A **pharyngeal fricative** is produced by constriction of the vocal tract, or constriction between the retracted tongue and pharynx to create frication, and is usually substituted for fricatives. A **nasal snort** involves forced nasal air emission, in contrast to the obligatory error of **nasal emission** which is a passive loss of air, and is usually substituted for [s, ʃ]. These errors represent attempts to valve the airstream and create an acoustic event prior to loss of air pressure through the velopharyngeal region. Similarly, the compensatory errors associated with fistulae represent attempts to produce sounds prior to loss of air through the fistula, thus the tongue retraction. In most cases, manner of articulation and voicing features (voice or voiceless) are preserved, and it is only the place of articulation that is in error (Golding-Kushner, 1989, 1995).

There is no question that maladaptive compensatory errors can only be corrected using speech therapy. However, there is controversy regarding the appropriate sequencing of speech therapy and physical correction of velopharyngeal insufficiency with prosthetics or surgery. The prevalent view has long been that the VPI must be treated first, followed by speech therapy in the presence of adequate velopharyngeal closure (McWilliams et al., 1990). However, recent studies have demonstrated that VPI and compensatory articulation errors have a bidirectional relationship. That is, the presence of VPI leads to the development of the compensatory speech pattern, but the production of these errors results in the exacerbation of VPI (Golding, 1981; Golding-Kushner, 1995; Henningsson & Isberg, 1986; Ysunza, Pamplona, & Toledo, 1992). Therefore, a view with growing acceptance is that compensatory articulation errors should be eliminated using speech therapy prior to secondary surgical procedures. When speech is hypernasal but free of compensatory articulation errors, the velopharyngeal muscles can be assumed to be performing at maximum efficiency and surgery can be performed, often with a less obstructive pharyngeal flap than appeared to be needed when compensatory articulation was present (Golding, 1981; Golding-Kushner, 1995; Ysunza, et al., 1992). Advocates of this approach stress that speech therapy should be centered strictly around the establishment of correct articulation production, and not at improvement of velopharyngeal function. Use of a speech bulb appliance may facilitate speech therapy for some patients (Golding-Kushner, Cisneros, & Le Blanc, 1995). Except in rare cases, velopharyngeal closure cannot be treated using therapy, and speech therapy to attempt to improve VP closure should never be attempted unless there is clear endoscopic evidence that it can be achieved in at least some phonetic contexts.

Articulation in Acquired Velopharyngeal Insufficiency.   Palatal defects and velopharyngeal insufficiency may be acquired after normal speech has developed. Gunshot wounds and the removal of tumors are two sources of acquired palatal defect. Adenoidectomy may result in VPI, especially in a patient with a submucous cleft palate that was undetected prior to surgery. Neurologic disorders resulting from disease (such as a cerebrovascular accident, myotonic dystrophy, muscular dystrophy, and so on) or accidents causing traumatic brain injury may also result in VPI. When a palatal defect or VPI are acquired after normal speech has developed, obligatory errors often result but compensatory errors do not occur. Treatment in such cases is usually limited to prosthetic or surgical management of VPI.

INSTRUMENTATION

The most important advances in the diagnosis and treatment of velopharyngeal dysfunction and related speech disorders over the last 20 to 30 years have resulted from the availability and use of increasingly sophisticated technology to visualize the vocal tract during unimpeded speech. Instru-

ments used in the assessment of velopharyngeal dysfunction may be categorized according to whether they provide direct examination or indirect assessment. If the purpose of examination is to determine a need for physical management and plan the most appropriate course of action, there is no question that direct visualization of velopharyngeal closure is imperative. If the clinician's purpose is for screening or for providing feedback to a patient during speech therapy, indirect techniques, which provide information about consequences of velopharyngeal motion but not about the motion itself, may, under some circumstances, be useful.

Direct Visualization

The earliest direct observations of velopharyngeal closure were made without the use of instruments by a physician through an ablative facial defect of a patient. Velopharyngeal closure cannot be visualized using intra-oral examination because it is out of view. Currently, direct observations of velopharyngeal closure during speech may be made using endoscopic and radiographic techniques.

Endoscopy.   The original viewing devices were panendoscopes—oral telescopes that could be rotated upward to provide an inferior view of velopharyngeal motion. However, only low vowels could be produced during examination because of the panendoscope's placement in the mouth. Nasal endoscopy, the use of a viewing endoscope inserted through one nostril, was introduced by Pigott (1969), and provided a way to observe velopharyngeal motion during unimpeded speech. The original endoscopes were rigid and uncomfortable, even with the nose anesthetized. Most examinations are now performed using flexible fiberoptic endoscopes introduced in Japan in 1974 (Matsuya, Miyazaki, & Yamaoka, 1974). These endoscopes have been manufactured with increasingly smaller diameters and are now as small as 2 mm and 3 mm, which allows for a much more comfortable examination and better scope maneuverability. The endoscope is inserted into one nostril following application of a mild topical anesthetic if necessary, and velopharyngeal motion can be observed from above while the patient repeats phrases or performs other speech tasks. The viewing end of the endoscope may be moved to various levels between the nasopharynx and larynx, providing a comprehensive examination of morphology (structure) and physiology (movement patterns) in the vocal tract (Figure 9.12). The endoscope is connected to an external cold light source, and may also be coupled to a video camera and monitor for recording and simultaneous viewing by the endoscopist and patient. Endoscopy provides the best possible view of velar morphology, which is necessary to diagnose occult submucous cleft palate and other anatomic abnormalities. The main limitation of endoscopy is that when velar motion occurs, it often obstructs observation of lateral pharyngeal wall motion. Therefore, both nasoendoscopy (or nasopharyngoscopy) and multiview videofluoroscopy, described in the next section, are necessary for a comprehensive diagnostic examination.

Radiography.   Early examinations of velopharyngeal closure relied on the use of static lateral cephalographs, usually taken during production of sustained [*s*]. This is not a useful type of examination because it does not provide information about dynamic velopharyngeal motion during speech, and also because it affords a view limited to the relationship between the velum and posterior pharyngeal wall. Successful physical management of velopharyngeal dysfunction, whether surgical or prosthetic, is dependent on examination of the lateral pharyngeal walls. Lateral cineradiography, which used film to record lateral views of the region during speech, addressed the need for observing the region in motion, but not the inability to view lateral pharyngeal wall motion. In the same year as endoscopy was introduced, Skolnick (1969) described a radiographic technique for observing velopharyngeal motion during unimpeded speech using multiple views with videotape recording. Referred to as multiview videofluoroscopy (MVF), it remains the technique of choice for examination of velopharyngeal closure, to-

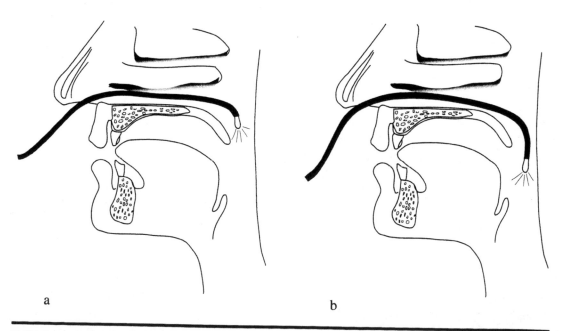

a   b

FIGURE 9.12 Sketch of flexible fiberoptic endoscope in place for nasopharyngoscopic examination. Note range of possible scope positions for examination.

gether with nasopharyngoscopy. MVF requires less radiation exposure than the earlier cineradiographic technique. The original three views described by Skolnick that are necessary to establish a three-dimensional concept of velopharyngeal motion are the lateral, frontal, and base views (Figure 9.13). Lateral view shows the velum and posterior pharyngeal wall. Frontal view allows observation of the movement of the lateral pharyngeal walls. Base view is an *en face* (head on) view of the "sphincter" from below, the exact opposite of the endoscopic view. Since Skolnick's original paper, additional views have been described that are useful under some conditions. Oblique views allow observation of one lateral wall and one side of the palate (or lateral edge of a pharyngeal flap, if present) (Shprintzen et al., 1980; Shprintzen & Golding-Kushner, 1989). This view is useful in patients with structural pharyngeal asymmetry, with asymmetry of velopharyngeal motion, and in patients with persistent hypernasality following pharyngeal flap surgery. The Towne view is an *en face* view from above, comparable to nasopharyngoscopy (Stringer & Witzel, 1986, 1989).

Indirect Techniques

Indirect techniques attempt to quantitatively or qualitatively describe the sequelae of VPI, such as hypernasal resonance or nasal air escape (Shprintzen & Golding-Kushner, 1989). Indirect techniques range from simplistic to very complex. Nasal emission may be detected using devices such as mirrors or stethoscopes held under the nose. Accelerometers can provide information on nasal vibrations. Other techniques are much more sophisticated, and have appeal because results are computerized. Two such techniques are pressure-flow and nasometry.

Pressure-flow. In 1964, Warren and DuBois described an aerodynamic procedure to estimate velopharyngeal orifice size. This is often referred to as the pressure-flow technique, because it is based on a concept from the field of physics that the area of an orifice can be determined by measuring the air flow through an orifice and the resulting changes in air pressure across it. Many adaptations and refinements in the technique have been described in the last 30 years, but the basic procedure has not changed (Warren, 1979; Warren, Dalston, Trier, & Holder, 1985). Nasal airflow is measured through a catheter in one nostril, and the difference in nasal and oral air pressure is calculated using information obtained from catheters in the other nostril and mouth (Figure 9.14). A computer estimates the size of the velopharyngeal orifice during the a target

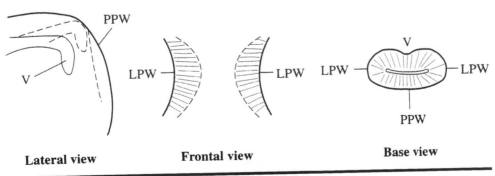

Lateral view   **Frontal view**   **Base view**

FIGURE 9.13 Multiview videofluoroscopy: lateral, frontal, and base views. Lateral view shows the degree of motion of the velum (V) and posterior pharyngeal wall (PPW), and tongue activity. Frontal view shows movement of both lateral pharyngeal walls (LPW). Base view shows the entire sphincter. The solid lines represent rest positions, and the dotted lines represent the position during speech.

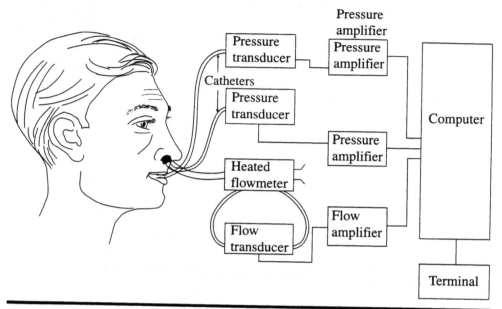

FIGURE 9.14 Equipment used to record intra-oral and nasal pressures for pressure-flow technique. (From Dalston, R. M., Warren, D. W., Morr, K. E., & Smith, L. R. (1988). Intraoral pressure and its relationship to velopharyngeal inadequacy, *Cleft Palate Journal, 25,* 212. Reprinted with permission from the American Cleft Palate-Craniofacial Association.)

sound, often [*p*], which should be produced with complete velopharyngeal closure. A major limitation of the pressure-flow technique is that the results relate to function in terms of the respiratory requirements for speech but do not actually evaluate speech performance (Dalston & Warren, 1986). Also, results interpreted as differences in size of a velopharyngeal gap may be influenced by extraneous factors such as respiratory effort, fistulae, and nasal patency. More importantly, there is a very low correlation between estimated orifice size based on pressure-flow studies and observed orifice size using multi-view videofluoroscopic examinations, raising significant questions about the validity of aerodynamic studies for purposes of clinical management (McWilliams et al., 1981).

Nasometer.   The nasometer is a computer-based instrument that computes a ratio between nasal and oral acoustic energy. It was based on an ear-

lier acoustic measure described by Fletcher and Bishop (1970) called TONAR (The Oral-Nasal Acoustic Ratio). In nasometry, microphones are positioned at the nose and mouth on either side of a shield which acts as a sound separator, and the data are fed into a computer and displayed on a monitor (Figure 9.15). The difference between the nasal energy and oral energy is referred to as a *nasalance score.* As with the pressure-flow technique, extraneous factors may affect test results, including positioning of the two microphones and nasal patency. Even the speech sample used during the procedure may affect the nasalance score. Importantly, the nasalance score is an acoustic measurement, not a physical measurement. There is not a direct correlation between the size of a velopharyngeal gap and the degree of perceived hypernasality. Therefore, while use of a nasometer may, in some cases, provide a quantified "measure" of hypernasality, it cannot be used to make valid inferences about the size, shape, or lo-

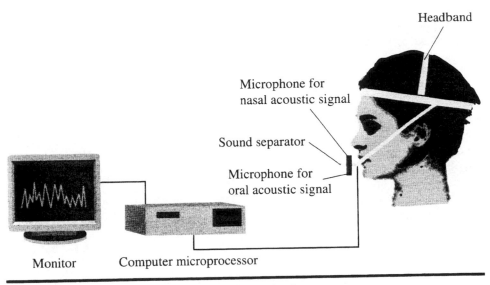

FIGURE 9.15   Equipment used for nasometric examination.

cation of a velopharyngeal gap. Furthermore, agreement between nasometer measures of nasalance and clinical ratings of hypernasality is often poor and may be strongly influenced by the phonetic make up of the speech sample used (Watterson, McFarlane, & Wright, 1993; Karnell, 1995).

With any assessment technique, an instrument's utility cannot exceed the skill of the examiner. A speech-language pathologist at a large medical center performed a nasometric examination on a patient who was severely dysarthric following a stroke. The patient had very weak respiratory support and his speech was barely audible. The nasometer registered a high oral pressure, but no nasal signal. This could have been due to nasal congestion, improper headgear placement, or the impaired underlying respiratory pressure. The speech-language pathologist concluded that the patient's palate was "paralyzed in the closed position." The speech-language pathologist was so caught up in the objectivity of a computerized analysis that he failed to recognize the physiologic impossibility of his conclusion. This anecdote should serve as a strong reminder that prior to attempting to diagnose a disorder,

one must completely understand normal anatomy and physiology, the possible consequences of abnormality, injury, or illness, and the appropriate application of technology.

SPEECH–LANGUAGE MANAGEMENT

When a language delay or disorder is diagnosed, treatment is no different than for children without cleft palate. In fact, there are few special techniques for treating this population. The areas of greatest concern are resonance, which 99 percent of the time requires surgical or prosthetic management, and the compensatory errors that comprise cleft palate speech. Elimination of a compensatory articulation disorder requires intensive, individual therapy three to five times per week, and a direct, traditional articulation therapy approach (Hoch, Golding-Kushner, Sadewitz, & Shprintzen, 1986; Golding-Kushner, 1995). Nonspeech activities such as blowing, sucking, gagging, icing, palatal massage, exercises to increase palatal or lingual strength or range of motion, and so on, do not result in improvement in either articulation or velopharyngeal closure (Powers & Starr, 1974; Ruscello, 1982; Starr,

1990). Therefore, time, effort, and finances should not be wasted on trying these or similar activities.

Velopharyngeal closure is sometimes inconsistent in patients with hypernasality, and the pattern and source of inconsistency must be determined to select the most appropriate treatment. Two special types of inconsistent velopharyngeal closure are **phone-specific velopharyngeal insufficiency** and **phone-specific velopharyngeal closure.** In these two special conditions, velopharyngeal closure is achieved on all sounds except one (usually [s]), or on no sounds except one (also usually [s]). These types of VPI, especially phone-specific VPI, also occur among noncleft patients, some of whom are apraxic. Unlike other types of VPI, these two disorders are actually articulation errors, and usually respond well to speech therapy, visual biofeedback therapy using nasopharyngoscopy, or speech-bulb reduction therapy. Two types of borderline velopharyngeal closure have been described (Morris, 1972, 1984). They are *sometimes but not always* (SBNA) and *almost but not quite* (ABNQ). Patients with SBNA may be candidates for the therapy modalities used in phone-specific problems. However, patients with ABNQ show no evidence of closure, and require physical management of VPI.

Major Points of Chapter

- Craniofacial anomalies including cleft lip and/or palate may occur either in isolation or as part of a wider genetic syndrome.
- Craniofacial anomalies may affect any of the facial structures, including the lips, and the hard and/or soft palate.
- Craniofacial anomalies are frequently associated with feeding difficulties and diseases of the middle ear and can result in specific kinds of articulatory and voice defects.
- Treatment varies according to the kind and extent of the cleft, and can include surgical repair of the palate, prosthestic and dental management, and orthodontistry, in conjunction with speech and language services.

Discussion Guidelines

1. Compare and contrast the craniofacial characterics of a genetic syndrome and a chromosome disorder.
2. Describe the different surgical management options available for a child born with a complete unilateral cleft of the hard and soft palates.
3. Explain why a team approach is essential in the management of a child born with a cleft palate.

REFERENCES

Argamaso, R. V., Levandoski, G. J., Golding-Kushner, K. J., & Shprintzen, R. J. (1994). Treatment of asymmetric velopharyngeal insufficiency with skewed pharyngeal flaps. *Cleft Palate and Craniofacial Journal, 31,* 287–294.

Argamaso, R. V., Shprintzen, R. J., Strauch, B., Lewin, M. L., Daniller, A., Ship, A. G., & Croft, C. B. (1980). The role of lateral pharyngeal wall motion in pharyngeal flap surgery. *Plastic and Reconstructive Surgery, 66,* 214.

Bardach, J., & Salyer, K. E. (1995). Cleft palate repair: Anatomy, timing, goals and principles, and techniques. In J. Bardach and R. J. Shprintzen (Eds.), *Cleft palate speech management: A multidisciplinary approach.* (pp. 102–136). St. Louis: Mosby-Year Book.

Berry, G. A. (1889). Note on a congenital defect of the lower lid. *Royal London Ophthalmic Hospital Reports, 12,* 255–257.

Cohen, M. M., Jr. (1982). *The child with multiple birth defects.* New York: Raven Press.

Cohen, M. M., & Bankier, A. (1991). Syndrome delineation involving orofacial clefting. *Cleft Palate Journal, 28,* 119–120.

Croft, C. B., Shprintzen, R. J., & Rakoff, S. J. (1981). Patterns of velopharyngeal valving in normal and cleft palate subjects: A multi-view videofluoroscopic and nasendoscopic study. *Laryngoscope. 91,* 265.

Dalston, R., & Warren, D. (1986). Comparison of Tonar II, pressure flow, and listener judgements of hypernasality in the assessment of velopharyngeal function. *Cleft Palate Journal, 23,* 103.

Dickson, D. R., & Maue-Dickson, W. (1972). Velopharyngeal anatomy. *Journal of Speech and Hearing Research, 15,* 372.

Dickson, D. R., & Maue-Dickson, W. (1980). Velopharyngeal structure and function: A model for biomechanical analysis. In N. J. Lass, (Ed.). *Speech and language advances in basic research and practice.* Vol 3. 168.1. New York: Academic Press.

Fletcher, S. G., & Bishop, M. E. (1970). Measurement of nasality with TONAR. *Cleft Palate Journal, 7,* 610.

Gereau, S. A., Stevens, D., Bassila, M., Sher, A. E., Sidoti, E. J., Jr., Morgan, M., Oka, S. W., & Shprintzen, R. J. (1988). Endoscopic observations of Eustachian tube abnormalities in children with palatal clefts. In D. J. Lim, C. D. Bluestone, J. O. Klein, & J. D. Nelson (Eds.). *Symposium on otitis media.* (pp. 60–63). Toronto: B. C. Decker.

Golding, K. J. (1981, May). *Articulation and velopharyngeal insufficiency: A rationale for pre-surgical speech therapy.* Fourth International Congress on Cleft Palate and Related Craniofacial Anomalies, Acapulco, Mexico.

Golding-Kushner, K. J. (1989). *Speech therapy for compensatory articulation errors in patients with "cleft palate speech."* Videotape produced by the Center for Craniofacial Disorders, Montefiore Medical Center, Bronx, New York.

Golding-Kushner, K. J. (1991). Craniofacial morphology and velopharyngeal function in four syndromes of clefting. Unpublished doctoral dissertation. The Graduate School and University Center, City University of New York, New York.

Golding-Kushner, K. J. (1995). Treatment of articulation and resonance disorders associated with cleft palate and VPI. In R. J. Shprintzen & J. Bardach (Eds), *Cleft palate speech management: A multidisciplinary approach* (pp. 327–351). St. Louis: C. V. Mosby.

Golding-Kushner, K. J., Argamaso, R. V., & Mitnick, R. (1994, May). *Pharyngeal flaps in patients with velo–cardio–facial syndrome.* American Cleft Palate-Craniofacial Association. Toronto, Canada.

Golding-Kushner, K. J., Argamaso, R. V., Cotton, R. T., D'Antonio, L., Grames, L. M., Henningsson, G., Isberg, A., Jones, D. L., Karnell, M. P., Klaiman, P. G., Lewin, M. L., Marsh, J. L., McCall, G. N., McGrath, C. O., Muntz, H. R., Nevdahl, M. T., Pigott, R. W., Rakoff, S. J., Shprintzen, R. J., Sidoti, E. J., Skolnick, L., Vallino, L. D., Volk, M.,

Williams, W. N., Witzel, M. A., Wood, V. L., & Ysunza, A. (1990). Standardization for the reporting of nasopharyngoscopy and multi-view videofluoroscopy: A report from an international working group. *Cleft Palate Journal, 27*(4), 337–347.

Golding-Kushner K. J., Cisneros, G., & LeBlanc, E. (1995). Speech bulbs. In R. J. Shprintzen & J. Bardach (Eds.), *Cleft palate speech management: A multidisciplinary approach* (pp. 352–363). St. Louis: C. V. Mosby.

Golding-Kushner, K. J., LeBlanc, S., & Tantillo, M. (1990, November). *The speech therapy team: Redefining the concept.* American Speech and Hearing Association, Seattle, Washington.

Golding-Kushner, K. J., Weller, G., & Shprintzen, R. J. (1985). Velo-cardio-facial syndrome: language and psychological profiles. *Journal of Craniofacial Genetics and Developmental Biology, 5,* 259–266.

Gorlin, R. J., Cohen, M. M., & Levin L. S. (1990). *Syndromes of the head and neck* (3rd Ed.). New York: Oxford University Press.

Graber, T. M. (1954). The congenital cleft palate deformity. *Journal of the American Dental Association, 48,* 375.

Greene, J. C., Vermillion, J. R., Hay, S., Gibbens, S. F., & Kerschbaum. (1964). Epidemiologic study of cleft lip and palate in four states. *Journal of the American Dental Association, 68,* 387.

Hagerty, J. (1965). Embryology, anatomy and growth of the orofacial complex. *ASHA Report #1,* 5–17.

Hall, C., & Golding-Kushner, K. J. (1989). Long term follow-up of 500 patients after palate repair prior to 18 months of age. *Sixth International Congress on Cleft Palate and Craniofacial Anomalies.* Abstract.

Hall, C. D., Golding-Kushner, K. J., Argamaso, R. V., & Strauch, B. (1991). Pharyngeal flap surgery in adults. *Cleft Palate Journal, 28*(2), 179–182.

Hallok, G. G. (1985). In utero lip repair in A/J mice. *Plastic and Reconstructive Surgery, 75,* 785.

Henningsson, G., & Isberg, A. (1986). Velopharyngeal movements in patients alternating between oral and glottal articulation: A clinical and cineradiographical study. *Cleft Palate Journal, 23,* 1.

Hoch, L., Golding-Kushner, K. J., Sadewitz, V., & Shprintzen, R. J. (1986). Speech therapy. In B. J. McWilliams (Ed.), *Seminars in speech and language: Current methods of assessing and treating children with cleft palates.* New York: Thieme.

Iglesias, A., Kuehn, D. P., & Morris, H. L. (1980). Simultaneous assessment of pharyngeal wall and velar displacement for selected speech sounds. *Journal of Speech and Hearing Research, 23,* 429.

Isberg, A., & Henningsson, G. (1987). Influence of palatal fistulas in velopharyngeal movements: A cineradiographic study. *Journal of Plastic and Reconstructive Surgery, 79,* 525.

Jensen, B. L., Kreiborg, S., Dahl, E., & Fogh-Anderson, P. (1988). Cleft lip and palate in Denmark, 1976–1981: Epidemiology, variability, and early somatic development. *Cleft Palate Journal, 25,* 258.

Johnston, M. C. (1975). The neural crest in abnormalities of the face and brain. In D. Bergsma (Ed.), Morphogenesis and malformation of the face and brain. *Birth defects: Original article series II, 7,* 1.

Johnston, M. C., & Sulik, K. K. (1984). Embryology of the head and neck. In D. Serafin & N. G. Georgiade (Eds.), *Pediatric plastic surgery* (p. 184). St. Louis: C. V. Mosby.

Jones, K. L. (1988). *Smith's recognizable patterns of human malformation.* Philadelphia: W. B. Saunders.

Kapp, K. (1979). Self-concept of the cleft lip and/or palate child. *Cleft Palate Journal, 16,* 171.

Karling, J., Larson, O., Leanderson, R., & Henningsson, G. (1993). Speech in unilateral and bilateral cleft palate patients from Stockholm. *Cleft Palate Journal, 30*(1), 73–77.

Karnell, M. P. (1995). Nasometric discrimination of hypernasality and turbulent nasal airflow. *Cleft Palate Journal, 32,* 145–148.

Kernahan, D. A., & Stark, R. B. (1958). A new classification for cleft lip and cleft palate. *Journal of Plastic Reconstructive Surgery, 22,* 435.

Kriens, O. (1990). Documentation of cleft lip, alveolus, and palate. In J. Bardach & H. Morris (Eds.), *Multidisciplinary management of cleft lip and palate* (pp. 127–133). Philadelphia: W. B. Saunders.

Krogman, W. M. (1973). Craniofacial growth and development: An appraisal. *Journal of the Americn Dental Association, 87,* 1037.

Krogman, W. M. (1979). Craniofacial growth: prenatal and postnatal. In H. K. Cooper, R. L. Harding, W. M. Krogman, M. Mazaheri, & R. T. Millard, (Eds.), *Cleft palate and cleft lip: A team approach to clinical management and rehabilitation of the patient* (p. 23). Philadelphia: W. B. Saunders.

Lindsay, W. K., LeMesurier, A. B., & Farmer, A. W. (1962). A study of the speech results of a large series of cleft palate patients. *Journal of Plastic and Reconstructive Surgery, 29,* 273.

Lipson, A. (1995). The changing phenotype and extraordinary variability of VCF: 200 cases from down under. *First annual meeting of the velo-cardio-facial Syndrome Educational Foundation,* Bronx, N. Y.

Lipson, A. H., Yuille, D., Angel, M., Thompson, P. G., Vanderwood, J. G., & Beckenham, E. J. (1991). Velo–cardio–facial syndrome: An important syndrome for the dysmorphologist to recognize. *Journal of Medical Genetics 28,* 596–604.

Long, N., & Dalston, R. (1983). Comprehension abilities of one-year-old infants with cleft lip and palate. *Cleft Palate Journal, 20,* 303.

Matsuya, T., Miyazaki, T., & Yamaoka, M. (1974). Fiberoptic examination of velopharyngeal closure in normal individuals. *Cleft Palate Journal, 11,* 286.

McGrath, C., & Anderson, M. (1990). Prosthetic treatment of velopharyngeal incompetence. In J. Bardach, & H. Morris (Eds.), *Multidisciplinary management of cleft lip and palate.* Philadelphia: W. B. Saunders.

McWilliams, B. J., Bluestone, C. D., & Musgrave, R. H. (1969). Diagnostic implications of vocal cord nodules in children with cleft palate. *Laryngoscope, 79,* 2072.

McWilliams, B. J., Glaser, E. R., Philips, B. J., Lawrence, C., Lavorato, A. S., Beery, Q. C., & Skolnick, M. L. (1981). A comparative study of four methods of evaluating velopharyngeal adequacy. *Journal of Plastic and Reconstructive Surgery, 68,* 1.

McWilliams, B. J., Lavorato, A. S., & Bluestone, C. D. (1973). Vocal cord abnormalities in children with velopharyngeal valving problems. *Laryngoscope, 83,* 1745.

McWilliams, B. J., Morris, H. L., & Shelton, R. L. (1990). *Cleft palate speech* (2nd Ed.). Philadelphia, B. C. Decker.

Morley, M. E. (1973). *Cleft palate and speech.* (7th Ed., reprinted). Edinburgh, Scotland, Churchill Livingstone.

Morris, H. L. (1962). Communication skills of children with cleft lip and palate. *Journal of Speech and Hearing Research, 5,* 79.

Morris, H. L. Cleft palate. (1972). In A. J. Weston (Ed.), *Communicative disorders: An appraisal.* Springfield, IL.: C. C. Thomas.

Morris, H. L. (1984). Types of velopharyngeal incompetence. In H. Winitz (Ed.), *Treating articulation disorders: For clinicians by clinicians.* Baltimore: University Park Press.

Oberg, K. C., Evans, M. L., Nguyen, T., Peckham, N. H., Kirsch, W. M., & Hardesty, R. A. (1995). Intra-uterine repair of surgically created defects in mice (lip incision model) with a microclip: Preamble to endoscopic intrauterine surgery. *Cleft Palate Journal, 32*(2), 129–137.

Oka, S. W. (1979). Epidemiology and genetics of clefting: With implications for etiology. In H. K. Cooper, R. L. Harding, W. M. Krogman, M. Mazaheri, & R. T. Millard (Eds.), *Cleft palate and cleft lip: A team approach to clinical management and rehabilitation of the patient* (p. 108). Philadelphia: W. B Saunders.

Olin, W. H. (1960). *Cleft lip and palate rehabilitation.* Springfield, IL: C. C. Thomas.

Ortiz-Monasterio, F., & Micolo, I. T. (1990). Multidisciplinary management of cleft lip and palate in Mexico. In J. Bardach & H. Morris, (Eds.), *Multidisciplinary management of cleft lip and palate* (pp. 57–68). Philadelphia: W. B. Saunders.

Paradise, J. L., & Bluestone, C. D. (1974). Early treatment of the universal otitis media of infants with cleft palate. *Pediatrics. 53,* 48.

Paradise, J. L., Bluestone, C. D., & Felder, H. (1969). The universality of otitis media in 50 infants with cleft palate. *Pediatrics. 44,* 35.

Pecyna, P., Feeny-Giacoma, M., & Neiman, G. (1987). Development of the object permanence concept in cleft lip and palate and noncleft lip and palate infants. *Journal of Communication Disorders, 20,* 233.

Peters, J. P. & Chinsky, R. R. (1974). Sociological aspects of cleft palate adults: I: marriage. *Cleft Palate Journal, 11,* 443.

Peterson-Falzone, S. J. (1990). A cross sectional analysis of speech results following palatal closure. In J. Bardach & H. Morris (Eds.), *Multidisciplinary management of cleft lip and palate* (pp. 750–757). Philadelphia: W. B. Saunders.

Peterson-Falzone, S. J. (1995). Speech outcomes in adolescents with cleft lip and palate. *Cleft Palate Journal, 32*(2), 125–128.

Pigott, R. W. (1969). The nasendoscopic appearance of the normal palatopharyngeal valve. *Journal of Plastic and Reconstructive Surgery, 43,* 19–24.

Powers, G., & Starr, C. (1974). The effects of muscle exercises on velopharyngeal gap and nasality. *Cleft Palate Journal, 11,* 28.

Richman, L. C. (1978). The effects of facial disfigurement on teachers' perception of ability in cleft palate children. *Cleft Palate Journal, 15,* 155.

Richman, L. C. & Harper, D. C. (1978). Observable stigmata and perceived maternal behavior. *Cleft Palate Journal, 15,* 215.

Ruscello, D. M. (1982). A selected review of palatal training procedures. *Cleft Palate Journal, 18,* 181.

Scambler, P. J., Kelly, D., Lindsay, E., Williamson, R., Goldberg, R., Shprintzen, R. J., Wilson, D. I., Goodship, J. A., Cross, I. E., & Burn, J. (1992). Velo-cardio-facial syndrome associated with chromosome 22 deletions encompassing the DiGeorge locus. *Lancet, 339,* 1138–1139.

Schechter, B., Golding, K. J., Shprintzen, R. J., & Rakoff, S. (1977). A new approach to the placement of the prosthetic speech bulb in velopharyngeal inadequacy (abstract). *Cleft Palate Journal, 14*(4), 361.

Schweckendiek, W. (1978). Primary veloplasty: long-term results without maxillary deformity. A twenty-five year report. *Cleft Palate Journal 15,* 268.

Shames, G. & Rubin, H. (1979). Psycholinguistic measures of language and speech. In K. Bzoch (Ed.), *Communicative disorders related to cleft lip and palate.* Boston: Little, Brown and Company.

Shprintzen, R. J. (1988). Pharyngeal flap and the pediatric upper airway. *International Anesthesiology Clinics, 26,* 74–83.

Shprintzen, R. J. (1992). The implications of the diagnosis of Robin sequence. *Cleft Palate Journal, 29,* 205–209.

Shprintzen, R. J. (1995). *The history of the delineation of Velo-cardio-facial syndrome (VCF).* First Annual Meeting of the Velo-cardio-facial Syndrome Educational Foundation, Bronx, N. Y.

Shprintzen, R. J., Croft, C. B., Berkman, M. D., & Rakoff, S. J. (1979). Pharyngeal hypoplasia in Treacher Collins syndrome. *Archives of Otolaryngology, 105*(3), 127–131.

Shprintzen, R. J., Croft, C. B., Berkman, M. D., & Rakoff, S. J. (1980). Velopharyngeal insufficiency in the facio-auriculo-vertebral malformation complex. *Cleft Palate Journal, 17,* 132–137.

Shprintzen, R. J., & Goldberg, R. (1995). The genetics of clefting and associated syndromes. In R. J. Shprintzen & J. Bardach (Eds.), *Cleft palate speech management: A multidisciplinary approach.* (pp. 16–43). St. Louis: Mosby-Yearbook.

Shprintzen, R. J., Goldberg, R. B., Golding-Kushner, K. J., & Marion, R. (1992). Late onset psychosis in the velo-cardio-facial syndrome: A clinical and genetic analysis. *American Journal of Medical Genetics, 42,* 141–42.

Shprintzen, R. J., Goldberg, R. B., Lewin, M. L., Sidoti, E. J., Berkman, M. D., Argamaso, R. V., & Young, D. (1978). A new syndrome involving cleft palate, cardiac anomalies, typical facies, and learning disabilities: Velo-cardio-facial syndrome. *Cleft Palate Journal, 15,* 56.

Shprintzen, R. J., & Golding-Kushner, K. J. (1989). Evaluation of velopharyngeal insufficiency. In G. Healy & E. Friedman (Eds.), *Otolaryngologic clinics of North America* (pp. 519–536). Philadelphia: W. B. Saunders.

Shprintzen, R. J., Lewin, M. L., Croft, C., Daniller, A., Argamaso, R. V., Ship, A., & Strauch B. A. (1979). Comprehensive study of pharyngeal flap surgery: Tailor made flaps. *Cleft Palate Journal, 16,* 46.

Shprintzen, R. J., McCall, G. N., Skolnick, M. L., & Lencione, R. M. (1975). Selective movement of the lateral aspects of the pharyngeal walls during velopharyngeal closure for speech, swallowing, and whistling in normals. *Cleft Palate Journal, 12,* 51.

Shprintzen, R. J., Siegel-Sadewitz, V. L., Amato, J., & Goldberg, R. (1985). Anomalies associated with cleft lip, cleft palate, or both. *American Journal of Medical Genetics, 20*(4), 585–595.

Skolnick, M. L. (1969). Video velopharyngography in patients with nasal speech, with emphasis on lateral pharyngeal motion in velopharyngeal closure. *Radiology, 93,* 747–755.

Skolnick, M. L., & Cohn, E. R. (1989). *Videofluoroscopic studies of speech in patients with cleft palate.* New York: Springer-Verlag.

Skolnick, M. L., & McCall, G. N. (1972). Velopharyngeal competence and incompetence following pharyngeal flap surgery: A videofluoroscopic study in multiple projections. *Cleft Palate Journal, 9,* 1.

Skolnick, M. L., McCall, G. N., & Barnes, M. (1973). The sphincteric mechanism of velopharyngeal closure. *Cleft Palate Journal, 10,* 286.

Spriestersbach, D., Darley, F., & Morris, H. (1988). Language skills in children with cleft palate. *Journal of Speech and Hearing Research, 1,* 279.

Stark, R. B. (1941, 1977). Embryology of cleft palate. In J. M. Converse (Ed.), *Plastic and reconstructive surgery: principles and procedures in connection, reconstruction, and transplantation.* (Vol. 4, 2nd ed.) Philadelphia: W. B. Saunders.

Starr, C. (1990). Treatment by therapeutic exercises. In J. Bardach & H. Morris (Eds.), *Multidisciplinary management of cleft palate.* Philadelphia: W. B. Saunders.

Strauss, R. P., & Broder, H. (1990). Psychological and sociocultural aspects of cleft lip and palate. In J. Bardach, & H. Morris (Eds.), *Multidisciplinary management of cleft lip and palate* (pp. 831–837). Philadelphia: W. B. Saunders.

Stringer, D. A., & Witzel, M. A. (1986). Velopharyngeal insufficiency on videofluoroscopy: A comparison of projections. *American Journal of Radiology, 146,* 15–19.

Stringer, D. A., & Witzel, M. A. (1989). Comparison of multi-view videofluoroscopy and nasopharyngoscopy in the assessment of velopharyngeal insufficiency. *Cleft Palate Journal, 26,* 88.

Trost, J. E. (1981). Articulatory additions to the classical description of the speech of persons with cleft palate. *Cleft Palate Journal, 18,* 193.

Vanderas, A. P. (1987). Incidence of cleft lip, cleft palate, and cleft lip and palate among races: A review. *Cleft Palate Journal, 24,* 216.

Warren, D. W. (1979). PERCI: A method for rating palatal efficiency. *Cleft Palate Journal, 16,* 279.

Warren, D. W., & DuBois, A. B. (1964). A pressure-flow technique for measuring velopharyngeal orifice size during continuous speech, *Cleft Palate Journal, 1,* 52.

Warren, D. W., Dalston, R. M., Trier W. C., & Holder, M. B. (1985). A pressure-flow technique for quantifying temporal patterns of palatopharyngeal closure. *Cleft Palate Journal, 22,* 11.

Watterson, T. L., McFarlane, S. C., & Wright, D. S. (1993). The relationship between nasalance and nasality in children with cleft palate. *Journal of Communication Disorders, 26,* 13–28.

Webster's college dictionary. (1991). New York: Random House.

Wilhelmsen, H. R., & Musgrave, R. H. (1966). Complications of cleft lip surgery. *Cleft Palate Journal, 3:* 223.

Ysunza, A., Pamplona, C., & Toledo, E. (1992). Changes in velopharyngeal valving after speech therapy in cleft palate patients: A videonasopharyngoscopic and multi-view videofluoroscopic study. *International Journal of Pediatric Otorhinolaryngoly, 24,* 45.

10

STRUCTURAL AND FUNCTIONAL ASPECTS OF NORMAL AND DISORDERED SWALLOWING

JERI A. LOGEMANN

This chapter reviews the anatomy and physiology of normal swallowing, including the effects of age on the normal swallow, beginning at birth and extending through old age. The systematic changes in the normal swallow with the characteristics of the incoming food are described, as are changes resulting from volitional control. Symptoms of swallowing disorders are outlined. Evaluation techniques to define the anatomic or physiologic reason(s) for the swallowing disorder in a particular patient are described. These include videofluorographic examination, videonasendoscopic assessment, manometric measures, ultrasound and scintigraphic evaluation procedures, and electromyography and ultrafast computerized tomography. Procedures for treating swallowing disorders are also described. The role of the multidisciplinary team in swallowing evaluation and treatment is also discussed. Finally, the speech–language pathologist's involvement in evaluation and treatment of swallowing is reviewed.

Dysphagia, or difficulty swallowing, can occur as a result of damage to the structures of the head and neck or because of problems with neuromuscular control. It may occur in newborn infants, young children, and adolescents, as well as throughout the adult years (Logemann, 1983, 1993). Because of the wide range of medical etiologic factors causing dysphagia, the occurrence of swallowing disorders is high. It has been estimated that 13 to 15 percent of patients in acute care hospitals are dysphagic, 30 to 35 percent of patients in rehabilitation settings are dysphagic, and 40 to 50 percent of patients in nursing homes are dysphagic (Groher & Bukatmun, 1986).

Speech–language pathologists have been involved in the evaluation and treatment of swallowing disorders since the 1930s (Miller & Groher, 1993). At that time, the focus of intervention was on methods of feeding children with cerebral palsy. As the role of speech–language pathology grew in medical settings in the 1970s, speech–language pathologists were called upon to apply their expertise in the anatomy and physiology of the head and neck to the evaluation and treatment of swallowing disorders in patients with neurologic disorders and those who had undergone surgery for head and neck cancer. Since that time, speech–language pathologists and speech scientists have been leaders in research on normal swallowing physiology and neurophysiology, and in the evaluation and treatment of swallowing disorders.

The importance of speech–language pathologists' involvement in dysphagia is based upon their knowledge of the anatomy and physiology of the upper aerodigestive tract and the frequent co-occurrence of speech and swallowing disorders. The upper aerodigestive tract is unique, as it serves three functions: respiration, swallowing, and speech production. Treatment for a disorder in one function, such as swallowing, may inadvertently affect another function of the mechanism either negatively or positively. It is critical that speech–language pathologists be familiar with the entire range of physiology of the upper aerodigestive tract in order to effectively treat patients with speech and/or swallowing disorders. The purpose of this chapter is to introduce the student in speech–language pathology to the anatomy and physiology of normal and abnormal swallow and to the role of the speech–language pathologist in the evaluation and treatment of patients with **dysphagia** (swallowing disorders).

ANATOMY AND PHYSIOLOGY OF NORMAL SWALLOWING

In order to serve the functions of respiration, swallowing, and speech production efficiently and safely, the upper aerodigestive tract must be able to switch rapidly between an open airway for respiration and a closed airway for swallowing. It must also shift the position of the structures within the oral cavity, pharynx, and the larynx to operate differently during respiration, deglutition (swallowing), or phonation. These switches between functions occur rapidly (within 100ths of a second) and efficiently, such that aspiration (i.e., the entry of food into the airway below the true vocal folds) occurs rarely in normal individuals, and airway maintenance is optimal.

The gross anatomy of the upper aerodigestive tract is presented in Figure 10.1. The **upper aerodigestive tract** includes the structures forming the nasal cavity, the oral cavity, the pharynx, the larynx, and the cervical esophagus. In the oral cavity, the lips, anteriorly, serve to keep food in the mouth during chewing and swallowing. The tongue is the

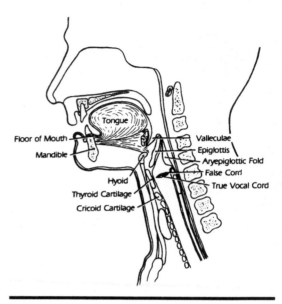

FIGURE 10.1   Drawing of the upper aerodigestive tract in the midsagittal plane.

most mobile structure within the upper aerodigestive tract and for swallowing is divided into the oral tongue and the pharyngeal tongue. The oral tongue is utilized in speech articulation and extends approximately from the tongue tip to the back, adjacent to the soft palate. The tongue base or pharyngeal aspect of the tongue extends approximately from the soft palate to the hyoid bone and valleculae. The **valleculae** is the space between the tongue base and the epiglottis. The oral portion of the tongue functions during the oral stage of swallowing, propelling the bolus backward, while the tongue base functions during the pharyngeal stage, applying pressure to the food to propel it through the pharynx.

The entry to the nose from the pharynx (the velopharyngeal valve) is comprised of the soft palate and the lateral and posterior pharyngeal walls and is open during nose breathing, but closes during selective speech sound productions, as well as during some aspects of swallowing. The airway is comprised of the larynx and the trachea as well as the bronchi and lungs. Situated at the top of the airway, the primary biologic function of the larynx is to protect the airway during swallow. The larynx contains three valves that close during swallow: the true vocal folds, the arytenoid cartilages with the false vocal folds and the base of the epiglottis, and the epiglottis. The larynx closes during a swallow in order to protect the airway from the entry of food or liquid. Similarly, the airway closes at the vocal folds during the production of some speech sounds. The pharynx is comprised of the superior, medial, and inferior pharyngeal constrictor muscles laterally and posteriorly, and which attach to the skull base, soft palate, tongue base, and larynx anteriorly. The pharynx remains open during respiration and phonation but closes for a brief period (i.e., approximately .25 to .30 of a second) during swallowing. As the pharyngeal constrictors attach to the larynx, they form two recesses or pockets, known as the pyriform sinuses. (See Figure 10.2.) Together, the valleculae and pyriform sinuses are known as the pharyngeal recesses or spaces and form the normal pathway for food through the pharynx during swallowing.

During a swallow, the food moves backward in the mouth with oral tongue propulsion and enters the valleculae. The food then passes from the valleculae around the epiglottis to the **pyriform**

sinuses and from the pyriform sinuses into the esophagus. Three valves in the upper aerodigestive tract must open or close appropriately during swallow to direct food into the esophagus: (1) the velopharyngeal valve, which closes to prevent food from entering the nose; (2) the airway, which closes at three levels to prevent food from entering; and (3) the upper esophageal sphincter (UES), which opens to allow food into the esophagus.

The upper esophageal sphincter (UES) or **cricopharyngeal (CP)** region is situated at the bottom of the pharynx, posterior to the larynx, and serves as a valve into the esophagus. The upper esophageal sphincter's primary biologic function is to prevent the inhalation of air into the esophagus during the inhalation portion of the respiratory cycle. The upper esophageal sphincter is comprised of the cricopharyngeal muscle (the inferior portion of the inferior constrictor) attached to the posterior portion of the cricoid cartilage, as shown in Figure 10.3. The cricoid cartilage is the only laryngeal cartilage forming a complete ring and is the most inferior cartilage within the larynx. Thus, the cricopharyngeal region or upper esophageal sphincter is a musculoskeletal sphincter, comprised of both cartilage and muscle.

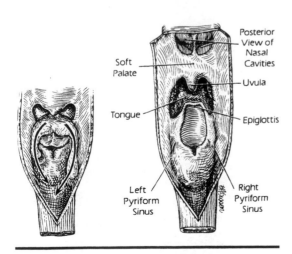

FIGURE 10.2 Posterior view of the pharynx illustrating the attachment of the pharyngeal constrictors to the larynx.

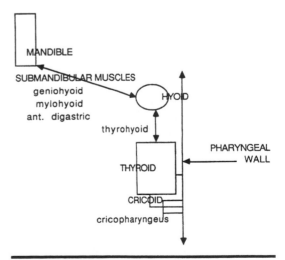

FIGURE 10.3 Diagram of the upper esophageal sphincter (UES) from a superior view.

Below the larynx, the airway is comprised of the trachea, which contains tracheal rings made of cartilage. These tracheal rings are three-fourths round so that the posterior wall of the trachea is comprised of soft tissue rather than cartilage. This soft tissue posterior wall of the trachea is known as the *common wall* because it serves as both the back wall of the trachea and the anterior wall of the esophagus.

Valves in the Upper Aerodigestive Tract

The upper aerodigestive tract may be defined as a series of tubes and valves that must open or close at appropriate times during the swallow (see Figure 10.4). It is critical that the speech–language pathologist be knowledgeable about these valves and their physiology because patients frequently exhibit disorders in these valve functions. Moving anteriorly to posteriorly, the lips are most anterior valve. The lips close to keep food in the mouth during chewing and swallowing. The tongue can be called a valve because it can make complete contact with the roof of the mouth or it can maintain a varying degree of space between itself and the hard palate. The third valve is the velopharynx, which closes momentarily during the swallow to prevent food from entering the nose, but is usually open during respiration. The fourth valve is the larynx, which closes momentarily during swallow (.30 to .60 seconds) in order to prevent the entry of food or liquid into the airway. The fifth valve is the upper esophageal sphincter (UES) or cricopharyngeal region. This valve is normally closed except during the moment of swallowing. However, as the bolus (i.e., the material being swallowed) approaches, the UES opens to allow the bolus to enter the esophagus.

The Physiology of Normal Swallowing

Normal swallowing consists of a set of behaviors resulting in food moving from the mouth to the stomach. Normal swallowing varies systematically with the characteristics of the food to be swallowed and the degree of volitional control to

THE VOCAL TRACT AS A SYSTEM OF VALVES

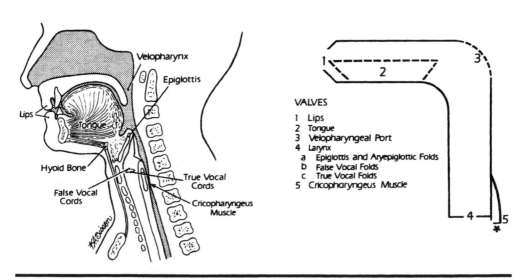

FIGURE 10.4   Diagram of the upper aerodigestive tract as a series of tubes and valves.

be exerted (Logemann, 1993). The swallow is often described as containing four phases: (1) Oral Preparation; (2) the Oral Stage; (3) the Pharyngeal Stage; and (4) the Esophageal Stage. These stages vary in their relationships to one another depending on the bolus characteristics. The oral preparatory stage is characterized by chewing and the breakdown of food to a consistency appropriate for swallowing. During chewing, lip closure keeps food in the mouth anteriorly, while rotary lateral motion of the jaw and rotary lateral motion of the tongue controls food, places it on the teeth, mixes it with saliva, and replaces it onto the teeth. A certain degree of facial tone must be present to prevent food from lodging in the lateral **sulcus,** i.e., the space between the teeth and facial musculature. During oral preparation the soft palate may be pulled downward and forward to help keep food in the mouth posteriorly. However, during active chewing there is frequently no soft palate to back tongue contact, allowing premature spillage of food from the oral cavity into the pharynx, where it rests until the remainder of the food is chewed and the oral stage of swallow begins. At the end of oral preparation, food is subdivided by the tongue and formed into a ball or bolus that can be swallowed easily. The tongue then holds the bolus of food to be swallowed either on the surface of the tongue with the sides and anterior portion of the tongue tip sealed against the alveolar ridge, or on the anterior floor of the mouth in front of the tongue. If the bolus is held on the anterior floor of the mouth, the tongue must then pick up the bolus and place it in the superior position.

If liquid or other food does not require chewing when it is placed in the mouth, the soft palate is typically pulled down and forward against the back of the tongue to hold the liquid or other foods in the oral cavity until the swallow is initiated. Again, the bolus or ball of food is held on the tongue with the sides and tip of tongue sealed against the alveolar ridge, or the bolus is held on the anterior floor of the mouth and is picked up and put in the superior position on the tongue.

The oral stage of swallow is initiated when the tongue tip and lateral margins of the tongue

are sealed against the alveolar ridge and the midline of the tongue applies pressure to the food bolus. The midline tongue action propels the bolus backward until it reaches the region of the faucial arches at the posterior oral cavity. The sensory information from the tongue motion (as well as the moving bolus of food), sends nerve impulses to the nucleus tractus solitarius in the brainstem and to the cortex regarding the need to trigger the pharyngeal stage of swallowing. The exact nature of the sensory input needed to trigger the pharyngeal swallow is not known. However, it is clear that tongue action which stimulates deep proprioceptive sensory receptors in the tongue is an important part of that sensory stimulus.

The neuromotor components of the pharyngeal stage of swallowing are programmed in the nucleus ambiguus in the medulla (lower portion) of the brainstem. The sensory input from the oral cavity and pharynx is thought to be integrated and decoded at the nucleus tractus solitarius adjacent to the nucleus ambiguus. The motor components of the pharyngeal swallow include the elevation and forward motion of the hyoid bone and larynx. These movements contribute to the functioning of other adjacent structures during the pharyngeal stage of swallow. The velopharyngeal port closes as the bolus passes to prevent food from entering the nose. As the bolus passes the tongue base, the propulsion of the food, which is initiated by the oral tongue, continues as the base of the tongue moves backward and the contraction of the lateral and posterior pharyngeal walls moves them inward to meet the backward-moving tongue base.

Airway closure to prevent the entry of food or liquid occurs at essentially the same time as the upper esophageal sphincter opens. Airway closure is thought to progress from bottom (true vocal folds) to top (the airway entrance at the arytenoid cartilages which are lifted by laryngeal elevation and tilt forward to meet the thickening epiglottic base and the epiglottis). Airway closure is facilitated by the elevation of the larynx, which brings the arytenoids closer to the base of the epiglottis (Logemann, et al., 1992). During the moment of airway closure, which lasts approximately .30 to .70 of a sec, respiration ceases.

The opening of the upper esophageal sphincter is accomplished as the cricopharyngeal muscle relaxes, enabling the forward motion of the larynx, particularly the cricoid cartilage, to open the sphincter (Jacob, Kahrilas, Logemann, Shah, & Ha, 1989). Thus, the upper esophageal sphincter is opened biomechanically by the forward motion of the larynx. As the food is propelled to the upper esophageal sphincter and through the sphincter to the esophagus, the pressure of the bolus of food itself widens the cricopharyngeal opening. As the food enters the esophagus, the peristaltic action in the esophagus takes over bolus propulsion, pushing the food through the esophagus and through the lower esophageal sphincter into the stomach.

The esophagus is a collapsed muscular tube comprised of circular muscle fibers. These fibers contract sequentially (top to bottom) to propel food, liquid, or air through the esophagus and through the lower esophageal sphincter. The lower esophageal sphincter is a muscular valve that is contracted until food approaches. As food approaches, the muscle fibers comprising the valve relax to allow the food to pass into the stomach. The purpose of the lower esophageal sphincter is to prevent food and stomach acid from backflowing out of the stomach and into the esophagus. Backflow of food or liquid from the stomach is called reflux. (See Chapter 11 for a discussion on the effects of reflux on the vocal folds.)

Changes in Normal Swallow with Age

In infants who suck from a bottle or a breast, the tongue and jaw move vertically as a unit against the nipple to pump liquid into the oral cavity. As the baby matures, the tongue moves independently of the jaw. The pumping action expresses milk from the nipple into the back of the oral cavity or into the valleculae, where it collects after each small pump. When the bolus of liquid is large enough, the pharyngeal swallow is triggered and the liquid moves from the oral cavity or valleculae into the esophagus. The bolus collects in

the esophagus with repeated pharyngeal swallows until an esophageal peristaltic wave or contraction wave occurs. Thus, in the infant, the oral stage, the pharyngeal stage, and the esophageal stage are separated from each other with collection of food into a larger bolus before the pharyngeal swallow or the esophageal swallow is triggered. If the infant is given a single bolus of liquid such as from a spoon, the normal adult pattern of oral to pharyngeal to esophageal activity with no delay is observed. In infancy and early childhood, the lower esophageal sphincter is not mature, resulting in frequent backflow from the stomach into the esophagus or even into the pharynx or oral cavity.

With normal aging, the esophageal contraction becomes uncoordinated and less efficient, so that after age 60 many normal individuals experience increasing episodes of reflux. After age 60, holding the bolus on the anterior floor of the mouth prior to initiating the oral stage of swallow is commonplace. As a result, oral transit times (the time to propel a bolus through the oral cavity) are longer because the tongue must pick up the bolus and bring it onto the anterior surface of the tongue. Typically, in adults over age 60, the pharyngeal swallow is slightly delayed in triggering. As a result, the food progresses further down the tongue base before the pharyngeal swallow is triggered. This is thought to result from a slower neural processing time.

As normal adults (particularly men) reach their 80s and 90s, they exhibit reduced laryngeal and hyoid movement. These changes do not significantly affect the efficiency or safety of the swallow, as long as the individual is healthy. However, if the individual becomes ill or physically weak, these changes in the oropharyngeal swallow may decrease the individual's swallow efficiency and increase the risk of aspiration.

Systematic Changes in Normal Swallow with Bolus Characteristics

In recent years it has become apparent that normal swallowing is not a single physiologic event, but a set of behaviors that together result in moving food or liquid from the mouth to the stomach. These behaviors differ significantly in their temporal characteristics. Understanding the various normal swallow behaviors is important for the speech–language pathologist in understanding the nature of the dysphagic patient's swallowing difficulties. A number of systematic changes in oropharyngeal swallow occur as a result of changes in the characteristics of the food to be swallowed (Kahrilas & Logemann, 1993). As the volume of the food increases, the oral and pharyngeal stages of swallow increasingly overlap, rather than occurring in a sequence. For example, during a small volume swallow, such as saliva (approximately 1 ml), the oral stage of swallow is followed in sequence by the pharyngeal stage and then the esophageal stage. However, in swallows of 20 ml, such as a drink of water from a cup, the oral and pharyngeal stage occur simultaneously. The pharyngeal propulsion of the bolus by the tongue base and pharyngeal walls occurs later, as bolus volume increases in order to accommodate the passage of the larger bolus. The durations of closure of the airway and opening of the cricopharyngeal or upper esophageal sphincter increase systematically as bolus volume increases in order to accommodate the larger volume.

As viscosity (stickiness) of the bolus increases, the degree of muscle activity increases and the pressure exerted on the bolus increases. Only bolus volume and viscosity have been studied in normal individuals. Other bolus characteristics such as taste have not been examined in terms of their influence on normal swallow physiology. Certain tastes may result in faster or slower swallowing.

Changes in Swallow with Voluntary Control

A great deal of volitional control can be exerted over oropharyngeal swallow behavior. Volitional control allows some dysphagic patients to change selected aspects of their swallow physiology in order to improve their swallow. For example, the airway can be closed volitionally at the vocal folds or at the entrance to the airway prior to and during a swallow. A patient with reduced closure of the airway entrance can enhance that closure when taught to do so voluntarily. Also, the duration of laryngeal elevation can be controlled volitionally, as can the degree of muscle effort exerted during a swallow (Kahrilas, Logemann, Krugler, & Flanagan, 1991). These volitional controls are used in dysphagia treatment, but are also used by normal individuals in the course of a variety of different swallows. For example, many normal adults hold their breath before and during a large volume liquid swallow from a cup, perhaps as added protection for the airway. Additional studies of the effects of voluntary control are needed to increase our knowledge of normal swallow behaviors and, potentially, to identify other aspects of swallow physiology that can be placed under voluntary control.

SWALLOWING DISORDERS

Disorders in the oropharyngeal swallow can include unilateral or bilateral abnormalities in any one or a combination of the anatomic, motor, or sensory components of the normal oropharyngeal swallow described earlier (Logemann, 1993). This includes lip closure; facial tone; oral tongue motion for chewing and propelling food backward in the mouth; jaw motion; soft palate motion downward; velopharyngeal closure; triggering of the pharyngeal swallow; and the motor components of the pharyngeal swallow, including laryngeal and hyoid upward and forward movement, pharyngeal wall contraction, airway closure, upper esophageal sphincter opening, and tongue base movement. For example, lip closure can be damaged resulting in drooling, the lateral motion of the tongue for chewing can be impaired, the triggering of the pharyngeal swallow can be delayed so that food arrives in the pharynx too early, the motor activity of the pharyngeal walls can be damaged unilaterally or bilaterally, leaving food clinging to the pharyngeal wall(s) after the swallow, and so forth. The responsibility of the swallow therapist is to evaluate the control of each of the separate anatomic, sensory, and motor components involved in the oropharyngeal swallow and to identify those anatomic structures, motor components, or sensory deficits that are present in an individual patient. Treatment for oropharyngeal swallowing disorders is based upon the clinician's knowledge of the patient's swallow physiology, not on the symptoms of their disorders. In most cases, the swallowing therapist is a speech–language pathologist. But in some settings, the role of the swallowing therapist is taken by another professional such as an occupational therapist, a physical therapist, a nurse, or other professional.

Symptoms of Swallowing Disorders

Symptoms of swallowing disorders range from perceived difficulty eating to coughing during meals, slow eating, apparent physical difficulty manipulating food, and so on. In some dysphagic patients there are no visible symptoms even when food or liquid is entering the airway. The entry of food into the airway below the true vocal folds, which may or may not result in a cough, is known as aspiration. If the food enters the airway entrance but does not go below the true vocal folds, it is known as penetration. If the swallow is inefficient and food remains in the mouth or the pharynx, it is known as residue or residual food. Generally, patients will swallow repeatedly to clear residual food because they have sensory awareness of the food lodging in their mouth or pharynx. Some patients do not have this sensory input and therefore do not dry swallow or attempt to swallow multiple times. **Aspiration, penetration** and **residue** are all symptoms of a swallowing disorder. In order to plan effective treatment, the clinician must determine the abnormal anatomy and/or physiology that is causing these symptoms.

For example, the patient with a brainstem (medullary) stroke may exhibit severe symptoms of a swallowing disorder at one week poststroke, including coughing and a severe gurgly voice quality. These symptoms indicate the need for a more in-depth physiologic evaluation of the oropharyngeal swallow. A radiographic (videofluoro-scopic) assessment of the patient's swallow reveals a unilateral paresis of the pharyngeal wall and reduced laryngeal anterior and vertical movement resulting in reduced cricopharyngeal (upper esophageal) opening. As a result of these physiologic disorders, very little food enters the esophagus. Instead, the food collects in the pyriform sinus on the weak side of the pharynx, where it regularly overflows into the airway, causing the symptoms of coughing and gurgly voice. Treatment of this patient would be directed at improving laryngeal movement with exercise and eliminating the damaged side of the pharynx from the bolus path with postural change.

Patient Groups Experiencing Swallowing Disorders

A large number of patients who have sustained sudden or progressive neurologic disorders exhibit swallowing problems. Included in this population are those who have suffered a stroke, a head trauma, or a spinal cord injury. Patients with progressive neurologic disease will usually experience swallowing problems at some point in the course of their disease, sometimes as the initial symptom. Diseases such as Parkinson's disease, amyotrophic lateral sclerosis, myasthenia gravis, multiple sclerosis, and post-polio syndrome, can cause oropharyngeal swallowing problems. Patients who have sustained trauma to the head or neck, such as a gunshot or knife wound, also usually exhibit oropharyngeal swallowing problems. The patient who has a tumor of the head and/or neck that requires radiation or surgical treatment will also exhibit swallowing impairment. Patients with systemic disease, such as scleroderma, dermatomyositis, rheumatoid arthritis, or diabetes may also have swallowing problems. Children with cerebral palsy, dysautonomia, Werdnig-Hoffman disease and other congenital and acquired neurologic disorders are also prone to oropharyngeal swallowing problems. Because the esophagus becomes less functional with age, the older patient who suffers a stroke or head injury may acquire oropharyngeal swallowing problems as a result of the neurologic damage in addition to their age-related pre-existing esophageal dysfunction. Also, children with congenital neurologic disorders exhibit a higher incidence of esophageal problems (in addition to their oropharyngeal swallowing problems) than normal children.

Evaluation of Swallowing Disorders

Evaluation of swallowing disorders begins with a bedside or clinical assessment of the patient's history, and a physical examination of the vocal tract or upper aerodigestive tract (Logemann, 1983). History-taking includes gathering information about the patient's medical history and medical diagnosis as well as medications taken and particular symptoms of the swallowing problem. Medical consultations that have taken place since the onset of the patient's swallowing problems are also reviewed. Then, the swallow therapist conducts a physical examination of the anatomy and physiology of the oral cavity, pharynx, and larynx, in order to define the normalcy of structure and any obvious physical impairments. In general, oral structures and function can be adequately assessed in the clinical examination. However, because of its complexity and relative invisibility, the pharyngeal aspects of swallow physiology are not easy to visualize in the physical examination. For this reason, most swallowing therapists use various imaging procedures to examine the pharyngeal aspects of swallow including videofluorography, videonasendoscopy, ultrasound, scintigraphy, and ultrafast computerized tomography. Videofluorography is generally the procedure of choice.

Videofluorographic Examination of Swallow. The most commonly used imaging procedure for the study of oropharyngeal swallowing is videofluorography or moving x-ray (Logemann, 1993). This procedure enables evaluation of most of the motor components of the pharyngeal swallow including laryngeal motion, hyoid motion, oral tongue and tongue base motion, pharyngeal wall movement, closing of the airway and opening of the esophageal sphincter, as well as closure of the

velopharyngeal port. The movement of the bolus is imaged in relation to the movement of the structures. During the radiographic examination, the patient is usually given a variety of food types such as thin liquid, thick liquid, pudding, and a food requiring chewing (in both premeasured amounts as well as unrestricted amounts) in order to define oropharyngeal physiology under these circumstances. This study is usually initiated with the patient viewed in the lateral plane, as shown in Figure 10.5. Several swallows of each bolus type and volume are usually repeated. Then, several bolus types that are difficult for the patient are also visualized in the anterior–posterior plane to define the symmetry of the swallow. Figure 10.6 shows an anterior–posterior view of the pharynx with structures outlined with barium after the swallow.

If the patient exhibits swallow impairments that significantly affect the safety or efficiency of the swallow, treatment strategies are usually introduced to assess their effectiveness in improving the efficiency and safety of the patient's swallow. Thus, the radiographic study is both an assessment of the anatomy and physiology of the oral cavity and pharynx in order to define the underlying anatomic or physiologic disorder, and a study of treatment effects or efficacy. In approximately 80 percent of the patients who aspirate or get food in the airway during the videofluorographic study, positive benefit from treatment strategies can be defined immediately. Thus, the goal of the radiographic study is to define both the patient's swallowing disorder and to determine effective treatment strategies so that the patient can proceed with some oral intake immediately after the study. Usually, this test is conducted by the swallowing therapist in conjunction with a radiologist. The report from such an examination will also indicate the nature of the treatment plan.

When recorded on videotape, the fluoroscopic study can be analyzed by playback in slow motion or frame-by-frame. Videotape records at 60 fields (separate pictures) per second. Events in the pharyngeal swallow can be measured from the videotape in terms of their duration, e.g., the length of time that the airway is closed or the tongue base is

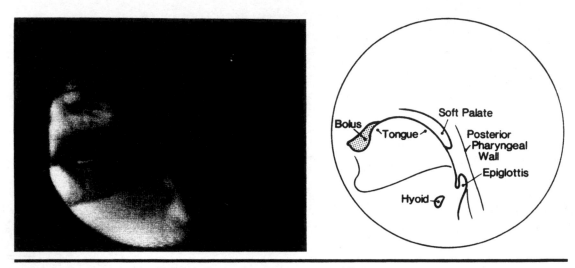

FIGURE 10.5   Lateral videofluorographic view of the upper aerodigestive tract.

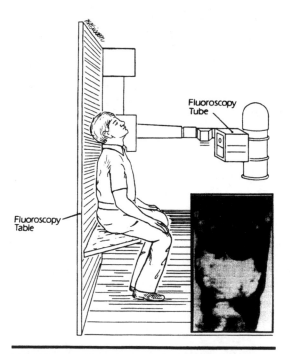

FIGURE 10.6   Posterior–anterior view of the upper aerodigestive tract with structures coated with barium.

in contact with the posterior pharyngeal wall. Computer analysis of the video images allows measurement of the range and timing of structural movement during the pharyngeal swallow (Logemann, Kahrilas, Begelman, & Pauloski, 1989). For computer analysis, selected video fields are digitized into the computer using a video digitizing board and stored in the computer's memory. When all video fields of interest are stored, each field is recalled from memory and structural landmarks of interest are marked with the mouse, e.g., the anterior superior corner of the hyoid bone. Software allows each marked point to be stored according to its x–y coordinates. When all structural points of interest on all fields are marked and stored, the software enables plotting of the movement of each structure over time, as shown in Figure 10.7. This type of analysis permits the study of the coordination of the swallow, i.e., the way in which each movement relates in time to every other movement, and to identify disorders of coordination. Videofluorography has the disadvantage of providing radiation exposure to the patient. Generally, this is a very low dose of radiation exposure since the procedure takes less than

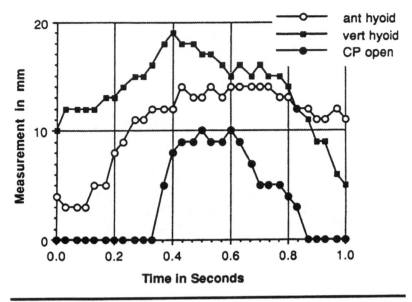

FIGURE 10.7 Graph of the anterior and vertical hyoid movement and cricopharyngeal opening over time on a swallow of 5 ml liquid barium.

five minutes. Videofluorography does not enable the measurement of pressures generated during the swallow. However, the speed and efficiency of the movement of the food through the mouth and pharynx indirectly indicate the adequacy of the pressure on the bolus.

Videonasendoscopy. Videonasendoscopy involves the placement of a flexible fiberoptic tube approximately 3 mm in diameter through the nose, over the soft palate, and into the pharynx as shown in Figure 10.8 (Bastian, 1993). A light topical anesthetic is placed in the nostril to facilitate easy placement of the tube. With the fiberoptic tube in place, the pharynx can be observed from above, before and after a swallow. If the end of the tube is placed behind the soft palate, as shown in Figure 10.8, the base of tongue, valleculae, and pharyngeal walls are visible. The vocal folds are only partially visible. Because the pharynx and larynx close during the swallow, the physiology during a swallow cannot be observed. Events oc-

curring before the swallow as well as the amount of food left in the pharynx after the swallow or aspirated after the swallow can be seen. Unfortunately, because of the placement of the tube through the nose, the oral stage of swallowing is also not visible. Because of its invasive nature, i.e., the placement of the tube through the nose, and because swallowing is not directly observable, nasendoscopy has limited application to the thorough evaluation of swallow physiology. If the tube is lowered slightly so that the tip is just below the epiglottis, the larynx is visible (see Figure 10.9), but the valleculae, tongue base, and pharyngeal walls are not visible. Thus, the patient's ability to follow instructions to volitionally close the airway before the swallow at the vocal folds and/or at the entryway between the arytenoid, the base of epiglottis, and the false vocal folds can be assessed.

Manometry. Manometry is a technique that measures pressures during swallowing. Measuring pressures during pharyngeal swallowing involves

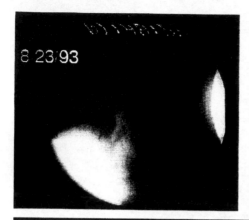
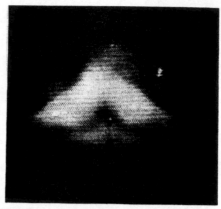

FIGURE 10.8 Lateral radiographic view of the upper aerodigestive tract with an endoscopic tube in place with the tip at the level of the uvula (left) and the structures visible with the tube at this level (right).

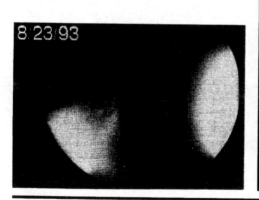

FIGURE 10.9 Lateral radiographic view of the upper aerodigestive tract with an endoscopic tube positioned with the tip at the level of the epiglottis (left) and the structures viewed with the tube at that level (right).

the placement of a flexible 3 to 4 mm diameter tube through the nose. The tube contains 3 to 4 solid state pressure sensors that are positioned in the pharynx at the level of the tongue base and upper esophageal sphincter, as shown in Figure 10.10, so that pressures within the food bolus can be measured as it passes through the pharynx. Similarly, the timing of pharyngeal wall contraction can also be measured as the contraction passes the sensors. The pressure sensors are wired to an external amplifier in a polygraph that writes out the pressure changes. Without concurrent videofluoroscopy, it is difficult if not impossible to interpret manometry in the pharynx because it is not possible to identify the source of the pressure changes seen on the polygraph without simultaneous videofluorography (Ergun, Kahrilas, & Logemann, 1993). Thus, by itself, manometry in the pharynx is not sufficient to provide data on the anatomy and physiology of the oral pharyn-

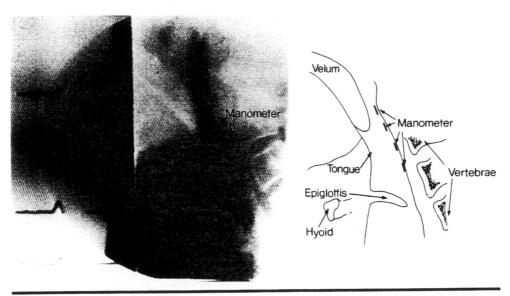

FIGURE 10.10   Lateral radiographic view of the upper aerodigestive tract with a manometric tube placed transnasally.

geal swallow. Also, as an invasive technique involving placement of a tube into the nose, this procedure is not widely applicable.

Ultrasound.   Ultrasound is an imaging technique utilizing high frequency sound waves to define soft tissue structures (Shawker, Sonies, Hall, & Baum, 1984). Currently, ultrasound does not provide good images of the pharynx. However, ultrasound does define tongue motion during swallow so that the oral phase of swallowing can be imaged. The duration of oral transit of the bolus, as well as patterns of tongue movement, have been defined with ultrasound. However, ultrasound cannot image the pharynx and has not been widely used as a diagnostic procedure in swallowing.

Scintigraphy.   Scintigraphy is a nuclear medicine test in which the patient swallows measured amounts (usually 10 ml) of galium, which is a radioactive liquid (Muz, Mathog, Rosen, & Borrero, 1987). A computer camera takes photographs of the galium bolus during swallow and calculates the exact amount of galium swallowed at any one

time. If there is aspiration, the amount of aspiration can be quantified. If there is residual food left in the mouth or the pharynx, this can also be measured by the galium computer camera. Scintigraphy, then, takes pictures of the food being swallowed, not the motions of the structures creating the swallow. From scintigraphy, physiologic and/or anatomic swallow disorders cannot be clearly identified. However, if the goal of the study is to define the amount of aspiration or residue, scintigraphy would be the procedure of choice.

Ultrafast Computerized Tomography.   Ultrafast computerized tomography takes pictures of a particular level in the body at a rate of 17 per second. Ultrafast computerized tomography has been used to measure pharyngeal dimensions during swallow by setting the level of photograph at the midpharynx and taking 17-frame-per-second pictures of the pharynx during swallow (Ergun, Kahrilas, Lin, Logemann, & Harig, 1993). Using a ruler to account for magnification in the viewing area, the pharyngeal dimensions during swallow can be defined, as can the volume of the bolus during swallow. Studies using ultrafast computerized tomography have defined the proportion of air swallowed with a bolus. The larger the amount of food swallowed, the smaller the amount of air swallowed. However, on average, normal adults swallow a large volume of air during eating, usually in the range of 10 to 15 ml per swallow.

Electromyography.   Electromyography is an instrumental technique that has been utilized to study selected muscle activity during swallow (Perlman, 1993). With electromyography, an electrode is placed on the surface of the neck, or a hooked wire is placed into selected muscles in the oral cavity or pharynx, and the electrical activity of these muscles is monitored throughout the swallow. Surface electrodes have been used to define the onset or occurrence of a swallow in some research studies. Surface electrodes are usually placed on the muscles under the chin (the submandibular muscles; i.e., mylohyoid, geniohyoid, anterior belly of digastric) or above the larynx. These muscles are some of the first muscles to contract during swallowing, so that the electromyographic signal serves as a marker for the swallow. Hooked wire electrodes have been used to study muscle contractions in the pharyngeal wall during swallowing and other muscle activities. Hooked wire electrodes have also been used to study the laryngeal muscles and tongue and lip musculature during speech production. While these studies are interesting, they do not provide enough diagnostic information to define the components of the oropharyngeal swallow that are damaged in a dysphagic patient. Electromyography has also been used for biofeedback, particularly in patients with reduced lip closure or reduced laryngeal elevation. It has also been used to monitor the degree of muscle effort used during swallow in order to encourage patients to swallow with greater effort.

Treatment for Swallowing Disorders

Treatment for swallowing disorders takes a number of forms (Logemann, 1983). Treatment may be compensatory in that it is designed to eliminate the symptoms of the swallowing disorder without necessarily changing swallowing physiology. This type of treatment is often used when a patient is likely to recover functional swallow spontaneously, and the compensation allows the patient to eat orally under defined conditions with the compensation until their swallow normalizes. Or, treatment can involve active exercise programs to alter swallow physiology and muscle function. In general, the clinician's approach to treatment of a dysphagic patient begins, when possible, with compensatory strategies because they work quickly and can be utilized with a wide range of patients. Since they are largely under the clinician's control, they can be used with infants and children, as well as patients with poor cognitive ability. Compensatory strategies also have the advantage of not increasing muscle effort so that patients do not fatigue easily when using them.

Compensations include changes in the head or body posture of the patient, increasing sensory input, changing bolus volume or viscosity, and modifying the feeding strategies of the patient. Changing the patient's head or body posture can change the direction of food flow and change oral pharyngeal dimensions (Rasley, et al., 1993). Five postural techniques have been defined in terms of their systematic effects on bolus flow and pharyngeal dimensions, and, on that basis, the swallowing disorder(s) for which they are effective. The chin-down posture narrows the airway entrance, widens the valleculae, and pushes the epiglottis and tongue base posteriorly. The chin-up posture facilitates oral drainage of food into the pharynx by gravity. When a patient has a unilateral weakness of the pharyngeal wall, head rotation to the weak side of the pharynx closes the side to which the head is rotated, directing food down the opposite, stronger side. Tilting the head toward the stronger side of the mouth and pharynx facilitates food flow to the location where stronger muscles can best control it. Lying the patient down on the back or the side changes the directional effect of gravity on residual food, often keeping food from falling directly into the airway after the swallow. These postures are applied selectively to various swallowing disorders based upon their systematic effects on bolus flow and pharyngeal dimensions. Postural techniques alone can be quite effective in eliminating aspiration and allowing patients to eat by mouth safely. For example, the patient who suffers a medullary stroke may get sufficient benefit from head rotation to the damaged side of the pharynx to enable oral intake on thin and thick liquids until spontaneous recovery occurs. A patient who has suffered a knife wound to one side of the neck may also be able to return to oral intake by swallowing with the head rotated to the side of the injury.

Increasing sensory input to the patient's oral cavity prior to a swallow attempt often facilitates the speed and efficiency of the swallow (Logemann, et. al., 1995). This can be done by stimulation of the faucial arches by a cold laryngeal mirror (thermal/tactile stimulation); by delivering a bolus with a sour taste; by increasing the downward pressure of the spoon on the tongue as the food is being presented; by allowing the patient to self-feed (which utilizes arm and hand control as a preliminary stimulus); or by encouraging the patient to chew a bolus as an additional oral sensory stimulus, even though the food may not require chewing.

For many patients with dysphagia, the particular volume or viscosity of the bolus provides increased sensory input and results in an improved swallow. In the videofluorographic study of the oropharyngeal swallow, patients are usually given a liquid bolus of various volumes from 1 to 10 ml, as well as foods of various viscosities, such as thick liquid, pudding, and a piece of a cookie.

Changing the way patients are fed can either facilitate their swallow or make it more unsafe or inefficient. Many patients require time between swallows in order to swallow three to four times on a single bolus. Some patients require placement of food in a more sensitive area of the mouth. Other patients require visualization of the food before they can initiate an adequate swallow. If they are fed too much too quickly, the food can literally back up in their pharynx and be aspirated, particularly if their swallow is slightly slowed or discoordinated. The speech–language pathologist will evaluate the way in which the patient is fed and instruct the patient's caregivers regarding optimal feeding strategies.

Swallowing Therapy. Swallowing therapy involves active muscle exercise designed to change the physiology of the swallow (Logemann, 1983, 1993). The kinds of exercise used include stretching a particular structure through its full range of motion. Range of motion exercises usually involve moving the structure as far as possible in the desired direction and holding the structure in its extreme range of motion for one second, then relaxing. Range-of-motion exercises can be done for the tongue, lips, jaw, and vocal folds and laryngeal elevation. Exercises for chewing also can be utilized to improve both the range and coordination of tongue and jaw motion during chewing. These exercises are particularly helpful in patients who have had surgical treatment for head and neck cancer.

Swallowing **maneuvers** involve applying voluntary control to selected elements of the pharyngeal swallow. There are currently four swallow maneuvers utilized in therapy: (1) the supraglottic swallow, which is a voluntary breath-hold before and during the swallow; (2) the super-supraglottic swallow, which involves a voluntary breath hold with effort or bearing down before and during the swallow; (3) the effortful swallow, which involves swallowing with a great deal of muscular effort; and (4) the Mendelsohn maneuver, which requires the patient to swallow normally, but during the swallow to maintain laryngeal elevation for several seconds longer than normal. Each of these maneuvers changes specific elements in the pharyngeal swallow. The supraglottic swallow closes the true vocal folds before and during the swallow, thus protecting the larynx or airway early. The super-supraglottic swallow closes the entrance to the airway between the arytenoid and the base of the epiglottis and false vocal folds before and during the swallow. This adds to the strength of airway protection. The effortful swallow increases the tongue-base motion posteriorly during the swallow and increases the pressure generated on the bolus in the pharynx during the swallow. The Mendelsohn maneuver increases laryngeal elevation and the duration of laryngeal elevation during the swallow, which prolongs cricopharyngeal opening, since laryngeal motion is the major force in opening the cricopharyngeal region. The patient mentioned earlier who suffered the medullary stroke may need the Mendelsohn maneuver to facilitate oral intake or as an exercise.

Any of these exercises can be done without food to keep the patient safe from aspiration, if they are regularly getting food or liquid into the lungs during swallow. When these exercises are done without food, the procedure is known as *indirect therapy,* and the patient is practicing the swallow coordination while maintaining safety. These exercises can also be done with food, which is known as *direct swallowing therapy.* Most often, these exercises are given for one to two weeks, and up to one to two months, and then the patients recovers oral intake. However, there are some patients who require swallow maneuvers permanently in order to safely and efficiently swallow.

Multidisciplinary Team. The speech–language pathologist's involvement in the evaluation and treatment of swallowing disorders has grown dramatically in the past 20 years. In order to be successful with dysphagic patients, speech–language pathologists must have a thorough working knowledge of the anatomy and physiology of the upper aerodigestive tract and swallowing, as well as speech, the various imaging and instrumental procedures utilized in the assessment of oral pharyngeal swallowing, and the various treatment procedures appropriate for specific types of patients. Two patients with the same swallowing physiology may require different treatment approaches because of the varying etiologies of their swallowing problems. The patient with motoneuron disease cannot tolerate active exercise programs, while the patient who has undergone surgical procedures for head and neck cancer must utilize active exercise programs to improve swallowing range-of-motion and coordination. The speech–language pathologist involved in swallowing management must also be familiar with multidisciplinary team interaction as well as efficient interaction with physicians. Because swallowing problems can be complex, many patients need referral for a consultation with a specialty physician including an otolaryngologist (ear, nose, and throat specialist), a gastroenterologist (esophagus and gastrointestinal tract specialist), a neurologist (central nervous system specialist), a gerontologist (aging and diseases of the elderly specialist), or a pulmonologist (pulmonary specialist). Other nonphysician specialists may be needed, including a doctor who specializes in evaluating and managing nutrition, an occupational therapist (OT) who develops assistive devices to facilitate the patient's self-feeding, and the physical therapist, who facilitates positioning of the patient. Other physicians and nonmedical professionals may also be needed by some patients. Generally, the speech–language pathologist serves as the coordinator of the multidisciplinary team.

In the currently changing health care system, in which there is a de-emphasis on specialists, it may be difficult to get approval to refer a patient to every professional on the multidisciplinary swallowing team. Therefore, the speech–language pathologist needs to prioritize referrals, sending the patient first to the physician-specialist most likely to provide important information to the patient's diagnosis. Experience with a number of swallowing centers has shown that the patient who presents with a swallowing disorder of no known etiology usually has some type of neurologic problem. It may be a progressive neurologic disease such as Parkinson's disease, amyotrophic lateral sclerosis, or myasthenia gravis (any of which may begin with swallowing disorders), or a brain tumor, or other neurologic problem. On this basis, a patient with a significant dysphagia of unknown medical etiology should first be referred to a neurologist.

The speech–language pathologist's role in the evaluation and treatment of swallowing disorders is critical to a patient's successful recovery from dysphagia. When speech–language pathologists examine a dysphagic patient, it is important to follow the mechanism's physiologic hierarchy, i.e., beginning with respiration, then swallowing, and then speech, which is an overlaid function. Respiration is paramount for survival. If respiration is impaired, both swallowing and speech will be affected. Respiration may be negatively affected by swallowing (which requires airway closure and momentary cessation of respiration) and by speech (which requires prolongation of exhalation). Concerns about establishing effective communication should be addressed after the patient's respiratory status is determined and after swallowing has been examined. If communication is assessed first and the patient has respiratory difficulties, the patient may experience respiratory distress.

Major Points of Chapter

- Swallowing disorders occur frequently in children and adults with neurologic or structural problems that are either congenital or acquired.
- The structure and physiology of the normal swallow provides a basis for identifying and diagnosing swallowing abnormalities.
- Assessment may include physical examination of the vocal tract, medical history, and behavioral observation.
- Instrumentation to assess pharyngeal swallow is essential, and includes videofluorography, videonasendoscopy, manometry, ultrasound, scintigraphy, and electromyography.
- Swallowing treatment involves applying voluntary control to selected elements of swallow, as well as providing compensatory movements and positions to facilitate swallow.

Discussion Guidelines

1. Describe the structure of the five valves in the upper aerodigestive tract, and provide the functions of each valve.
2. How does videonasendoscopy compare with videofluoroscopy? Describe the advantages

and disadvantages of each technique with respect to the specific aspects of swallowing that can be assessed by each.
3. The bedside or clinical evaluation of a patient with dysphagia typically assesses some aspects of the patient's function but cannot evaluate others. Discuss those aspects that can and cannot be evaluated in the typical bedside clinical examination.

REFERENCES

Bastian, R. W. (1993). The videoendoscopic swallowing study: An alternative and partner to the videofluoroscopic swallowing study. *Dysphagia, 8,* 359–367.

Ergun, G. A., Kahrilas, P. J., & Logemann, J. A. (1993). Interpretation of pharyngeal manometric recordings: Limitations and variability. *Dis Esoph, 6,* 11–16.

Ergun, G. A., Kahrilas, P. J., Lin, S., Logemann, J. A., & Harig, J. M. (1993). Shape, volume and content of the deglutitive pharyngeal chamber imaged by ultrafast CT. *Gastroenterology, 105,* 1396–1403.

Groher, M. E., & Bukatmun, R. (1986). The prevalence of swallowing in two teaching hospitals. *Dysphagia, 1,* 3–6.

Jacob, P., Kahrilas, P., Logemann, J., Shah, V., & Ha, T. (1989). Upper esophageal sphincter opening and modulation during swallowing. *Gastroenterology, 97,* 1469–1478.

Kahrilas, P. J., & Logemann, J. A. (1993). Volume accommodations during swallowing. *Dysphagia, 8,* 259–265.

Kahrilas, P. J., Logemann, J. A., Krugler, C., & Flanagan, E. (1991). Volitional augmentation of upper esophageal sphincter opening during swallowing. *American Journal of Physiology, 260,* G450–456.

Logemann, J. A. (1983). *Evaluation and treatment of swallowing disorders.* Austin, TX: Pro-Ed.

Logemann, J. A. (1993). *A manual for videofluoroscopic evaluation of swallowing (2nd ed).* Austin, TX: Pro-Ed.

Logemann, J., Kahrilas, P., Begelman, J., & Pauloski, B. R. (1989). Interactive computer program for biomechanical analysis of videofluorographic studies of swallowing. *AJR, 153,* 277–280.

Logemann, J. A., Kahrilas, P. J., Cheng, J., Pauloski, B. R., Gibbons, P. J., Rademaker, A. W., & Lin, S. (1992). Closure mechanisms of the laryngeal vestibule during swallow. *American Journal of Physiology, 262,* G338–G344.

Logemann, J. A., Pauloski, B. R., Colangelo, L., Lazarus, C., Fujiu, M., & Kahrilas, P. J. (1995). Effects of a sour bolus on oropharyngeal swallowing measures in patients with neurogenic dysphagia. *Journal of Speech and Hearing Research, 38(3),* 556–563.

Miller, R. M., & Groher, M. E. (1993). Speech–language pathology and dysphagia: A brief historical perspective. *Dysphagia, 8,* 180–184.

Muz, I., Mathog, R., Miller, P., Rosen, R., & Borrero, J. (1987). Detection and quantification of laryngotracheopulmonary aspiration with scintigraphy. *Laryngoscope, 97,* 1180–1185.

Perlman, A. L. (1993). Electromyography and the study of oropharyngeal swallowing. *Dysphagia, 8,* 351–355.

Rasley, A., Logemann, J. A., Kahrilas, P. J., Rademaker, A. W., Pauloski, B. R., & Dodds, W. J. (1993). Prevention of barium aspiration during videofluoroscopic swallowing studies: Value of change in posture. *AJR, 160,* 1005–1009.

Shawker, T., Sonies, B., Hall, T., & Baum, G. (1984). Ultrasound analysis of tongue hyoid and larynx activity during swallowing. *Invest Radiol, 19,* 82–86.

11

STRUCTURALLY RELATED AND NEUROGENIC VOICE DISORDERS

CAROLE T. FERRAND

The voice is one of the most unique aspects of human ability and behavior. The voice is not only the carrier of verbal speech, but also is strongly linked to self concept. Most individuals have a very good idea of what their voices feel like and sound like, what experts in the field of voice call "vocal image" or "vocal self perception" Haskell (1987). In addition, voice is strongly related to emotional status. For instance, most individuals have experienced their voice quivering as they talked about some deeply felt situation or episode. Anger or excitement tend to result in a voice that is louder and higher pitched. Voice also gives strong clues to listeners as to external identity, that is, socioeconomic status, educational status, and personality type.

This close relationship between voice, self-concept, and emotional state makes voice therapy both challenging and, occasionally, frustrating. Voice therapy involves dealing not just with a larynx and a pair of vocal folds, but with an individual who brings to the therapy situation a unique cluster of emotional, social, educational, and personal characteristics, all of which are closely intertwined with voice.

The field of voice disorders has grown dramatically over recent years. This growth has re-

sulted from advances in the knowledge of the structure and function of the vocal folds of the larynx, as well as advances in the use of computerized equipment. These two types of advances have come together to produce improved surgical treatment for many diseases and disorders of the larynx and vocal folds—treatment that focuses on the preservation of voice as an important objective. In addition, specialists from different areas have become more interested in working together to develop and promote the study of voice, including singing teachers, otolaryngologists, speech pathologists, voice scientists, singers, actors and others. So much new knowledge has become available that many experts are advocating a separate specialty of voice, called "vocology," or "vocal arts medicine" (e.g., Benninger, Jacobson, & Johnson, 1994).

This chapter explores different types of structurally related and neurogenic voice problems in children and adults. First, a review of normal laryngeal anatomy and physiology is provided, as a thorough understanding of different types of voice problems and clinical management is not possible without a basis of comparison. Emphasis is placed on recent developments in laryngeal anatomy and physiology, and the way in which this expanded

247

understanding has influenced the clinical management of voice problems. The way that the vocal mechanism grows and changes over the course of the lifetime is discussed. Descriptions of different types of disorders are presented together with explanations of the effect of the disorder on the voice. The final section describes different treatments for various disorders, from well-established behavioral voice therapy procedures to the most current surgical techniques. Throughout the chapter, and particularly in the final section, the need for an interdisciplinary approach to voice management, one that draws on the expertise of all professionals interested in the care of the voice, is emphasized.

ANATOMY AND PHYSIOLOGY OF THE VOCAL MECHANISM

The vocal mechanism includes the laryngeal skeleton plus the joints, three pairs of folds, and the extrinsic and intrinsic muscles.

The Laryngeal Skeleton

The laryngeal skeleton is made up of a single bone and nine cartilages. The **hyoid bone** is a small U-shaped bone that forms the attachment for the tongue. The larynx is suspended from this bone by a sheet of membrane (hyothyroid membrane). The hyoid bone consists of the **body** in the front, and the major horns that form the long sides of the *U*. Projecting slightly upward from each major horn is a small protrusion, the minor horn.

The largest cartilage of the larynx is the thyroid. This structure is formed by two plates of cartilage (the laminae) that are fused in the front. The fusion of these plates occurs at an angle, which is more acute in men than in women. It is this protrusion which is known as the Adam's apple, and which, because of the different angles, is generally more prominent in men than in women. A small, V-shaped notch (the thyroid notch) is apparent at the top surface of the laryngeal protrusion. Two long projections (the superior cornua), one at either side and toward the back of the thyroid, extend upward and connect, by means of

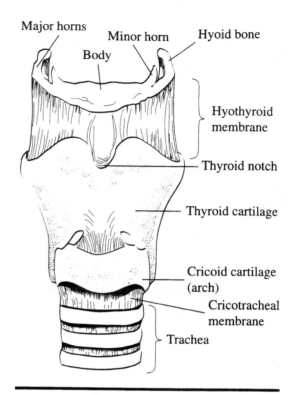

FIGURE 11.1 Front view of larynx.

various ligaments, to the hyoid bone. Two shorter projections (the inferior cornua) extend downward and articulate with the sides of the cricoid cartilage. The back aspect of the thyroid is open. The vocal folds are attached (like the point of a *V*) to the inner surface of the thyroid, just below the thyroid notch, at the **anterior commissure.**

The **cricoid cartilage** (Latin for "signet ring") is so-called because of its shape, being narrow in the front (the arch), and flaring to a larger, squarish plate in the back. The shape of this posterior plate explains its name—the **quadrate lamina.** The cricoid is surrounded by the thyroid, and is located just above the first ring of the trachea. Both the thyroid and cricoid cartilages are composed of hyaline cartilage. This type of cartilage is bluish-white in color, and somewhat transparent. It tends to ossify (become bony) with age.

The **epiglottis** is the last unpaired cartilage of the larynx. Unlike the thyroid and cricoid carti-

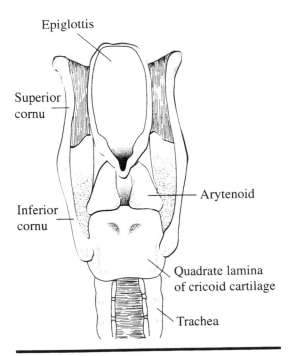

FIGURE 11.2 Back view of larynx.

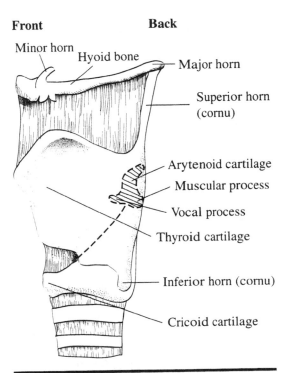

FIGURE 11.3 Side view of larynx.

lages, it is composed of elastic cartilage which is yellowish in color, opaque rather than transparent, more flexible than hyaline cartilage, and does not ossify. The epiglottis is a broad cartilage shaped like a leaf. It is attached by means of the **thyroepiglottic ligament** to the inner surface of the thyroid cartilage, just below the thyroid notch. It also attaches to the body of the hyoid bone by way of the hyoepiglottic ligament. The epiglottis performs an important function during swallowing, by folding down over the entrance to the larynx and acting as a bridge to direct food and liquids to the esophagus. It is less important in the production of voice.

The paired **arytenoid cartilages** are small hyaline cartilages that are located on top of the back aspect of the cricoid. They are pyramidal in shape, being broad and flattish at their base, and extending upward to more of a point at their apex. Two projections extend from their base. The **vocal process** on each arytenoid protrudes anteriorly, toward the thyroid cartilage. Each **muscular process** projects laterally and slightly posteriorly. The

arytenoids play a crucial role in phonation, as the vocal folds are attached to the vocal processes. Many intrinsic muscles of the larynx attach to the muscular processes, and have the effect of pivoting the arytenoids in various ways. In turn, this allows the vocal folds to be opened and closed, permitting vocal fold vibration.

There are several cartilages that do not appear to play an important role in voice production. The paired **corniculate cartilages** are located at the tip of the arytenoids, but may not be present in all individuals. The paired **cuneiform cartilages** are small elastic rods of cartilage, located within the aryepiglottic folds. Their primary function may be to stiffen these folds.

Joints of the Larynx

There are two joints in the larynx, both crucial in the production of a normal voice. The **cricoarytenoid joint,** as its name indicates, is formed by the articulation between the base of each arytenoid and the top surface of the cricoid. There are two cricoarytenoid joints, one on either side of the back of the cricoid. This joint allows two types of movement of the arytenoid cartilages: a limited gliding motion of the cartilages toward each other, and a fairly unrestricted back and forth rocking motion of the arytenoids (Dickson & Dickson, 1982).

Since the vocal folds are connected to the vocal processes of the arytenoids, any movement of the arytenoids must necessarily have an effect on the positioning of the vocal folds. When, through the action of intrinsic laryngeal muscles, the muscular processes of the arytenoids are swung away from each other, the vocal processes are forced toward each other, pulling the attached vocal folds along and closing them (**adduction**). Conversely, when other laryngeal muscles pull the muscular processes toward each other, the vocal processes and the attached vocal folds are separated (**abduction**). Thus, the cricoarytenoid joints are instrumental in vocal fold opening and closing.

The **cricothyroid joints** are located between each inferior **cornu** of the thyroid, and the lateral surface of the cricoid cartilage. This joint allows the thyroid cartilage to tilt downward over the front of the cricoid, or allows the cricoid cartilage to tilt upward so the front of the cricoid comes closer to the thyroid. Movement of either the cricoid or thyroid in this way increases the distance between the arytenoid cartilages in the back and the thyroid cartilage in the front. Recall that the vocal folds are attached to the vocal processes of

TABLE 11.1   Structures of the Laryngeal Skeleton

Hyoid bone
Thyroid cartilage
Cricoid cartilage
Epiglottis
Arytenoids (2)
Corniculate (2)
Cuneiform (2)
Cricothyroid joints (2)
Cricoarytenoid joints (2)

the arytenoids at the back, and at the anterior commissure of the thyroid in front. Thus, increasing the distance between these two points has the effect of stretching the vocal folds, making them more tense and thin. When the vocal folds are elongated, stretched, and tense, they vibrate more rapidly, resulting in a higher pitch. The cricothyroid joints, then, are the main agents of pitch change in the human voice.

Cavities of the Larynx

The larynx can be thought of as a tube, within which there are three cavities. The **vestibule** extends from the entrance to the larynx (the **aditus laryngis**) to the ventricular (false) vocal folds. The ventricular folds lie parallel to, but superior to, the true vocal folds. Between the true and false vocal folds is a small space, known as the **laryngeal ventricle** (or ventricle of Morgagni). This space contains mucous glands, which are important in maintaining the lubrication of the vocal folds. The space below the true vocal folds is the **atrium,** also known as the **inferior division** (Dickson et al., 1982), or the **subglottal cavity** (Colton & Casper, 1990). The inferior boundary of the atrium, and thus of the larynx, is the first tracheal ring.

Structures within the Larynx

There are three primary structures within the larynx, all of which consist of folds (bundles) of different types of tissue.

The **aryepiglottic folds** run from the sides of the epiglottis to the apex of each arytenoid cartilage. They form the lateral boundaries of the aditus laryngis. They are sheets of connective tissue and muscle that contract in a circular (sphincter) action to close the entrance of the larynx during swallowing (for further discussion see Chapter 10).

The **ventricular folds** or false folds lie just above and parallel to the true vocal folds, but do not extend out to the midline as far as the true folds. They are not as richly supplied with muscles as are the true folds, and thus are only capable

TABLE 11.2 Structures within the Larynx

STRUCTURE	LOCATION	FUNCTION
Aryepiglottic folds	Sides of epiglottis to apex of each arytenoid	Close entrance to larynx during swallowing
False vocal folds	Parallel and superior to true vocal folds	Close during swallowing, lifting
True vocal folds	Anterior commissure to each vocal process	Close for swallowing and phonation, open for inhalation of air

of limited movement. They close during swallowing, during effortful activities such as lifting heavy objects, and during natural functions such as excretion or childbirth.

The true **vocal folds** are the most complex structures in the larynx. It is only recently that the extraordinary nature and degree of their complexity has been determined, primarily due to the work of Hirano and his colleagues. It has been known for a long time that the vocal folds consist of various layers, including the thyroarytenoid muscle, a layer of mucous membrane surrounding the muscle, and a layer of epithelium covering the mucous membrane. Recent research using highly sophisticated technology such as electron microscopy has revealed the different cellular compositions and the different mechanical properties of these layers. The outermost layer of the vocal folds is the **epithelium.** This is an extremely thin layer of cells that contains very soft, almost fluid-like tissue (Titze, 1994). Beneath the epithelium is a mucous membrane (called the **lamina propria**), which itself is composed of three layers. The superficial layer of the lamina propria (also known as **Reinke's space**) consists of loosely organized elastin fibers. Elastin is a kind of connective tissue made up of fibers that are very flexible and stretchable. This layer has an almost gel-like consistency. The intermediate layer of the lamina propria is also composed of elastin fibers, as well as some collagen fibers. Collagen is a connective tissue, but unlike elastin, the fibers do not stretch. In the intermediate layer, the fibers are more densely packed than in the superficial layer, and are arranged in a more linear fashion. This layer is more

dense and less flexible than the superficial layer, and its composition has been compared to soft rubber bands (Colton et al., 1990). The final layer of the lamina propria, the deep layer, consists of densely packed and well-organized collagen fibers, somewhat like cotton thread (Colton et al., 1990). Again, this layer is less flexible than the intermediate layer.

The final structure that makes up the vocal folds is the thyroarytenoid muscle. This is the main mass of the vocal folds, and is considerably thicker and denser than the other layers. Colton and Casper (1990) suggested that this layer can be likened to a bundle of stiff rubber bands. These five layers of the vocal folds have been reclassified by Hirano and his colleagues on the basis of the differing degrees of the stiffness of the layers. Hirano's model of the vocal folds is known as the *cover-body* model. The **cover** consists of the epithelium and the superficial layer of the lamina propria. The **transition,** or **vocal ligament,** encompasses the intermediate and deep layers of the lamina propria. The thyroarytenoid muscle forms the body of the vocal folds. This grouping of structures demonstrates the different vibrating properties of each layer. The cover, being most loose and pliable, is the portion of the vocal fold that vibrates most strongly. The vocal ligament is stiffer than the cover, with its own mode of vibration, and the body is the stiffest of all. Clearly, the vocal folds are a multilayered and extremely complex vibrator. This structural complexity gives rise to a sound wave that is extremely complex, and that in turn results in a rich and resonant human voice.

TABLE 11.3   Structure of the True Vocal Folds, and Hirano's Cover-Body Model

Epithelium	Cover—	Epithelium
Lamina propria		Superficial layer
Superficial layer	Transition—	Intermediate layer
Intermediate layer		Deep layer
Deep layer	Body—	Thryoarytenoid muscle
Thyroarytenoid muscle		

The space between the true vocal folds is the **glottis,** divided into the membraneous glottis and the cartilaginous glottis. The membraneous glottis, which forms approximately three-fifths of the entire length of the glottis, is bounded by the vocal ligament on either side. The vocal processes form the lateral edges of the cartilaginous glottis, which accounts for about two-fifths of the glottis.

Muscles of the Larynx

The muscles of the larynx are divided into **extrinsic muscle** and **intrinsic muscle** groups. The extrinsic muscles (also known as the "strap muscles") are those that have one point of attachment to the larynx (actually to the hyoid bone) and the other point of attachment to another structure outside the larynx, such as the sternum or the cranium. The extrinsic muscles, in turn, are subdivided into the infrahyoids and the suprahyoids. The infrahyoids have their external point of attachment at structures below the hyoid bone (sternum and scapula), and the other point of at-

tachment on the hyoid bone. The suprahyoids have one point of attachment to structures located above the hyoid bone (mandible, temporal bone) and the other to the hyoid bone. The infrahyoids, when they contract, pull the entire larynx downward. Contraction of the suprahyoids pulls the entire larynx upward in the neck. These large up-and-down movements of the larynx occur mainly during swallowing.

There are five intrinsic muscles of the larynx. These muscles have both their origin and their insertion within the larynx itself. Two of the five muscles function to close (adduct) the vocal folds. The lateral cricoarytenoids (LCA) arise from the upper border of the cricoid (one on either side), and insert into the muscular process of the arytenoids. When they contract, they swing the muscular processes away from each other, bringing the vocal processes toward each other. The vocal folds, attached to the vocal processes, are also brought toward each other, closing the membraneous glottis. The other adductor, the interarytenoid (IA), consists of two parts: the transverse, which

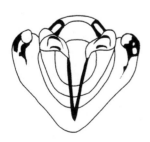
Quiet breathing

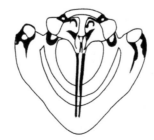
Normal phonation

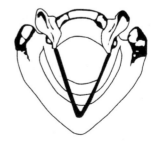
Forced inhalation

FIGURE 11.4   Vocal fold positions.

runs horizontally across the backs of the two arytenoid cartilages, and the oblique, which forms a cross between the back portions of each arytenoid. The cross is formed by fibers originating at the base of each arytenoid and inserting into the apex of the opposite arytenoid. When the interarytenoid muscle contracts, it glides the arytenoid cartilages toward each other, closing the posterior portion of the glottis. There is only one intrinsic muscle that opens the vocal folds—the posterior cricoarytenoid (PCA). This is a large, fan-shaped muscle that originates on the back aspect of each cricoid cartilage, and inserts into the muscular process of the corresponding arytenoid cartilage. Upon contraction, the muscular processes are rotated toward each other, which in turn has the effect of swinging the vocal processes away from each other and opening the vocal folds. The paired cricothyroid (CT) muscle is also divided into two parts. The pars recta originates at the upper surface of the sides of the cricoid cartilage. Its fibers run at an almost upright angle to insert into the lower border of the thyroid cartilage. The pars oblique originates at the same place as the pars recta, but, as its name implies, its fibers run in a more angled

direction, and insert near the inferior horn of the thyroid cartilage. This muscle functions as the primary pitch changer. When it contracts, the front of the thyroid cartilage is tilted down toward the cricoid, thus increasing the distance between the anterior commissure of the thyroid and the arytenoid cartilages. Recall that the vocal folds are attached at both the anterior commissure in the front, and the arytenoids at the back. Increasing the distance between these points, therefore, stretches and elongates the vocal folds, and makes them thinner and more tense. This increases the rate at which they vibrate, resulting in a higher pitch.

Finally, the thyroarytenoid (TA) forms the main mass of the true vocal folds. This is a paired muscle, coursing from the anterior commissure to the arytenoids. One part of the muscle, the muscularis, inserts into the muscular process of each arytenoid. The other part, the vocalis, inserts into each vocal process. This thyroarytenoid muscle is passively opened, closed, tensed, and relaxed by the force of the other intrinsic muscles. It can also, however, exert a more active internal tension that stiffens it and helps to increase the rate of vibration.

TABLE 11.4   Intrinsic Muscles of the Larynx

MUSCLE	LOCATION	FUNCTION	INNERVATION
Lateral cricoarytenoid	Lateral portion of cricoid to muscular process	Adductor	RLN
Interarytenoid			
Transverse	Back of arytenoids: Side of one arytenoid to side of other arytenoid	Adductor	RLN
Oblique	Back of arytenoids: Base of one arytenoid to apex of opposite arytenoid	Adductor	RLN
Posterior cricoarytenoid	Back aspect of cricoid to muscular process	Abductor	RLN
Cricothyroid			
Pars recta	Side aspect of cricoid to inferior border of thyroid	Tensor	SLN
Pars oblique	Side aspect of cricoid to inferior cornu	Tensor	SLN
Thyroarytenoid	Anterior commissure to vocal process	Body of vocal folds; internal tension	RLN

ADDUCTORS

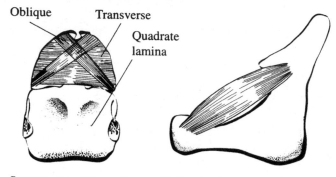

ABDUCTOR

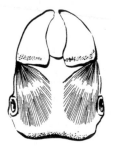

TENSORS

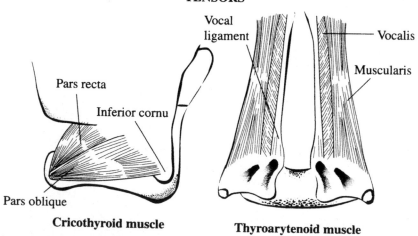

FIGURE 11.5   Intrinsic muscles of the larynx.

Innervation of the Larynx

It is important to understand how the vocal folds receive information from the nervous system (innervation). Damage to the nervous system from any cause has predictable effects on vocal fold function, depending on the site of the lesion.

The larynx is innervated primarily by the **vagus nerve** (Cranial nerve X). The cell bodies of the vagus originate in the nucleus ambiguus in the medulla oblongata. The nerve branches into three divisions as it extends downwards. The first branch is the pharyngeal nerve, which supplies motor impulses to various muscles of the soft palate. The second branch is the superior laryngeal nerve (SLN), which further subdivides into the internal and external branches. The internal branch provides sensory information to the larynx. The external branch innervates one sole muscle of the larynx—the cricothyroid. The last division of the vagus is called the recurrent laryngeal nerve (RLN). This is a particularly interesting nerve for several reasons. First, it does not go directly to the larynx, but winds under the heart and then loops back up to the larynx. Second, it is not symmetrical on the right and left sides. On the right side, the RLN passes under the subclavian artery of the heart, before coursing back up to the larynx. On the left, the RLN descends much further, winding under the arch of the aorta and then back up to the larynx. The RLN innervates all intrinsic muscles of the larynx except the cricothyroid. The RLN (particularly on the left side) is very susceptible to injury because of its length, and because of its proximity to the heart. In fact, Stemple, Glaze, & Gerdeman (1995) pointed out that a patient with an unexplained paralysis of the vocal folds should be evaluated for cardiac problems that could be affecting the RLN.

VOICE PRODUCTION

Myoelastic–Aerodynamic Theory of Phonation

The vocal folds act as a sound generator by vibrating the air coming through the larynx from the lungs, thus setting up a sound wave in the vocal tract. The **myoelastic–aerodynamic theory** of phonation, proposed in the 1950s, is the most widely accepted model of voice production. This model describes voice production as a combination of muscle force (myo), tissue elasticity (elastic), and air pressures and flows (aerodynamic). In order to initiate vocal fold vibration, the vocal folds must close. This is achieved by the LCA and IA muscles, which exert a force called medial compression. When medial compression holds the vocal folds closed at the midline, the pressure of the air beneath the folds (**subglottal pressure**) begins to increase. When the subglottal pressure is strong enough, it overcomes the resistance of the closed vocal folds and forces them apart. A puff of air escapes into the vocal tract, setting the air within the tract into vibration. Meanwhile, the vocal folds have begun to close again, due to the interaction of two forces. First, the vocal folds begin to recoil back to the midline, due to their natural elasticity. As they begin to close, they form a narrow channel. Second, the air passing through this constriction formed by the closing vocal folds becomes negative in pressure, due to an aerodynamic force known as the **Bernoulli Principle.** This principle states that air passing through a narrow channel increases in velocity and decreases in pressure. This decrease in pressure further helps to close the folds completely.

Recently, Titze (1994) has extended this model to include the influence of the air pressures above the level of the glottis. The air in the vocal tract gets alternately compressed and rarefied as the pressure puffs are released through the vocal folds, and as the pressures within the vocal folds become positive and negative. As the air within the vocal tract gets compressed, the pressure within the vocal tract becomes positive; as the air becomes rarefied, the pressure becomes negative. This causes a top-down effect that influences the pressure within the vocal folds. The positive pressure in the vocal tract plays a role in forcing the vocal folds apart once they have been closed, and correspondingly, the negative pressure in the vocal tract contributes to closing the vocal folds once they have been blown apart. Thus, the vocal tract pressures help in the maintenance of vocal fold vibration. Once again, subglottal pressure begins to build up, and the whole process repeats itself. One such opening and closing of the folds constitutes one cycle of vocal fold vibration.

As previously mentioned, because of their layered structure, the vocal folds vibrate in an extremely complex fashion. Rather than opening and closing as a whole, the folds open from bottom to top and close from bottom to top in an undulating way. This undulating, or rolling, wavelike motion is particularly evident in the loose and pliable cover layer of the folds, and has been termed the **mucosal wave.** This flexibility of motion is crucial for the production of a normal voice. Disturbance or disruption of the mucosal wave interferes with voice production and results in various types of vocal problems.

The vocal folds vibrate for as long as the individual is producing a voiced sound. For a voiceless sound, or to inhale, the vocal folds are opened by the PCA. The rate of vibration depends on the length, mass, and tension of the folds, and is related to pitch. The greater the length and mass, and the less the tension and stiffness, the slower the vocal folds vibrate, and the lower the person's pitch, and vice versa. Rate of vibration of the vocal folds is called **fundamental frequency** (FO), and is measured in cycles per second, or Hertz (Hz). Children, with their small vocal folds, tend to have a high frequency of vibration (around 250–300 Hz for boys and girls prior to puberty). Adult females have an average FO of 180–250 Hz, and adult males, who generally have longer and more massive vocal folds, range in FO between approximately 80–150 Hz.

Changing Pitch and Loudness

The cricothyroid (CT) muscle is primarily responsible for pitch change. The CT muscle tilts the thyroid downward toward the cricoid, thus stretching and elongating the vocal folds. This decreases the mass of the folds per unit area, and increases their stiffness and tension. As a result, they vibrate more quickly, resulting in a higher FO and higher pitch. The thyroarytenoid (TA) muscle may also play a role in increasing the internal stiffness of the folds and helping to speed up the rate of vibration. To lower pitch, the vocal folds relax and become more massive per unit area, thus decreasing the vibratory rate.

Loudness depends on the interaction between medial compression and subglottal pressure. To increase loudness, more medial compression is exerted by the LCA and IA muscles. The vocal folds are held together at the midline more tightly. The amount of subglottal pressure necessary to overcome the medial compression is therefore greater, and takes longer to build up. When the subglottal pressure is sufficient, it blows the folds open with more force. The folds are blown apart more widely, causing a stronger burst of air to enter the vocal tract, and creating a higher intensity sound wave. After this high-energy opening, the vocal folds close again with correspondingly greater collision force.

During speech, the vocal folds continuously modify their tension characteristics to change pitch and loudness in accordance with the verbal message. These continuously varying changes give rise to the prosody (melody) of language—the rising and falling inflections that signal linguistic meaning (such as whether an utterance is a question or a statement), mood, and emotion.

GROWTH AND DEVELOPMENT OF THE LARYNX THROUGH THE LIFESPAN

Like other structures and systems in the body, the larynx and vocal folds change with growth, maturity, and aging, in a continuous process from birth to senescence. Not surprisingly, the larynx of the newborn infant is different than that of the adult, both in its structure and in its position in the neck. Whereas the adult larynx is situated at the level of the seventh cervical vertebrae, the infant larynx is positioned much higher—between the first and third cervical vertebrae. The larynx gradually descends in the neck, reaching the level of C6 at around age 5, and the level of C7 around age 15–20. Interestingly, the larynx continues to descend gradually throughout life, leading to a corresponding lowering of pitch. The infant larynx is also much smaller than the adult version, and the vocal folds are much shorter.

Kahane (1978, 1983, 1988) and Hirano (1974, 1977) have measured larynges of cadavers of various ages. Based on these measurements, it has been determined that the length of the membraneous vocal folds in infants is around 2–3 mm, with the cartilagineous vocal folds measuring another 2 or 3 mm. The membraneous vocal folds grow at a rate of 0.4 mm per year for females, and 0.7 mm per year for males, resulting in an adult length of approximately 16 mm for males, and 10 mm for females (Titze, 1994). The cartilaginous vocal folds do not show as great an increase in length, increasing just a few millimeters by adulthood. Total vocal fold length in adult males is around 17–23 mm, and in females is, on the average, 12–17 mm (Sataloff, 1991). The composition of the vocal folds also demonstrates significant changes during childhood. In infants, the vocal ligament is not well-differentiated; it starts to develop its complex layered structure at around age three or four (Hirano, 1981). The infant larynx is not well-developed neurologically, and the infant does not have fine control over vocal fold function. The birth cry has been reported to have a FO of approximately 500 Hz, so it sounds extremely high pitched. With growth of the larynx, and its descent in the neck, the average FO lowers to around 275 Hz for both boys and girls, and remains at that level until puberty.

With puberty come dramatic changes in laryngeal growth, particularly for boys. The cartilages of the larynx enlarge, including the epiglottis, which becomes flatter and less bulky (Sataloff, 1991). The angle of the thyroid cartilage decreases in males to around 90°, but remains at a greater angle of 120° in females, resulting in the more prominent Adam's apple in males. The laryngeal mucosa become stronger and thicker, and

in males, the thyroarytenoid muscles increase in bulk. At puberty, the vocal folds grow markedly. Male vocal folds grow 4–8 mm in length; those of females grow 1–3.5 mm (Sataloff, 1991). The pitch of the voice decreases correspondingly, lowering about one octave in males, to around 130 Hz, with less of a decrease in females (about 2.5 semitones, to about 220 Hz). These prepubertal and pubertal changes occur within the context of sociocultural changes. Ferrand and Bloom (1996) found that changes in intonation patterns emerged at around seven to eight years for boys, but not for girls. They suggested that boys at that age start to mirror adult male vocal patterns of less contrastive pitch change, while girls of the same age maintain their more highly contrastive pitch patterns. By age 18, the voice in both males and females has reached its mature stage.

The process of aging takes its toll on the laryngeal mechanism as it does on most bodily structures and functions. Laryngeal cartilages ossify, leading to loss of flexibility and fine control. The ossification process is a gradual one, and interestingly, the cartilages ossify at different rates. The thyroid and cricoid ossify during the early twenties, while the arytenoids ossify in the late thirties. The entire laryngeal skeleton (except for the epiglottis, which is composed of elastic cartilage) is ossified by approximately age 65 (Sataloff, 1991). Other degenerative changes that have been noted include thinning and atrophy of the vocal fold muscles, bowing of the vocal folds, disorganization of the fibers in the lamina propria, and a decrease in the amount and quality of mucous secretions in the larynx, resulting in loss of lubrication (Chodzko-Zajko & Ringel, 1987; Kahane, 1987). These and other changes can lead to a perceptual change in the older voice, which has been referred to as the "senescent voice" (Mueller, Sweeney, & Baribeau, 1984). In fact, stereotypes of the older voice are common, including descriptions of older voices as quavery, tremulous, weak, hoarse, or breathy. However, not all older individuals show this kind of deterioration in vocal function. Research has shown that the physiological health of the person is more influential in determining their vocal quality and vocal health than is chronological age (Hollien, 1987). Older people in good shape often sound younger than younger people in poor physiological condition.

THE PREVALENCE OF STRUCTURALLY RELATED AND NEUROGENIC VOICE DISORDERS

The number of people afflicted with structurally related and/or neurogenic voice disorders has not been clearly established. Estimates of school-aged children with voice disorders range from 6 percent to almost 24 percent. Stemple et al. (1995) noted that the generally accepted figure for children is 6 percent. The incidence for adults appears to be similar, 5 percent for adult females, and 7.2 percent for adult males (LaGuaite, 1972, cited in Stemple et al., 1995). Herrington-Hall, Lee, Stemple, Niemi, and McHone (1988) investigated a group of 1262 patients with various types of vocal complaints, and found that vocal nodules were the most prevalent (21.6 percent), followed by edema (14.1 percent), polyps (11.4 percent), cancer (9.7 percent), vocal fold paralysis (8.1 percent), no visible pathology (7.9 percent), laryngitis (4.2 percent), and leukoplakia (4.1 percent).

TYPES OF STRUCTURALLY RELATED VOICE DISORDERS

Structurally related disorders are those that affect the structures of the larynx and vocal folds. They may occur at any age, in both sexes, singly, or in combination with other disorders. They may affect a person's ability to produce a normal voice to a great degree, or not at all. Many of these disorders affect the airway, and some can be life-threatening. Some of the problems are more prevalent in childhood, while others tend to occur more often in adult life. Yet others may occur in either children or adults. Some may be congenital (occurring at or shortly after birth), and others may be caused by trauma or illness. Those disorders that

occur more commonly in children are presented first, followed by those that occur more often in adults.

Terminology

Vocal terminology has been rather confusing, due to the subjective nature of evaluating the voice, and due to the many different terms that people use to describe the same or similar types of disorders. For instance, vocal characteristics have been described as rough, raspy, strident, shrill, hoarse, harsh, light, tinny, shrieky, breathy, husky, weak, and so on. The list is almost endless, and reflects the multidimensional nature of the voice, as well as the subjective way in which most individuals judge voice quality. These terms all refer to the perceptual aspect of voice—the voice that is heard by a listener. They are not good descriptors of how well the vocal folds are actually working, nor are they satisfactory in describing the acoustic characteristics of the vocal signal generated by vocal fold vibration. Acoustic measures are those that describe the dimensions of the voice output, such as frequency and intensity, in more objective terms.

The current trend in speech–language pathology is to use only those perceptual terms that have a firm basis in vocal fold physiology and acoustics. This narrows the list to a few major perceptual characteristics: hoarseness, breathiness, harshness, and tremor. **Hoarseness** is the voice quality heard in laryngitis, and reflects a lack of regularity in the vocal fold vibration. The mucosal wave is not being generated efficiently, resulting in an acoustic signal which is aperiodic (noisy). This noise in the signal is perceived as hoarseness. **Breathiness** is the perception of air escaping through vocal folds that are not closing properly. This escaping air sets up turbulence in the airstream passing through the vibrating vocal folds. **Harshness** refers to a voice that sounds strained and tense, and reflects the excessive tightness of the vocal folds as they vibrate. **Tremor** relates to rhythmic changes in frequency and/or amplitude of vocal fold vibration, perceived as a quavery quality in the voice. Other terms refer to deviations in pitch, loudness, resonance, and breathing. Pitch may be too high, too low, may lack variety (monopitch), or may sound like two pitches occurring simultaneously (diplophonia). Loudness level may be too great, not great enough, lack variety (monoloudness), or occur in jerky bursts. Resonance disorders usually include hypernasality (too much air resonated in the nasal cavities on nonnasal sounds), and hyponasality (too little air being resonated in the nasal cavities on nasal sounds). When the airway is compromised, stridor (noisy breathing) may be heard.

Laryngomalacia

Laryngomalacia is one of the most common congenital voice disorders. The larynx above the glottis lacks normal stiffness, due to a lack of calcium. The epiglottis lacks cartilaginous support, resulting in a characteristic omega shape. The glottis itself and the area of the larynx below the glottis are normal. There may also, however, be similar flaccidity of the trachea (tracheomalacia). The main vocal characteristic is **stridor** (noisy breathing), resulting from the aryepiglottic folds being drawn into the glottis on inhalation. This condition and the associated stridor usually resolves by age two, but may persist until age four.

Laryngomalacia can occur either as an isolated phenomenon, or together with other problems (McClurg & Evans, 1994), such as pharyngeal hypotonia (weakness of the pharynx), vocal fold paralysis, subglottic stenosis (to be discussed), and macroglossia (tongue too large for mouth). Surgical intervention is usually not necessary, unless there is complete or nearly complete collapse of the glottis on inspiration, which seriously compromises the airway. Surgical management may also be indicated if there is a complication from the obstruction, such as feeding difficulties or severe gastroesophageal reflux. **Gastroesophageal reflux** is a condition in which the contents of the stomach escape into the esophagus and pharynx. The acidity of these contents can irritate and inflame the sensitive tissues in the pharyngeal and laryngeal areas (McClurg & Evans, 1994). When

required, surgical techniques involve trimming the excess or collapsing tissue from the supraglottic larynx with a laser.

Laryngeal Web

In order for a normal glottis to develop, the vocal folds must separate by the 10th week of embryonic development (Stemple et al., 1995). Lack of separation results in webbing anywhere along the length of the glottis. A web is a thin sheet of connective tissue that attaches the two vocal folds. The effect of a web on voice depends on the length and thickness of the tissue. A tiny web at the anterior commissure will probably have minimal effect on voice, whereas a longer web can result in severe hoarseness and breathiness. Treatment consists of surgically dividing the web. If the web is complete, it is called **congenital laryngeal atresia.** The infant born with this condition must have immediate surgery to establish an airway.

Papilloma

Recurrent respiratory papillomatosis (RRP) is, according to Doyle, Gianoli, Espinola, and Miller (1994), one of the most difficult and frustrating benign diseases treated by otolaryngologists. It is also the most common benign neoplasm of the larynx. Papillomas are wart-like growths on the epithelium, which typically begin at the anterior portion of the vocal folds and then spread to include the aryepiglottic folds, the ventricular folds, and other structures within the larynx. The etiology is believed by most authorities to be the human papillomavirus (HPV), although some experts maintain that RRP is hormonally related.

The symptoms of RRP include hoarseness, stridor, **aphonia,** and respiratory distress. Different types of treatments have been tried over the years, including radiation therapy, cryosurgery, hormone therapy, and many others. The current treatment of choice is laser excision of the papilloma (Doyle et al., 1994). A minority of speech–language pathologists working in voice believe that behavioral voice therapy is indicated as the primary treatment for RRP, however, most oto-laryngologists and speech–language pathologists recommend some form of medico–surgical management in conjunction with voice therapy to maintain the best possible voice.

While RRP is more common in juveniles, it can be found in all age groups and in both genders. The disease may be aggressive or nonaggressive. Doyle et al. (1994) defined RRP as aggressive in patients requiring a total of 10 or more removal procedures, with three or more procedures over a one-year period. The disease is also considered aggressive if it spreads to the subglottic region, trachea, or bronchi. The nonaggressive form was defined by Doyle et al. (1994) as less than a total of 10 procedures, with no more than three procedures in a one-year period, and the absence of spread to other regions. The disease seems to be more aggressive in children, who also tend to have more complications than adult patients. Complications include anterior and posterior commissure webbing; glottic, subglottic, and tracheal stenosis; and even cardiac arrest.

Subglottic Stenosis

Stenosis refers to a narrowing or closing of tissues. Subglottic stenosis can be congenital or acquired, and reflects a narrowing of the larynx below the level of the vocal folds. This may occur from either thickened or narrowed cartilage, or from thickened soft tissues. The subglottis can be damaged (with a resulting narrowing) from many different causes, such as accident, surgical trauma, radiation therapy, local or systemic disease, paralysis of the RLN, lesions affecting the central nervous system, benign or malignant neoplasms, scarring, infectious granulomas caused by syphillis, tuberculosis, chronic subglottic laryngitis, and improperly performed tracheotomy (Figi, 1940). Recently, gastroesophageal reflux disease (GERD) has been associated with subglottic stenosis (Jindal, Milbrath, Shaker, Hogan, & Toohill, 1994). Stenoses can differ in degree, character, and extent, and can therefore have differing effects on both vocal and respiratory function. Current treatment employs

endoscopic laser therapy to excise the tissue or cartilage. For children who are unresponsive to this kind of therapy, the widely accepted treatment is reconstruction of the affected area using cartilage taken from the ribs (April & Marsh, 1993).

Cricoarytenoid Joint Fixation

Fixation (ankylosis) of the cricoarytenoid joint may be related to rheumatoid arthritis (RA), or gouty arthritis (GA), in which case it tends to occur in later adulthood. Fixation can also arise from trauma, which can occur at any age.

Rheumatoid Arthritis. Rheumatoid arthritis is a heterogeneous group of disorders in which the major symptom is inflammation in multiple joints (Krane & Simon, 1986). According to Krane and Simon, the etiology is unknown, but is probably a parvovirus (small DNA virus).

While the disease may occur at any age, it is more common in the third or fourth decade of life. Symptoms include pain in the affected joint at rest as well as with motion, swelling, limitation of motion, and difficulty in using the joint, usually due to pain and muscle weakness secondary to inflammation and disuse. The swelling may be due to edema, thickening of the synovial membrane (membrane that lines the joint) and other soft tissues, increased vascularity of the synovium, or the presence of synovial effusion (Krane & Simon, 1986). Reddened joints are less common, and may be present in individuals whose disease is of acute onset. Swelling in RA rarely extends far beyond the joint margin, in contrast to disorders such as connective tissue disease, in which swelling may extend beyond the confines of the joint. Extensive inflammation and pain often lead to disuse of joints and consequent muscle atrophy. In severe cases, bone and cartilage become eroded.

Since the cricoarytenoid (CA) joint is a synovial joint, it can develop RA. Arthritis involving the CA joints may be acute or chronic, and unilateral or bilateral. In acute CA arthritis, there may be tenderness over the larynx, bright red swelling over the arytenoids, as well as hoarseness, pain on swallowing with radiation to the ear (due to irritation of the vagus nerve), labored breathing (dyspnea), and stridor (Leicht, Harrington, & Davis, 1987). There may also be a feeling of fullness in the throat. This is often aggravated by speaking or swallowing. The hoarseness varies with the degree of joint **ankylosis** and inflammation. The severity of dyspnea varies with the degree of acute airway obstruction. If the joint becomes immobilized, the vocal folds become fixed, and this can compromise the airway. Many patients with upper airway obstruction from ankylosis are misdiagnosed as having asthma or being psychoneurotic (Leicht, Harrington, & Davis, 1987).

In the chronic stage, pain is usually minimal or absent. There is no redness or edema. There may be slight thickening and roughness of the mucosa over the arytenoids. The symptoms depend on the degree and position of joint fixation. Unilateral fixation of the joint in the abducted position may result only in dyspnea on moderate exertion. Hoarseness is usually absent or minimal. Bilateral ankylosis on abduction allows for an adequate airway, but produces hoarseness and perhaps dyspnea on moderate exertion. When the joint is fixed in a position that keeps the vocal folds more adducted, dyspnea may occur with even the slightest exertion. Leicht, Harrington, and Davis (1987) noted that the stridor resulting from a narrowed glottis can be the most alarming symptom. The stridor can be a result of the adduction alone, or it can be due to swelling and secretions, or both. Stridor can also result from upper respiratory infections superimposed on preexisting ankylosis. There is a range of severity from stridor at night while sleeping, to respiratory failure, acute life-threatening airway obstruction, and even cardio-pulmonary arrest.

According to Guerra, Lau, and Marwah (1992), cricoarytenoid involvement occurs in as many as 25 to 35 percent of patients with RA, and is present in the majority of cases at autopsy (45 to 86 percent of RA patients). Treatment consists of oxygen, cool humidification of the patient's environment, anti-inflammatories, and steroids. If there is severe airway obstruction, surgical intervention may be necessary. Arytenoidectomy (removal of the arytenoid cartilage) is performed to clear the airway obstruction.

Gouty Arthritis. Cricoarytenoid arthritis can also be associated with gouty arthritis (GA). Acute GA is an inflammatory response to too much uric acid, and is extremely painful. Gout used to be associated with wealth, as it results from a meat- and fat-rich diet. In bygone days, only the wealthy could afford such a diet. The current prevalence of gout in the U.S. is small (0.2 percent). Ninety-five percent of cases occur in men, with most incidences in the fifth decade (Guttenplan, Townsend, Hendrix, & Balsasa, 1991). In chronic GA, any joint, including the temporomandibular joint and the CA joint, may be affected. Symptoms include pain, dysphagia, and hoarseness. There may be cricoarytenoid fixation. Treatment for gout includes diet control and anti-inflammatory agents (e.g., indomethacia).

Trauma. Any kind of injury to the larynx, particularly blunt injury to the neck or injury to the larynx due to endoscopic examination and intubation can damage the CA joints, or even dislocate the arytenoid cartilage. Clearly, arytenoid injury can affect vocal fold vibration, resulting in hoarseness, dyspnea, and dysphagia. One of the primary problems with joint trauma is the development of fibrosis in and around the affected joint (Jie, Rong, & Chang, 1991). Proliferation of fibrous tissues limits joint recovery and joint movement. In fact, the recovery of vocal fold movement may depend on whether fibrosis of the joint occurs. Jie et al. (1991) proposed that if the acute inflammatory reaction to the trauma subsides without fibrous tissue proliferation, vocal fold function can be expected to return. If fibrosis of the joint occurs, complete restoration of vocal fold function is impossible.

Sulcus Vocalis (SV)

Sulcus vocalis is a benign disorder in which a fine longitudinal furrow or groove exists along the medial edge of the vocal fold. The length and depth of the groove varies with the individual. Only a short, shallow segment of the fold may be involved, or the sulcus could extend over the entire length of the fold. Nakayama, Ford, Brandenburg, and Bless (1994) classified sulcus lesions of laryngeal specimens into three groups based on the depth and shape of the groove (invagination): (I) Superficial type: sulcus confined to the superficial layer of the lamina propria (Reinke's space); (IIa) Deep type: sulcus penetrates the superficial layer and approximates the intermediate and deep layers (vocal ligament); (IIb) Pouch type: deep type in which the sulcus exhibits a pouch shaped configuration.

Etiology is uncertain, but could be congenital or acquired. According to Nakayama et al. (1994), the case for a congenital problem is strengthened by the fact that some sulcus patients have been dysphonic for as long as they can remember, and lesions have been identified in some children. However, SV might also be acquired in later life, given the high incidence of SV in the geriatric population, and the frequent concurrence of SV with laryngeal inflammatory disease, such as acute or chronic laryngitis and vocal fold polyps. SV may result in mild or moderate **dysphonia.** Other clinical findings include bowed folds and excessive ventricular fold adduction.

NEUROGENIC VOICE DISORDERS

The term *neurogenic voice disorders* refers specifically to disorders resulting from damage to the parts of the central and peripheral nervous system that deal with voice production. The disorders discussed in this chapter include those that affect primarily the laryngeal mechanism. Neurogenic disorders that affect other speech subsystems (respiration, articulation, resonation), but which also have a laryngeal component (e.g., Parkinson's disease), are included in Chapter 8.

Vocal Fold Paralysis

Vocal fold paralysis is the most common neuropathology of the larynx, and, depending on the spe-

cific site of damage to the nerve supply, can be either unilateral or bilateral, and of the abductor or adductor types. In unilateral paralysis, only one of the folds is paralyzed. Bilateral paralysis affects both vocal folds. Abductor paralysis means that the fold(s) cannot open—it is paralyzed at or close to the midline. Conversely, adductor paralysis leaves the folds unable to close. With damage to the recurrent laryngeal nerve (RLN) only, abduction and adduction are affected, but pitch control is relatively intact. Damage to only the superior laryngeal nerve (SLN) causes problems in pitch, but does not affect the opening and closing of the vocal folds. If the pharyngeal nerve is affected, hypernasality will be present.

Causes of damage to the vagus nerve and its branches are varied, and include trauma, viral infection, nerve degeneration from a progressive neurological disease, damage during surgery (e.g., thyroid gland surgery), heart problems, and other causes. The idea that heart problems can result in damage to the RLN may sound surprising, but knowing the anatomy of the RLN makes the connection clear. As previously discussed, the RLN, unlike most other nerves, does not run straight from its cell body to the larynx. Rather, the right RLN descends into the chest and winds under the subclavian artery of the heart, before turning upwards and running into the larynx. The left RLN descends into the chest, loops under the arch of the aorta, and then ascends to the larynx. Both RLNs, because of their close proximity to the heart, may be affected by cardiac problems such as heart congestion. When the cause of the problem is unknown, the resulting paralysis is called ideopathic.

According to Crumley (1994), when the RLN is injured, the acute effects are immediate flaccidity of the vocal fold on the same side as the nerve, loss of abduction and adduction, severe dysphonia, and often, aspiration of food and drink into the trachea. Crumley noted that the acute phase may last several weeks, and is generally followed by an intermediate phase, characterized by a slight improvement in vocal quality. This partial recovery may result from compensation by the intact fold, and by reinnervation on the paralyzed side. The chronic phase begins in the fourth or fifth month. Usually by this time regeneration of the damaged vagus nerve has begun, and there may be some clinical evidence of improvement.

The degree of vocal impairment depends on whether the paralysis is unilateral or bilateral, and the distance the folds are fixed from the midline. Typically, a bilateral problem results in more severe problems than a unilateral problem. However, much depends on the position of the paralyzed folds. Two paralyzed folds that are fixed fairly close to the midline may be passively vibrated by air going through the glottis, and the voice may sound nearly normal. On the other hand, when one fold is normal, but the other is paralyzed far from the midline, the unimpaired fold will not be able to make closure against the fixed fold, and the resulting voice will be extremely weak and breathy, or possibly even aphonic. Usually, with vocal fold paralysis, the individual has a weak and "mushy"-sounding cough, because the folds cannot close firmly enough to build up the necessary subglottal pressure (Hegde, 1995). Dysphagia may also be present.

PATHOLOGY RESULTING FROM VOCAL ABUSE

Behaviors are abusive when they irritate the vocal folds. Constant slamming and rubbing together of the vocal folds result in inflammation and swelling of the delicate epithelium and mucosal layers of the folds. This kind of abuse can lead to actual structural changes of the folds, which can often be ameliorated with behavioral voice therapy, but sometimes may necessitate surgical removal.

Examples of abusive vocal behaviors include yelling, screaming, hard glottal attack, speaking over noise, habitual coughing and throat clearing, using inappropriately high or low pitch levels, smoking, talking in a smoky environment, vocalizing toy and animal noises, grunting or talking during strenuous exercise, and singing without proper training. There are three primary types of growths which occur as a result of vocal abuse.

Nodules

Nodules (often called *singer's nodes*) are benign growths originating from the epithelium. When they first start to develop, they are soft, reddish, vascular, and pliable. With continued abuse they become more fibrous and hard, and appear whitish in color. Typically, nodules are bilateral, as the striking of one nodule against the opposite fold causes irritation at the same spot on the opposite fold. Nodules occur at the location on the folds where vibration is most vigorous. The vocal characteristics of the voice include low pitch, hoarseness, and breathiness.

Polyps

Polyps, like nodules, are benign tumors of the mucosa. Polyps are generally more pliable and softer than nodules, and are therefore often found only on one fold. Unlike nodules, polyps can result from a single episode of severe abuse, or they can also develop over time. Also unlike nodules, polyps can arise from causes other than vocal abuse (e.g., allergies), and are not necessarily located at the same place on the vocal folds. Polyps can occur either on the folds themselves, or above or beneath the folds. There are three types of polyps. *Sessile* polyps have a broad base, while *pedunculated* polyps are perched on a thin stalk. Polyps may also be *diffuse,* and affect the entire length of the vocal fold (called *polypoid degeneration*). The voice is typically low pitched, hoarse, and breathy.

Contact Ulcer

Contact ulcers differ from both nodules and polyps, as they do not directly affect the membraneous portion of the folds themselves. Rather, the mucosal covering of the tips of the vocal processes become eroded. Sometimes, rough grainy tissue called *granulation tissue* develops around the ulcer. Contact ulcers are often bilateral. They can be caused by speaking loudly at very low pitches and other forms of abuse.

Traditionally, these kinds of ulcers have been connected with a particular personality stereotype—that of the aggressive, ambitious male in his 40s, who speaks with an "authoritative" low-pitched voice which places strain on the posterior portion of the folds. However, recent research (Watterson, Hansen-Magorian, & McFarlane, 1990) indicates that while this disorder affects men in their 40s, females also develop contact ulcers (although more males than females do seem to be affected). Also, individuals at ages younger and older than their 40s may develop ulcers. This study also found that while half of the individuals spoke with a very low pitch, the other half did not. It has also recently been suggested that contact ulcers may be related to gastroesphageal reflux (Lumpkin, Bishop, & Katz, 1989), or may result from intubation trauma to the larynx when a person has general anesthesia.

A major symptom of contact ulcer is pain, which may radiate to the ear. The voice may or may not be affected. If the voice is affected, it may sound breathy and hoarse. These characteristics result from the individual's attempt to prevent pain during phonation, rather than from irregularity of vocal fold vibration due to the ulcer itself.

ASSESSMENT

Stemple et al. (1995) noted that "the primary objectives of the diagnostic voice evaluation are to discover the etiologic factors associated with the development of the voice disorder and to describe the deviant vocal symptoms" (p. 97). The information from the assessment is then used to construct an individualized treatment plan.

The assessment process draws on the expertise of the speech–language pathologist, otolaryngologist, and other professionals as appropriate (e.g., vocal coach, neurologist, psychologist, allergist, endocrinologist). Laryngologists examine the laryngeal mechanism and diagnose the pathology. They also decide what type of treatment is best for the patient, whether it be medical, surgical, behavioral, or a combination of treatments. The speech–language pathologist evaluates the

vocal symptoms and establishes and carries out a treatment regimen to improve vocal function. For people who use their voices for their livelihood, such as actors and singers, a vocal coach or singing instructor assesses the efficiency and correctness of performance techniques and suggests modifications as needed (Stemple, et al., 1995).

For many years, assessment and diagnosis of voice problems relied heavily on subjective evaluations about the quality, pitch, and loudness characteristics of the voice. Listening to the sound of the voice remains an important part of the complete diagnostic examination, and yields important information about overall severity of the vocal problem. However, the traditional role of subjective perceptual judgments has been supplemented over the past 10 years, by a more objective evaluation of physiological and acoustic factors related to the disorder. This has been made possible by the development of sophisticated computerized instrumentation that allows clear visualization of the vocal folds as they vibrate in the larynx, plus the measurement of the sound wave generated by the vocal folds.

These instrumental measures provide crucial information about laryngeal physiology and about changes in laryngeal physiology as voice behavior is manipulated by the patient in conjunction with the speech–language pathologist. Table 11.5 presents a brief summary of a few different types of instrumental measures and the kinds of information they provide. For a more complete description of instrumentation, see the chapter on instrumental measurement of voice in Stemple et al. (1995).

Behavioral Measures

Behavioral measures refer to those strategies designed to assess the vocal characteristics of the patient's voice, as well the efficiency of the patient's voice usage. This part of the assessment is usually performed by the speech–language pathologist, either before or after the otolaryngologist's examination of the patient's larynx. An important part of this assessment is obtaining a thorough case history. The case history should include medical as-

TABLE 11.5 Types of Instrumental Techniques Available for Vocal Assessment

TECHNIQUE	TYPE OF INFORMATION PROVIDED
Videostroboscopy	Symmetry of vocal fold movement
	Periodicity of vocal fold vibration
	Glottic configuration
	Mucosal wave
Endoscopy	Vocal fold mobility
	Mucosal abnormalities
	Mass lesions
Acoustic measures	Fundamental frequency (pitch)
	Frequency range
	Frequency/amplitude perturbation
	Harmonics/noise ratio
	Intensity (loudness)
	Dynamic range
Aerodynamic measures	Airflow volume and rate
	Subglottic pressure
Electroglottography	Vocal fold contact area
Electromyography	Electrical activity generated by muscle contraction

pects of the patient's life that might impact on voice, such as allergies or hormonal problems. Professional considerations can influence voice either directly or indirectly. For instance, individuals who rely on their voice for their livelihood, such as a teacher, might use their voice excessively, resulting in pathologies such as nodules or polyps. Work-related stress can indirectly affect voice by causing the individual to talk with a tense and strained laryngeal mechanism. Similarly, educational and social factors influence how people uses their voice and how efficiently they use it.

Following the case history, the speech–language pathologist typically performs an oral–peripheral examination, noting such factors as laryngeal area tension, swallowing difficulties, and the presence of laryngeal sensations such as tickling, dryness, or burning. To evaluate the vocal characteristics of the patient's voice, the speech–language pathologist may use a commercially available dysphonia rating scale, or may develop an appropriate scale. Typically, the vocal aspects that are assessed include pitch level, loudness level, and quality. The speech–language pathologist also notes the presence of any stridor.

In order to evaluate pitch, loudness, and quality, the patient performs various vocal tasks, such as sustaining isolated vowels for as long as possible, producing vowels at the highest and lowest pitches to determine pitch range, and counting to 200 to establish endurance and fatigue limits. Other tests include evaluation of dynamic range (the softest and loudest voice levels the patient can produce), and forceful coughing to assess the adequacy of glottal closure.

CLINICAL MANAGEMENT

Clinical management of an individual with a voice problem is a team endeavor in which different professionals are responsible for different aspects of treatment. As with any team activity, the professionals involved must communicate with each other in order to provide the patient with an integrated and intelligent plan of treatment. Any medical, surgical, or pharmacological treatment is provided by an otolaryngologist or other medically qualified physician, such as an allergist, pulmonary specialist, or endocrinologist. Teaching the individual strategies to modify incorrect singing or acting techniques is usually the domain of the singing teacher or acting coach. The speech–language pathologist has the responsibility of working with the patient to develop the most efficient and effective ways of using the laryngeal mechanism. Voice difficulties related to psychological problems may necessitate the services of a counselor or psychotherapist.

Clinical management strategies can be broadly divided into two categories: medico–surgical, and behavioral voice therapy. Medico-surgical treatments consist of any type of drug therapy and different types of surgical procedures. Behavioral voice therapy focuses on such areas as educating patients about the larynx and their disorders, instituting programs of vocal hygiene, and teaching patients strategies for altering various aspects of voice production. These two types of treatments are not mutually exclusive; they often go hand-in-hand to provide the patient with the best possible care. For instance, patients who have polyps surgically removed from their vocal folds need to be taught a less abusive way of using the vocal mechanism, in order to prevent the recurrence of the problem. Or, children whose vocal folds are scarred from frequent removals of papilloma, must be encouraged to make the most efficient use of their vocal capacity.

Phonosurgery

Phonosurgery is the name given to a group of different surgical procedures that have as their aim the removal of the underlying cause of the problem, as well as the preservation or restoration of the patient's best possible voice. This aim represents a departure from previous surgery in terms of vocal philosophy. Until quite recently, the actual vocal characteristics of the patient's voice were of secondary importance, if taken into consideration at all. With the advent of new information regarding vocal fold structure and function, the explosion of sophisticated new technology, and the emphasis on the team approach, has come a strong interest in maintaining, preserving, or restoring the patient's vocal quality. This is particularly true in the case of

TABLE 11.6 Types of Phonosurgical Procedures

PROCEDURE	EFFECT ON LARYNGEAL STRUCTURE/FUNCTION
Laryngeal framework surgery	Adjust position and/or tension of vocal folds
Laryngeal injection techniques	Increase mass of affected vocal fold; passive displacement of medial edge of fold to midline
Microsurgical techniques	Remove benign tumors from vocal fold
Laryngeal reinnervation techniques	Transplanted nerves provide innervation to affected vocal fold

singers and other professionals who depend on their voices, but it also applies to nonprofessionals.

There are several different types of phonosurgical procedures, including laryngeal framework surgery, laser surgery, laryngeal injection techniques, and laryngeal reinnervation techniques. Table 11.6 presents a summary of these procedures.

Laryngeal Framework Surgery. The major innovator in this area has been Isshiki, who developed a surgical means of indirectly shifting the position of the vocal folds, either medially towards the midline, or laterally away from the midline. The shape and tension of the vocal folds can also be altered with this kind of surgery. These techniques, in which some kind of synthetic implant is inserted into the larynx through a "window" in the thyroid cartilage, are called **thyroplasty.**

According to Blaugrund (1991), laryngeal framework surgery represents a significant advance in phonosurgery, because the vocal folds can be modified without directly operating on them. This reduces problems of accidental injury to the delicate tissues of the vocal folds during surgery, and reduces vocal fold scarring, while allowing the membraneous vocal folds to be left intact, thus preserving the mucosal wave that is such an essential component of proper vibration and phonation. Leder and Sasaki (1994) pointed out that even a small insult to the free margins of the vocal folds can result in a large deterioration in vocal quality, due to disruption of the mucosal wave.

The most common type of laryngeal framework surgery is medialization (Type I), aimed at improving vocal fold closure in cases of unilateral vocal fold paralysis, vocal fold atrophy, vocal fold bowing, and so on. Netterville, Stone, Luken, Civantos, and Ossoff (1993) described a procedure for medializing a paralyzed vocal fold. Local anesthetic is used. The larynx is exposed through a small incision over the midportion of the thyroid cartilage. A template is used to identify a window parallel to the lower border of the thyroid cartilage. The thyroarytenoid muscle (the main body of the vocal fold) is medialized while the patient phonates, in order to identify the best possible voice. When this is achieved, the surgeon carves an implant from a synthetic material (**Silastic**) which best fits the patient's specifications. The implant has the effect of pushing the affected fold towards the midline (Leder & Sasaki, 1994). The vocal folds are then able to achieve better closure, resulting a voice that is less breathy and hoarse.

Another kind of laryngeal framework surgical procedure is arytenoid adduction. This procedure may be more effective than just a Type I thryoplasty in certain cases, as when the immobile fold is fixed at a great distance from the intact fold, and when the impaired fold is positioned at a higher level than the unimpaired fold in the area of the vocal processes (Blaugrund, 1991). In this case, the thyroid cartilage is again the means of entering the larynx. The arytenoid cartilage itself is rotated to an appropriate position which will result in the most advantageous location of the vocal fold.

Leder and Sasaki (1994) reported on five women with unilateral vocal fold paralysis who received Type I thyroplasty. The women were followed up to four years, four months postoperatively. The authors measured fundamental frequency (FO), intensity, maximum phonation time, and breath groups. FO was significantly higher after the procedure (191.4 Hz compared to 135.1 Hz). The women were also able to sustain vowels for longer intervals after the surgery (9.8 seconds compared to 5.7 seconds), resulting in improved breath support for speech production.

Laryngeal Injection Techniques. Injection of various substances (commonly Teflon) into a paralyzed vocal fold has been the most common means of effecting improved closure. The rationale for this kind of procedure is that the filler substance will passively displace the medial edge of the impaired fold toward the midline (Ford, 1991). Theoretically, this allows the uninvolved fold to close against the impaired fold, thus improving closure and decreasing breathiness and hoarseness. Ford (1991) noted that with this technique, not only should vocal function be improved (i.e., reduction in the effort required for phonation, increased vocal intensity, increased phonation time), but choking and aspiration problems should be reduced.

The injection can be done either via the mouth (transorally) using direct laryngoscopy, or through the cricothyroid membrane to the thyroarytenoid muscle (transcutaneously) using a flexible fiberscope. Ford (1991) described the steps involved in an injection. First, the material is injected just lateral to the tip of the vocal process. If necessary, further sites are injected in the membranous fold, until adequate closure is achieved.

The filler material may be either an alloplastic (such as Teflon) or bioimplants (such as fat or collagen). These materials have different characteristics. Alloplastics permanently change the structure of the vocal fold, and should therefore not be used in cases in which a return of vocal function is possible. Bioimplants do not just displace the host tissue, but actually become a part of the tissue. Teflon is currently the main FDA-approved substance (Ford, 1991). However, problems can occur with the use of Teflon, such as inflammatory tissue reactions that can result in the formation of granuloma tissue, and migration of tiny particles to the lymph nodes, lungs, kidneys, and spleen (Ossoff, Koriwchak, Netterville, & Duncavage, 1993). Another problem with Teflon is that unless the material is buried deep in the thyroarytenoid muscle, the vocal fold cover can become stiffened to the point where a mucosal wave is not able to occur.

The bioimplant used most often is cross-linked bovine collagen, with the trade name Phonagel, or Zyplast (Ford, 1991). The preferred site of injection for collagen is in the deep layer of the lamina propria, which itself is composed of dense collagen fibers. Unlike Teflon, collagen should not be implanted into the thyroarytenoid muscle, because in that kind of tissue it will be re-sorbed into the host tissue, and not have the de-sired effect of medializing the vocal fold.

Microsurgery.   Microsurgical techniques are em-ployed very commonly in the treatment of many different types of laryngeal problems, including the removal of polyps, nodules, cysts, sulcus vo-calis, and so on. With the advent of sophisticated instruments such as operating microscopes and various microlaryngeal surgical instruments, these techniques have become a viable way of both re-storing the vocal folds to a healthier state, and, im-portantly, of preserving the vocal fold cover to ensure the preservation of the patient's voice. Sur-gery is performed through a laryngoscope under general anesthesia (Bouchayer & Cornut, 1991). Total voice rest is usually prescribed for some in-terval after surgery, in order for healing to occur. Voice therapy is usually indicated postoperatively, in order to evaluate the patient's vocal function, and to promote the most efficient use of the indi-vidual's vocal mechanism.

Laryngeal Reinnervation Techniques.   These techniques may be useful in cases in which there is asymmetry in the muscle mass and tension of the two folds, as often happens in cases of unilat-eral vocal fold paralysis. Recurrent laryngeal nerve (RLN) regeneration after partial injuries sometimes results in a reinnervation of the mus-cles by the ipsilateral RLN. However, because ad-ductor nerve fibers often reinnervate abductor muscle fibers, and vice versa, the movements of the vocal folds may become jerky and uncoordi-nated. This can result in inappropriately timed

movements of the vocal folds during breathing and phonation (Crumley, 1994). Laryngeal injec-tion would not be appropriate in this kind of situa-tion, because the muscle mass of the vocal fold is likely to be near normal, and the injection would further increase the mass and stiffness of the fold, disrupting vocal quality.

Laryngeal reinnervation techniques are either nerve-to-muscle transplants, or nerve-to-nerve transplants. These techniques are based on the principle that transplanted blocks of muscle, or transplanted nerves, can provide a flow of nerve impulses to the paralyzed fold. As one might pre-dict, the characteristics of the donor muscle or nerve will be transmitted to the host muscle. As Stemple et al. (1995) pointed out, it is therefore most important that the characteristics of donor and host are similar, in order to prevent jerky and discoordinated movements of the reinnervated muscle. Stemple et al. (1995) also noted that other medialization procedures may be necessary after the reinnervation, to facilitate vocal fold closure and increase vocal fold mobility.

Behavioral Voice Therapy

While the medical specialist performs medical and surgical treatments, it is generally the speech–language pathologist who has the primary respon-sibility for choosing and implementing behavioral techniques to improve vocal function. Karnell (1991) defined voice therapy as a "behavioral ma-nipulation of physiological processes with the in-tent of improving or providing optimal vocal function. It may be the primary procedure, or it may be used to complement phonosurgical, phar-macological, or psychotherapeutic treatment" (p. 213). The type of treatment provided depends on the nature of the voice problem. Purely struc-tural diseases such as cancer require medico–surgical treatment. Voice problems resulting from psychological problems will not, of course, re-spond to medical treatment, but would probably be best served by some form of counseling. Many voice problems, such as polyps, may be appropri-ately treated by a combination of medico–surgical

(surgical removal) and behavioral (voice therapy) techniques.

Karnell (1991) developed five classifications of behavioral therapy techniques. Many of these techniques were developed and have been used for a long time by experts in the field of voice such as Boone, Aronson, Bless, and others. The first category consists of techniques designed to counter vocal misuse, and typically have **hyperfunction** (excessive effort and muscular strain) of the vocal folds as a primary component. These techniques generally focus on reducing the force of vocal fold closure during vibration. Commonly used techniques include easy onset of voice to prevent hard glottal attacks at voice initiation; phonating with a slightly breathy quality; the yawn–sigh technique to relax the intrinsic and extrinsic laryngeal musculature; the chewing technique also aimed at muscular relaxation; and the massage and manipulation of the external larynx to reduce tension.

The second category suggested by Karnell (1991) comprises strategies to counter **hypoadduction,** in which the vocal folds are not adducting with enough force. The resulting weak, breathy-sounding voice may result from vocal fold paral-

TABLE 11.7 Classification of Behavioral Voice Therapy (Based on Karnell, 1991)

CATEGORY	FOCUS OF TREATMENT
1	Techniques to counter hyperfunction and vocal misuse; reduce force of vocal fold closure
2	Techniques to counter hypofunction; increase force of vocal fold closure
3	Techniques to minimize vocal abuse; patient education, elimination of vocally abusive situations
4	Techniques to optimize vocal endurance; performance techniques, breath support
5	Techniques to optimize voice quality; relaxation, modification of pitch and loudness

ysis, sulcus vocalis, thin vocal folds that have atrophied (as happens with advanced age), or psychological problems. Techniques are aimed at increasing the force of vocal fold closure, and include isometric exercises such as pushing down strongly on a chair while simultaneously phonating; using a hard glottal attack to initiate phonation; or using coughing or throat clearing (which both use high levels of muscular energy) as preparatory strategies to initiate phonation. Karnell (1991) noted that these types of techniques focus on either strengthening muscles normally used for phonation, or activating accessory muscle groups that are generally not involved in voice production, or a combination of both.

The third category involves techniques to minimize vocal abuse. Vocal abuse tends to be prevalent in individuals who also misuse the voice by exerting excessive muscular strain and tension on the laryngeal mechanism. Vocal abuse includes any behavior that causes the vocal folds to be slammed together with excessive force, such as shouting and screaming, habitual coughing and throat clearing, talking over loud noise, and so on. Vocal abuse also includes habits such as smoking and/or excessive drinking, both of which irritate the delicate tissues of the vocal fold cover, often resulting in inflammation. The focus in these kinds of strategies is twofold. First, the patient needs to be educated about the nature of the vocal folds and vibration, and the effects of abuse on the vocal mechanism. Second, vocally abusive situations relevant to the individual must be identified, and reduced or eliminated. Strategies should be designed by the patient and the therapist to compensate for the abusive behaviors, and less abusive behaviors should be substituted.

The next category includes strategies to optimize vocal endurance, particularly in those situations in which individuals need to use their voices for long periods of time. Such people include professionals who rely on their voices for their livelihood, such as singers, actors, teachers, preachers, and others. Techniques to increase vocal endurance include performance preparation, such as warm-up and cooldown exercises. A simple way of optimizing vocal endurance is to increase fluid intake and eliminate fluid-robbing substances (e.g., alcohol, caffeine). Vocal endurance depends heavily on adequate respiratory support, so techniques include breathing exercises to optimize vocal output.

Finally, techniques are available to optimize voice quality. Basically, success with any of the other four categories should have the effect of optimizing voice quality. However, there may be some specific techniques that can help to facilitate a client's best voice (see, for instance, Boone and McFarlane, 1994, for a complete description of voice facilitating techniques). These exercises include modifying pitch and/or loudness levels, and using relaxation strategies and biofeedback techniques.

The recent expansion of knowledge about vocal fold structure and function, in conjunction with the increasingly sophisticated technology that is available, has resulted in dramatic changes in the way that laryngeal problems are evaluated and treated by laryngologists, speech–language pathologists, and other professionals interested in the care of voice. Together with behavioral techniques, these different strategies allow a wide variety of choices to be combined, so that individual patients receive the best possible treatment for their voice problem.

Major Points of Chapter

- Advances in sophisticated acoustic and physiologic instrumentation have resulted in greatly increased knowledge of the complex structure and function of the vocal folds.
- Structurally related and neurogenic voice disorders may arise from a variety of causes, and may be congenital or acquired.
- Use of instrumentation has augmented traditional behavioral measures of vocal function.
- Treatment requires a team approach to integrate modern phonosurgical techniques and behavioral voice therapies.

Discussion Guidelines

1. Compare and contrast an organic voice disorder that is likely to be present in a young

child with one that is more likely to be present in an older adult.
2. Explain the ways in which acoustic and physiologic instrumentation can supplement the voice evaluation.
3. Identify four types of phonosurgical techniques, and describe the voice disorders for which each technique is most useful.

REFERENCES

April, M. M., & Marsh, B. R. (1993). Laryngotracheal reconstruction for subglottic stenosis. *Annals of Otology, Rhinology, and Laryngology, 102,* 176–181.

Benninger, M. S., Jacobson, B. H., & Johnson, A. F. (1994). The multidisciplinary voice clinic. In M. S. Benninger, B. H. Jacobson, & A. F. Johnson (Eds.), *Vocal arts medicine: The care and prevention of professional voice disorders.* New York: Thieme Medical Publishers, Inc.

Blaugrund, S. M. (1991). Laryngeal framework surgery. In C. N. Ford & D. M. Bless (Eds.), *Phonosurgery: Assessment and surgical management of voice disorders* (pp. 183–199). New York: Raven Press.

Boone, D. R., & McFarlane, S. C. (1994). *The voice and voice therapy* (5th ed.). Englewood Cliffs, NJ: Prentice-Hall.

Bouchayer, M., & Cornut, G. (1991). Instrumental microscopy of benign lesions of the vocal folds. In C. N. Ford & D. M. Bless (Eds.), *Phonosurgery: Assessment and surgical management of voice disorders* (pp. 143–165). New York: Raven Press..

Chodzko-Zajko, W. J., & Ringel, R. L. (1987). Physiological aspects of aging. *Journal of Voice, 1,* 18–26.

Colton, R. H., & Casper, J. K. (1990). *Understanding voice problems: A physiological perspective for diagnosis and treatment.* Baltimore, MD: Williams and Wilkins.

Crumley, R. L. (1994). Unilateral recurrent laryngeal nerve paralysis. *Journal of Voice, 8,* 79–83.

Dickson, D. R., & Dickson, W. M. (1982). *Anatomical and physiological bases of speech.* Austin, TX: Pro-Ed.

Doyle, D. J., Gianoli, G. J., Espinola, T., & Miller, R. H. (1994). Recurrent respiratory papillomatosis: Juvenile versus adult forms. *Laryngoscope, 104,* 523–527.

Ferrand, C. T., & Bloom, R. L. (1996). Gender differences in children's intonational patterns. *Journal of Voice, 10,* 284–291.

Figi, F. A. (1940). Chronic stenosis of the larynx with special consideration of skin grafting. *Annals of Otology, Rhinology, and Laryngology, 49,* 394–409.

Ford, C. N. (1991). Laryngeal injection techniques. In C. N. Ford & D. M. Bless (Eds.), *Phonosurgery: Assessment and surgical management of voice disorders* (pp. 123–141). New York: Raven Press.

Guerra, L. G., Lau, K. Y., & Marwah, R. (1992). Upper airway obstruction as the sole manifestation of rheumatoid arthritis. *Journal of Rheumatology, 19,* 974–976.

Guttenplan, M. D., Townsend, M. J., Hendrix, R. A., & Balsara, G. (1991). Laryngeal manifestations of gout. *Annals of Otology, Rhinology, and Laryngology, 100,* 899–902.

Haskell, J. A. Vocal self-perception: The other side of the equation. *Journal of Voice, 1,* 172–179.

Hegde, M. N. (1995). *Introduction to communicative disorders* (2nd ed.). Austin, TX: Pro-Ed.

Herrington-Hall, B., Lee, L., Stemple, J., Niemi, K., & McHone, M. (1988). Description of laryngeal pathologies by age, sex, and occupation in a treatment seeking sample. *Journal of Speech and Hearing Disorders, 53,* 57–65.

Hirano, M. (1974). Morphological structure of the vocal cord as a vibrator and its variations. *Folia Phoniatrica, 26,* 89–94.

Hirano, M. (1977). Structure and vibratory behavior of the vocal folds. In M. Sawashima, & S. C. Fanklin (Eds.), *Dynamic aspects of speech production* (pp. 13–30). Tokyo: University of Tokyo Press.

Hirano, M. (1981). Structure of the vocal fold in normal and disease states: Anatomical and physical studies. In C. Ludlow & M. Hart (Eds.), ASHA Reports No. 11, Proceedings of the Conference on the Assessment of Vocal Pathology (pp. 11–30). Rockville, MD: American Speech-Language-Hearing Association.

Hollien, H. (1987). "Old voices": What do we really know about them? *Journal of Voice, i,* 2–17.

Jie, X. J., Rong, X. T., & Chang, X. Q. (1991). Laryngeal pathological findings following trauma to cricoarytenoid joint. *Journal of Voice, 5,* 252–256.

Jindal, J. R., Milbrath, M. M., Shaker, R., Hogan, W., & Toohill, R. J. (1994). Gastroesophageal reflux disease as a likely cause of "ideopathic" subglottic stenosis. *Annals of Otology, Rhinology, and Laryngology, 103,* 186–191.

Kahane, J. (1978). A morphological study of the human prepubertal and pubertal larynx. *American Journal of Anatomy, 151,* 11–20.

Kahane, J. (1983). A survey of age-related changes in the connective tissues of the human adult larynx. In D. M. Bless & J. Abbs (Eds.), *Vocal fold physiology* (pp. 44–49). San Diego, CA: College-Hill Press.

Kahane, J. (1987). Connective tissue changes in the larynx and their effects on voice. *Journal of Voice, 1,* 27–30.

Karnell, M. P. (1991). Adjunctive measures for optimal phonosurgical results: The role of voice therapy. In C. N. Ford & D. M. Bless (Eds.), *Phonosurgery: Assessment and surgical management of voice disorders* (pp. 213–224). New York: Raven Press.

Krane, S. M., & Simon, L. S. (1986). Rheumatoid arthritis: Clinical features and pathogenic mechanisms. *Medical Clinics of North America, 70,* 263–280.

Leder, S. B., & Sasaki, C. T. (1994). Long-term changes in vocal quality following Isshiki Thyroplasty Type I. *Laryngoscope, 104,* 275–277.

Leicht, M. J., Harrington, T. M., & Davis, D. E. (1987). Cricoarytenoid arthritis: A cause of laryngeal obstruction. *Annals of Emergency Medicine, 16,* 885–887.

Lumpkin, S. M. M., Bishop, S. G., & Katz, P. O. (1989). Chronic dysphonia secondary to gastroesophageal reflux disease (GERD): Diagnosis using simultaneous dual-probe prolonged pH monitoring. *Journal of Voice, 3,* 351–355.

McClurg, F. L., & Evans, D. A. (1994). Laser laryngoplasty for laryngomalacia. *Laryngoscope, 104,* 247–252.

Mueller, P. B., Sweeney, R. J., & Baribeau, L. J. (1984). Acoustic and morphologic study of the senescent voice. *Ear Nose and Throat Journal, 63,* 292–295.

Nakayama, M., Ford, C. N., Brandenburg, J. H., & Bless, D. M. (1994). Sulcus vocalis in laryngeal cancer: A histopathologic study. *Laryngoscope, 104,* 16–24.

Netterville, J. L., Stone, R. E., Luken, E. S., Civantos, F. J., & Ossoff, R. H. (1993). Silastic medialization and arytenoid adduction: The Vanderbilt experience. *Annals of Otology, Rhinology, and Laryngology, 102,* 413–424.

Ossoff, R. H., Koriwchak, M. J., Netterville, J. L., & Duncavage, J. A. (1993). Difficulties in endoscopic removal of Teflon granulomas of the vocal fold.

Annals of Otology, Rhinology, and Laryngology,
102, 405–412.

Sataloff, R. (1991). The effects of age on the voice. In
R. T. Sataloff (Ed.), *Professional voice: The sci-
ence and art of clinical care* (pp. 141–151). New
York: Raven Press.

Stemple, J. C., Glaze, L. E., & Gerdeman, B. K. (1995).
Clinical voice pathology: Theory and management
(2nd ed.). San Diego, CA: Singular Publishing
Group.

Titze, I. R. (1994). *Principles of voice production.* Englewood Cliffs, NJ: Prentice-Hall.

Watterson, T., Hansen-Magorian, H. J., & McFarlane,
S. C. (1990). A demographic description of laryngeal contact ulcer patients. *Journal of Voice, 4,* 71–
75.

12

ALARYNGEAL SPEECH REHABILITATION

DIANNE SLAVIN

Much has changed since the first total laryngectomy was successfully performed in 1873 by Theodore Billroth, in Vienna, Austria. At that time, due to the high risk of infection, aspiration pneumonia, and the recurrence of disease, removal of the larynx was a very risky procedure. Mortality rates were very high and remained high through the turn of the century (Bailey, 1985). Gradually, surgical techniques improved and survival rates began to improve. Surgical removal of the larynx as a treatment for laryngeal cancer was not accepted as an efficacious approach until the mid-1920s (Rosenberg, 1971).

For the next approximately 30 years, total laryngectomy was considered by most members of the medical community to be the only viable treatment for laryngeal cancer. Since then, alternative treatment methods, both surgical and nonsurgical, have been developed as diagnostic procedures improved and understanding of cancer development increased (Pressman, 1956; Bailey, 1985). In recent years, medical advances have resulted in improved mortality rates. This improvement can be attributed to the perfection of surgical procedures, the maintenance of reliably high levels of sterilization and cleanliness in operating rooms, and the administration of antibiotics to stave off infections (Doyle, 1994).

In addition, technological advances have resulted in early detection of malignancies. Early detection has lead to earlier treatment and generally improved long term survival rates for many types of cancer including laryngeal cancer (American Cancer Society, 1990). As patients live longer, issues other than the disease itself have become rehabilitation concerns. The identification of physical, physiological and social changes that result from removal of the larynx has lead to a multidisciplinary approach to post laryngectomy rehabilitation.

The speech–language pathologist (SLP) is an integral part of the rehabilitation team. In order to function effectively, the speech–language pathologist should acquire a comprehensive understanding of all aspects of the rehabilitative process. As we move into the twenty-first century, changes in the health care system continue to impact on the rehabilitative process generally and on post-laryngectomy rehabilitation specifically. Treatment options have increased so the speech–language pathologist will probably see more patients who have had more than one surgery or have undergone a combination of treatments such as radiation therapy and surgery. Hospital stays are shorter so more post laryngectomy rehabilitation is done either in the form of home care or on an out-patient basis. Also, health care professionals including speech–language pathologists must work more efficiently to maximize the value gained by clients during the treatment period for which they have medical coverage.

The primary focus of the speech–language pathologist is to aid the patient in the acquisition of an alternative means of verbal communication. In order to accomplish this goal, the speech–language pathologist must understand the multidimensional nature of the rehabilitative process. The purpose of this chapter is to provide students in speech–language pathology with a comprehensive overview of postlaryngectomy rehabilitation. The chapter begins with a review of normal laryngeal function, then proceeds with a discussion of various aspect of laryngeal cancer. This is followed by an explanation of the medical, anatomical, physiological and psychosocial aspects of postlaryngectomy rehabilitation. The chapter concludes with a description of the specific nature of the various forms of alaryngeal speech.

THE LARYNX

The laryngeal mechanism serves two very important functions. Biologically, the laryngeal structures serve as a valve to protect the airway. During swallowing, the vocal folds close tightly, and the epiglottis tips backward, covering the **laryngopharynx** (Daniloff, Schuckers, & Feth, 1980). Food and drink are directed into the esophagus, thus securing the trachea from aspiration. Loss of this valving function would compromise the airway and could result in death. (See Chapter 10 for a detailed discussion.)

Laryngeal structures (including the cricoid, thyroid, and arytenoid cartilages along with the intrinsic and extrinsic laryngeal muscles) have evolved to serve a distinctly different purpose from the biological one, enabling humans to develop a melodic and sustainable voice. The laryngeal mechanism provides an easily produced voice that may be initiated and halted with amazing precision. This precision in the onset and offset of voice is manifested in the ability to make

the voice–voiceless contrasts in sounds like /p/ and /b/, or /s/ and /z/, to yell and whisper, to sing, to speak, to pause, and to speak again. Speech is such a natural, seemingly automatic process that people tend to take it for granted. The sound of an individual's voice is part of their identity. Indeed, each human voice is as unique to the individual as fingerprints. Thus, loss of voice results in a loss of part of the self. (See Chapter 11 for more detailed information on laryngeal structure and function.)

Individuals who lose their larynx due to trauma or surgery need to communicate using some form of **alaryngeal speech.** Alaryngeal speech refers to a form of oral communication produced without the larynx. This form of speech seldom develops naturally and is rarely heard in children. Usually, alaryngeal speech must be taught. It is the desirable outcome when the larynx has been surgically removed. The procedure used to remove the larynx, called a **laryngectomy,** is performed only when the larynx is so severely damaged by trauma or disease that its valving function, which is crucial to survival, is lost. When this occurs, the team approach is the favored model of service delivery. The speech–language pathologist is a central participant in a team of specialists involved in the rehabilitation of laryngectomized patients. The speech–language pathologist is concerned primarily with the establishment of an alternative form of oral communication. Therefore, speech–language pathologists must understand the events leading up to the laryngectomy, the personality of the patient, and the patient's reaction to being laryngectomized. These factors influence the specific options and techniques involved in the acquisition of alaryngeal speech.

LARYNGEAL CANCER

The most common reason for someone to undergo a total laryngectomy is laryngeal cancer. Laryngeal cancer, according to statistics compiled by the American Cancer Society (1990), is typically diagnosed in adults between 50 and 70 years of age. Laryngeal cancer is more common in males but research has shown a narrowing in the ratio of males and females developing laryngeal cancer over time. For instance, Robin et. al (1989), using data compiled in the cancer registry of Birmingham and West Midlands, Great Britain, calculated a 10:1 male to female ratio between 1957 and 1961 as compared to a 5.3:1 ratio between 1977 and 1981. Similarly, Bailey (1985) reported that the relative incidence of laryngeal cancer in males to females in the United States went from 12:1 to 6:1 in the 20 years between 1965 and 1985.

According to an American Cancer Society (1994) report, approximately 12,500 new cases of laryngeal cancer were projected to occur in the United States in 1994. Of these, it was estimated that 9,800 would be male and 2,700 female. The death rate from laryngeal cancer for both sexes is approximately 30 percent. For African Americans, however, the incidence and mortality rates associated with laryngeal cancer are higher than those reported for Caucasians (Ries, Hankey, & Edwards, 1990). This may be explained, in part, by a higher exposure to suspected causative agents. In the inner city, or in rural areas, there may be environmental pollutants in the air, water, or food supply, or exposure to smoke, radiation, or drugs (Union Internationale Centre le Cancer [UICC], 1987). Socioeconomic factors also play a role. Economically disadvantaged individuals with laryngeal cancer may not seek medical intervention until the disease is more advanced.

Early identification and treatment of laryngeal cancer is crucial to survival. Medical advances in diagnostic and surgical techniques over the past 40 years have resulted in high cure rates when the disease is diagnosed in its early stages (Gates, Ryan, & Lauder, 1982). Bailey (1985) stated that when treated early, "laryngeal cancer is the most frequently cured malignancy of the aerodigestive tract" (p. 257).

Causal Factors

Excessive smoking, particularly in combination with excessive alcohol consumption, has been shown to increase the risk of developing laryngeal cancer. Wynder, Covey, Marbuchi, Johnson, and Muschinsky (1976) found that people who smoked more than 35 cigarettes and consumed more than seven ounces of alcohol daily were 22 times more likely to develop laryngeal cancer than those who did not smoke and drink. Additionally, they reported that excessive smoking alone increased the risk factor seven times above the risk to nonsmokers. However, excessive drinking in the absence of smoking has not been found to increase the risk of laryngeal cancer (Lawson, Biller, & Suen, 1989). Environmental factors, such as exposure to asbestos, are suspected but as yet are unproved risk factors.

Types of Laryngeal Cancer and Associated Symptoms

Malignant tumors may originate in the area above the glottis (supraglottic), below the glottis (subglottic), or on the vocal folds (glottic). Symptoms vary depending on the location of the lesion in the larynx. Supraglottic lesions frequently cause swallowing difficulty or dysphagia. Other symptoms include weight loss, neck swelling, pain to the ipsilateral ear, and inspiratory stridor (breathing noise). Glottic lesions cause a disruption in the vibratory pattern of the vocal folds resulting in hoarseness. Persistent hoarseness in the absence of any other known cause such as an upper respiratory infection or vocal abuse is one of the danger signs associated with laryngeal cancer. Inspiratory and/or expiratory stridor also may be present. Subglottic lesions frequently cause **dyspnea** (breathing difficulty); as subglottic tumors may obstruct the airway, stridor also is a common symptom.

The most common form of laryngeal cancer is squamous cell carcinoma. The vocal folds are covered by a layer of epithelium made up of squamous (flat) cells. In its early stages, the lesion appears as an irregular thickening of the epithelial surface of the vocal fold. Histological analysis reveals the cellular structure of the lesion. Cell structure may be described as poorly, moderately, or well-differentiated. Using a grading system first developed by Broders (1926), evaluators calculate the ratio of tumor cells to those of the host or "normal" cells. As the proportion of tumor cells increases relative to the host cells, the tumor is considered to be more well-differentiated. The well-differentiated cell structure is associated with a better prognosis, because tumors composed of this cell type are usually more clearly contained and usually grow more slowly. Therefore, these types of tumors are more easily targeted and eradicated with treatment. Conversely, less differentiated tumors with poor cell structure may spread more rapidly and tend to be more difficult to treat (Doyle, 1994).

Less common forms of laryngeal cancer called *chondrocarcinoma* and *chondrosarcoma* may arise from the laryngeal cartilages rather than from the various glottic areas. Pain, stridor, hoarseness, and shortness of breath may result from these tumors depending upon their size and location within the larynx.

Diagnostic Techniques

When carcinoma of the larynx involves one or both of the vocal folds it may result in vibratory and perceptual changes similar to those that result from vocal polyps and papilloma. Therefore, it is impossible to diagnose this condition on a perceptual or acoustic basis. Routine laryngeal examination including indirect laryngoscopy may reveal such clinical signs of cancer as enlarged lymph nodes in the neck, fullness in the cricothyroid or thyroid membrane, and visible lesions in the laryngeal area. Direct laryngoscopy utilizing fiberoptic techniques may be useful in assessing the degree to which vocal fold movement is impaired and provide an initial impression of the tumor type, size, and location. Additional information regarding the size and location of tumor within the neck may be obtained from magnetic resonance imaging (MRI) and computerized axial tomography (CT) scans. These procedures are becoming more popular because of their diagnostic value and noninvasive nature.

Carcinomas do not suddenly appear. They develop slowly over a long period of time. Malignant tumors begin as small lesions at a particular site. When diagnosed at this early stage, they are referred to as **carcinoma in-situ.** If untreated, the malignancy will grow and may eventually invade adjacent tissue and/or spread through the blood or the lymphatic system to other parts of the body. **Metastasis** refers to tumors that have spread through the body from the site of the primary tumor.

In order to describe the extent to which a malignancy has spread, a staging system was developed in 1983 by the American Joint Committee for Cancer Staging and End Results Reporting. The system, called the *TMN system,* is presented in Table 12.1. *T* signifies the location of the primary tumor. A tumor in-situ would be identified at *TIS.* Tumors also are numerically rated from zero to four. *T0* means a primary tumor is not evident. *T4* signifies a massive tumor extending well beyond the site of origin.

The *N* in this system refers to the extent to which the lymph nodes near the tumor are involved. A numerical rating of zero to three is applied. *N0* means that cancer is not present in the nodes. *N3* signifies unilateral and/or bilateral lymph node involvement.

Finally, the *M* stands for metastasis. *M0* means no metastasis and *M1* indicates that metastasis has occurred. An *X* may follow the *T, N* or *M* to indicate that assessment at that level was not possible or not completed.

Treatment of Laryngeal Cancer

The earlier laryngeal cancer is diagnosed, the more treatable it is by nonsurgical means. Studies have shown that radiation therapy alone is 85 to 95 percent successful in treating unilateral supraglottic and glottic tumors (Brady & Davis, 1988). Although some surgeons would prefer to eliminate the disease through a form of partial laryngectomy (to be discussed later in this section), Dickens, Cassisi, Million, and Boa (1983) compared outcomes for 139 patients and found cure rate with radiation only to be comparable to that of surgery. Radiation as the sole treatment for T1

TABLE 12.1 TNM Staging System for Cancer

STAGING	
Primary Tumor (T)	
T_x	Tumor that cannot be assessed by rules
T_0	No evidence of primary tumor
Supraglottis	
TIS	Carcinoma in-situ
T_1	Tumor confined to region of origin with normal mobility
T_2	Tumor involving adjacent supraglottic site(s) or glottis without fixation
T_3	Tumor limited to larynx with fixation and/or extension to involve postcricoid area, medial wall of pyriform sinus, or preepiglottic space
T_4	Massive tumor extending beyond the larynx to involve oropharynx, soft tissues of neck, or destruction of thyroid cartilage
Glottis	
TIS	Carcinoma in-situ
T_1	Tumor confined to vocal cord(s) with normal mobility (including involvement of anterior or posterior commissures)
T_2	Supraglottic and/or subglottic extension of tumor with normal or impaired cord mobility
T_3	Tumor confined to the larynx with cord fixation
T_4	Massive tumor with thyroid cartilage and/or extension beyond the confines of the larynx
Subglottis	
TIS	Carcinoma in-situ
T_1	Tumor confined to the subglottic region
T_2	Tumor extension to vocal cords with normal or impaired cord mobility
T_3	Tumor confined to the larynx with cord fixation
T_4	Massive tumor with cartilage destruction or extension beyond the confines of the larynx, or both
Nodal Involvement (N)	
N_x	Nodes cannot be assessed
N_0	No clinically positive nodes
N_1	Single clinically positive homolateral node less than 3 cm in diameter
N_2	Single clinically positive homolateral node 3 to 6 cm in diameter or multiple clinically postivie homolateral nodes, none over 6 cm in diameter
N_{2a}	Single clinically positive homolateral node, 3 to 6 cm in diameter
N_{2b}	Multiple clinically positive homolateral nodes, none over 6 cm in diameter
N_3	Massive homolateral node(s), bilateral nodes, or contralateral node(s)
N_{3a}	Clinically positive homolateral nodes, none over 6 cm in diameter
N_{3b}	Bilateral clinically positive nodes (in this situation, each side of the neck should be staged separately; that is, N_{3b}: right, N_{2a}: left, N_1)
N_{3c}	Contralateral clinically positive node(s) only
Distant Metastasis (M)	
M_x	Not assessed
M_0	No (known) distant metastasis
M_1	Distant metastasis present

continued

TABLE 12.1   Continued

STAGE GROUPING	
Stage I	$T_1 N_0 M_0$
Stage II	$T_2 N_0 M_0$
Stage III	$T_3 N_0 M_0$
	T_1 or T_2 or T_3, N_1, M_0
Stage IV	T_4, N_0 or N_1, M_0
	Any T, N_2 or N_3, M_0
	Any T, any N, M_1
Residual Tumor (R)	
R_0	No residual tumor
R_1	Microscopic residual tumor
R_2	Microscopic residual tumor

Source: Reprinted with permission from *American Joint Committee for Cancer Staging and End Results Reporting: Manual for stages of cancer* (pp. 38–39), Philadelphia: J. B. Lippincott.

and T2 tumors may also be preferred because vocal quality is minimally affected. Often, however, a combination of treatment modalities including radiation, surgery (such as partial laryngectomy), and/or chemotherapy are used to eradicate more extensive lesions.

Surgical Options.   Various surgical options are available, depending on the size and location of the tumor.

Cordectomy.   Cordectomy may be recommended for unilateral T1 and T2 lesions that are well defined and superficial. The surgery involves the resection of the tissues containing the tumor and the margins of healthy tissue around it. Essentially, the diseased vocal fold is removed. As would be expected, postsurgical voice is breathy, weak, and hoarse.

Partial Laryngectomy.   Partial laryngectomy includes procedures referred to as *hemilaryngectomy* and *vertical partial laryngectomy.* Typically, these procedures result in the removal of at least half of the thyroid cartilage, the arytenoid cartilage, and the membranous tissues on the involved side, including the vocal fold. These procedures are recommended for T2 and T3 lesions involving one side of the larynx with

intact vocal fold mobility (Silver, 1981). Vocal function is altered by this procedure, resulting in voice quality that is hoarse and breathy. Swallowing difficulty may also ensue, but usually resolves following a short course of dysphagia therapy.

Supraglottal Laryngectomy.   This surgical procedure is most appropriate for tumors confined to the epiglottis and ventricular folds. In order for this kind of procedure to be successful, the cancer must not involve the base of the tongue, the pyriform sinus, or the arytenoid body. This surgery involves removal of much of the hyoid bone, the ventricular folds, the epiglottis, and a section of thyroid cartilage. The removal of parts of the hyoid bone superiorly and the thyroid cartilage anteriorly are considered necessary to provide an adequate margin of resection. As the true vocal folds are not involved, phonation after this procedure is unaffected.

Near Total Laryngectomy.   Near total laryngectomy may be considered for larger unilateral tumors (T3 and T4). This procedure, introduced by Pearson and associates (1980, 1986), requires the removal of the entire larynx, leaving only a narrow strip of tissue on the side contralateral to the tumor, connecting the trachea with the pharynx. Since the entire larynx is removed, a permanent tracheostoma is created in the neck. The strip of tissue is reconstructed into a shunt (channel) through which pulmonary air may be directed into the pharynx when the tracheostoma is occluded. (See Figure 12.1.) This speaking shunt provides a vibratory source for voice. DeSanto, Pearson, and Olsen (1989) reported the results of near total laryngectomy performed on 29 patients with non-glottal upper aerodigestive system cancers. The majority of these cases were rehabilitated without loss of voice or altered respiration.

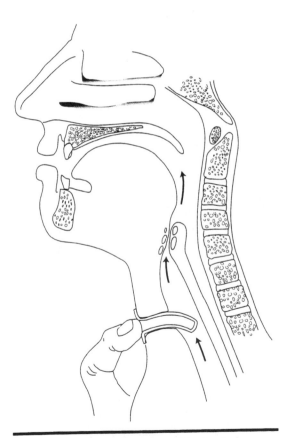

FIGURE 12.1   Saggital section of the healed postoperative neck following extended hemilaryngectomy. The tracheotomy must be valved with a finger to shunt air up into the pharynx.

The success of the surgical procedures described above decreases as the size of the tumor and the extent of the resections increases. The risks associated with the more extensive procedures, particularly hemilaryngectomy and near total laryngectomy, include **stenosis** or narrowing of the reconstructed larynx, pain, swelling, infection, improper healing, swallowing difficulty, aspiration, and recurrence of the disease (Ward, 1988). When these surgeries fail to halt the progression of the disease, a total laryngectomy will be recommended. Consequently speech–language pathologists are likely to treat patients for whom the laryngectomy is a salvage procedure. This has important implications for rehabilitation, because these patients may have faced a second diagnosis of cancer and have undergone a second, more extensive, body-altering surgery. In view of the different medical and surgical approaches that are now performed depending on the location of the laryngeal cancer, considerable variation exists in the postsurgical anatomy and physiology of these patients. Therefore, the speech–language pathologist must carefully evaluate the postoperative function of the remaining structures related to alaryngeal speech production (Doyle, 1994).

Total Laryngectomy. This procedure is most commonly performed in cases in which laryngeal cancer has been diagnosed and other forms of treatment, such as radiation therapy or the less radical surgeries previously described, have been ruled out. Total laryngectomy may be the preferred course of treatment because of the extent of the disease or because alternative treatments have been unsuccessful in halting the progression of the disease. Total laryngectomy involves the removal of the entire laryngeal framework, including the hyoid bone superiorly and usually the upper tracheal rings inferiorly. The removal of the body's protective valving mechanism necessitates that the surgical site be isolated from the digestive tract so that food and drink can be ingested normally. Respiratory function is then maintained by tipping the top of the trachea forward and sewing it to the base of the neck, where a permanent

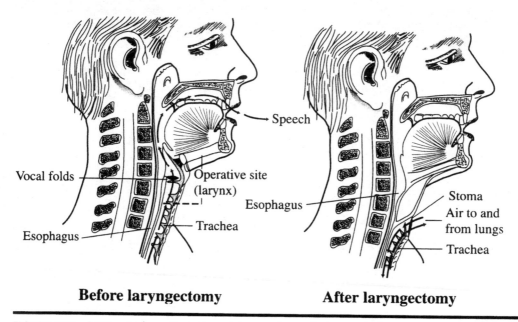

FIGURE 12.2   Anatomical configuration of the vocal tract before and after total laryngectomy.

opening called a **tracheostoma** (or **stoma**) is created. Pulmonary air no longer passes through the pharynx, oral, or nasal cavities. Rather, air passes directly into the trachea. As a result, these patients become neck breathers. The changes in the anatomical configuration of the vocal tract are illustrated in Figure 12.2.

THE REHABILITATION TEAM

Speech–language pathologists play an integral role on a team of specialists involved in the rehabilitation of people who have undergone treatment for laryngeal cancer. In cases where the larynx has been spared, the speech–language pathologist assesses the integrity of the laryngeal mechanism in regard to its valving function as well as its phonatory function. Individualized treatment plans are developed to address dysphagia and/or dysphonia. The speech–language pathologist collaborates with the patient, the family members, the physician, and the nurses to maximize improvement in laryngeal functions for swallowing as well as for voicing.

In cases where a total laryngectomy was performed, a more comprehensive rehabilitation plan is required. The rehabilitation team typically consists of a physician, a surgeon, nurses, a speech–language pathologist, a social worker or rehabilitation counselor, and possibly a radiologist, a physical therapist, a psychologist, and a vocational counselor.

The physician, either an internist, an **otolaryngologist,** or a cancer specialist (**oncologist**), is usually in charge of case management. The physician makes medical decisions regarding the overall medical status of the patient.

The surgeon, an otolaryngologist or head and neck surgeon, performs all the surgical procedures deemed necessary to improve the patient's chances for survival. The surgeon also monitors the patient's recovery and rehabilitation in the absence of another primary care physician.

The radiologist may be involved either before or after removal of the larynx. The radiologist helps in the assessment of the patient's condition and in the application of radiation therapy as prescribed by the physician.

Nurses help the patient through the initial postsurgical period. They aid the patient in acquiring the new hygienic practices, including clearing the stoma, using a suctioning machine, and in some cases, learning to maintain a tracheostomy tube. If the patient begins to use a speech aid while still in the hospital, nurses can be very helpful in encouraging its use. As nurses tend to have most postsurgical contact with patients, it is important that the speech–language pathologist educate the nursing staff regarding the different forms of alaryngeal speech. Nurses should be familiar with the types of alaryngeal speech their patients are most likely to use (Casper & Colton, 1993).

A social worker may be involved in the assessment of personal problems regarding finances, home care, and vocational status. The social worker may be available to family members to provide emotional support and information regarding community resources.

A physical therapist will be consulted if surgery and/or radiation have resulted in a reduction in the range-of-motion of the head, neck, or arms. Stiffness and swelling in the neck may restrict or preclude the patient's ability to use one or more forms of alaryngeal speech.

Ideally, a rehabilitation counselor or psychologist also will be part of the rehabilitation team. These professionals are trained to assess the patient's emotional reaction to the occurrence of cancer, the loss of voice, the altered anatomy, and the impact these events may have on families, friends and coworkers. If psychological services are deemed necessary, recommendations will be made for individual and/or group counseling. The patient might also be provided with information regarding local self-help groups.

The Role of the Speech–Language Pathologist

It is important for the speech–language pathologist to be fully informed about the medical status of the patient as well as about the patient's communication needs. No matter how well-informed a patient may seem to be about the surgery and the changes it brings, the actual impact of the laryngectomy cannot be anticipated. The speech–language pa-

thologist needs to be sensitive to the emotional adjustment patients must make to this disability.

The role of the speech–language pathologist is to facilitate the restoration of oral communication through the use of alaryngeal speech. Three forms of alaryngeal speech are available. Artificial larynges or speech aids generate an extrinsic sound source that is introduced into the vocal tract at the level of the neck or mouth. Intrinsic forms of alaryngeal speech include (1) esophageal speech, produced when air pushed into the upper esophagus is forced through a reconstructed neoglottis; and (2) tracheoesophageal speech, which is generated when pulmonary air is shunted into the esophagus through a prosthesis. Each mode of alaryngeal speech will be discussed more fully later in the chapter.

In order to provide the best services for a patient, including determining which type of alaryngeal speech is best, the speech–language pathologist must be completely familiar with and comfortable with the physical and psychosocial factors that influence postlarygectomy rehabilitation decisions. Specifically, the speech–language pathologist should become knowledgeable regarding the following:

Medical Status. Medical status includes knowledge of the presence and severity of coexisting medical conditions and diseases such as cancer, pulmonary disease, diabetes, heart disease, high blood pressure, emotional illness, substance addictions, and dementia. This information is important because it may affect the prognosis for the development of some forms of alaryngeal speech. For example, patients with a pulmonary disease such as emphysema may be unable to sustain the pulmonary air pressure needed to generate tracheoesophageal speech. Other medical conditions, like heart disease, may leave the patients so weak that they are not motivated or able to focus on acquiring alaryngeal voice.

Communicative Needs. The speech–language pathologist needs to know how important verbal communication is to the patient. Because the loss of voice affects so many social, occupational, and psychological functions, it is considered by many to be the biggest challenge faced by laryngectomized individuals. Hunt (1964) questioned 84 patients regarding their concerns following laryngectomy and found that loss of voice was of greater concern to them than the diagnosis of cancer. This finding was substantiated by Blanchard (1982) who, reporting on responses solicited from 115 members of laryngectomee clubs in the United States, found loss of voice and difficulty learning esophageal speech to be the foremost problem.

The extent to which patients rely on oral communication in activities of daily living may impact on their motivation to learn a new method of speaking. People who are motivated to speak may overcome many obstacles to do so (Davis, 1981). Conversely, patients who become withdrawn and depressed as a result of the laryngectomy tend to be less receptive to attempts to establish an alternative form of verbal communication (Bisi & Conley, 1965; Gardner, 1961; Gates, Ryan, Cantu, & Hearne, 1982).

Patient Reaction to Alaryngeal Speech. Patients will resist learning and using a form of alaryngeal speech that they find unacceptable. All forms of alaryngeal speech sound different than the laryngeal voice the individual has lost. Several studies have documented the particular difficulty that women have in accepting alaryngeal voice because of the hoarseness and masculine quality associated with the lowered pitch (Gardner, 1966; Gilmore, 1961; Stoll, 1958). However, individuals of both sexes may have difficulty adjusting to alaryngeal forms of speaking. King, Fowlks, and Pierson (1968) reported that half of their subjects, regardless of the form of communication they used (including esophageal speech, artificial larynx, and writing), never used it outside the house. In view of reports such as these, it is important for the speech–language pathologist to help the patient through the adjustment process. Acceptance of the new voice may come slowly.

Adjustment to the Disability. Laryngectomy poses a number of physical and emotional challenges to the patient. The degree to which individuals are disturbed by any or all of the life changes resulting from their altered condition may affect their ability to learn or accept alaryngeal speech. Becoming a neck breather is among the biggest physical challenges faced by the laryngectomee. The creation of a tracheostoma means that the person must breathe through the neck. Inhaled air will no longer be warmed and filtered through the nose and other structures comprising the upper respiratory tract. The body's defensive response to the unwarmed air taken directly into the trachea is to produce more mucous. Newly laryngectomized individuals often experience tracheal congestion that may be so severe that suctioning of the trachea is necessary to clear the airway. This condition usually resolves within a few months, but may be quite distressing for a period of time. Covering the stoma with a bib and layers of clothing, particularly in cold weather, helps to alleviate this condition.

Neck breathing also may result in changes in the patient's sense of smell and taste. Blowing one's nose becomes difficult and coughed-up phlegm is expelled through the stoma, instead of the mouth. The loss of the valving function provided by the larynx also precludes stabilization of the thorax during lifting. This may particularly affect patients with jobs involving manual labor. Additionally, patients must learn to take precautions when bathing or showering to keep water out of the stoma. Swimming and chin-high soaks in a Jacuzzi are no longer options.

Perhaps the most important psychological challenge a person must confront after a laryngectomy is the loss of voice. The loss of voice means more than the loss of verbal communication. Sounds of laughter, crying, and other vocal expressions of emotion are lost or significantly changed following laryngectomy. The feelings of grief associated with the loss of the sound of one's voice may impact on the willingness of patients to accept alaryngeal speech.

Other psychosocial challenges may include the reaction of loved ones to the physical changes in the patient, or the patient's own reaction to an altered self-image. Individuals may also be concerned about the possible loss of their job or the fear that new physical limitations will preclude continued employment or career advancement.

Finally, fear that the cancer will reoccur may be a constant threat. Patients who express an unrelenting fear or become depressed following laryngectomy should be referred for psychological evaluation and be encouraged to contact local self-help and support groups.

Support Groups.   The International Association of Laryngectomies (IAL) is a parent organization that has chapters in many communities across the country. The IAL publishes a quarterly newsletter containing updates regarding medical and therapeutic interventions available to laryngectomized individuals, their families and speech–language pathologists. Local support groups, sometimes called "Lost chord clubs," may be affiliated with the IAL. Information regarding the location of affiliate members is available through the IAL. The IAL also sponsors an annual meeting as well as a voice institute, where laryngectomied people and their families can become acquainted. They also may meet with speech–language pathologists and other professionals to share concerns and learn about new developments regarding **laryngectomee** rehabilitation.

THE REHABILITATIVE PROCESS

Preoperative Consultation

One might think that a preoperative consultation between a speech–language pathologist and a person scheduled for a laryngectomy would be routine and commonplace. However, in a survey of laryngectomized individuals and their spouses, Salmon (1986a) found that such a consultation occurred only about one-third of the time. The survey also revealed that most preoperative information was supplied by the surgeon and/or nurses. Spouses were often present at the preoperative consultation with the surgeon, but were infrequently included in the consultations between the patient and the nurse or the speech–language pathologist. Reportedly, the surgeons discussed mostly the surgical procedure and provided little information about the rehabilitation process.

The majority of the laryngectomees and most of the spouses who responded to the questionnaire felt that they were not well-prepared for the surgery. When asked what information should be provided to others before laryngectomy, the laryngectomized respondents in the Salmon survey most often indicated that information about the different ways to communicate after surgery, information about the surgical procedure, and information regarding their prognosis for recovery should be provided. They also believed it would be important to supply information about the anatomical and physiological changes associated with such functions as laughing and coughing, the feeding tube, swallowing problems, the stoma, the mucus, the impaired sense of taste and smell, the inability to blow the nose or to sneeze, and the altered appearance.

The spouses surveyed by Salmon (1986a) reportedly were most concerned preoperatively with the details of the operation, the anticipated outcome and prognosis, what to expect the patient to look like in the intensive care unit, and how to care for the patient immediately after surgery when nurses are not available. They were specifically interested in learning about the care of the stoma, the use of the suction machine, and the feeding tube. The spouses also desired information regarding possible emotional reactions that patients and spouses may have to the altered anatomy, disease, and so on.

Ideally, the speech–language pathologist should meet with the patient, family members, and/or close friends shortly after the diagnosis of cancer has been made. The speech–language pathologist can serve as a source of information and support to the patient, family, and friends. The speech–language pathologist can provide assurance that many people continue to live normal lives following laryngectomy, and that most people are able to adjust well to the resulting physical changes.

It is important at the onset for the speech–language pathologist to find out what the patient has been told, so that information may be reinforced or expanded upon—particularly information related to the surgery and what to expect immediately after it. New information may also be provided about alaryngeal speaking options. The speech–language pathologist may demonstrate an electrolarynx and/or offer to introduce the future laryngectomee to another laryngectomized person. If voice restoration is planned as part of the primary surgery, information about tracheoesophageal speech should be offered. (This option will be discussed more fully in a later section.)

Other information that may be useful to the speech–language pathologist can also be acquired at this time. For example, it is advantageous for the speech–language pathologist to observe the patient's laryngeal voice and habitual speech patterns. The presence of a foreign accent or regional dialect should be noted, as these differences could make it difficult for listeners to understand the patient's mouthed or whispered speech postoperatively. Additionally, screening of cognitive status, manual dexterity, and auditory acuity may be conducted as appropriate (Casper et al., 1993).

Postoperative Consultation

The postoperative consultation between the newly laryngectomized individual and the speech–language pathologist is devoted firstly to finding out how the patient is coping and how much information the person has been given. Having a family member or close friend present may be helpful. It is important, however, for the speech–language pathologist to address the patient directly and to be supportive of communicative efforts. It is a good idea to have paper and pencil available if lip reading the patient proves too difficult.

Also, at this time speech aids (such as different types of electrolarynges) may be demonstrated and made available. Some time should be spent reviewing speech options and the opportunity to visit with an esophageal and/or tracheoesophageal speaker can be offered to the patient. Finally, literature regarding postlaryngectomy rehabilitation should be provided so that the patient and family may review it at their leisure. When interacting with the patient and family, it is important to re-

member that a traumatic surgery has been performed. The patient and family will need time to adjust to these events. It is important to support the patient during the recovery process and to be optimistic regarding the reestablishment of oral communication.

ALARYNGEAL SPEECH

Reestablishment of one or more forms of oral communication may be the most important part of the rehabilitation process. The speech–language pathologist, together with the patient, as well as other members of the rehabilitation team, will select the form(s) of alaryngeal speech available given the patient's anatomical status and psychosocial needs. There are currently three major forms of alaryngeal speech available: the artificial larynx, esophageal speech, and tracheoesophageal (TP) speech.

Artificial Larynx

There are two types of artificial larynges: pneumatic and electronic. Each type of device provides a sound source that is introduced into the vocal tract either at the level of the neck or the oral cavity.

Pneumatic Devices. The pneumatic device is a hand held apparatus consisting of a tube that houses a reed or membrane that vibrates when air passes across it. At one end of the tube is a cup that is placed over the tracheostoma to provide an airtight seal, ensuring that pulmonary air flows through the tube. At the other end of the tube is a mouthpiece.

Speech is produced when the patient's exhaled pulmonary air passes through the vibratory source. Sound is generated and the person articulates with the mouthpiece placed in the oral cavity above the tongue. The sound generated by pneumatic devices is low in pitch but does not sound mechanical. Phrasing of speech is normal and patients easily learn to coordinate the initiation of sound with articulation. However, these devices are cumbersome. They require access to an un-covered stoma and the use of two hands, one to hold the cup securely over the stoma and the other to hold the mouthpiece in place. For these reasons, pneumatic devices are not popular.

Electrolarynges. The **electrolarynx** is one of the most accessible and popular forms of oral communication. There are a number of styles and models available from a variety of manufacturers. These handheld devices provide a sound source that is either applied to the neck so sound is con-ducted through the vocal tract transcervically, or funneled through a tube directly into the oral cav-ity where the sound is resonated. As the person ar-ticulates, audible speech is produced.

The most popular intraoral device is the Cooper-Rand, pictured in Figure 12.3. This instru-ment consists of a battery-operated pulse genera-tor connected with a wire to a handheld tone generator, into which a small plastic tube is in-serted. The battery and pulse generator are housed in a small case that can be clipped to clothing or slipped into a pocket. At the top of the case are two dials controlling pitch and loudness. These are usually set to levels judged by the patient and speech–language pathologist to be comfortable, and remain unchanged during conversational speech.

The plastic tube is placed in the mouth. Sound is introduced into the mouth by pressing an on–off switch on the tone generator. With prac-tice, patients learn to appropriately time voicing with speech and to place the tube so that it inter-feres minimally with articulatory movements. This intraoral device is desirable because it can be used immediately after surgery. As this form of speech is usually readily learned, patients often prefer it to writing as a means of communication. Depending on the response of the patient, this form of alaryngeal speech may be used only dur-ing the immediate postsurgical period, or may be adopted as either a secondary or primary means of oral communication.

Neck devices are the most popular kind of ar-tificial larynx. These are battery-operated instru-ments that generate sound via a transducer or by the action of a piston hitting a diaphragm. They are small, lightweight, wireless, handheld instru-ments. Speech is generated when the patient places the vibrating head of the device securely against the neck and activates an on–off switch that generates a tone. The sound travels through the pharynx into the oral cavity, where it is further modified by articulatory movements.

In order to use a neck device, the neck tissue on at least one side must be soft and supple so the sound can penetrate through it into the pharynx. The laryngectomized person must also have the manual dexterity to press the on–off switch, and to time the activation of the device with the initiation and termination of speech.

Electrolarynges are manufactured by several companies. Specific features regarding pitch and loudness capabilities, size, shape, and weight vary

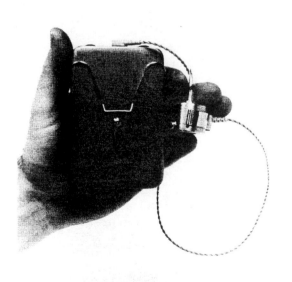

FIGURE 12.3 Cooper-Rand intraoral artificial larynx.

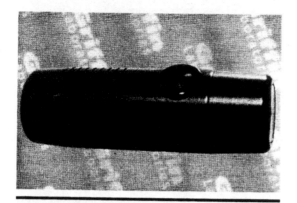

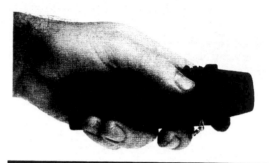

FIGURE 12.6   Servox artificial larynx.

FIGURE 12.4   Western Electric artificial larynx.

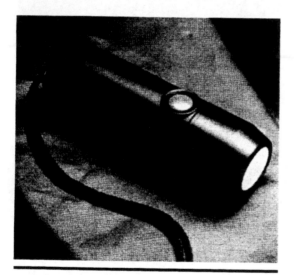

FIGURE 12.5   AT&T artificial larynx (discontinued by manufacturer but may still be in use).

somewhat from model to model. The Western Electric (Figure 12.4), the AT&T (Figure 12.5), and the Servox (Figure 12.6) are among the most commonly utilized handheld instruments in the United States. A comprehensive history of artificial larynges and descriptions of those currently available can be found in Keith and Darley (1986).

The electrolarynx is an easy-to-use and reliable sound source, requiring little maintenance. Even if the laryngectomized person develops an-

other form of alaryngeal speech, it is recommended that an electrolarynx be kept accessible. In emergency situations, these devices enable the person to call attention to themselves and to obtain assistance if they became unable to utilize alternative speech skills.

In addition to the above reasons why laryngectomized persons should be encouraged to use an artificial larynx, Lerman (1991) includes the following: (1) Using an artificial larynx may reduce anxiety and tension in the patient and the family, thereby creating a less stressful environment; (2) the artificial larynx provides opportunities to practice skills such as compensatory movements for articulation and reduction of stoma noise that must be acquired for production of acceptable esophageal speech; (3) it gives laryngectomees (after some training) viable, understandable speech early in the management process so that effective communication can be used while they are attempting to learn esophageal speech; (4) it is economically beneficial for some patients who must return to work immediately; (5) use of the artificial larynx reduces both the possibility of acquiring whispered or buccal speech and the need to communicate by writing; and finally, (6) it allows individuals who may never be able to use esophageal speech an acceptable method of verbal communication.

There are two primary disadvantages to using an artificial larynx. The most common complaint is that they sound artificial and robotic. The second complaint is that one hand must be available to operate the device. Despite these disadvantages, the artificial larynx remains a viable, readily available means of oral communication that can be used as a primary or secondary method of speaking.

Esophageal Speech

Esophageal speech is an intrinsic form of alaryngeal speech that utilizes the laryngectomized individual's reconfigured anatomy. Since excision of the larynx necessitates the creation of a permanent tracheostoma, pulmonary air bypasses the vocal tract completely, making it inaccessible for speech purposes. Therefore, a different air reservoir must be created to drive an alternative sound source.

At the entrance to the esophagus is a sphincter composed of fibers of the cricopharyngus and inferior pharyngeal constrictor muscles. Because of its location between the pharynx and the esophagus, it is called the **pharyngoesophageal sphincter (P–E sphincter)**. This sphincter is vibrated in esophageal speech, producing sound, and is therefore often called the neoglottis.

The P–E Sphincter.   Following the removal (**extirpation**) of the larynx and the repositioning of the trachea, the pharynx and upper esophageal regions must be reconstructed. During surgery, many of the extrinsic laryngeal muscles are cut from their points of attachment on the thyroid cartilage and hyoid bone. The cricopharyngeus is among the muscles in which attachments must be reconstructed. In reconstruction, the detached ends of the various muscles are connected in an opposing manner, creating a new anatomical area. Because the muscles are attached to each other, it is difficult to isolate the contraction of any specific muscle. Further, the way in which the muscles are reconnected may vary from patient to patient. Consequently, it is not always possible to determine which muscles comprise the neoglottis.

Most often, the P–E segment is composed of tissue derived from the cricopharyngeus and inferior pharyngeal constrictor muscles. The sphincter is in a constant state of contraction. However, weakened contractions of the cricopharyngeus

muscle have been described postsurgery (Kirschner, Scatliff, Dey, & Shedd, 1963; Winans, Reichback, & Waldrop, 1974) probably because of its separation from its original attachment. The characteristics of the reconstructed tissue that constitutes the P–E segment is highly variable. Damste (1979) observed that the P–E segment may vary "from wide to narrow, from long to short, and its shape can be flat, round and predominant" (p. 55).

The location of the P–E sphincter may also vary from individual to individual. In their classic study, Diedrich and Youngstrom (1966) reported that the location of the P–E segment varied between cervical vertebrae four and seven (C4–C7), but was most frequently located between C5 and C6. Diedrich and Youngstrom also reported a range for length of the P–E segment from 18 to 23 mm during phonation of different vowels. Average length was found to be 21 mm based on cineflurograms and 29 mm based on spot films.

The P–E sphincter functions much differently from the vocal folds. Unlike the larynx, which houses several paired muscles which adduct, abduct, and which are capable of pretuning and fine motor adjustments, the P–E sphincter is composed of an unpaired ring of muscle fibers. Shipp (1970) investigated the degree of control esophageal speakers had over muscle activation of the P–E sphincter. He was able to identify particular patterns of muscle activation in his subjects when they took air into the esophagus. During voicing, however, the patterns of muscle activation appeared to be unique to each individual. This finding led Shipp to conclude that ". . . each individual utilizes a method of alaryngeal phonation that is most efficient for him consistent with his post-operative anatomy and physiology" (pp. 191–192). Not surprisingly, the variability inherent in the reconstructed aerodigestive tracts of alaryngeal speakers results in a tone of varying acoustic properties.

Acoustic Characteristics of Esophageal Voice. Given the variability in the size, shape, length, mass, and location of the P–E sphincter, it is not surprising that the tone generated by this structure varies from person to person. There have been many investigations regarding the acoustic properties of esophageal voice. On average, the esophageal voice has a fundamental frequency (f0) of 65 Hz—approximately one octave below that of a male laryngeal voice. However, individual fundamental frequencies may range from about 20 to 150 Hz (Hoops & Noll, 1969; Robbins, 1984; Shipp, 1967; Snidecor & Curry, 1960; Weinberg & Bennett, 1972).

Differences in mean f0 between males and females have been reported by Weinberg and Bennett (1972), who acoustically analyzed speech samples of 15 female and 18 male esophageal speakers. They found statistically significant differences between the mean f0s exhibited by the two groups. Specifically, the women had mean f0s approximately seven semitones higher than the men. However, examination of the individual f0s of the men and the women revealed a great deal of individual variability. Mean f0s for the 15 females ranged from 33 to 200 Hz. Mean f0s for the males ranged from 34 to 83 Hz. Eight of the females exhibited f0s above the upper limit set by the males in this study. Interestingly, listeners asked to identify the sex of these speakers via audiotape recordings were 90 percent accurate in their identification of the men and 80 percent accurate in identification of the women (Weinberg & Bennett, 1971).

Esophageal speakers also demonstrate intensity levels that average 10 dB below that of normal speakers. Weinberg, Horii, and Smith (1980) calculated mean dB sound pressure levels (SPLs) of 61.9 to 69 dB among the esophageal group, as compared to 74.5 dB for the normal speakers. These findings were substantiated by Slavin and Ferrand (1995), in a study of 26 proficient esophageal speakers. Their subjects had mean intensities of 64 to 80 dB with a group mean of 69 dB. These results are also similar to those of Robbins, Fisher, Blom, and Singer (1984), who reported a mean intensity of 73.8 dB for 15 esophageal subjects.

Researchers have also found that esophageal speakers vary in their rate of speech. Even among superior esophageal speakers, rate has been found to range from 85 to 129 words per minute (Snidecor & Curry, 1959). These speaking rates are considerably slower than the normal speech rate of 150 to 190 words per minute. Esophageal speech rate is determined in part by the extent to which the speaker is able to control air as it passes through the neoglottis. This is referred to as **transneoglottic air flow.** The faster the air stored in the upper esophagus is depleted, the more often the speaker must pause to replenish it. The typical esophageal speaker is able to say three to five words per air charge as compared to the 12 of a laryngeal speaker. Decreased phrase length leads to an increased pause time that slows the overall speech rate. The need to repeatedly replenish the air supply also reduces the rate of speech. However, this reduced rate of speech may not necessarily have an unfavorable effect on perceptual ratings of speech proficiency. The 26 highly proficient esophageal speakers studied by Slavin and Ferrand (1995) demonstrated total speaking times that ranged from approximately 82 to 188 words per minute during oral readings. It appears that as long as speech intelligibility is intact, a wide range of speech rates may be acceptable to listeners. These acoustic research studies are important because they show that there is no one ideal form of esophageal speech. Individual esophageal speakers adapt to their altered phonatory systems in individualized ways to maximize the physiological resources available to them.

Methods of Air Intake. Some people with intact larynges have learned that by pushing air into their esophagus, they can belch voluntarily. This is the basis for esophageal voice. Air is pushed through the P–E sphincter into the esophagus and immediately released back (**eructated**) through the sphincter into the vocal tract. The P–E sphincter becomes the new vibratory source (neoglottis) driven by the force of subsphincteric air. Recall that the P–E sphincter is usually closed. In order for air to flow through the sphincter and into the esophagus, it is necessary to overcome the resistance of the sphincter. Air may be injected into the esophagus using methods that create air pressure differences (either above or below the neoglottis) great enough to overcome the resistance of the closed P–E sphincter. This pool of air, temporarily stored in the upper third of the esophagus for the purpose of voicing, may be referred to as the *air reservoir* or the *neolung*. The various means by which air is injected into the esophagus are called injection techniques. Three methods of air injection that may be employed to fill (**insufflate**) the upper esophagus include glossal press, consonant injection, and inhalation.

Glossal Press. Glossal press is achieved in three steps: (1) air is trapped in the oral cavity; (2) the dorsum of the tongue is pushed against the palate; and (3) with a piston-like motion, the air within the oropharynx is compressed raising the air pressure above the P–E sphincter. When the air pressure exceeds the resistance of the sphincter, it will open and air will pass through it.

Consonant Injection. The consonant injection method takes advantage of the intraoral buildup of pressure that occurs during the production of consonants such as plosives and affricates. The patient is simply instructed to say words or C–V syllables beginning with these sounds. The intraoral pressure increase may be great enough to overcome the sphincteric resistance.

Inhalation. The method of inhalation is more difficult to describe. It is achieved by decreasing the pressure below the neoglottis rather than increasing the pressure above it, as in the previously described methods. This increase in negative pressure may be achieved by asking the patient to inhale. Inhalation through the tracheostoma may result in more than doubling the negative pressure values within the esophagus (Duguay, 1991). If the P–E sphincter tension is not too great, the inhalation will result in airflow into the esophagus to equalize the pressure.

A number of studies have shown that insufflation of the upper esophagus may be easier following laryngectomy because of a reduction in the normal pressure of the P–E sphincter (Kirschner

et al., 1963; Welch, Gates, Luckmann, Ricks, & Drake, 1979; Winans, Reichback, & Waldrop, 1974). This pressure reduction may also contribute to an individual's ability to quickly and easily release the trapped air into the vocal tract.

Esophageal speakers may learn to utilize one or a combination of all three of the methods just described in the attainment of ongoing speech. During the course of esophageal speech therapy, practice usually begins with single words or syllables and gradually expands to include phrases, sentences, and ultimately, conversational speech. Mastery of more than one insufflation technique is desirable since frequent recharging of the air supply is necessary. The volume of air contained in the upper esophagus is tiny when compared to the air capacity of the lungs. Isshiki and Snidecor (1965) reported that the capacity of the upper esophagus is limited to approximately 50 cc (five tablespoons according to Salmon, 1986b), while lung capacity ranges from 2,000 to 4,000 cc (Zemlin, 1988). Therefore, rapid, unobtrusive air injection and expulsion will contribute to speech fluency and the overall perception of speech acceptability.

Pros and Cons of Esophageal Speech. Some of the limitations of esophageal speech are obvious. As stated previously, the esophagus cannot hold much air. In order for esophageal speech to become functional, the speaker must learn to inject and return air quickly and easily. The air reservoir must be adequate to support several syllables of speech and the speech must be loud enough and clear enough in quality to be intelligible. As one begins to speak, the air reserve becomes depleted quickly and needs to be replenished if audible speech is to be continued. This small air reserve also limits loudness capability, making speaking particularly difficult in noisy environments. In an effort to overcome limited loudness, some people may attempt to speak more loudly by pushing pulmonary air out through the stoma. The resulting **stoma blast** is a noisy rush of air that may further interfere with speech intelligibility.

The voice generated by the neoglottis does not sound normal. It is low in pitch and often sounds raspy and hoarse. Since the acoustics of the altered vocal tract are similar in men and women, this lowered vocal pitch may be especially disturbing to women.

While these limitations are significant, the primary problem with esophageal speech is that only one-third to one-half of all laryngectomized individuals are able to develop an esophageal voice that is good enough to be functional for daily living. The inability to acquire esophageal speech may be related to physical and/or psychosocial factors. Physically, the patient must be able to achieve the pressure differential above and below the P–E segment necessary to move air from the pharynx into the upper esophagus. In addition, the tension of the P–E segment must be such that air pressure can overcome it fairly easily. If the P–E segment is strongly contracted or subject to spasms, smooth, reliable phonation will be impossible. The esophagus also must be capable of holding the air charge. A patient suffering from sphincteric or gastrointestinal problems may be at risk for esophageal speech failure. The causes of failure are not always easily diagnosed or resolved once identified. Therefore, the majority of laryngectomized patients must rely on other forms of alaryngeal speech, including voice restoration procedures, particularly **trachoesophageal speech.**

For those who do acquire esophageal speech, there are some clear advantages. Esophageal speech can be a readily accessible and effective intrinsic means of oral communication. It requires no instrumentation or maintenance other than practice. People who develop proficient esophageal speech can sound quite natural in terms of the intonational or prosodic features of speech. Research has shown that although esophageal voice is noisier than laryngeal voice, esophageal speakers are often able to effectively manipulate the frequency, intensity, and duration of the vocal signal to mark lexical, syntactic, and contrastive stress (Gandour & Weinberg, 1983; Gandour, Weinberg, & Garzione, 1983; McHenry, Reich, & Minifie, 1982). This ability is an important aspect of overall intelligibility and communicative effectiveness.

Voice Restoration Following Laryngectomy

Between 1950 and 1980, several surgical procedures were attempted to restore speech following laryngectomy. The goal of these procedures was to create a means whereby pulmonary air could be accessed by the speaker for voice production. Some surgeons sought to achieve this by constructing an air shunt between the trachea and either the esophagus or the pharynx (Calcaterra & Jafek, 1971; Conley, DeAmestre, & Pierce, 1958; Curry, Snidecor, & Isshiki, 1973; Taub & Bergner, 1973). Others sought to reestablish voice through the use of a combination of an air shunt and a mechanical voicing source between the trachea and pharynx (Weinberg, Shedd, & Horii, 1978). The results of these surgeries were promising but outcomes were mixed. Postoperative complications associated with these procedures included aspiration, stenosis of the air shunt, inadequate healing, and difficulty managing salivary leakage. Consequently, these operations were performed on a very selective basis.

Tracheoesophageal Puncture

In 1979, an otolaryngologist named Marc Singer, in collaboration with a speech–language pathologist named Eric Blom, developed a surgical technique that revolutionized the concept of voice restoration following total laryngectomy (Singer & Blom, 1980). In this procedure, pulmonary air is diverted into the esophagus through a **fistula** (small hole) created by the surgeon in the tissue wall separating the trachea from the esophagus. The fistula is kept open by the insertion of a silicone prosthesis. The prosthesis acts as a one-way valve. When the stoma is occluded, the air from the lungs is diverted through the prosthesis into the esophagus at a point below the P–E sphincter. The prosthesis is constructed to allow air from the trachea to pass through it into the esophagus, while food and liquid from the esophagus are unable to pass through into the trachea. Air from the lungs is thus directed into the pharynx and expelled through the P–E sphincter, resulting in trachoesophageal (TE) voice.

Perceptually TE voice sounds similar to esophageal voice because it is a form of esophageal voice. Specifically, the sound is produced by the vibratory effect of pulmonary air passing into the esophagus and up through the P–E sphincter. It is low pitched, with a limited pitch range relative to laryngeal speakers. Since the air supply is readily available and plentiful, the TE voice has greater loudness capability and allows for near normal rate and phrasing of speech. Acoustically, TE speakers produce mean f0s comparable to adult male voices of 100 Hz (Robbins, et al. 1984). Amplitude measures also reported by Robbins (1984) and Robbins et al. (1984) were higher (perceptually louder) than normals during oral reading (88 versus 77 dB). This is attributed to the higher resistance levels within the esophageal airway (Weinberg et al., 1982).

The tracheoesophageal puncture (TEP) procedure has undergone some modifications in recent years (Spofford, Jafek, & Barcz, 1984; Stewart & Sherwen, 1987) and has become popular over the past decade. TEP has become an attractive alternative form of alaryngeal speech for a number of reasons. First, postsurgical complications are minimized by careful subject selection. Second, voice is readily attained by most patients, restoring fluent speech ability with a minimum of instruction. Third, the procedure may be performed at the time of the laryngectomy or at any time thereafter if the patient is deemed to be a viable candidate. There are a number of physical and psychosocial factors that must be considered when selecting candidates for this procedure.

Physical requirements include a history free of drug and alcohol dependency. Candidates must be competent to maintain the prosthesis over a long period of time. They also must have an adequate healing capacity. Heavily irradiated tissue, or previously reconstructed areas of the neck, pharynx, esophagus, or tongue may preclude the fistulazation procedures. Coexisting diseases that impede healing (e.g., diabetes) may also disqualify people. In addition, the TEP candidate must

have an adequately large stoma size to house the prosthesis. The stoma must, however, also be small enough to be easily occluded with a finger or pressure valve. Another physical prerequisite is that candidates must possess adequate visual ability and manual dexterity to maintain the prosthesis. The prosthesis has to be removed, cleaned, and replaced on a regular basis. Adequate pulmonary support to overcome neoglottic resistance for a sustained period of time is also crucial to success. This is important so that phonation is not inappropriately interrupted.

A final physical determinant for candidacy is insufflation testing. The purpose of this test is to determine the ease with which TE speech can be produced. Prior to the surgery, a rubber catheter is passed through the nose into the esophagus. A valve (to which one end of the catheter is attached) is placed into the stoma so that the patient is able to blow pulmonary air through the catheter into the upper esophagus. The increased air pressure built up below the P–E segment should readily overcome sphincteric resistance and be released back up through the P–E segment, producing sound. The ease with which the sound is generated, as well as its quality, are then assessed. Sometimes the P–E segment spasms with a sudden increase in subneoglottic pressure. People with this problem will be unable to sustain phonation. For the insufflation test to be considered successful, the prospective candidate should be able to maintain continuous phonation for at least eight seconds (Blom, Singer, & Hamaker, 1985).

Psychosocial requirements include the motivation to undergo the surgery and to maintain the prosthesis, the cognitive capacity to understand the nature of the surgery and the maintenance required for the prosthesis, and emotional stability. If a patient meets all of the above criteria, the procedure may be performed and the prosthesis may be inserted.

Establishment of Tracheoesophageal Speech
Fitting the Prosthesis. At the time of the surgery, the fistula is maintained by the insertion of a catheter until healing has occurred. The initial evaluation and prosthesis fitting may take place any time

between two days and two weeks after the surgery, depending upon whether the procedure was done as a primary procedure or as a secondary one.

At the time of the first postoperative visit, the speech–language pathologist must spend time speaking to the patient and family regarding the anatomical and physiological changes that have occurred. It is important to find out how the patient and family are reacting to these changes. Additionally, the patient may be experiencing discomfort or distress about issues related to feeding, the management of secretions from the tracheostoma, and pain and/or stiffness in the neck (particularly if the TEP was performed as a part of the primary surgery). These issues should be addressed before fitting of the prosthesis is attempted. Silicone prostheses are available from three manufacturers, including Inhealth Technologies, who distribute the original Blom–Singer prosthesis, American V. Muellar, and Bivona. These companies produce a variety of prostheses designed to meet the specific requirements of the patient. The one-way valving devices are tube-like appliances with an opening at the tracheal end to allow the flow of pulmonary air, and a valve consisting of a slit (duck bill) or a hinge at the end that is inserted into the esophagus. (See Figure 12.7.) A collar or flange usually surrounds the

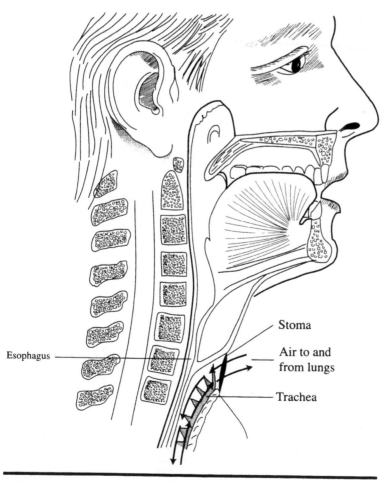

Esophagus

Stoma

Air to and from lungs

Trachea

FIGURE 12.7 Tracheoesophageal puncture.

valved end of the prosthesis. The prosthesis is pushed into the esophagus just past the flange. The flange helps hold the prosthesis in place and keeps it from slipping out of the fistula if the patient should cough.

The length of prostheses range from 1.4 to 3.6 cm. The prosthesis must extend from just inside the edge of the tracheostoma to just beyond the tracheoesphageal wall. Depths differ from person to person. A prosthesis that is too long may become buried in the far (distal) wall of the esophagus and may occlude the valve, impeding airflow into the esophagus. Other features of the prosthesis also must be considered. The amount of resistance presented by the prosthesis changes with the length and diameter of the tube as well as the nature of the valve. Air pressure required to force open the duck-bill valve may range from 2 to 25 cm H_2O depending on the rate of airflow from the lungs (Weinberg & Moon, 1984). For patients who have difficulty sustaining the air pressure necessary to overcome this resistance, a low-pressure valved prosthesis has been developed. (See Figure 12.8). The prosthesis best for the individual will be the one that permits easy flow of air into the esophagus and does not take up too much space within the tracheostoma.

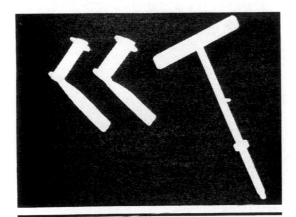

FIGURE 12.8 Low pressure tracheoesophageal puncture voice prosthesis (right) and duckbill voice prosthesis (left) with insertion devices attached.

Once a prosthesis is chosen, the patient must be instructed regarding its insertion and maintenance. Instruction is provided by the speech–language pathologist, and should take place in a well-lit area. If the patient wears glasses, they should be wearing them. As in all cases when the speech–language pathologist may come into contact with a patient's bodily fluids, surgical gloves must be worn. The catheter placed through the fistula at the time of the surgery will be removed by the speech–language pathologist. The patient should be given several trials reinserting the catheter into the fistula. Then, practice inserting and removing the prosthesis may begin. Once removed, the patient must be warned that the tracheoesophageal fistula may close quite rapidly (often within 30 minutes) if not dilated. If this occurs, another surgery would be needed to reestablish it.

The prosthesis, once inserted, is secured to the outside of the tracheostoma with tape. At this point the patient should be instructed in occlusion of the stoma to divert pulmonary air into the esophagus. Ideally, if the prosthesis fits well, sound will be generated readily. If sound is not forthcoming or is intermittent, the speech–language pathologist must do some trouble shooting to determine if the problem is the result of a physical obstruction like sphincter spasm, or whether the prosthesis is an inappropriate length, or a combination of the two.

A patient who adapts well to the prosthesis may also want to be fitted with an air pressure valve. This device is fitted into the tracheostoma and occludes it automatically when pulmonary air pressure reaches the level necessary for speech purposes. This feature is desirable as it frees both hands during speech. Such a device is pictured in Figure 12.9. A kit is available to aid the speech–language pathologist in determining the proper resistance of the air pressure valve. This is important, as the valve must stay open for normal breathing as well as for heavier breathing, such as that required for climbing stairs or playing tennis. Some pressure valves are now self-adjustable, enabling the individual to vary pressure requirements at will.

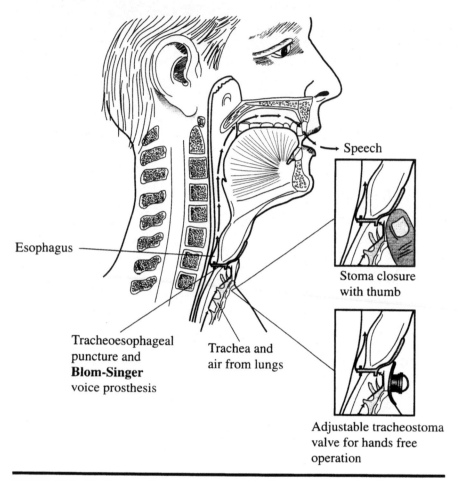

→ Speech

Esophagus

Stoma closure
with thumb

Tracheoesophageal
puncture and
Blom-Singer
voice prosthesis

Trachea and
air from lungs

Adjustable tracheostoma
valve for hands free
operation

FIGURE 12.9   Tracheoesophageal puncture with Blom–Singer prosthesis and
adjustable tracheostoma air pressure valve in place.

Recent Advances in Prosthetic Design.   A new type of prosthesis has recently been introduced that makes it possible for patients who previously would have been deemed poor candidates for TEP (because of poor eyesight or lack of manual dexterity) to develop TE speech. The prosthesis is placed in the fistula tract and can remain there for prolonged periods of time, as it does not require daily cleaning. Because this device can remain in the fistula tract for long periods before replacement is necessary, it is referred to as an *indwelling, semipermanent prosthesis.* This device further increases the options for patients undergo-

ing laryngectomy and increases the likelihood of voice restoration for many.

Pros and Cons of Tracheoesophageal Puncture.
With careful selection, risk of complications is minimal and success rates are high. Many TEP patients can speak with minimum instruction after the prosthesis has been inserted. TE speech is desirable because it may be the most natural-sounding alaryngeal speech. Particularly for males, TE speech is an attractive speech alternative.

There are several disadvantages to this method of alaryngeal speech. First, patients need to undergo an additional surgical procedure if it was not performed at the time of the laryngectomy. Patients often are not anxious to undergo another hospitalization. Second, the prosthesis requires regular maintenance. The ritual of removing, cleaning, and reinserting the prosthesis may continue for many years. Also, if the patient does not use a pressure valve, one hand must be free to occlude the stoma. Finally, some patients encounter difficulty speaking while eating. However, this is a problem for all alaryngeal speakers.

Perceptual Characteristics of Alaryngeal Speech

Individuals learn to adapt to their reconfigured aerodigestive tracts in highly individualized ways. The degree of speech proficiency attained by laryngectomized individuals varies along a continuum from poor to superior. Some people master the use of an electrolarynx, or esophageal speech, or TE speech. Some become proficient speakers, while others may be judged as fair or good communicators using one or more forms of alaryngeal speech.

A number of studies have been conducted to determine listeners' perceptions of the three forms of alaryngeal speech. In studies in which listeners are asked to assess the speech intelligibility of alaryngeal speech, electrolarynx speech is typically the least well understood form of alaryngeal speech. This reduction in intelligibility results largely from the speaker's inability to make voice/ voiceless contrasts. The split-second timing necessary to signal voiceless sounds like *s, f, p,* or *t* simply is not possible with an electrolarynx (Shames, Font, & Matthews, 1963; Weiss & Basili, 1985).

TE speech also has been compared to other forms of alaryngeal speech. Clark and Stemple (1982) reported that listeners found TE speech to be the most pleasant sounding when compared to esophageal and electrolarynx speech. However, Trudeau (1987) and Sedory, Hamlet, and Conner (1989) reported that some esophageal speakers were rated by listeners as equally acceptable or more acceptable than TE speakers, despite the fact

that the TE speakers exhibited longer mean phonation times, increased intensity, and more syllables/ breath than the esophageal speakers. Behaviors such as nonspeech noises, audible inhalations, slurring of words, and poor loudness control may detract from the speech intelligibility of TE speakers (Sedory et al., 1989).

Taken together, the literature provides no clear indication that one form of alaryngeal speech is best (Casper et al., 1993). All three forms can be effective sources of speech communication. Largely because of their low pitch, all three forms tend to be viewed as abnormal, particularly for women. Generally the f0 of TE speech is higher than that of esophageal speech. It is important to remember that individual speakers may obtain f0s above those generally obtained. The acoustic characteristics of any given esophageal or TE speaker are difficult to predict.

EVALUATING THE LARYNGECTOMIZED PATIENT

In an effort to reduce medical costs, laryngectomized patients typically stay in the hospital only about 10 days. By the time of discharge from the hospital, these patients may have had a pre- and/or postoperative consultation and sometimes a limited amount of speech therapy. However, most alaryngeal speech therapy is done as part of a home care program or on an outpatient basis.

The type of alaryngeal speech chosen for a particular patient is be based on an evaluation of patient need and medical status. When evaluating people who have been recently laryngectomized, it is important for the speeech–language pathologist to speak directly to them and lip read if possible. The speeech–language pathologist should not hesitate to ask them to repeat what cannot be understood. The use of an electrolarynx should be encouraged. When a friend or family member accompanies the patient, the speeech–language pathologist should avoid letting that person speak for the patient. These clinical strategies may reassure patients that they are respected as mature adults who still have a capacity to communicate.

One of the first things the speeech–language pathologist needs to find out is how the patient is currently communicating. They may be mouthing their speech or speaking forcefully, causing air to rush out from the stoma, resulting in a noisy distraction called a stoma blast. They may be communicating solely by writing, or they may have begun to use an electrolarynx. A few patients, when speaking conversationally, may have spontaneous injections of air into the esophagus, resulting in intermittent esophageal phonation. A smaller number of patients come in talking, having taught themselves what they need to do to maintain esophageal speech.

As the speech–language pathologist inquires about the patient's background and history, it is important to informally observe the patient's articulatory patterns and note the presence of undesirable behaviors like stoma blasts, excessive breathing noise, and facial grimacing, as well as spontaneous injections and esophageal voicing.

Medical History

It is important to find out what patients can relate about their medical history including pre-existing medical conditions, preoperative symptoms, hospital admissions, radiation treatment or chemotherapy, as well as any prior laryngeal surgery. This questioning will provide insight into the involvement of patients in their own care, the level to which they have been educated, and the amount of detail regarding their condition they can handle. This is helpful in treatment planning. The speech–language pathologist can begin to assess patients' acceptance of the disability and their motivational level. Responses to these questions may also provide insight regarding the extent to which educational and emotional counseling is needed.

Present Status

Present status refers to the patient's current ability to manage self-care, including tracheal secretion management, discomfort associated with the surgery, and eating. Signs of postoperative depres-

sion may include passivity in regard to self-care. Referral for counseling should be discussed and acted upon as indicated.

Communication Needs

Vocational status can impact on motivation and thus on prognosis for the attainment of alaryngeal speech. Patients who plan to resume careers have communication needs that must be addressed. Retired patients also have social and personal communication requirements and activities they may wish to resume. The degree to which verbal communication is important to the patient is a crucial factor in helping the patient develop one or more forms of alaryngeal speech.

Family status may also affect the type of alaryngeal speech best suited to the individual. The degree of self-sufficiency required of the patient may influence communication options. For example, patients considering TEP may require some assistance inserting the prosthesis or securing the device. Such assistance would necessitate the availability of a supportive living companion. Patients living alone may prefer to become proficient electrolarynx users so they are confident in their ability to readily communicate with others by phone or face-to-face without assistance from others.

Beyond the Case History

Assessment of the peripheral oral mechanism is of particular importance. Dentition may be lost as a result of radiation therapy and tissue shrinkage may also occur. Patients may need to be fitted with dentures or may be in the process of adjusting to dentures. Lingual strength and mobility are also crucial to articulation clarity and the ability to inject air into the esophagus. Both skills should be assessed.

All forms of alaryngeal speech should be discussed, demonstrated, and/or described. As individuals may acquire esophageal speech at different rates, an individual's potential for development of esophageal speech may not be readily apparent. Therefore, the patient should be reassured if initial attempts at air injection are unsuccessful. Conversely, the patient who shows initial success insufflating the esophagus may not develop functional esophageal speech.

At the end of the evaluation, the patient should be given some printed material about postlaryngectomy rehabilitation, self-care, and alaryngeal speech options to reinforce information that was presented verbally. A treatment schedule should also be confirmed at this time.

SUMMARY

Living with a laryngectomy presents many challenges—some physical, some emotional. Fortunately, many laryngectomized individuals are successful in meeting these challenges. The speech–language pathologist plays a key role in the rehabilitation process by facilitating the acquisition of alaryngeal speech. Enhanced communication may result in the retention of self-esteem, decreased feelings of isolation, and may speed the rehabilitative process. The speech–language pathologist who chooses to work with this population must be a skilled instructor and a well-informed, sensitive practitioner. A suggested list of do's and don'ts is provided in Table 12.2. These may be

helpful when interacting with a laryngectomized person.

Major Points of Chapter

- Recent medical advances have resulted in improved long-term survival rates in people with laryngeal cancer.
- The type and extent of laryngeal cancer determines the appropriate surgical technique.
- There are surgical and nonsurgical options for the treatment of laryngeal cancer.
- Medical status and social and communicative needs are among the critical factors influencing postlaryngecomy rehabilitation.
- The rehabilitation process includes preoperative and postoperative consultations with the patient and rehabilitation team.
- Postlaryngectomy rehabilitation includes artificial larynx, esophageal, and tracheoesophageal speech options.

Discussion Guidelines

1. Discuss the medical and psychosocial factors that may impact on a patient's decision whether or not to undergo a tracheoesophageal puncture one year following total laryngectomy.

TABLE 12.2   Suggestions for Interacting with a Laryngectomized Speaker

DON'Ts
DON'T raise your voice to a laryngectomized individuals unless you know they are deaf. (Many are not.)
DON'T talk down to them or treat them like children. (They're not.)
DON'T make assumptions about them. (Find out what they feel.)
DON'T put words in their mouths. (Do your best to understand what they are saying.)
DON'T be negative about their efforts. (They're too good at that themselves.)
DON'T expect too much (or too little) of them. (Find out where each person is.)

DOs
DO relate to laryngectomized individuals as individuals and learn their strengths.
DO make sure you know their limitations and try to imagine how they feel.
DO show them respect and your desire to understand.
DO look directly at them when they speak and watch their lips.
DO ask them to repeat when you don't understand what they say.
DO treat them as dignified adults with intact intelligence.

2. Compare and contrast the anatomical, physiological, perceptual, and acoustic characteristics of esophageal speech and tracheoesophageal speech.

3. Describe the purpose of the preoperative consultation. What information should be provided to the patient, and what information should a speech–language pathologist learn about the patient?

REFERENCES

American Cancer Society. (1990). *Cancer facts and figures—1990.* American Cancer Society, Atlanta, GA.

American Cancer Society (1994). *Cancer facts and figures-1994.* Atlanta, GA.

Bailey, B. J. (1985). Glottic carcinoma. In B. J. Bailey & H. F. Biller (Eds.), *Surgery of the larynx* (pp. 257–278). Philadelphia: W. B. Saunders.

Bennett, S., & Weinberg, B. (1973). Acceptability ratings of normal, esophageal, and artificial larynx speech. *Journal of Speech and Hearing Research, 16,* 608–615.

Bisi, R. H., & Conley, J. J. (1965). Psychologic factors influencing vocal rehabilitation of the postlaryngectomy patient. *Annals of Otology, Rhinology, and Laryngology, 74,* 1073–1078.

Blanchard, S. L. (1982). Current practices in the counseling of the laryngectomy patient. *Journal of Communication Disorders, 15,* 233–241.

Blom, E. D., Singer, M. I., & Hamaker, R. C. (1985). An improved esophageal insufflation test. *Archives of Otolaryngology, 111,* 211–212.

Brady, L. W., & Davis, L. W. (1988). Treatment of head and neck cancer by radiation therapy. *Seminars in Oncology, 15,* 29–38.

Byrne, J., Kessler, L. G., & Devesa, S. S. (1992). The prevalence of larnygeal cancer among adults in the United States: 1987. *Cancer, 69,* 2154–2159.

Calcaterra, T. C., & Jafek, B. W. (1971). Tracheo-esophageal shunt for speech rehabilitation after total laryngectomy. *Archives of Otolaryngology, 94,* 124–128.

Casper, J., & Colton, R. H. (1993). *Clinical manual for laryngectomy and head/neck cancer rehabilitation.* San Diego: Singular Publishing Group.

Clark, J. G., & Stemple, J. C. (1982). Assessment of three methods of alaryngeal speech with a synthetic sentence identification (SSI) test in varying message-to-competition ratios. *Journal of Speech and Hearing Research, 25,* 333–338.

Conley, J. J., DeAmesti, F., & Pierce, M. D. (1958). A new surgical technique for the vocal rehabilitation of the laryngectomized patient. *Annals of Otology, Rhinology, and Laryngology, 67,* 655–664.

Curry, E. T., Snidecor, J. C., & Isshiki, N. (1973). Fundamental frequency characteristics of Japanese Asai speakers. *Laryngoscope, 83,* 1759–1763.

Damste, P. H. (1979). Some obstacles in learning esophageal speech. In R. L. Keith & F. L. Darley (Eds.). *Laryngectomee rehabilitation* (pp. 49–61). San Diego: College Hill Press.

Daniloff, R., Schuckers, G., & Feth, L. (1980). *The physiology of speech and hearing: An introduction.* Englewood Cliffs, NJ: Prentice-Hall.

Davis, P. (1981). Rehabilitation after total laryngectomy. *Medical Journal of Australia, 1,* 396–400.

DeSanto, L. W., Pearson, B. W., & Olsen, K. D. (1989). Utility of neartotal laryngectomy for supraglottic pharyngeal, base of tongue, and other cancers. *Annals of Otology, Rhinology and Laryngology, 98,* 2–7.

Dickens, W. J., Cassisi, N.J., Million, R. R., & Boa, F. J. (1983). Treatment of early vocal cord carcinoma: A comparison of apples and apples. *Laryngoscope, 93,* 216–219.

Diedrich, W. M., & Youngstrom, K. A. (1966). *Alaryngeal speech.* Springfield, IL: Charles C. Thomas.

Doyle, P. C. (1994). *Foundations of voice and speech rehabilitation following laryngeal cancer.* San Diego, CA: Singular Publishing Group, Inc.

Duguay, M. J. (1991). Esophageal speech training: The initial phase. In S. J. Salmon & K. H. Mount (Eds.). *Alaryngeal speech rehabilitation* (pp. 47–78). Austin, TX: Pro-Ed.

Gandour, J., & Weinberg, B. (1983). Perception of intonational contrasts in alaryngeal speech. *Journal of Speech and Hearing Research, 26,* 142–148.

Gandour, J., Weinberg, B., & Garzione, B. (1983). Perception of lexical stress in alaryngeal speech. *Journal of Speech and Hearing Research, 26,* 418–424.

Gardner, W. H. (1961). Problems of laryngectomees. *Rehabilitation Record, 2,* 15–19.

Gardner, W. H. (1966). Adjustment problems of laryngectomized women. *Archives of Otolaryngology, 83,* 31–42.

Gates, G. A., Ryan, W., Cantu, E., & Hearne, E. (1982). Current status of laryngectomee rehabilitation: II.

Causes of failure. *American Journal of Otolaryngology, 3,* 8–14.

Gates, G. A., Ryan, W., & Lauder, E. (1982). Current status of laryngectomee rehabilitation: IV. Attitudes about laryngectomee rehabilitation should change. *American Journal of Otolaryngology, 3,* 97–103.

Gilmore, S. I. (1961). Rehabilitation after laryngectomy. *American Journal of Nursing, 61,* 86–89.

Hoops, H. R., & Noll, J. D. (1969). Relationship of selected acoustic variables to judgments of esophageal speech. *Journal of Communication Disorders, 2,* 1–13.

Hunt, R. B. (1964). Rehabilitation of the laryngectomee. *Laryngoscope, 74,* 382–395.

Isshiki, N., & Snidecor, J. C. (1965). Air intake and usage in esophageal speech. *Acta Otolaryngologica, 59,* 559–574.

Keith, R. L., & Darley, F. L. (1986). *Laryngectomee rehabilitation* (2nd ed.). Austin, TX: Pro-Ed.

King, P. S., Fowlks, E. W., & Pierson, G. A. (1968). Rehabilitation and adaptation of laryngectomy patients. *American Journal of Physical Medicine, 47,* 192–203.

Kirschner, J. A., Scatliff, J., Dey, F. L., & Shedd, D. P. (1963). The pharynx after laryngectomy. *Laryngoscope, 73,* 18–33.

Lawson, W., Biller, H. F., & Suen, J. Y. (1989). Cancer of the larynx. In E. N. Myers & J. Y., Suen, *Cancer of the head and neck* (2nd ed.). New York: Churchill Livingstone.

Lerman, J. W. (1991). The artificial larynx. In S. J. Salmon & K. H. Mount (Eds.). *Alaryngeal speech rehabilitation for clinicians by clinicians.* (pp. 27–46). Austin, TX: Pro-Ed.

McHenry, M., Reich, A., & Minifii, F. (1982). Acoustic characteristics of intended syllabic stress in excellent esophageal speakers. *Journal of Speech and Hearing Research, 25,* 554–564.

Neel, H. B., Devine, K. D., & DeSanto, L. W. (1980). Laryngofissure and cordectomy for early cordal carcinoma: Outcome in 182 patients. *Otolaryngology—Head and Neck Surgery, 88,* 79–84.

Pearson, B. W. (1986). Office examination of the laryngectomee. In R. L. Keith & F. L. Darley (Eds.), *Laryngectomy rehabilitation,* (pp. 253–262). San Diego: College Hill Press.

Pearson, B. W., Woods, R. D., & Hartman, D. E. (1980). Extended hemilaryngectomy for T3 glottic carinoma with preservation of speech and swallowing. *Laryngoscope, 90,* 1950–1961.

Pressman, J. J. (1956). Submucosal compartmentalization of the larynx. *Annals of Otology, Rhinology, and Laryngology, 65,* 766–773.

Ries, L. A., Hankey, B. F., & Edwards, B. K. (Eds.). (1990). *Cancer Statistics Review, 1973–1987.* (NIH Publication No. 90—2789). National Cancer Institute, Bethesda, MD.

Robbins, J. (1984). Acoustic differentiation of laryngeal, esophageal, and tracheoesophageal speech production. *Journal of Speech and Hearing Disorders, 49,* 202–210.

Robbins, J. A., Fisher, H. B., Blom, E. D., & Singer, M. L. (1984). A comparative acoustic study of normal, esophageal, and tracheoesophageal speech production. *Journal of Speech and Hearing Disorders, 49,* 202–210.

Robin, P. E., Powell, J., Holme, G. M., Waterhouse, J. A. H., McConkey, C. C., & Robertson, J. E. (1989). *Cancer of the larynx: Clinical cancer monograph, Volume 2.* London: MacMillan Press.

Rosenberg, P. J. (1971). Total laryngectomy and cancer of the larynx. *Archives of Otolaryngology, 94,* 313–316.

Salmon, S. J. (1986a). Pre and postoperative conferences with the laryngectomized and their spouses. In R. L. Keith & F. L. Darley (Eds.). *Laryngectomy rehabilitation,* (pp. 277–290). San Diego: College Hill Press.

Salmon, S. J. (1986b). Factors that may interfere with esophageal speech, In R. L. Keith and F. L. Darley (Eds.). *Laryngectomy rehabilitation,* (pp. 357–364) San Diego: College Hill Press.

Sedory, S. E., Hamlet, S. L., & O'Connor, N. P. (1989). Comparisons of perceptual and acoustic characteristics of tracheoesophageal and excellent esophageal speech. *Journal of Speech and Hearing Disorders, 54,* 209–214.

Shames, G. H., Font, J., & Matthews, J. (1963). Factors related to speech proficiency of the laryngectomized. *Journal of Speech and Hearing Research, 28,* 273–278.

Shipp, T. (1967). Frequency, duration and perceptual measures in relation to judgment of alaryngeal speech acceptability. *Journal of Speech and Hearing Research, 10,* 417–427.

Shipp, T. (1970). EMG of pharyngoesophageal musculature during alaryngeal voice production. *Journal of Speech and Hearing Research, 13,* 184–192.

Silver, C. E. (1981). *Surgery for cancer of the larynx and related structures.* New York: Churchill-Livingston.

Singer, M. I., & Blom, E. D. (1980). An endoscopic technique for restoration of voice after laryngectomy. *Annals of Otology, Rhinology and Laryngology, 89,* 529–533.

Slavin, D., & Ferrand, C. T. (1995). Acoustic characteristics of proficient esophageal voice: Toward a multidimensional model. *Journal of Speech and Hearing Research, 38,* 467–478.

Snidecor, J. C., & Curry, E. T. (1959). Temporal and pitch aspects of superior esophageal speech. *Annals of Otology, Rhinology, and Laryngology, 68,* 1–14.

Snidecor, J. C., & Curry, E. T. (1960). How effectively can the laryngectomee expect to speak? *Laryngoscope, 70,* 62–67.

Spofford, B., Jafek, B., & Barcz, D. (1984). An improved method for creating tracheoesophageal fistulas for Blom-Singer or Panje voice prostheses. *Laryngoscope, 94,* 257–258.

Stewart, I. A., & Sherwen, P. J. (1987). Trachoesophageal puncture simplified. *Laryngoscope, 97,* 639–640.

Stoll, B. (1958). Psychological factors determining the success or failure of the rehabilitation program of laryngectomized patients. *Annals of Otology, Rhinology, and Laryngology, 67,* 550–557.

Taub, S., & Bergner, L. H. (1973). Air bypass voice prosthesis for vocal rehabilitation of laryngectomees. *American Journal of Surgery, 125,* 748–756.

Trudeau, M. D. (1987). A comparison of the speech acceptability of good and excellent esophageal and tracheoesophageal speakers. *Journal of Communication Disorders, 20,* 41–49.

Union Internationale Contre le Cancer (UICC). (1987). *Manual of clinical oncology.* Berlin: Springer-Verlag.

Ward, P. H. (1988). Complications of laryngeal surgery: etilogy and prevention. *Laryngoscope, 98,* 54–57.

Weinberg, B., & Bennett, S. (1971). A study of talker sex recognition of esophageal voices. *Journal of Speech and Hearing Research, 14,* 391–395.

Weinberg, B., & Bennett, S. (1972). Selected acoustic characteristics of esophageal speech produced by female laryngectomees. *Journal of Speech and Hearing Research, 15,* 211–216.

Weinberg, B., Horii, Y., Blom, E. D., & Singer, M. I. (1982). Airway resistance during esophageal phonation. *Journal of Speech and Hearing Disorders, 47,* 194–199.

Weinberg, B., Horii, Y., & Smith, B. E. (1980). Long time spectral and intensity characteristics of esophageal speech. *Journal of the Acoustical Society of America, 67,* 1781–1784.

Weinberg, B., & Moon, J. (1984)). Aerodynamic properties of four tracheoesophageal puncture prostheses. *Archives of Otolaryngology, 110,* 673–675.

Weinberg, B., Shedd, D. P., & Horii, Y. (1978). Reed-fistula speech following pharyngolaryngectomy. *Journal of Speech and Hearing Disorders, 43,* 401–403.

Weiss, M. S., & Basili, A. G. (1985). Electrolaryngeal speech produced by laryngectomized subjects: Perceptual characteristics. *Journal of Speech and Hearing Research, 28,* 294–300.

Welch, R. W., Gates, G. A., Luckmann, K. F., Ricks, P. M., & Drake, S. T. (1979). Change in the force-summed pressure measurements of the upper esophageal sphincter prelaryngectomy and postlaryngectomy. *Annals of Otolaryngology, 88,* 804–808.

Winans, C. S., Reichback, E. J., & Waldrop, W. F. (1974). Esophageal determinants of alaryngeal speech. *Archives of Otolaryngology, 99,* 10–14.

Wynder, E. L., Covey, L. S., Marbuchi, K., Johnson, J., & Muschinsky, M. (1976). Environmental factors in cancer of the larynx, a second look. *Cancer, 38,* 1591–1601.

Zemlin, W. R. (1988). *Speech and hearing science: Anatomy and physiology.* (3rd ed.) Englewood Cliffs, NJ: Prentice-Hall.

13

SPASMODIC DYSPHONIA

CELIA F. STEWART, MITCHELL F. BRIN, AND ANDREW BLITZER

Spasmodic dysphonia is a rare voice disorder that starts when patients are in early adulthood (Aronson, Brown, Litin, & Pearson, 1968a; Brin, Fahn, Blitzer, Ramig, & Stewart, 1992). Unlike other voice disorders, the symptoms of spasmodic dysphonia usually disappear when patients sustain vowels, cough, clear their throats, yawn, sigh, laugh, or sing. The structure of the larynx is normal. There are two types of spasmodic dysphonia: **adductor** and **abductor** (Aronson, 1985). Adductor is the more common form. With **adductor spasmodic dysphonia,** the voice is produced with increased **expiratory effort** and the prominent vocal symptoms are a **strained-strangled,** rough voice quality with sudden intermittent **voice arrests** and decreased loudness. **Abductor spasmodic dysphonia** is characterized by a breathy or whispered voice quality with sudden intermittent voice arrests and a rough voice quality. Some patients with abductor spasmodic dysphonia hyperventilate when they talk or speak on both **inspiration** and expiration.

Clinical management of individuals with spasmodic dysphonia may be challenging. Izdebski and Dedo (1981) stated that "any patient with voice problems suggestive of spasmodic dysphonia may present a diagnostically difficult task be-cause diagnosis must be based on symptoms alone" (p. 1090). Characteristics to be taken into account in confirming the diagnosis include assessment of the perceptual and acoustic speech symptoms, review of the case history, visualization of the laryngeal structures, and assessment of neurological control of movement of the body. No one professional can be responsible for all these evaluations. Therefore, diagnosis of spasmodic dysphonia requires a team of professionals including a speech–language pathologist, an otolaryngologist, and a neurologist. Each member of the team brings a unique perspective to the evaluation and treatment. The synergetic effect of the different perspectives enables the patient to have a thorough evaluation and ensures that appropriate therapy is provided. The role of the speech–language pathologist is to assess the presence or absence of **dysphonia,** to identify the severity of the dysphonia, to take part in planning treatment, to provide voice therapy if it is appropriate, and to educate the patient about the disorder and its treatment.

This chapter presents information that will develop an understanding of the nature and treatment of spasmodic dysphonia. The chapter is divided into three sections. The first section describes changes in theory and practice over the past 120 years, including psychological and neurological models of etiology. The second section delineates the onset, voice, and **vocal fold** characteristics that are unique to spasmodic dysphonia. The third section examines methods to use when evaluating and rehabilitating patients with spasmodic dysphonia.

HISTORICAL PERSPECTIVE

Spasmodic dysphonia was first identified by Traube in 1871 in a brief case study of a woman described as having a "spastic form of nervous hoarseness" (translated by Schaefer & Freeman, 1987, p. 162). The woman was reported to speak with increased effort and a rough voice quality. She intermittently produced falsetto voice. Traube described the vocal folds as closing spastically, with one fold overlapping the other. He attributed the voice disorder to nervousness but no evidence was given to confirm that the voice disorder was psychogenic. Traube's explanation appears to have been the catalyst for identifying spasmodic dysphonia as a psychogenic disorder.

In contrast, Schnitzler (1875, translated by Schaefer & Freeman, 1987) named the disorder *aphonia spastica* and described two patients who had symptoms of "cramping of the vocal cords and forced voice" (page 162). In addition, Schnitzler reported that involuntary movements occurred in the face, arms, and legs during speech. Schnitzler attributed the voice disorder and other involuntary movements to a physical cause. The contrasting perspectives of Traube and Schnitzler began the ongoing debate about the underlying etiology of spasmodic dysphonia.

Over the past 120 years spasmodic dysphonia has been given at least 11 different names. (See Table 13.1) The name changes when new theories about the cause of the disorder are developed or when new symptoms are discovered. The term *spasmodic* is used because "the neurologic evidence . . . is chiefly in the extrapyramidal realm. It is also our observation that the strained voice quality in this disorder waxes and wanes from

TABLE 13.1 Names for Spasmodic Dysphonia

NAME	AUTHOR
nervous hoarseness	Traube 1871
spastic dysphonia	Schnitzler 1875
coordinated laryngeal spasm	Nothnagels 1896
mogiphonia	Fraenkel 1887
lalophobia	Coen 1886
psychophonasthenia	Greene 1938
inspiratory speech	Critchley 1939
stuttering with the vocal cords	Bellussi 1952
hysterical aphonia	Maximov 1961
spasmodic dysphonia	Aronson et al. 1968b
focal laryngeal dystonia	Blitzer & Brin 1986

moment to moment in a spasmodic fashion" (Aronson, Brown, Litin, & Pearson, 1968b). Consequently, the most commonly used name currently is spasmodic dysphonia. The newest name is **focal laryngeal dystonia.** This name reflects the understanding that most cases of spasmodic dysphonia are a focal **dystonia** resulting from impairment to the central nervous system (Blitzer, Brin, Fahn, & Lovelace, 1988). The involuntary movements of the vocal folds are believed to be elicited by the action of speaking.

PSYCHOGENIC PERSPECTIVE

Historically, physicians believed that spasmodic dysphonia was psychogenic, caused by psychological factors that were untreatable. The term *psychogenic* has been defined as a disorder "originating in the mind or in mental or emotional conflict" (Nicolosi, Harryman & Kresheck, 1983, p. 193). Aronson (1990) noted that psychogenic disorders "exist in the absence of organic laryngeal pathology" (p. 120) and occur either during a prolonged period of stress or after a stressful event. Psychogenic voice disorders affect women more frequently than men (Aronson, Peterson, & Litin, 1960; Butcher, Elias, Raven, & Yeatman, 1987, Greene & Mathieson, 1989). Aronson,

Brown, Litin and Pearson (1968b) described four types of psychogenic voice symptoms: (1) patient is mute and does not move the articulators, (2) patient whispers and has normal articulation, (3) patient has an intermittent breathy voice quality, and (4) patient has a consistent voice disorder. Patients with spasmodic dysphonia may show the voice symptoms described in types 2, 3, and 4.

The symptoms of neurogenic and psychogenic voice disorders are similar. Both psychological and neurological voice symptoms may appear bizarre and may be mimicked by individuals who do not have the disorder. For example, an individual with spasmodic dysphonia can produce a clear voice on short responses such as *Hi* or *No,* yet have strangled or breathy voice in connected speech. Consequently, identifying a symptom as either neurogenic or psychogenic depends on looking at the onset and course of the development of the disorder, the pattern of all speech symptoms, the consistency with which the symptoms are produced, the response to therapy, and the structure and function of the larynx.

Determining if a "sign or symptom is psychogenic is usually based on indirect, circumstantial, and impressionistic evidence" (Aronson, et al., 1968b, p. 168). Voice disorders that appear after an important life change such as a traumatic event, an illness, a change in the job, or the death of a loved one, have been attributed to psychological problems (Aronson, 1985; Brodnitz, 1976; Heaver, 1959; Rabuzzi & McCall, 1972). However, life for adults is full of anxiety-producing events—loved ones develop cancer, people lose their jobs, and so on. If these kinds of events were necessary and sufficient to cause spasmodic dysphonia, there would be an epidemic. However, spasmodic dysphonia remains a rare disorder.

Some psychogenic voice disorders develop suddenly after an illness such as a cold, laryngitis, or flu (Aronson, et al., 1968b). Spasmodic dysphonia has two patterns of onset. The more common pattern occurs when spasmodic dysphonia develops slowly and worsens over time. The less common pattern occurs when the disorder develops abruptly. Both patterns of onset also occur

with neurological disorders. Dysarthrias that result from a stroke have an abrupt onset and dysarthrias that result from a progressive neurological disease develop slowly. Consequently, the speed of onset does not necessarily suggest whether a disorder has a psychogenic or neurogenic cause.

If the voice problem allows patients to gain socially acceptable reasons for not fulfilling their social obligations or vocational roles, then it is suspected to have a psychogenic component (Heaver, 1959). Consequently, it is important to learn if changes in status accompanied the onset of spasmodic dysphonia. If the patient "gains" in some way by having a voice disorder, it is possible that the disorder may be attributed to a psychogenic cause. However, patients who have spasmodic dysphonia often report that the disorder makes it difficult for them to talk and as a result they talk less and feel isolated. Isolation may be a social or vocational gain for some individuals, but most people continue to work in spite of their disability.

A psychogenic cause is suspected when patients' affect does not match the attitude expressed in their words. If a patient smiles when telling about the disorder or has a flat facial expression, then the cause of the disorder may be hypothesized to be psychological. Persons with spasmodic dysphonia generally have appropriate affect. At times, an individual with spasmodic dysphonia will exert force to produce voice and generate extraneous muscle activity in the face, neck, shoulders, or chest. This extraneous muscle activity may change facial expression and make the speaker appear angry or impatient. Therefore, a change in facial expression is not always a signal that the voice disorder is psychogenic.

Some researchers have speculated that if they see no pathology on the vocal folds, then the voice disorder must have a psychogenic cause (Heaver, 1959; Rabuzzi & McCall, 1972). This assumption ignores the fact that a laryngeal pathology may not be revealed under the conditions of the examination. If the examination is done in a different way, the pathology may be visible. If a patient with spasmodic dysphonia sustains vowels during a laryngeal examination, the larynx will typically appear normal. However, if the patient says connected meaningful utterances while the larynx is visualized, the laryngeal movements will be abnormal (Hartman & Vishwanat, 1984).

Voice disorders are frequently surmised to be caused by a psychological disorder if the severity of the voice disorder improves when the patient drinks alcohol. Many individuals with spasmodic dysphonia report that their voice improves when they drink alcohol (Aronson, et al., 1968b). Alcohol has psychological effects; it decreases inhibitions and helps the drinker feel friendlier and more gregarious. Some people use alcohol to relax, to stimulate their appetite, and to gain a mild sense of euphoria. On the other hand, alcohol also has another effect. It is a central nervous system depressant that acts like other tranquilizing and hypnotic drugs to depress the functions of the lungs and heart. Alcohol changes the way the brain functions and controls movement, including the movements of the vocal folds.

The lack of sustained improvement from therapy is cited as a classic symptom of psychogenic voice disorders (Aronson et al., 1968b; Heaver, 1959; Rabuzzi & McCall, 1972). Patients who have spasmodic dysphonia generally do not make sustained progress in voice therapy or psychotherapy (Segre 1951; Boone, 1971; Brodnitz, 1976; Izdebski & Dedo, 1981). However, another therapy is effective. When spasmodic dysphonia is treated with injections of **botulinum toxin** (BTX), most patients have sustained benefit. BTX is a neuromuscular treatment that "causes paralysis by blocking the presynaptic release of acetylcholine at the neuromuscular junction" (ANN, 1990, p. 2). Therefore, spasmodic dysphonia may be a neurological disorder.

NEUROGENIC PERSPECTIVE

Currently, the most widely held belief is that spasmodic dysphonia is a symptom of central nervous system impairment (Blitzer & Brin, 1991; Blitzer, Lovelace, Brin, Fahn, & Fink, 1985; Brin, Fahn, Blitzer, Ramig, & Stewart, 1992; Dedo, 1976; Robe, Brumlik, & Moore, 1960). It is classified as a "type of dystonia (laryngeal dystonia) that may present focally or in association with other dystonic movements" (Blitzer et al., 1985, p. 594). Brin et al. (1992) have noted that "dystonia is characterized by abnormal involuntary movements that are typically action-induced. In spasmodic dysphonia, the action is that of speaking" (p. 245).

Several types of evidence support the idea that dystonia is a neurological disorder of central motor control characterized by abnormal involuntary muscle contractions frequently resulting in inappropriate movements of the body. (See Chapter 8 for further discussion.) Dystonia can involve any voluntary muscle. When the individual is at rest, the anatomic structures appear normal. However, when the person performs a specific task such as speaking, involuntary movements emerge. Specific motor acts typically activate the dystonic movements. While these dystonic movements are usually slow, they may also be quick and repetitive, or jerky (Blitzer & Brin, 1991; Blitzer, Brin, Fahn, Lovelace, 1988; Brin, Blitzer, Fahn, Gould, & Lovelace, 1989; Brin et al., 1992).

Dystonia may affect muscles in the limbs, trunk, neck, and face. Dystonic movements may be restricted to one muscle group (focal dystonia); may involve a contiguous group of muscles, such as one or two limbs, or the neck and one limb (segmental dystonia); or may be widespread (generalized dystonia) (Blitzer & Brin, 1991; Brin, et al., 1992; Fahn, 1988). Dystonia usually begins as a **focal** disorder. If the dystonia begins in adulthood, it tends to remain in that one muscle group, but if the onset begins in childhood the dystonia can spread to other regions of the body (Marsden, 1991).

Examples of focal dystonia include uncontrolled eye blinking (blepharospasm), movements of the jaw, tongue, and mouth (oromandibular dystonia); spasms twisting the neck (spasmodic torticollis); and spasms of the hand and forearm during writing (graphospasm) (Blitzer & Brin, 1991,

Fahn, 1988). Meige's disease, a combination of blepharospasm and oromandibular dystonia, is an example of segmental dystonia because it involves two regions. Focal dystonic movements are usually observable only when a person performs a specific movement. For example, graphospasm is usually absent at rest, but may be activated by writing, typing, or playing a musical instrument; oromandibular dystonia may be elicited by speaking or eating. Like other types of dystonia, a skilled movement activates spasmodic dysphonia—the motor act of speaking. Vocal tasks like sustaining vowels, crying, moaning, singing, laughing, coughing, and yawning usually do not elicit the symptoms and so performance of non-speech sounds typically remains unimpaired (Arnold, 1959; Blitzer et al., 1988; Brodnitz, 1976).

Although spasmodic dysphonia typically occurs in isolation as a focal dystonia, other dystonic symptoms may accompany spasmodic dysphonia, resulting in multifocal, segmental, or generalized dystonia (Brin et al., 1989). Dystonic symptoms including Meige (Jacome & Yanez, 1980), blepharospasm (Aminoff, Dedo, & Izdebski, 1978; Brin et al., 1992), idiopathic torsion dystonia (Marsden & Sheehy, 1982), torticollis (Aronson, Brown, Litin, & Pearson, 1968a), and oromandib-

ular, graphospasm (Aminoff, Dedo, & Izdebski, 1978) are observed in about 25 percent of the patients with spasmodic dysphonia (Blitzer & Brin, 1990; Blitzer, et al., 1985).

Dystonia has both primary and secondary causes. Table 13.2 lists some primary and secondary causes. Primary dystonia is idiopathic, either with a hereditary pattern or without a hereditary pattern (Marsden, 1988). In families that have a hereditary pattern of dystonia, various relatives may have different types of focal, segmental, or generalized dystonia. Patients without a hereditary pattern have no evidence by history, examination, or lab studies of any identifiable cause for the dystonia. Secondary dystonia develops as a symptom of other neurological disorders, psychological disorders, or exposure to environmental causes such as trauma, infections, tumors, toxic chemicals, or medication (Brin et al., 1992). Primary dystonias are typically action-induced; symptoms are enhanced with use of the affected body part and usually improve or disappear when the action is not performed. By contrast, secondary dystonias may result in fixed postures of the affected muscles or in extensive dystonia limited to one side of the body (Brin et al., 1992).

TABLE 13.2 Causes of Dystonia

PRIMARY (IDIOPATHIC)	SECONDARY
Without a hereditary pattern (No identifiable cause)	Symptom of other neurologic syndromes (Wilson's Disease, Leigh's Disease, Huntingtons's Disease)
With a hereditary pattern	Environmental Cause (Head trauma, brain lesions, infection, brain tumor, multiple sclerosis, medications such as Phenothiazine, chemical toxins)
	Parkinsonism
	Psychogenic
	Pseudodystonia (Arnold Chiari Malformation, congenital muscular torticollis, and congenital postural torticollis)

Note: This table is modified from that presented by Fahn, 1988, Marsden, 1988, and Calne & Lang, 1988.

Dystonic movements of the vocal folds are activated by connected speech. Conversely, vocal fold movements are usually normal during non-speech sound production, such as sustaining vowels, laughing and coughing (Aronson et al., 1968a, Hartman & Vishwanat, 1984, McCall, Skolnick, & Brewer, 1971). During connected speech, the vocal folds approximate too closely and forcefully, or the false vocal folds close and obstruct the view of the true vocal folds. In some cases, the forceful closure may pull the arytenoid cartilages forward toward the pediole of the epiglottis.

No consistent pathological brain finding is associated with spasmodic dysphonia, but the organic basis of spasmodic dysphonia is supported by laboratory investigation. Some individuals with spasmodic dysphonia have delayed reaction times when initiating voicing. That is, if individuals who have spasmodic dysphonia are asked to say a word as soon as possible after hearing a tone, some will react more slowly and say the word later than individuals who do not have spasmodic dysphonia (Reich & Till, 1993). This delay in the initiation of words may be a mechanical response to the forceful contraction of the vocal folds. As expected, a similar delay is not observed when patients produce nonspeech sounds, including throat clearing or inspiratory **phonation** (Reich & Till, 1993). This prompt initiation is probably related to the normal movements of the vocal folds on nonspeech sounds.

Other laboratory tests support the idea that individuals with spasmodic dysphonia may have subtle impairments in central auditory processing. Some patients perform synthetic sentence identification with and without ipsilateral competing messages and staggered spondaic word tests with less accuracy than expected (Hall, 1981). Auditory brainstem response (ABR) evaluates retrocochlear function through evoked potentials and is used for site of lesion testing. ABR testing of some patients with spasmodic dysphonia has revealed abnormally large increments in wave five, prolonged inter-peak latencies, and increased amplitude on acoustic reflexes (Feldman, Nixon, Finitzo-Hieber, & Freeman, 1984; Finitzo-Hieber,

Freeman, Gerling, Dobson, & Schaefer, 1982; Hall, 1981; Schaefer, Finitzo-Hieber, Gerling, & Freeman, 1983). These differences may represent a subtle variation in central nervous system function. However, these differences are not usually observed clinically.

Some patients with spasmodic dysphonia have abnormal cephalic-gastric and cephalic-cardiac reflexes. The cephalic-gastric reflex occurs when stomach acid is secreted in reaction to seeing, smelling, tasting, chewing, or swallowing food, or in response to physical and chemical reactions in the stomach. Some patients with spasmodic dysphonia secrete a decreased amount of gastric acid in response to sham feedings (where subjects chew food for 30 minutes but do not swallow it) (Feldman et al., 1984; Schaefer, 1983). The cephalic-cardiac reflex occurs when a cold stimulus applied to the face causes a reflexive change in the heart rate. In some people with spasmodic dysphonia, fluctuations in heart rates are reduced from the level expected of normal individuals (Schaefer, 1983; Feldman et al., 1984). Schaefer (1983) hypothesized that some people with spasmodic dysphonia have problems at the level of the brainstem because both these reflexes are controlled at the level of the brainstem.

Developments in brain imaging have led to greater understanding of the function of the brain. Magnetic Resonance Imaging (MRI) produces computerized pictures of the brain using radio waves and magnetism. Brain Electrical Activity Mapping (BEAM) uses Electroencephalography (EEG) and evoked potential data to graphically display a transaxial section of the brain in real time. In BEAM, colors are used to identify active and inactive parts of the brain during various tasks. Single Photon Emission Computed Tomography (SPECT) is designed to measure functional changes such as regional blood flow, by detecting gamma ray emissions from intravenous injected radioisotopes. Finitzo and Freeman (1989) found 23 percent of their patients with spasmodic dysphonia had brain lesions when imaged with MRI, 56 percent had abnormal BEAM responses, and 76 percent had abnormal hypoperfusion on SPECT. These neurological differences support the argument for an organic basis for spasmodic dysphonia.

CHARACTERISTICS OF SPASMODIC DYSPHONIA

Spasmodic dysphonia is a rare voice disorder. The onset pattern, voice symptoms, and movements of the vocal folds are unlike those observed with organic structural modifications that influence voice. (See Chapter 11.) Because the patterns are unique to spasmodic dysphonia, the disorder appears unusual. Nevertheless, when one gains familiarity with the characteristics of spasmodic dysphonia, it is not difficult to identify.

Onset and Course of the Disorder

Spasmodic dysphonia affects men and women without warning. Blitzer and Brin (1990) reported that the clinical characteristics of spasmodic dysphonia and other types of dystonia are similar. They noted that "as with other forms of cranial dystonia, most patients present in adulthood" (p. 346). The average age of onset is 38 years (Blitzer & Brin, 1991). Nevertheless, the disorder can begin when individuals are as young as three years or as old as 85 years (Brin et al., 1992). Blitzer and Brin (1991) found that 58 percent of their patients were female. No geographic, environmental, or occupational pattern has been identified with the onset of spasmodic dysphonia (Izdebski & Dedo, 1981a). Although the etiology of spasmodic dysphonia is obscure, trauma, exposure to phenothiazine drugs, and a genetic predisposition have been identified as potential causes (Brin, et al., 1992; Gordon, Brin, Giladi, Hunt, & Fahn, 1990). The onset of spasmodic dysphonia has also been associated with head colds, flu, laryngitis, and upper respiratory infections (Aronson, Brown, Litin, & Pearson, 1968a; Robe, Brumlik, & Moore, 1960).

As discussed earlier, spasmodic dysphonia has two general patterns of development. The more common pattern occurs when the dysphonia begins as a mild, intermittent problem and gradually worsens over one to three years. The patient is frequently unaware of the exact date of the onset. Subsequently, the disorder becomes chronic and the **overall severity** reaches a plateau, but fluctuations continue in day-to-day and minute-to-minute severity. The second, less common pattern of development, occurs when a patient identifies an abrupt onset followed by a chronic voice disorder. The voice disorder may worsen or improve over time or may remain at the initial level of severity (Aronson et al., 1968a; Izdebski & Dedo, 1981b, 1984; Wolfe, Ratusnik, & Feldman, 1979). Once spasmodic dysphonia begins, the overall severity of the disorder may fluctuate but the disorder rarely resolves (Aronson et al., 1968a).

Voice, Speech, and Associated Somatic Symptoms

Speakers with spasmodic dysphonia describe their voices as a burden to both themselves and their listeners (Izdebski, Dedo, & Boles 1984). The voices sound unusual (strained–strangled or whispered) and may distract the listeners from paying attention to the content of the message. In addition, **speech intelligibility,** rate, and fluency are generally decreased (Aronson et al., 1968b; Bloch, Hirano, & Gould, 1985; Ludlow & Connor, 1987). The voice characteristics of spasmodic dysphonia are apparent during connected speech in the habitual pitch range, but are usually not apparent on isolated words or sounds (Izdebski & Dedo, 1981a). However, Segre (1951) and Robe et al. (1960) noted that when the condition is severe, voice symptoms such as a strained–strangled or breathy quality may occur even on isolated words and sounds.

The day-to-day or minute-to-minute fluctuations in severity may be mild or may be so severe that the voice is only mildly dysphonic at times and severely dysphonic at other times. The fluctuations may be random. When patients are aware of fluctuations, they cannot always identify the stimuli that ameliorate or aggravate the voice disorder. Nevertheless, symptoms are usually exacerbated by stressful situations such as talking on the telephone or to groups of people (Izdebski & Dedo, 1981b). Symptoms may also worsen when the speaker is ill, tense, or fatigued. Some patients have brief periods of improved or normal phonation when they first wake up in the morning, speak to a physician, or feel anger, joy, or alcoholic intoxication (Aronson et al., 1968b; Izdebski & Dedo, 1981a; Segre, 1951). Voice production is generally normal when speakers perform nonspeech tasks such as laughing, shouting, whispering, singing, yawning, sighing, coughing, sustaining vowels, producing falsetto, or clearing their throats (Arnold, 1959; Aronson et al., 1968a; Bloch et al., 1985; Finitzo & Freeman, 1989, Izdebski & Dedo, 1981a, Ludlow & Connor, 1987). In addition, speakers with spasmodic dysphonia generally produce segments of normal voice during short responses (Bloch et al., 1985, Brodnitz, 1976). This pattern of improvement is not typically seen with other types of organic structural modifications that influence voice.

Another disabling symptom of spasmodic dysphonia is increased effort (Aronson et al., 1968a). Patients feel effort in their articulators, strangulation, burning in their throats, and tightness across their chests and abdomens when speaking. The level of effort becomes more normal during nonspeech tasks such as sustaining vowels in falsetto, laughing, and singing (Aronson et al., 1968b). If an unreasonable amount of physical exertion is required to speak, people may smile or nod to avoid speaking.

Most patients try to find a way to improve their voice quality or to reduce effort, such as speaking on inhalation, speaking quietly, or laughing (Bloch et al., 1985; Robe et al., 1960; Sapir & Aronson, 1985). Some people attempt to increase speech intelligibility by speaking slowly (Aronson et al., 1968a; Bloch, 1965; Bloch et al., 1985; Ludlow & Connor, 1987; Robe et al., 1960). Nevertheless, these compensatory techniques offer only partial, temporary relief and are not adequate for conversational speech.

Classifications of Spasmodic Dysphonia (SD)

There are three classifications of spasmodic dysphonia: adductor, abductor, and mixed (Aronson, 1985).

Adductor SD. Adductor spasmodic dysphonia is most common, occurring in approximately 84 percent of speakers with spasmodic dysphonia (Blitzer & Brin, 1991). Speakers with adductor spasmodic dysphonia have increased expiratory effort or struggle during connected speech, and a choked, rough, strained–strangled voice quality. Abrupt initiation and termination of voice results in intermittent **aphonia,** voice breaks of varying length in vowels, staccato stutter-like **phonatory** blocks, and delayed phonation onset (Aronson et al., 1968a; Bloch, Hirano, & Gould, 1985; Ludlow & Connor, 1987; Robe et al., 1960; Sapir & Aronson, 1985). Vocal tremors (oscillatory types of movements) occur frequently and are characterized perceptually as a quavering voice quality that may make the patient sound old (Aronson et al., 1968a; Bloch, 1965; Bloch et al., 1985; Finitzo & Freeman, 1989; Rabuzzi & McCall, 1972). Individuals with adductor spasmodic dysphonia may speak with limited loudness, monopitch, monoloudness, altered inflection patterns, and intermittent bursts of loudness (Arnold, 1959; Aronson et al., 1968a; Bloch, 1965; Bloch et al., 1985; Brodnitz, 1976; Ludlow & Connor, 1987; Robe et al., 1960; Sapir & Aronson, 1985). Some patients strain so severely to produce voice that nonspeech sounds such as grunts and groans are produced involuntarily (Bloch et al., 1985; Brodnitz, 1976; Ludlow & Connor, 1987).

Abductor SD. Abductor spasmodic dysphonia has been called the antithesis of adductor spasmodic dysphonia (Zwitman, 1979). Patients with abductor spasmodic dysphonia exhibit a normal or breathy voice quality interrupted by abrupt termination of voicing (Aronson, 1985; Brin et al., 1992, Blitzer & Stewart, 1993; Wolfe & Bacon, 1976). These abrupt voice terminations are triggered by voiceless consonants and result in effortful aphonic whispered segments of speech (Aronson, 1985) and brief periods of silence between initial consonants and adjacent vowels (Zwitman, 1979). These speakers frequently have vocal tremor and reduced overall speech intelligibility (Aronson, 1985). In addition, patients have difficulty increasing the loudness of their voices and may be misunderstood in noise (Zwitman, 1979). When patients push large quantities of air through their vocal tracts in an attempt to produce voice, they may hyperventilate and feel dizzy and lightheaded.

Mixed SD.   When patients have a combination of adductor and abductor symptoms, they display the third classification, mixed spasmodic dysphonia. Speakers with mixed spasmodic dysphonia have a mixture of strained–strangled, rough sounds, and breathy breaks (Cannito & Johnson, 1981). The characteristics of the mixed type lie along a continuum with some patients having predominately adductor symptoms and others with predominantly abductor symptoms.

At times individuals with spasmodic dysphonia will overcompensate for their voice symptoms, making it difficult to determine if they have adductor or abductor spasmodic dysphonia. For instance, speakers with adductor spasmodic dysphonia may consciously produce breathy or whispered voices to ease the strong adductor contractions of their vocal folds. The opposite compensation occurs when patients with abductor spasmodic dysphonia use increased effort to constrict the laryngeal area, thus increasing expiratory drive and producing strained voices. Because of these compensatory techniques, diagnosis of the particular type of spasmodic dysphonia may be difficult.

Vocal Fold Effects

During optimal phonation, exhalation is initiated and the true vocal folds are stiffened and adducted by the intrinsic laryngeal muscles to a **phonation-neutral** position (the vocal folds are adducted closely enough to vibrate but the **glottis** remains slightly open) (Lieberman, 1968). Air passes between the vocal folds, and the vocal folds move toward the **midline** due to a slight negative pressure created by the air passing through the narrow opening. The vocal folds are sucked together, closing the glottis and blocking the airway. As air pressure builds up below the vocal folds, the vocal folds are blown apart. The elastic recoil of the vocal folds and the suction created by the air moving between them bring the vocal folds back together (Liebermann, 1968, Zemlin, 1988). Phonation results from the rapid vibration of the vocal folds. (See Chapter 11.) During optimal phonation the **ventricular vocal folds** are not adducted (Liebermann, 1968; Zemlin, 1988), but during disordered phonation, the pattern of vibration may be altered in various ways.

The vocal folds may be inspected by holding the patient's tongue, placing a laryngeal mirror in the back of the patient's mouth, and then having the patient breathe quietly or say a sustained vowel. This method of observation, known as *indirect laryngoscopy,* is used for structural assessment of the vocal folds during **respiration** without phonation and during production of sustained vowels. Connected speech cannot be assessed with indirect laryngoscopy because people cannot talk when a mirror is in the back of their mouths (Arnold, 1959; Dedo, 1976). Individuals with spasmodic dysphonia generally produce sustained vowels without difficulty. Consequently, when the vocal folds of speakers with spasmodic dysphonia are viewed by indirect laryngoscopy, they often appear normal (Arnold, 1959; Dedo, 1976; Robe et al., 1960; Segre, 1951).

In order to view the vocal folds during connected speech, a flexible fiber-optic tube is inserted through the nose and positioned above the vocal folds. The image can be projected onto a television screen and videotaped. This procedure is called *flexible fiber-optic laryngoscopy.* Since the instrument is inserted through the nose and does not block the mouth, the patient can speak in sentences, sing, or sustain vowels during the evaluation. Flexible fiber-optic laryngoscopy in speakers with adductor spasmodic dysphonia has revealed adductor spasmodic movements of the true vocal folds and forceful adduction of the ventricular folds over the true vocal folds during speech (Parnes, Lavorato, & Myers, 1978). Aronson et al. (1968a) noted that "during spasms the ligamentous portions of the vocal folds at times are squeezed together so tightly that no line may be observed separating them. In many instances the ventricular or false vocal folds adduct and obscure the true vocal folds" (p. 204). These movements occur when patients produce connected speech and are usually absent on nonspeech tasks.

On the other hand, flexible fiber-optic laryngoscopy has revealed abrupt **glottal** widening during speech in speakers with abductor spasmodic dysphonia (Aronson, 1985; Parnes, Lavorato, & Myers, 1978; Woodson, Zwirner, & Murray, 1991). In these speakers, the vocal folds may adduct before phonation and then abruptly abduct during speech (Hartman & Vishwanat, 1984). The abrupt abduction of the vocal folds corresponds to aphonic segments of speech.

DIAGNOSIS AND TREATMENT

The diagnosis of spasmodic dysphonia may be difficult because there are no laboratory tests that are specific for the disorder. Diagnosis is based upon the clinical phenomenology and the exclusion of other disorders through a process of elimination. Spasmodic dysphonia is rare; practitioners may see only a few cases in their lifetime. Therefore, professionals may be unfamiliar with spasmodic dysphonia. Patients often see many specialists before they are accurately diagnosed (Aronson et al., 1968b; Segre, 1951). Consequently, spasmodic dysphonia is frequently misdiagnosed as "laryngitis, sinusitis, allergic rhinitis, multiple sclerosis, myasthenia gravis, Parkinson's disease, vocal abuse, and bronchial or tracheal infections" (ASHA, 1993b).

Evaluation

Evaluation and treatment of spasmodic dysphonia "requires the involvement of an interdisciplinary team, including an otolaryngologist, a speech–

language pathologist, a neurologist, and a physician skilled in regional electromyography" (ANN, 1990, p. 9). Other team members such as a geneticist, family physician, and radiologist may be helpful. These professionals bring their own unique perspective and knowledge to the evaluation in order to ensure that accurate diagnosis is made and that appropriate therapy is offered.

The speech–language pathologist performs an assessment "to diagnose a voice disorder, describe perceptual phonatory characteristics, measure aspects of vocal function, and examine phonatory behavior. Assessment may result in recommendations for treatment or follow-up, or in referral for other examinations or services" (ASHA, 1993a, p 69). Speech–language pathologists base their diagnosis of spasmodic dysphonia on the individual's history, perceptual symptoms, and ability to modify voice production. In addition, assessment of hearing acuity, articulation, fluency, language, and swallowing skills, and acoustic and aerodynamic measurements may be helpful in selected cases (ASHA, 1993a). The structure and movements of the vocal folds may be evaluated. Speech–language pathologists must match the data collected with their knowledge of the onset and course of various disorders, their knowledge of the vocal and acoustic symptoms associated with structural, neurologic, and psychogenic disorders, and their knowledge of the structure and movement of the vocal folds.

History.   Evaluation of the history of a patient with spasmodic dysphonia has two components: determining if the history matches the history associated with spasmodic dysphonia, and ruling out other voice disorders. A speech–language pathologist reviews the history to see if the patient's symptoms and history match the pattern of a known voice disorder, i.e., the patient's symptoms and dysphonia history must be compared with the profiles of other voice disorders. The speech–language pathologist needs information about the patient's prenatal, perinatal, and early developmental history. The patient may describe the onset, the course of the disorder, and the consistency of the symptoms. Information about medical evaluations, diagnoses, and treatment from neurologists and otolaryngologists may be elicited. Family history is important because up to 23 percent of patients with spasmodic dysphonia have a family history of dystonia (Blitzer & Brin, 1990). Information about previous therapy for the voice disorder may be explored. The way patients use their voice and the extent of their voice use may be investigated, as well as the effects of the voice disorder on patients' educational, vocational, and social performance. When the symptoms match a known pattern, diagnosis is simple. However, if the patient's symptoms and history do not correspond to the expected patterns, other alternatives must be considered. The patient may have misunderstood the questions, inappropriate voice samples may have been collected, or knowledge about this type of voice disorder may be incomplete (Aronson, 1985; Bridger & Epstein, 1983; Morrison, Nichol, & Rammage, 1986; Sapir & Aronson, 1987).

Perceptual Voice Evaluation. A perceptual voice evaluation is performed to determine the existence and severity of the disorder. On the surface, this task appears simple. However, a voice disorder may fluctuate and the symptoms may not be noticeable during the evaluation. Accordingly, the voice evaluation must be structured to elicit symptoms and to maximize the fluctuations in different speaking tasks so that the characteristics of the disorder can be identified.

Over the years, researchers have shown that good inter-rater reliability can be achieved among skilled judges for rating the overall severity of spasmodic dysphonia (Aronson & DeSanto, 1983; Izdebski, Dedo, Shipp, & Flower, 1981; Sapir & Aronson, 1985; Sapir, Aronson, & Thomas, 1986). One scale, The United Spasmodic Dysphonia Rating Scale (USDRS), has been standardized by consensual validation (Stewart, 1994). The USDRS includes voice and speech stimuli, a two-part rating form, definitions of the dimensions, a training tape, and directions for scoring the scale. All 15 dimensions are rated on a 7-point scale.

The dimensions include overall severity, rough voice quality, breathy voice quality, strained–strangled voice quality, abrupt voice initiation, voice arrest, aphonia, voice loudness, bursts of loudness, **voice tremor,** expiratory effort, **speech rate,** reduced speech intelligibility, and related movements and grimaces. In addition, six voice and speech tasks are used to elicit improvement in voice performance.

Movement Evaluation. Patients with spasmodic dysphonia should undergo a comprehensive neurological examination. This is in keeping with the observation that, in most cases, spasmodic dysphonia is a manifestation of a brain–motor control condition, i.e., neurological disease. A detailed neurological assessment is necessary to classify the neurologic condition. The neurological evaluation may include those tasks that classically bring out movement disorders. During the examination, one is looking particularly for evidence of dystonia involving segments of the body, in an effort to further characterize the patient's movement disorder. The neurological manifestations and associated findings should be documented. In most situations, this is facilitated by referral to a movement disorder center.

Vocal Fold Evaluation. Examination of the larynx in spasmodic dysphonia includes direct visualization of the laryngeal movements by stroboscopic endoscopy with a fiber-optic instrument inserted through the nose. This allows the patient to speak, since the dystonic symptoms are best seen in connected speech. Videotape recording of the endoscopy may be helpful because the record can be reviewed repeatedly or viewed by other consultants. This record may be used to monitor the progress of the disorder or the patient's response to therapy.

The stroboscope provides either a flashing light to simulate a slow motion of the vocal fold vibration, or it flashes at the fundamental frequency to simulate a frozen image in the vibratory cycle. The stroboscope has a microphone to sense the fundamental frequency and to coordinate the flashing light to the same frequency. This slowed motion allows assessment of the mucosal wave, which may be impaired by scarring, edema, and/ or subtle defects in the mucosa when there is a structural (nonneurological) abnormality. (See Chapter 11.) Stroboscopy also allows accurate evaluation of the closing and opening pattern of the larynx, and can sometimes indicate the probable underlying cause of the faulty closure or faulty opening.

Adductor spasms of the vocal folds are seen during connected speech at normal pitch and loudness. Adductor spasms can be classified according to the intensity of the inappropriate spasm. Table 13.3 lists the four types of closure. Type I hyperfunction describes the vocal folds coming together too tightly; Type II includes the vocal folds and the false vocal folds adducting too tightly; Type III involves the arytenoids being pulled anteriorly in addition to the over closure; and Type IV occurs when the arytenoids are pulled so far forward that they touch the pediole of the epiglottis, thereby completely closing the glottis (sphincteric).

Abductor spasms are best elicited with sentences that are loaded with voiceless consonants. The arytenoids are found to pull open during phonation, often producing a breathy voice and tremor.

TABLE 13.3 Types of Closure in Adductor Spasmodic Dysphonia

ADDUCTOR TYPE	SYMPTOMS
Type 1	The vocal folds come together too tightly
Type 2	The vocal folds and the false folds come together too tightly
Type 3	The arytenoid cartilages are pulled forward in addition to tight vocal fold closure
Type 4	The arytenoid cartilages are pulled so far forward they touch the pediole of the epiglottis and completely close the glottis

Approaches to Treatment

Providing optimal treatment requires the involvement of an interdisciplinary team. Team members evaluate those aspects of treatment that relate to their area, and help form the treatment plan. The role of the speech–language pathologist is to take part in planning treatment, to provide voice therapy when appropriate, to assess response to treatment, and to educate the patient about the disorder and its treatment.

Historically, different hypotheses about the cause of a disorder have led to a variety of treatments. Obviously, if a disorder is hypothesized to have a behavioral cause, treatment would address the behavioral issues; however, if the disorder is hypothesized to have a medical cause, treatment would address the medical issues (Segre, 1951). Consequently, over the years, both behavioral and medical treatments have been provided to ameliorate the symptoms of spasmodic dysphonia.

The results of behavioral therapies including psychotherapy, speech-language rehabilitation, hypnosis, relaxation, respiratory therapy, special diets, and biofeedback have been poor (Aronson, 1985; Aronson & DeSanto, 1983; Bloch, 1965; Heaver, 1959; Izdebski, Dedo, & Boles, 1984). Boone (1971) suggested that if speech therapy were attempted, a laugh may be used to produce easy phonation that is then integrated into speech. However, Boone (1971), Brodnitz (1976), and Izdebski & Dedo (1981b) have all reported that spasmodic dysphonia is highly resistant to voice therapy.

Medical treatments for spasmodic dysphonia have been directed at reducing the symptoms but not the underlying cause. In 1976, Dedo first described a surgical treatment for spasmodic dysphonia that involved cutting the **recurrent laryngeal nerve** on one side, resulting in flaccid paralysis of the ipsilateral vocal fold. Dedo reported that all the patients were pleased with the improvement in their voices, but that some patients had mild remnants of dysphonia. Some physicians have performed a recurrent laryngeal nerve crush rather than a clipping. In this procedure the nerve is only crushed and can regenerate so that the vocal fold is not permanently paralyzed.

However, the improvement from both recurrent laryngeal nerve clipping and crush appear to be only temporary (Aronson & DeSanto, 1981; Aronson & DeSanto, 1983). In 1981, Aronson and DeSanto evaluated the voices of 37 tape-recorded speakers with adductor spasmodic dysphonia before and one and one-half years following **recurrent laryngeal nerve section.** Immediately after surgery 97 percent had improved voice production; however, one and one-half years following surgery, 39 percent had reverted to their presurgical or to a worse level of functioning. The same speakers were reevaluated three years after surgery and 64% percent were found to have regressed to their previous level or to have worse voice than before surgery (Aronson & DeSanto, 1983). On the other hand, a study by Izdebski, Dedo, Shipp, and Flower (1981) found that 92 percent of the treated patients reported easier communication after surgery. These conflicting data appear to be the result of the way the two groups evaluated success: Aronson's group looked at clinicians' ratings and Dedo's group looked at patients' ratings of their own performance. Sapir, Aronson, and Thomas (1986) compared speakers' ratings of their own voices with the ratings that three speech–language pathologists made of the same speakers' voices. The three speech–language pathologists' ratings were consistent with each other, but the speakers' self-ratings were not consistent with those of the professionals. The speakers tended to rate their own dysphonia as less severe than did the speech–language pathologists. However, Dedo and Behlau (1991) found that 83 percent of patients had "effective conversational voices" (p. 276) up to 14 years after surgery. These conflicting results may be due to the different levels of severity of the patients in the different studies.

Patients with segmental and generalized dystonia, torticollis, and blepharospasm are occasionally treated with pharmacotherapy. Pharmacotherapy is usually initiated with either an anticholinergic, a benzodiazepine, or with baclofen. However, spasmodic dysphonia is rarely treated with drugs because only a small group of muscles is affected by the dystonia and the drug would affect all muscles in the body. In addition, the drugs may have undesirable side effects.

Botulinum toxin (BTX) is another therapy that treats the neurological symptoms. The bacterium *clostridia botulinum* is a potent poison found in contaminated food. If the bacterium is eaten, the toxin it produces can cause serious or fatal paralysis. BTX is a potent toxin that acts presynaptically to prevent the release of acetylcholine from the nerve endings at the neuromuscular junction (ANN, 1990; Kao, Drachman, & Price, 1976). "Advantage can be taken of this neuromuscular blocking effect to alleviate muscle spasms due to excessive neural activity of central origin or to weaken a muscle for therapeutic purposes" (ANN, 1990, p. 2). Injections of minute doses effectively relieve the hypercontraction of the muscles of the larynx. BTX has been approved by the Food and Drug Administration for the treatment of blepharospasm. The National Academies of Otolaryngology and Neurology have endorsed BTX as the treatment of choice for adductor spasmodic dysphonia.

Injections of BTX have resulted in improved voice production for both adductor and abductor spasmodic dysphonia (Blitzer & Brin, 1991; Blitzer et al., 1992; Blitzer et al., 1985; Brin et al., 1988, Brin et al., 1992; Ludlow, 1990; Ludlow, Naunton, Sedory, Schulz, & Hallett, 1988). BTX has been used to treat adductor spasmodic dysphonia since 1984 (Brin et al., 1988; Ludlow, 1990; Ludlow et al., 1988). The treatment is performed while the patient is awake. For adductor spasmodic dysphonia, BTX is injected into the thyroarytenoid muscles. The toxin is injected via a monopolar hollow core teflon-coated electromyographic (EMG) recording needle. The thyroarytenoid muscles are identified under EMG control to add precision to the procedure. To verify that the needle is in the thyroarytenoid muscle, the patient vocalizes a sustained /i/. If the EMG needle is in the appropriate location, the EMG machine will identify an increase in the amplitude of the signal during phonation. The toxin is then injected into the muscle.

The effect of the injection is temporary and the injection needs to be repeated every three-to-five months when the symptoms return. The strength of the response can be controlled by altering the level of the dose or by repeating injections. There are mild temporary side effects. For adductor spasmodic dysphonia, the transient side effects include mild choking on thin liquids, a breathy voice quality, and weakness when coughing, laughing, and yelling (Brin et al., 1988). Rashes and flu symptoms are two systemic side effects that affect less than one percent of the people who have BTX injections at the low doses used for the larynx. Treatment with BTX injections has been highly successful. Most patients with adductor spasmodic dysphonia evaluate their voices as reaching at least 90 percent of normal function (Brin et al., 1992; Ludlow, 1990).

For abductor spasmodic dysphonia, the BTX is injected into the posterior cricoarytenoid muscle via EMG control. To verify the location of the monopolar hollow core teflon-coated EMG recording needle, the patient is asked to sniff, because sniffing activates the posterior cricoarytenoid muscle. If the EMG needle is in the appropriate location, the EMG machine will show an increase in the amplitude of the EMG signal during sniffing. One side is injected at a time so that side effects are minimized. The mild temporary side effects include a stasis of food, shortness of breath, and vocal stridor on inhalation (Blitzer, Brin, Stewart, & Fahn, 1992). Some patients experience a worsening of their pre-existing vocal tremor. The mean overall level of improvement for patients with abductor spasmodic dysphonia is 70 percent of normal function (Blitzer et al., 1992).

Some patients with adductor and abductor spasmodic dysphonia can improve the quality of their voices and lengthen the benefits received from the injections by participating in short periods of voice therapy. If the breathiness following an injection for adductor spasmodic dysphonia is severe or lasts for an extended period of time, voice therapy can help. Before the injection, patients with adductor spasmodic dysphonia use increased expiratory drive to vibrate the stiffened vocal folds. After the BTX injections, the vocal folds are weak. Some patients do not decrease the expiratory drive. When the vocal folds are weakened, the excessive expiratory drive will blow the weak vocal folds apart and they will not vibrate.

Speech therapy helps some patients maximize the benefit of the BTX injections for both adductor and abductor spasmodic dysphonia. Therapy should be directed at decreasing expiratory drive, decreasing effort at the level of the vocal folds, and coordinating the expiratory drive with the stiffness of the vocal folds (Allen, personal communication, 1989). Control of the expiratory drive can be increased by improving posture and decreasing extraneous muscle activity in the upper body. If a patient has a quiet, breathy voice following BTX injection, reducing environmental noise and using an amplifier on the telephone can help the patient communicate (Blitzer & Stewart, 1993).

SUMMARY

Spasmodic dysphonia appears to be a focal laryngeal dystonia elicited by the motor act of speaking. Like other types of action dystonia, the dystonic movements of the vocal folds are usually aggravated during voluntary movement and are usually absent at rest. When an individual with spasmodic dysphonia is quiet, the vocal folds usually appear normal. However, when the person speaks, the involuntary movements of the vocal folds emerge. As a result, patients with spasmodic dysphonia sound bizarre because their voice is clear when they laugh but becomes disordered when they speak. In addition, the symptoms usually resolve when the patient sings.

Spasmodic dysphonia has two manifestations: adductor and abductor. Abductor is more rare. Patients with abductor spasmodic dysphonia exhibit a breathy weak voice quality interrupted by aphonic breathy breaks. Patients with adductor spasmodic dysphonia have a strained–strangled voice quality interrupted by intermittent strangled breaks and effort when speaking.

Spasmodic dysphonia is noticeable only when the patient is talking. When the patient laughs or sustains a high-pitched vowel, the symptoms usually disappear. Frequently, laryngeal examinations are performed while a patient sustains a vowel. Consequently, if a patient with spasmodic dysphonia has a laryngeal examination while sustaining a vowel, the vocal folds may appear normal. However, if the vocal folds are examined while the patient says a sentence, abrupt glottal widening may be seen with abductor spasmodic dysphonia and forced glottal closing may be seen with adductor spasmodic dysphonia.

The evaluation and treatment of spasmodic dysphonia require an interdisciplinary team approach. The speech-language pathologist is responsible for assessing the presence and severity of the voice disorder and for suggesting appropriate therapy. A new standardized scale is available to evaluate adductor spasmodic dysphonia. The current treatment of choice for both types of spasmodic dysphonia is injection of botulinum toxin. The injections have few side effects and the benefit lasts several months. Speech therapy is helpful for some patients following injections to reduce side effects or to lengthen the benefit of the injections.

Major Points of Chapter

- The traditional psychogenic perspective is contrasted with the more recent neurogenic perspective of spasmodic dysphonia.
- Types of spasmodic dysphonia include adductor, abductor, and mixed.
- Diagnosis of spasmodic dysphonia is usually made based on behavioral voice symptoms and through exclusion of other possibilities.
- Methods of treatment include behavioral voice therapy, and different surgical approaches.

Discussion Guidelines

1. What questions would be essential to include in an interview if you were going to evaluate a patient with spasmodic dysphonia?
2. During a voice evaluation it is essential to identify vocal tasks that a patient can perform appropriately as well as those performed inappropriately. Identify five vocal tasks that might improve the voice production of a patient with spasmodic dysphonia.
3. Outline the steps that should be taken in evaluating a patient with suspected spasmodic dyshonia. Include behavioral and instrumental measures.

REFERENCES

Allen, E. L. (1989). Personal communication in Voice Disorders class at New York University, New York.

American Speech-Language-Hearing Association (ASHA) (1993a). Preferred practice patterns for the professions of Speech-Language Pathology and Audiology. *ASHA Supplement No. 11, 35,* 69–70.

American Speech-Language-Hearing Association (ASHA) (1993b). *Spasmodic Dysphonia ASHA fact sheet...for People with Special Communication needs.* Rockville, MD: ASHA.

Aminoff, M. J., Dedo, H. H., & Izdebski, K. (1978). Clinical aspects of spasmodic dysphonia. *Journal of Neurology, Neurosurgery, and Psychiatry, 41,* 361–365.

ANN (1990). Assessment: the clinical usefulness of botulinum toxin-A in treating neurologic disorders. Report of the Therapeutics and Technology Assessment Subcommittee of the American Academy of Neurology. *Neurology, 40,* 1332–1336.

Arnold, G. E. (1959, April). Spastic Dysphonia. *Logos, 2,* 3–14.

Aronson, A. E. (1985). *Clinical voice disorders.* New York: Thieme.

Aronson, A. E. (1990). *Clinical voice disorders.* New York: Brian C. Dekker.

Aronson, A. E., Brown, J. R., Litin, E. M., & Pearson, J. S. (1968a). Spastic dysphonia. I. Voice, neurologic, and psychiatric aspects. *Journal of Speech and Hearing Disorders, 33,* 203–218.

Aronson, A. E., Brown, J. R., Litin, E. M., & Pearson, J. S. (1968b). Spastic dysphonia. II. Comparison with essential (voice) tremor and other neurologic and psychogenic dysphonias. *Journal of Speech and Hearing Disorders, 33,* 219–231.

Aronson, A. E., & DeSanto, L. W. (1981). Adductor spastic dysphonia: 1 1/2 years after recurrent laryngeal nerve resection. *Annals of Otology, Rhinology, and Laryngology, 90,* 2–6.

Aronson, A. E., & DeSanto, L. W. (1983). Adductor spastic dysphonia: Three years after recurrent laryngeal nerve resection. *Laryngoscope, 93,* 1–8.

Aronson, A. B., Peterson, H. W., & Litin, E. M. (1964). Voice symptomology in functional dysphonia and aphonia. *Journal of Speech and Hearing Disorders, 29,* 367–380.

Bassich, C. J. & Ludlow, C. L. (1986). The use of perceptual methods by new clinicians for assessing voice quality. *Journal of Speech and Hearing Disorders, 51,* 125–133.

Bellussi, G. (1952) Le disfonie ipercinetiche, Atti labor. Fonetica, *University Padova* (3) 1.

Blitzer, A., & Brin, M. F. (1986) Letters to the editor. *Laryngoscope, 96,* 1300–1301.

Blitzer, A., & Brin, M. F. (1990) Spasmodic dysphonia (laryngeal dystonia). In G. Gates (Ed.), *Current therapy in otolaryngology-head and neck surgery-4* (pp. 346–348). Toronto: B. C. Decker..

Blitzer, A., & Brin, M. F. (1991) Laryngeal dystonia: a series with botulinum toxin therapy. *Annals of Otology, Rhinology, and Laryngology, 100,* 85–89.

Blitzer, A., Brin, M. F., Fahn, S., & Lovelace, R. E. (1988, February). Localized injections of botulinum toxin for the treatment of focal laryngeal dystonia (spastic dysphonia). *Laryngoscope, 98,* 193–197.

Blitzer, A., Lovelace, R. E., Brin, M. F., Fahn, S., & Fink, M. E. (1985). Electromyographic findings in focal laryngeal dystonia (spasmodic dysphonia). *Annuals of Otology, Rhinology, and Laryngology, 94,* 591–594.

Blitzer, A. & Stewart, C. F. (1993) Abductor spasmodic dysphonia. In J. Stemple (Ed.) *Voice therapy: Clinical studies* (pp. 147–153). Mosby Year Book: Chicago.

Bloch, C. S., Hirano, M., & Gould, W. J. (1985). Symptom improvement of spastic dysphonia in response to phonatory tasks. *Annals of Otology, Rhinology, and Laryngology, 94,* 51–54.

Bloch, P. (1965). Neuro-psychiatric aspects of spastic dysphonia. *Folia Phoniatrica, 17,* 301–364.

Boone, D. R. (1971) *The voice and voice therapy.* Englewood Cliffs, NJ: Prentice-Hall.

Bridger, M. W. M., & Epstein R. (1983). Functional voice disorders: A review of 109 patients. *Journal of Laryngology and Otology, 97,* 1145–1148.

Brin, M. F., Blitzer, A., Fahn, S., Gould, W., & Lovelace, R. E. (1989). Adductor laryngeal dystonia (spastic dysphonia): Treatment with local injections of botulinum toxin (Botox). *Movement Disorders, 4,* 287–296.

Brin, M. F., Fahn, S., Blitzer, A., Ramig, L. O., & Stewart, C. F. (1992). Movement disorders of the larynx. In A. Blitzer, M. Brin, S. Fahn, C. T. Sasaki, & K. Harris, (Eds.), *Neurological disorders of the larynx.* New York: Thieme Medical Publishing.

Brin, M. F., Fahn, S., Moskowitz, C., Friedman, A., Shale, H. M., Greene, P. E., Blitzer, A., List, T., Lange, D., Lovelace, R. E., & McMahon, D. (1988). Localized injections of botulinum toxin for the treatment of focal dystonia and hemifacial spasm. *Advances in Neurology, 50,* 599–608.

Brin, M. F., Fahn, S., Moskowitz, C., Friedman, A., Shale, H. M., Greene, P. E., Blitzer, A., List, T., Lange, D., Lovelace, R. E., & McMahon, D. (1987). Localized injections of botulinum toxin for the treatment of focal dystonia and hemifacial spasm. *Movement Disorders, 2,* 237–254.

Brodnitz, F. S. (1976). Spastic dysphonia. *Annals of Otology, Rhinology, and Laryngology, 85,* 210–214.

Butcher, P., Elias, A., Raven, R., Yeatman, J., & Littlejohns, D. (1987). Psychogenic voice disorder unresponsive to speech therapy: Psychological characteristics and cognitive-behavior therapy. *British Journal of Communication Disorders, 27* (2) 137–158.

Cannito, M. P. & Johnson, J. P. (1981). Spasmodic dysphonia: A continuum disorder. *Journal of Communication Disorders, 14,* 215–223.

Calne, D. B., & Lang, A. E. (1988) Secondary dystonia. *Advances in Neurology, 50,* 9–33.

Cohen, R. (1886). *Pathologie und Therapie der Sprachanomalien.* Wien: Urban und Schwarzenberg.

Critchley, M. (1939). Spastic dysphonia ("inspiratory speech"). *Brain: A Journal of Neurology, 52,* 96–103.

Darley, F. L., Aronson, A. E., & Brown, J. R. (1975). *Motor speech disorders.* Philadelphia: W. B. Saunders

Dedo, H. H. (1976). Recurrent laryngeal nerve section for spastic dysphonia. *Annals of Otology, Rhinology, and Laryngology, 85,* 451–459.

Kao, I., Drachman, D. B., & Price, D. L.(1976). Botulinum toxin: Mechanism of presynaptic blockade. *Science, 193,* 1256–1258.

Fahn, S. (1988). Concept and classification of dysphonia. *Advances in Neurology 50*, 1–8.

Feldman, M., Nixon, J. V., Finitzo-Hieber, T., & Freeman, F. J. (1984). Abnormal parasympathetic vagal function in patients with spasmodic dysphonia. *Annals of Internal Medicine, 100*, 491–495.

Finitzo, T., & Freeman, F. (1989). Spasmodic dysphonia, whether and where: Results of seven years of research. *Journal of Speech and Hearing Research, 32*, 541–555.

Finitzo-Hieber, T., Freeman, F. J., Gerling, I. J., Dobson, L., & Schaefer, S. D. (1982). Auditory brainstem response abnormalities in adductor spasmodic dysphonia. *American Journal of Otolaryngology, 3*, 26–30.

Fraenkel, B. (1887) *Ueber beschaeftigungsneurosen der stimme.* Leipzig: G. Thieme.

Gordon, M. F., Brin, M. F., Giladi, N., Hunt, A., & Fahn, S. (1990). Dystonia precipitated by peripheral trauma. *Movement Disorders, 5*, 67.

Greene, J. S. (1938). Psychiatric therapy for dysphonia, aphonia, psychophonasthenia, falsetto. *AMA Archives & Otolaryngology, 28*, 213.

Greene, M., & Mathieson, L. (1989). *The voice and its disorders.* London: Whurr. 5th Edition.

Hall, J. W. III (1981). Central auditory function in spastic dysphonia. *American Journal of Otolaryngology, 2*, 188–198.

Hartman, D. E., & Vishwanat, B. (1984). Spasmodic dysphonia [Letter to the editor]. *Annals of Internal Medicine, 101*, 403.

Heaver, L. (1959). Spastic dysphonia. *Logos, 2*, 15–24.

Izdebski, K., & Dedo, H. H. (1981a). Selecting the side of recurrent laryngeal nerve section for spastic dysphonia. *Otolaryngology, Head and Neck Surgery, 89*, 423–426.

Izdebski, K., & Dedo, H. H. (1981b). Spastic dysphonia. In J. K. Darby (Ed.), *Speech evaluation in medicine* (pp. 105–127). New York: Grunet Stratton.

Izdebski, K., Dedo, H. H., & Boles, L. (1984). Spastic dysphonia: A patient profile of 200 cases. *American Journal of Otolaryngology, 5*, 7–14.

Izdebski, K., Dedo, H. H., Shipp, T., & Flower, R. M. (1981). Postoperative and follow-up studies of spastic dysphonia patients treated by recurrent laryngeal nerve section. *Otolaryngology, Head and Neck Surgery, 89*, 96–101.

Jacome, D. E., & Yanez, G. Y. (1980). Spastic dysphonia and Meige disease [Letter to the editor]. *Neurology, 30*, 349.

Lebrun, Y., Devreux, F., Rousseau, J., & Darimont, P. (1982). Tremulous speech, a case report. *Folia Phoniatrica, 34*, 134–142.

Liebermann, P. (1968) Direct comparison of subglottal and esophageal pressure during speech. *Journal of the Acoustal Society of America, 48*, 1159–1164.

Ludlow, C. L. (1990) Treatment of speech and voice disorders with botulinum toxin. *Journal of the American Medical Association, 264*, 2671–2676.

Ludlow, C. L., & Connor, N. P. (1987). Dynamic aspects of phonatory control in spasmodic dysphonia. *Journal of Speech and Hearing Research, 30*, 197–206.

Ludlow, C. D., Naunton, R. F., Sedory, S. E., Schulz, G. M., & Hallett, M. Effects of botulinum toxin injections on speech in adductor spasmodic dysphonia. *Neurology, 38* (8), 1220–1225.

Marsden, C. D. (1988). Investigation of dystonia. *Advances in Neurology, 50*, 35–44.

Marsden, C. D. (1991) *What is dystonia?* Vancouver, BC: Dystonia Medical Research Foundation.

Marsden, C. D., & Sheehy, M. P. (1982). Spastic dysphonia, Meige disease, and torsion dystonia [Letter to the editor]. *Neurology, 32*, 1202.

Maximov, I. (1961) De la symptomatologie des aphonias fonctionnelles. *Revue de Laryngologie, Otologie, Rhinologie, 82*, 896–905.

McCall, G. N., Skolnick, M. L., & Brewer, D. W. (1971). A preliminary report of some atypical movement patterns in the tongue, palate, hypopharynx, and larynx of patients with spasmodic dysphonia. *Journal of Speech and Hearing Disorders, 36*, 466–470.

Morrison, M. D., Nichol, H., & Rammage, L. A. (1986). Diagnostic criteria in functional dysphonia. *Laryngoscope, 96*, 1–8.

Nicolosi, L., Harryman, E., & Kresheck, J. (1983). *Terminology of communication disorders: Speech, language, hearing* (2nd ed.). Baltimore, MD: Williams & Wilkins.

Nothnagel (1881) referenced in Gerhardt, P. Bewegungstoerungen der stimmbaender. *Nothnagels Spesielle Pathologie und Therapie, 13.*

Parnes, S. M., Lavorato, A. S., & Myers, E. N. (1978). Study of spastic dysphonia using videofiberoptic laryngoscopy. *Annals of Otology, Rhinology, and Laryngology, 87*, 322–326.

Rabuzzi, D. D., & McCall, G. N. (1972). Spasmodic dysphonia: A clinical perspective. *Transactions of the American Academy of Opthalmology and Otolaryngology, 76*, 724–728.

Reich, A., & Till, J. (1983). Phonatory and manual reaction times of women with idiopathic spasmodic dysphonia. *Journal of Speech and Hearing Research, 26,* 10–18.

Robe, E., Brumlik, J., & Moore, P. (1960, March). A study of spastic dysphonia. *Laryngoscope, 70,* 219–245.

Sapir, S., & Aronson, A. E. (1985). Clinical reliability in rating voice improvement after laryngeal nerve section for spastic dysphonia. *Laryngoscope, 95,* 200–202.

Sapir, S., & Aronson, A. E. (1987). Coexisting psychogenic and neurogenic dysphonia: A source of diagnostic confusion. *British Journal of Disorders of Communication, 22,* 73–80.

Sapir, S., Aronson, A. E., & Thomas, J. E. (1986). Judgment of voice improvement after recurrent laryngeal nerve section for spastic dysphonia: Clinicians versus patients. *Annals of Otology, Rhinology, and Laryngology, 95,* 137–141.

Schaefer, S. D. (1983). Neuropathology of spasmodic dysphonia. *Laryngoscope, 93,* 1183–1184.

Schaefer, S. D., Finitzo-Hieber, T., Gerling, I. J., & Freeman, F. J. (1983). Brainstem conduction abnormalities in spasmodic dysphonia. *Annals of Otology, Rhinology, and Laryngology, 92,* 59–64.

Schaefer, S. D., & Freeman, F. J. (1987). Spasmodic dysphonia. *Otolaryngologic Clinics of North America, 20,* 161–178.

Schnitzler, J. (1895) *Klinescher atlas der laryngologie nebst anleitung zur diagnose und therapie der krankheiten des kehlokopfes und der luftrohre.* Wien: Braumuller, 215.

Segre, R. (1951). Spasmodic aphonia. *Folia Phoniatrica, 3,* 150–165.

Shulman, S. (1993) Symptom modification for abductor spasmodic dysphonia. In J. C. Stemple (Ed.). *Voice therapy: Clinical studies,* pp. 128–130. St. Louis, MO: Mosby Year Book.

Stewart, C. (1994). *Development of a standard evaluation of adductor spasmodic dysphonia.* Doctoral Dissertation, New York University, University Microfilms International.

Traube, L. (1871) *Zur lehre von den larynxaffectionen beim lleotyphus.* Berlin: Verlag Non August Hirschwald, 674–678.

Wolfe, V. I., & Bacon, M. (1976). Spectrographic comparison of two types of spastic dysphonia. *Journal of Speech and Hearing Disorders, 41,* 325–332.

Wolfe, V. I., Ratusnik, D. L., & Feldman, H. (1979). Acoustic and perceptual comparison of chronic and incipient spastic dysphonia. *Laryngoscope, 9,* 1478–1486.

Woodson, G. E., Zwirner, P., & Murray, T. (1991). Use of flexible laryngoscopy to classify patients with spasmodic dysphonia. *Journal of Voice, 5,* 85–91.

Zemlin, W. R. (1988). *Speech and hearing science: Anatomy and physiology* (3rd ed.). Englewood Cliffs, NJ: Prentice-Hall.

Zwitman, D. H. (1979). Bilateral cord dysfunctions: Abductor type spastic dysphonia. *Journal of Speech and Hearing Disorders,* 373–378.

14

COMMUNICATIVE MANAGEMENT OF PERSONS WITH MULTIPLE DISABILITIES

CAROL FLEXER, YVONNE GILLETTE, AND DENISE WRAY

Communicative management for persons with multiple disabilities is a challenging endeavor. Professional services need to be integrated into the person's lifestyle, encompassing school, work, and community involvement. Speech–language pathologists and audiologists no longer just "do therapy" or just "test hearing." Responsibilities are more global than in previous years. They are also more holistic, more interdisciplinary, more dynamic, and more challenging.

The purposes of this chapter are to provide a description of the populations of persons with multiple disabilities; explore role clarifications for the speech–language pathologist relative to direct or consultative service provision and management of assistive technology; emphasize the critical role of the audiologist in managing the integrity of the speech signal, hearing technologies, and the learning/acoustic environment; and discuss service provision strategies and the team members involved in multidisciplinary intervention.

DESCRIPTIONS OF PERSONS WITH MULTIPLE DISABILITIES

Individuals with multiple disabilities face challenges in two or more developmental skill areas: communication, cognition, motor, adaptive, and social skills. Populations commonly associated with multiple disabilities include persons with severe orthopedic impairments such as **cerebral palsy,** those with serious sensory impairment such as deaf–blindness, and those with serious health concerns, such as individuals with AIDS.

Historically, these individuals have been placed in institutions because of the limited support available to families for provision of adequate health, education, and social services. In the last quarter of a century, however, much has changed for these individuals. Advances in health care have made it possible for persons with multiple disabilities to survive various medical difficulties. Changes in the education system and family rights promoted by various federal laws such as the Rehabilitation Act and the **Individuals with Disabilities Education Act** have made meaningful education a real possibility. Through other laws, such as the **Americans with Disabilities Act** (ADA), society is beginning to offer individuals with multiple disabilities opportunities to take part in their communities by supporting access to the living and employment options that most of society takes for granted.

The prevailing concept motivating these changes is known as *normalization.* The notion of normalization prompted the community integration of persons who had previously been managed in state institutions. Normalization refers to practices such as the inclusion of special needs children in standard classrooms and programs such as the Special Olympics (Wolfensberger, 1995). While the original concern was with persons with mental retardation, the normalization movement also addresses the needs of persons with multiple disabilities. The concept of normalization guides the methods that professionals in communicative disorders use to provide appropriate assessment and intervention for persons with multiple disabilities. While the type of intervention chosen will vary depending upon the communication profile of each individual, all intervention should be designed to support the individual's health and education and to provide full access to their community.

NEUROMOTOR IMPAIRMENTS

Individuals may present neuromotor impairments resulting from various origins, including **neural tube** defects, muscular dystrophy, and cerebral palsy. Neural tube defects are **congenital** and refer to a range of malformations of the vertebrae and spinal cord, such as spina bifida and **myelomeningocele.** Muscular dystrophy refers to a group of progressive muscle diseases. Cerebral palsy is the neuromotor condition most likely to result in multiple disabilities, because the brain damage that results is frequently not confined to the motor regions of the brain.

Cerebral Palsy

Cerebral palsy refers to a group of brain damage **syndromes** that always result in movement disorder and may include mental retardation, seizures, sensory impairments, and communication disorders. When diagnosing cerebral palsy, physicians look for a nonprogressive condition with an onset in the developmental period. The origins of cerebral palsy vary, and many classifications for cerebral palsy exist. Incidence rates vary, but are generally cited as 1–2 cases per 1,000 live births.

Origins. Cerebral palsy is commonly diagnosed when brain damage occurs in the **prenatal** period, during labor and delivery, or in the **perinatal** period. Interestingly, labor and delivery complications used to be considered the most common cause of cerebral palsy; however, it is now documented that these difficult births are the result of pre-existing brain damage, rather than the cause of it. Approximately 44 percent of cases of cerebral palsy have prenatal origins, 19 percent relate to complications during labor and delivery, 13 percent are attributed to perinatal or early childhood causes, and 24 percent of cases do not have obvious origins (Hagberg & Hagberg, 1984).

Early Diagnosis. A diagnosis of cerebral palsy often takes up to two years to confirm, particularly in mild cases. Consequently, professionals monitor the first two years of development of infants known to be at risk for cerebral palsy, such as low birth weight infants (under 1500 grams), small for gestational age infants, and twins. (For a detailed discussion of risk factors, see Chapter 2.) Neuromotor movement tests are combined with developmental screening to detect early motor problems and possible related developmental delays. The motor delays associated with cerebral palsy are often the most obvious and therefore are diagnosed early. Confirmation of multiple disabilities in areas such as communication or cognitive abilities often takes longer to diagnose accurately.

Certain groups of behavioral symptoms can signal possible cerebral palsy in early infancy, including excessive sleeping, irritability when awake, weak cries, poor suck, and little interest in surroundings. The infant may rest in a floppy or extended position rather than the semiflexed position common to infants. Persistence of primitive reflexes, usually seen in the first six to twelve months of life, is also a characteristic. (See Batshaw and Perret, 1993, pp. 447–450 for further information on the reflexes.)

Types. The three types of cerebral palsy most commonly referred to include pyramidal (spastic), **extrapyramidal** (athetoid), and cerebellar (ataxic). Mixed types of cerebral palsy also exist.

Pyramidal (Spastic) Cerebral Palsy. In order for smooth voluntary movements to occur, nerve impulses must pass through the **pyramidal (direct) tract;** from the motor cortex located in the frontal lobe, through the brain stem, to the spinal cord, and on to a peripheral nerve. (See Chapter 8 for more detail about this pathway.) Damage along this path leads to spastic cerebral palsy, and various locations of the damage will result in different manifestations of the movement disorder. Spastic cerebral palsy presents as a "clasp-knife" resistance; that is, extreme rigidity of the limb, followed by a sudden "give."

Pyramidal cerebral palsy can be present in varied forms. **Diplegia,** a form of spastic cerebral palsy that affects the legs more than the arms, results from damage to the nerve fibers controlling leg movement. **Hemiplegia** presents as spasticity on one side of the body, and quadriplegia refers to movement difficulties affecting all four limbs. **Quadriplegia** frequently results in multiple disabilities because the brain damage is diffuse and often affects many systems, including communication and cognition. According to Eiben and Crocker (1983), hemiplegia is the most common form of pyramidal cerebral palsy, accounting for 45 percent of cases, followed by quadriplegia at 30 percent, and diplegia at 25 percent.

Extrapyramidal (Athetoid) Cerebral Palsy. The extrapyramidal (indirect) tract of the brain includes the **diencephalon** that lies beneath the cortex in the center of the brain. The diencephalon includes several structures, including the **basal nuclei** which have a role in modifying instructions from the motor cortex, which enhances posture and balance. The **cerebellum** also has a role in organizing movement by integrating impulses from the motor cortex and the basal nuclei (Capute & Accardo, 1991). Thus, smooth voluntary movement depends on the integration of nerve impulses from the cortex, basal nuclei, and cerebellum. Since all four limbs are involved in extrapyramidal cerebral palsy, **topographic** classification is not as useful as it is in spastic cerebral palsy. One characteristic of this type of cerebral palsy, known as **lead pipe rigidity,** involves increased tone that

persists through **flexion** and **extension** repeatedly. This type of hypertonicity is different than the clasp-knife characteristic of spastic cerebral palsy. Typically, upper extremities are more functionally involved than lower extremities. When upper extremities are severely impaired, this often poses a particular difficulty in life planning, since upper extremity function is essential to most vocational training.

The most common form of extrapyramidal cerebral palsy is the choreoathetoid type. In this form of cerebral palsy, the problem lies in regulating movement and maintaining posture. Choreoathetoid movements are abrupt and involuntary. (See Chapter 8 for detailed information on chorea.) Interestingly, muscle tone often appears normal, and involuntary movements are absent in sleep. Facial muscles are frequently affected in choreoathetoid cerebral palsy. Consequently, these individuals frequently have sucking, swallowing, drooling, and speaking difficulties. Individuals with athetoid cerebral palsy can sit and walk, but they must do so with extreme care because their muscles do not move smoothly, and tend to fluctuate unexpectedly during movement. Consequently these individuals may appear extremely clumsy in their movements and have difficulty with tasks that involve carrying objects or responding quickly, such as driving.

Other forms of extrapyramidal cerebral palsy are known as atonic or rigid. In atonic cerebral palsy, muscles are hypotonic or "floppy." Rigid cerebral palsy presents as a lead pipe or malleable rigidity.

Cerebellar (Ataxic) Cerebral Palsy. Several classification systems specify ataxic cerebral palsy as a separate disorder, rather than including it in the extrapyramidal category. The origin of **ataxia** is a dysfunction of the cerebellum which results in difficulty with posture and gait.

Mixed-Type Cerebral Palsy. Persons with mixed-type present characteristics of pyramidal and extrapyramidal cerebral palsy. Batshaw and Perret (1993) offer the example of a child with a right-side hemiplegia superimposed on generalized

choreoathetosis. Those with mixed-type cerebral palsy will frequently have mental retardation and other disabilities because of their extensive brain damage.

Associated Disabilities. All children with cerebral palsy have movement and posture disorders. Some children can walk, but have gait difficulties such as scissoring or toe walking. Many require orthotic devices such as braces or splints, walkers, crutches, and/or surgery along with physical and/or occupational therapy. These interventions are designed to maintain range-of-motion, promote stability, prevent contractures at certain joints, and control involuntary movements. Similar interventions may be required when the hand is involved. When children have limited walking skills, an individualized wheelchair is recommended.

Other concomitant disabilities can include mental retardation, visual and hearing deficits, speech–language disorders, and seizures. Testing for mental retardation is difficult to accomplish, since testing involves both motor and verbal responses. A commonly cited figure indicates that about two-thirds of children diagnosed with cerebral palsy are also mentally retarded. Visual problems are common and diverse and may include blindness, **nystagmus,** and/or **strabismus.** Nystagmus is a condition of random jerky eye movements that can co-occur with severe visual impairment. The same is true for strabismus, an imbalance in the eye muscles that interferes with focus. Spastic forms of cerebral palsy also carry a high incidence of seizure disorder. A seizure occurs when the brain's threshold for electrical activity is exceeded. (Further information on seizures is available in Chapter 26, Batshaw and Perret, 1993.) Cerebral palsy also can co-occur with behavioral and emotional problems.

Hearing, speech, and language problems are common. Since speech is a motor act, cerebral palsy affecting the articulators can result in **dysarthria.** Dysarthria results from weakness, paralysis, or incoordination of the speech musculature. Dysarthria can affect articulation, rate, loudness, pitch, prosody, stress, and nasality, depending

upon the type and severity of brain damage (Love & Webb, 1992). Dysarthria can be mild, or so severe that an augmentative device is required for intelligible communication. (For more information on dysarthria, refer to Chapter 8.) Language problems may be the result of mental retardation, or may be specific language disorders, depending upon the particular form of brain damage. Hearing problems are likewise diverse. Movement disorders related to the oral structures can result in feeding problems. (See Chapter 10.) Feeding problems can include **hypotonia,** weak suck, poor coordination for swallowing, **tonic bite,** hyperactive gag reflex, and exaggerated tongue thrust.

SENSORY IMPAIRMENTS

Sensory impairments frequently lead to multiple disabilities. While individuals with these disabilities are often described as blind, deaf, or deaf–blind, it is more common for individuals to have varying degrees of vision or **hearing impairment.** This section will familiarize the reader with information about visual impairment as a cause of multiple disability and dual sensory impairment.

Visual Impairment as an Origin of Multiple Disability

Visual impairment that originates at birth or within the first five years of life can result in multiple disabilities. Blindness occurring later in life does not have the same result, because visual information about the world has been gathered and can be drawn upon in learning and daily life. Persons without early visual experience do not have this advantage and must develop concepts based upon input from the other senses and any residual vision. Severe vision impairment is an origin of multiple disability because it can seriously impede growth in other domains. Concepts affected can cut across domains, influencing language, motor, social, and adaptive as well as cognitive skills.

The overall incidence of blindness in children is 1 in 3,000, with 46 percent born blind and an additional 38 percent losing sight in the first year of life. While 50 percent of these children have enough vision to read large print, 25 percent are totally blind and 25 percent have some light perception (Batshaw & Perret, 1993). A person who is legally blind can only see at 20/200 or less even with correction (Kirk, Gallagher, & Anastawiow, 1993). Vision of 20/200 means that a person can see only at 20 feet what someone with normal sight can see at 200 feet. Note that legal blindness does not mean that a person has absolutely no visual stimulation. The person may in fact be able to sense light and darkness and may have some visual imagery. A person who scores between 20/70 and 20/200 on tests of visual acuity, with corrective lenses, is legally partially sighted or described as experiencing low vision. Low vision is a term that refers to children and adults who can read print when assisted by a variety of devices. Visual impairments also can be defined using the educational terms of moderate, severe, and profound as a function of the adaptations that are necessary to assist these individuals in learning (Kirk et al., 1993). A moderate visual disability can be almost corrected with the help of visual aids; a severe visual disability can be helped only partially with visual aids (low vision); and a profound visual disability means that the person cannot use vision as an educational channel (legal blindness).

Factors such as the time of onset, the degree of blindness, and effects on other domains ultimately affect the individual's ability to function independently. The child's educational success and ultimate adult outcome is strongly related to the range of needs of each individual.

Origins of Blindness. Blindness can occur as an isolated phenomenon or as part of a complex **syndrome** involving many other disabilities. The most frequently occurring causes of blindness are **intrauterine** infections, such as rubella and **toxoplasmosis,** or malformations. Blindness due to **rubella** is often associated with congenital heart disease, hearing loss, cerebral palsy, and mental retardation. Other causes of blindness include **retinopathy of prematurity** (ROP), head trauma,

anoxia, eye infections, and tumors. ROP occurs in seven percent of infants weighing less than 2.5 pounds at birth and can be an isolated finding. The origin of ROP lies in the disruption of normal blood vessel development in the retina, coupled with oxygen treatments used when poor lung development results in bronchopulmonary dysplasia or more severe respiratory distress syndromes. (See Chapter 2 for more information on these conditions.)

Early Diagnosis of Blindness. Infants who are born prematurely and whose condition results in lung disorders are routinely tested for blindness due to the high correlation with ROP. Testing also occurs routinely when infants are born with multiple disabilities. Families often suspect blindness when an infant does not show interest in faces or bright colors, or if the eyes show unusual movement patterns, such as nystagmus or strabismus.

Associated Disabilities. Evaluation of the child with severe visual impairment is difficult because skill in vision is interwoven with every other skill domain. While children with severe visual impairment may have the muscle coordination to walk or perform fine motor tasks, they do not have the benefit of the visual feedback needed to perform these tasks accurately. When concepts are developed without the benefit of visual input, concept development can be distorted. For example, if the child is introduced to the concept of house, feeling a portion of the house acquaints the child with parts of the house, but not with the whole structure. Giving a toy replica of the house can assist, but only for the child with sufficient cognitive skill to differentiate between a real house and the more abstract toy—a concept that depends upon visual feedback. Many children need to be taught to generalize their experience with a newly learned concept to situations beyond the here and now. Such distortions affect not only conceptual development, but also language development. Communication is often affected because the child does not receive the benefit of nonverbal communication displayed by the speaker's body and face. Without the benefit of seeing the models of nonverbal communication, the child uses little of this form of message enhancement. Often blind children develop echolalia, which can be difficult to remediate. Echolalia may result from not being able to extract the gestalt of the communication act—the message exchange—which is highly tied to visual cues. They may also exhibit difficulty differentiating between the terms "you" and "I" and may have difficulty using them appropriately, because visual feedback assists in developing the notion of "self" as distinct from "other."

DUAL SENSORY IMPAIRMENT

According to demographic data on the population labeled deaf–blind, only 6.1 percent are actually totally deaf and blind. Approximately 3 percent are deaf with severe vision impairment, 48 percent are blind with severe hearing impairment, and 42.4 percent are severely hearing impaired and severely vision impaired (Goetz, Guess, & Stremmel-Campbell, 1987). The incidence of dual sensory impairment is low and difficult to determine because of the variability among states and reporting agencies in defining the disability. Figures reported by Fredricks and Baldwin (1986) suggest that 4,200 individuals with dual sensory impairment reside in the United States, and that while 94 percent of these 4,200 persons do have some residual hearing or vision, their ability to develop social/communicative interaction is seriously hindered. Helen Keller is perhaps the best known example of a person with acquired deafness and blindness.

Origins of Dual Sensory Impairment

Congenital rubella and Usher's syndrome are the major causes of dual sensory impairment in North America. When mothers contract rubella (German measles) in the first trimester of pregnancy, the disease can cause severe damage to the eyes, ears, and central nervous system of a developing fetus. In fact, an epidemic of rubella in the 1960s was the impetus for the development and delivery of many services to these individuals.

Usher's syndrome, which accounts for half of the individuals with dual sensory impairment in the United States, is genetically linked and characterized by sensorineural hearing loss and a progressive loss of vision from a condition known as **retinitis pigmentosa** (Batshaw & Perret, 1993). In Usher's syndrome, night blindness (an early symptom of retinitis pigmentosa) occurs in the first 10 years of life. Visual symptoms that develop later can include tunnel vision, decreased visual acuity, cataracts, **photophobia,** and problems with glare. Associated disabilities can include mental retardation, ataxia, and psychosis. Injuries or diseases may result in dual sensory impairment as well. This was the case with Helen Keller, whose disability resulted from a brain infection.

Early Diagnosis

Early diagnosis is more common today due to various health and education initiatives. Improved identification of children with sensory impairment results from newborn screening, follow-up clinics for premature and high-risk children, and early intervention mandates for the birth through five populations in many states.

Associated Disabilities

The disabilities associated with dual sensory impairment vary depending upon the origins of the disability, but can include mental retardation, emotional disorder, motor disability, and serious health concerns. It is obvious that even if all other systems are essentially intact, difficulties will persist because of the dependence upon the visual and hearing systems for learning and social skill development. Communicative disorders affect all individuals with dual sensory impairment and are difficult to surmount even with technological intervention, such as optic enlargers, **hearing aids,** and **assistive-listening devices.** Many individuals with dual sensory impairment continue to be educated in residential schools or in classrooms for students with multiple disabilities. The sensory abilities of individuals with less than total impairment assist considerably in extracting information from their surroundings and from their educational activities. However, the development of vocational or independent living skills requires considerable creativity on the part of educators, and the motivation of the individual and the family. While the ultimate goal for these individuals is independence, it is not achieved consistently as yet.

HEALTH IMPAIRMENTS

Many groups of individuals with health impairments (e.g., those who experience strokes that result in **aphasia,** or those with disabilities that affect the motor system, such as **amyotrophic lateral sclerosis [ALS]**), have long been served by professionals in communicative disorders. These disabilities are not the focus of this chapter. This section focuses on individuals with other diseases that are rare or new, and who are becoming more frequent consumers of speech–language pathology and audiology services.

For instance, many individuals with infectious diseases currently receive speech–language pathology and audiology services. In the 1993 ASHA Omnibus Survey, 20 percent of speech-language pathologists and audiologists reported that approximately 20 percent of their patients were infected with **cytomegalovirus (CMV),** 21.1 percent with hepatitis B virus (HBV), 17.9 percent with herpes simplex, 22.2 percent with human immunodeficiency virus (HIV) and 15.3 percent with tuberculosis (TB). Speech–language pathologists and audiologists must be aware of the ramifications of the diseases that may co-occur with the communicative disorders of some of their clients. A brief discussion of HIV illustrates this point.

Human Immunodeficiency Virus (HIV)

HIV is the causative agent of the acquired immunodeficiency syndrome (AIDS). HIV infects white blood cells, the brain, the bowel, the skin, and other tissues. Transmission occurs through blood, semen, or breast milk (Batshaw & Perret, 1993). The first cases were reported in 1980 and the first cases in children were reported a year later. In 1990, the Centers for Disease Control (CDC) reported a total of 160,000 cases in the United States, with one quarter reported in 1990. The CDC projected that by 1991 there would be 3,000 children with AIDS and 10,000 children with the HIV infection. HIV is considered an epidemic among homosexual men and intravenous drug users, but 1.7 percent of reported cases are among children under age 13.

Early Diagnosis. In adults, HIV can lie dormant for 8 to 10 years, making it difficult to detect unless specific tests are conducted. In children, the median incubation period is 12 months when the child is infected at birth, and 3.5 years when infection is a result of infected blood products. Adolescents will often acquire HIV from sexual contact or intravenous drug use and have a similar profile of incubation to adults. In many cases, the HIV infection remains undetected until symptoms begin to occur. Although HIV infection results in ultimate death, early diagnosis can allow an individual to receive life-extending treatments, such as zidovudine (AZT). There is some evidence to suggest that early treatment with AZT can help reduce the chance of developing the full-blown disease, improve the neurological outcome, or temporarily reverse some abnormalities. Eventually, disease control measures may be successful enough to move HIV infection into the status of a chronic disease.

Associated Disabilities. HIV infection is associated with a range of illnesses as well as with neurologic disabilities. (See Chapter 5 for a discussion of AIDS-related dementia.) Various forms of pneumonia are the most commonly associated illnesses. Other illnesses include bacterial infections, HIV-wasting syndromes, esophageal-wasting **candidiasis,** and **encephalopathy.** Failure to thrive, skin disease, diarrhea, and developmental delay are common and frequent presentations of HIV in children. A range of developmental outcomes have been described for children, from mild delays to frank regression. Neurologic dysfunction has been reported in 90 percent of advanced cases in children (Simonds & Rogers, 1992).

Communication disabilities that occur with HIV also vary depending on how the disorder manifests itself in a particular individual. Possible problems in the area of language include receptive and/or expressive language deficits, word finding/ retrieval difficulties, decreased levels of verbal expression, to name a few. Motor–speech problems can result from depressed respiratory support or from a weakening of speech musculature. Possible difficulties include dysarthria, other articulation problems, or voice problems such as hoarseness or hypernasality. (See Chapter 11.) Oral–motor and feeding problems can also occur. Some psychoneurological correlates can affect communication as well, including attention deficits, progressive apathy, and emotional lability.

THE ROLE OF THE SPEECH– LANGUAGE PATHOLOGIST

Speech–language pathologists (SLPs) provide services that are critical to the lives of individuals with multiple disabilities, including (1) identifying individuals who would benefit from communication skill intervention, whether the need is oral, written, or both; (2) diagnosing and appraising specific communication skills; (3) making referrals to other professionals when their interventions are needed to promote communication and related skills; (4) providing services and supports to promote communication skills or prevent communication impairments; and (5) providing counseling and guidance to clients, families, and interdisciplinary teams regarding communication skills.

Services and supports are available to individuals with disabilities and their families across their lifespan and typically include early intervention, preschool services and school-based services, followed by adult services that support

independent living and employment. The need for such services and the intensity of that need may vary during different aspects of the individual's life. Individuals and their families should be educated about the variety of options available to them, and then decide with their interdisciplinary team which services and supports are appropriate for them and how the service and support should be delivered. Since individuals with multiple disabilities have a wide spectrum of needs, speech– language services are generally delivered in an interdisciplinary context. Working with these individuals offers an opportunity for creative practice in speech–language pathology since speech– language services vary considerably depending upon the individual's communication profile, and the choices of the individual and the family.

A PHILOSOPHICAL APPROACH TO COMMUNICATION INTERVENTION

This section describes a philosophical approach to communication intervention with individuals who have multiple disabilities. Speech–language pathologists guided by the following philosophical principles are effective participants on interdisciplinary teams in a variety of service delivery models, addressing concerns of individuals with multiple disabilities (Gillette, DePompei, & Blosser, 1994, p. 6):

1. Communication is essential to successful outcomes in learning, socializing, employment, and independence.

2. All individuals can achieve some degree of competency in these areas regardless of their communication disability.

3. Individuals differ in the rate and means by which they achieve these outcomes.

4. Appropriate communication intervention requires an understanding of the unique speech– language disabilities present.

5. The mission of communication intervention is to facilitate the development of communication, language, and speech skills needed for learning, socializing, employment, and independence.

6. Communication partners hold a portion of the responsibility for successful communication.

7. Improving communication skills requires committing time, resources, and training to these communication partners.

8. Inclusion in the least restrictive environment is essential to developing the need to communicate.

9. Effective communication may require adapting the environment in which the individual must understand and be understood. These adaptations may include assistive technology.

10. Improvement in communication skills is incremental and dynamic.

Competencies for Speech–Language Pathologists

It is obvious that speech–language pathologists need disciplinary and interdisciplinary training and experience to implement this philosophy. Specific areas of competence needed include communication assessment (traditional and functional), communication intervention, assistive-technology selection and integration, team process skills, cultural diversity considerations, knowledge of etiology and related characteristics, and social values issues.

Communication Assessment. The goal of assessment is to provide direction for planning intervention programs. Speech–language pathologists must know how to select assessment methods appropriate for the needs of their clients. Due to physical or sensory disabilities, standardized instruments often need to be adapted to meet the needs of a particular client. The value of such assessments is that they typically provide a normative measure of the client's skills, allowing comparison to typical, age-matched individuals. Normative measures are often needed to justify services.

Traditional Assessment. A speech–language pathology assessment typically includes gathering a case history from the individual or a "significant other," choosing one or more diagnostic assessments to administer based upon the presenting problem, and obtaining a language sample from the client in a conversation with the speech–language pathologist or a "significant other." The speech–language pathologist chooses the assessments to administer based upon information gathered prior to the evaluation time. This includes information related to (1) the degree of intelligibility of the individual's speech; (2) the individual's receptive and expressive language skills in areas such as phonology, semantics, morphology, syntax, and pragmatics, and (3) any gap that may exist between the individual's ability to understand spoken language and to use spoken language. Many assessment tools exist to examine these characteristics of communication and the choice of assessment depends on the individual's age and abilities as well as the presenting problem. Harris and Shelton's *Desk Reference of Assessments in Speech–Language Pathology* (1993) is one source that begins to show the range of possibilities in the area of formal assessment.

Most assessment instruments assume that the senses are intact. Consequently, problems in administering formal assessments arise when persons have multiple disabilities. For example, tests of receptive vocabulary often require that the individual being tested point to the named picture from a range of choices. When an individual cannot point due to paralysis, adaptations must be made. The test may be cut apart so that the choices are sufficiently far apart for the individual to select the choice through eye gaze. Sometimes laser points or head pointers can be mounted on the head so the individual can use head movements to make choices. Most tests, whether receptive or expressive, depend upon pictures or objects to prompt a communication behavior. Individuals with visual impairments may need extra time to physically examine objects, or may need access to visual enlargement equipment in order to see the pictures. Individuals with health impairments may need to be tested in brief time periods over several sessions in order to stay alert and attentive to the tests when fatigue interferes with performance.

Similar considerations exist when the speech–language pathologist engages the individual in play or conversation to obtain a language sample. Children in wheelchairs will be less able to navigate from place to place to initiate play or conversation about topics of their choice. A child who is nonverbal may have much to express, but if the physical structures of speech are not functional, it is difficult to determine the extent of expressive language skill that potentially exists. Because of the complexities involved in testing persons with multiple disabilities, speech–language pathologists are highly dependent upon informants, such as families, social workers, teachers, and others who have ongoing relationships with the individual. These informants can assist the speech–language pathologist in making functional assessments of the individual's communication skills.

Functional Assessment. Methods for assessing communication skills within the context of daily life make a valuable contribution to an intervention plan. Here the speech–language pathologist can begin to answer the ultimate question of functional assessment: "How, what, and why does the individual communicate across persons and activities?" Such methods should include an assessment of communication patterns of important persons in the individual's life, as a base for determining behavior modifications in order to maximize the individual's communication attempts. The individual's message-sending skills may need to be assessed in a variety of modes—vocal, verbal, gestural, sign, or nonelectronic/electronic communication devices.

The speech–language pathologist must merge data from traditional and functional assessments in order to obtain a meaningful set of recommendations for intervention. The assessment cycle is complete when the speech–language pathologist integrates results and recommendations in a multidisciplinary plan developed with the family and the other members of the team.

Communication Intervention. Communication interventions are planned to achieve the outcomes determined by the multidisciplinary team. Intervention is often implemented within active experiences in the natural environment. Typical routines (e.g., changing diapers, riding on the school bus, arriving at work, or eating lunch) become the context of the training, and the partners as well as the individual with multiple disabilities receive training. Speech–language pathologists must incorporate appropriate modes of communication as well as appropriate messages in these interventions.

For example, individuals with AIDS may be intellectually capable of communicating information to their physician in complete sentences. However, if a person with AIDS has a low energy level, a speech–language pathologist may recommend preparation of a list of concerns prior to the physician's visit, which the individual can then supplement with brief expansions when more information is needed. Here the context for therapy is the visit to the physician, and the mode of communication is primarily written with brief verbal enhancement. The same method of communication can then be expanded to include more routines and partners, such as visits with family members, or trips to the pharmacy. A positive result of the communication intervention can lead to increased life participation due to conservation of the individual's energy.

Speech–language pathologists collect data to determine if outcomes are successfully met in targeted situations—at home, in school, and in social, employment, or living environments. Data sources can include direct observation, reports from the individual or significant others, and usually includes a combination of both. While the actual data collected depends on the individual's plan, examples of data include the number of conversations initiated successfully, the length and appropriateness of the conversation, and the intelligibility of the individual's messages to new and unfamiliar persons. Interventions are modified depending upon the results obtained (Gillette, 1989; also see section on Model Programs found in Appendix A).

Assistive Technology. Many types of assistive technology devices are now available to assist individuals with disabilities as they participate in their life experience. Speech–language pathologists are responsible for making the selection of augmentative alternative communication devices (AAC) with input from the client and team members. Since assistive technologies frequently interface with each other, speech–language pathologists must also be knowledgeable about other technologies such as **assistive listening devices,** environmental controls, power mobility systems, adapted play technology, and the use of switches and alternative keyboards for computer access and written communication.

Often, an AAC is one component of an individual's technology system. For example, an AAC that an individual requires for intelligible communication is mounted on a power wheelchair needed for independent mobility. The AAC can function as an alternative keyboard for the individual's desktop computer, which is used to complete written assignments. Selecting technology systems for disabilities is necessarily a team effort due to the intricate knowledge required and the expense involved. Selection of an appropriate device involves gaining a broad perspective on the client's skills, including a traditional speech and language assessment as well as literacy, motor, vision, and hearing evaluations. The individual's communication needs and desires for communication also enter in the decision for augmentative communication.

Once a communication device is selected and integrated into the individual's technology system, it is important for speech–language pathologists to provide training in the skills required for the successful use of augmentative communication, including operational, linguistic, social, and strategic competence (Light, 1989; also see section on Model Programs, Appendix A). Speech–language pathologists must incorporate augmentative communication devices in intervention plans.

Knowledge of computers is also an essential area of competence for the speech–language pathologist. In order to use computers effectively in assessment and intervention, skills in computer selection, awareness of adaptations for persons with disabilities, and familiarity with available peripherals are necessary. The use of appropriate criteria for software selection is essential in order to enhance communication skills such as socialization, receptive and expressive vocabulary, or literacy through the use of computers.

The Team Process. Speech–language pathologists must strive to ensure the cooperation of the individual and the multidisciplinary team. This cooperation is essential to the success of the

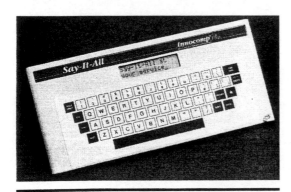

FIGURE 14.1 One example of an augmentative communication device, a Say-It-All, courtesy of Innocomp, Warrensville Heights, OH. Contact The Communication Aids Manufacturers Association (CAMA) for brochures on many devices (1-800-441-2262).

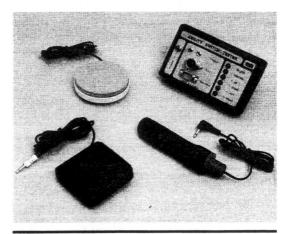

FIGURE 14.2 A switch tester and an array of switches which are used to operate some communication devices, as when an individual has motor difficulties, courtesy of TASH, Ajax, Ontario, Canada.

communication intervention plan, because communication is an essential component in almost every developmental skill area–cognitive, physical, social, and adaptive. The team must understand and accept the basic premise of functional communication intervention—that communication is not a separate activity of daily living that can be addressed in a one-to-one intervention session. Rather, communication needs to be addressed in naturally occurring activities of daily living if intervention is to be meaningful.

Speech–language pathologists may function as team members or team leaders, depending on the role assigned to them through team consensus. In either case, speech–language pathologists must understand the central role of the individual and the family to the team process. Plans must fit into the ongoing lives of families if they are to be implemented. Since speech–language pathology assessment and intervention plans include key roles for family and team members, their cooperation must be secured, often through a gradual trust-building partnership.

Consequently, successful speech–language pathologists are excellent communicators. They solicit questions, comments, and issues from the team prior to and during intervention, and continue to encourage input during the planning process. Their observations, recommendations, and oral or written reports must incorporate information from members of the team. Speech–language pathologists must be able to successfully communicate their recommendations to the team in order to bring about communicative change in the individual's daily living context. Ongoing contact with the team is required to document progress and make changes in plans based upon input.

Cultural Diversity.

The cultural background of the individual and the family will have an impact on the success of communication plans. When consulting with families, speech–language pathologists must consider the potential interpretation of a communication plan in light of the family's culture. They should understand the dimensions in which cultures differ, such as life demands, values, and supports. The success of communication intervention plans rests upon the success of the speech–language pathologist in assimilating the client's cultural perspective while planning and conducting interventions.

Etiology and Related Characteristics.

An effective speech–language pathologist demonstrates knowledge of the causes and characteristics of various types of problems. They know the diagnostic criteria associated with various disability groups. It is also important for speech–language pathologists to know sources they can access for further information on disability groups they may encounter. Such knowledge also greatly facilitates interaction with professionals from other disciplines.

Social Values Issues.

In order to serve the broadest needs of clients with multiple disabilities, speech–language pathologists must understand how society influences options for their clients. Societal influences include the impact of legislation and the interpretation of legislation on the lives of clients and on the services provided. Since models of service delivery stem directly from laws and their practice, speech–language pathologists must understand the models within which they provide service and must advocate for more appropriate models when needed. They must appreciate the important role advocacy groups play in influencing the laws and service systems. A broad understanding of human rights and privileges can help speech–language pathologists advocate more effectively for their clients when they see discrepancies between opportunities for able-bodied citizens and those with disabilities.

Clearly, the speech–language pathologist must bring a wide spectrum of knowledge and skills to the table in order to be effective. Since persons with multiple disabilities vary within and across groups, no step-by-step formulas for practice exist. The speech–language pathologist must pursue continuing education experiences in order to keep up with new programs, techniques, and technologies that address the concerns of these individuals.

THE ROLE OF THE AUDIOLOGIST

Any time speech is used to communicate or to teach, the assumption is that the person can "hear" and attend to the speaker. If an individual cannot hear clearly, or cannot attend to spoken communication, or if the environment is too noisy and distracting, then the major premise of the communicative situation is undermined.

Hearing is therefore a first-order event that must be identified and managed in order for spoken communication to occur. It could be argued that all persons with multiple disabilities have some type and degree of hearing or listening/focusing problem that requires audiologic management. Therefore, the audiologist is a critical member of an interdisciplinary team.

Hearing

Hearing loss is not an either/or phenomenon. A person is not normally hearing or deaf (Ross & Calvert, 1984). Rather, hearing impairment occurs along a broad continuum with over 96 percent of persons with hearing loss being more accurately described as hard-of-hearing rather than deaf. (See Chapter 15.) In fact, very few people have no remaining or **residual hearing** at all. Thus, the issue typically is not mere **audibility** of sound (is sound present or absent), but rather the ability to hear clearly one speech sound as distinct from another, even when wearing amplification.

The ability to identify word/sound distinctions is called **intelligibility.** An individual who cannot hear speech intelligibly due to a hearing problem, or due to being in a noisy environment, or due to having difficulty concentrating on the speaker, might hear *bake, cake, break, shake,* and *make,* all as *a.* Such mishearing could have dramatic and negative effects on a person's performance in home, school, and work environments. Unfortunately, because the individual demonstrates some audibility, the magnitude of the hearing problem is often underestimated. This underestimation of hearing and listening problems tends to occur even more with persons who have multiple disabilities, because

performance expectations may be lower, and the person's inappropriate responses may be attributed inaccurately to problems other than hearing.

The Acoustic Filter Effect

The **acoustic filter phenomenon** is a construct that can assist in understanding how even a "minimal" hearing impairment (such as one caused by ear infections—otitis media) can have detrimental developmental effects on spoken communication and learning if the hearing problem is not identified and managed. Hearing impairment can be described as an invisible acoustic filter that distorts, smears, or eliminates incoming sounds (Davis, 1990; Ling, 1989). The negative effects of the hearing impairment are apparent; the hearing loss itself is not. The primary negative effect of hearing problems of any type and degree is on the development of spoken communication. If speech sounds are not detected clearly (intelligibly), then spoken language will not develop and progress without intervention (Ling, 1989; Ross, Brackett, & Maxon, 1991). That is, we speak because we hear, not because we see. Reading, a secondary linguistic function, is built upon spoken language development (Simon, 1985). Thus, hearing is the basis of a whole chain of events leading to speaking, reading, academic performance, and ultimately to independent function.

Each individual with a hearing problem functions in a unique manner. There are many factors that influence how a person functions with a hearing problem, including the age of onset of the hearing impairment, the age of diagnosis, the type of hearing problem, the etiology, the degree of hearing impairment, the quality of audiologic management, other disabilities the person might experience, and the communication partners and patterns.

Computer Analogy

One helpful way to explain the potentially negative effects of any hearing problem on communicative function is to use a computer analogy. The basic concept of the computer analogy is that data input precedes data processing. An individual must have data (information) in order to learn. A primary way that information is entered into the brain is through the ears, i.e., hearing (Berg, 1987). If data are entered inaccurately or incompletely, analogous to having one's fingers on the wrong keys of a computer keyboard, or to having a malfunctioning keyboard, then the individual will have inaccurate or incomplete information to process.

Repairing the keyboard and enabling data to be entered correctly is analogous to using amplification technology that enables an individual to detect word/sound differences. However, all the previously entered inaccurate and incomplete information needs to be identified, and corrected data need to be reentered. Thus, the longer a person's hearing problem remains unrecognized and unmanaged, the more destructive the negative consequences of that hearing problem, and valuable intervention time is wasted.

Passive Learning and Distance Hearing

Another feature of hearing impairment is the impact of that hearing problem on **distance hearing.** Distance hearing is the distance over which speech sounds are intelligible and not merely audible (Ling, 1989). Hearing impairment of any type and degree reduces the distance over which speech sounds are intelligible, even with amplification. Typically, the greater the hearing loss, the greater the reduction in distance hearing. This reduction in distance hearing has far-reaching and negative consequences for classroom and life performance because distance hearing is linked to passive learning and casual listening (Ramsdell, 1978; Ross, Brackett, & Maxon, 1991).

An individual with a hearing problem, even a mild or unilateral hearing loss, cannot casually or passively overhear what people are saying, or the events that are occurring. Most persons with normal hearing seem to absorb passively information from their surroundings. Because hearing loss presents a barrier to the casual acquisition of information, persons with hearing problems often

seem oblivious to environmental events that are not directed actively to them. Therefore, because of this reduction in distance hearing and the elimination of passive listening and learning caused by hearing problems, persons with hearing loss need to be taught directly many skills and concepts that other persons learn incidentally (Erber, 1982).

Additional implications for reduction of distance hearing include lack of redundancy of instructional information, lack of access to social cues, and the need for assistive listening devices to expand earshot (Flexer, 1994). Distance hearing may be even more problematic for persons with multiple disabilities who may have difficulty focusing on any event not directed to them.

Amplification Devices

The audiologist can provide necessary hearing care management through the use of technology. The purpose of amplification technologies is to provide acoustic access to all learning and living environments. Different technologies may be appropriate for different communication situations.

Hearing Aids. Hearing aids are miniature public address systems, and are typically the initial, but not the only technology employed for persons who have hearing impairments. Hearing aid styles include behind-the-ear or ear-level (the most common and advantageous for children), in-the-ear (not usually suitable for children, due, in part, to inability of the hearing aid to attach to assistive listening devices), canal style (similar to in-the-ear only smaller), and body aid (which was typically prescribed for children, but is not as necessary now due to new, more powerful, ear-level hearing aids).

Hearing aids do not correct the hearing impairment. Rather, they function to amplify and shape the incoming sounds to make them audible to the person. Once sounds are detected by individuals, they must then have some listening experience to learn to make sense of those new incoming sounds.

Hearing aids are not designed to deal with all listening needs; they have limitations. One of the biggest limitations is that the microphone is on the wearer who may or may not be close to the speaker. The further the microphone is from the sound source, the poorer the ability to enhance the signal-to-noise ratio.

Signal-to-Noise Ratio.   Understanding the concept of **signal-to-noise ratio (S/N ratio),** also called Speech-to-Noise Ratio, is critical to understanding the need for assistive listening technology. S/N ratio refers to the relationship between the signal of choice, usually the speech of the communication partner and all other background sounds. Background sounds include the speech of other talkers, fans of heating or cooling systems, competing instructional sessions, hall noises, playground noises, workplace noises, computer noises, and so on. In order for a person with a hearing problem to hear the subtle differences among speech sounds, the speech signal must be 10 times more intense (+20 dB S/N) than all other background sounds (Hawkins, 1984). Persons with normal hearing require the S/N ratio to be about twice as intense (+6 dB S/N) as competing background sounds. Unfortunately, a favorable classroom has a S/N of +4 dB, which is unsuitable even for normal listeners (Berg, 1993). Therefore, since good intelligibility is essential for the development of spoken language, some means must be provided to enhance the S/N ratio for persons with multiple disabilities.

Ways to Enhance the S/N Ratio.   An obvious solution is to move closer to the person's ear so that the speaker's voice takes precedence over all background sounds. Sitting close beside a person rather than across would allow for a better S/N ratio. Having a child sit in one's lap allows one's voice to be directed into the child's ear or into the hearing aid microphone. Talking loudly from across the table or across the room promotes only audibility, not intelligibility, while an average loudness of speech very close to the person's ear facilitates intelligibility of that speech signal. A noisy room cannot possibly provide a favorable S/N ratio. In fact, typical home, workplace, and school noises

greatly interfere with the ability to hear a clear speech signal. If speech is being used as the communication medium for the person with multiple disabilities, then all professionals and communication partners must be mindful of the importance of enhancing the S/N ratio for the reception of spoken language.

Assistive Listening Devices (ALDs).   The term assistive listening device (ALD) represents a range of products designed to solve the problems of noise, distance from the speaker, and room reverberation or echo which cannot be solved with a hearing aid alone (Berg, 1987; Compton, 1993; Flexer, 1994). (For a detailed discussion of current technological options, refer to Chapter 15.) In other words, ALDs enhance the S/N ratio in order to improve the intelligibility of speech, thus enhancing a listening function. The two ALDs discussed here, personal FM systems and sound-field amplification, both use a **remote microphone** that can be placed close to the sound source. ALDs were never intended to replace hearing aids for those who use them, but rather to augment hearing aid function by adding the use of this remote microphone. Note that all amplification technology for persons with multiple disabilities must be fit by an audiologist.

An **FM unit** is a personal listening device comprised of a remote microphone transmitter that is placed near the desired sound source, and a receiver for the listener, who can be situated anywhere within 60 to 200 feet away (Berg, 1993; Flexer, 1994). There are no wires connecting speaker and listener because the unit is nothing more than a small FM radio that transmits and receives on a single frequency. This device creates a listening situation that is comparable to the speaker being within six inches of the person's ear at all times, thereby allowing for a favorable and constant S/N ratio. FM units are essential anytime a person with a hearing problem is in a noisy environment, a group learning situation such as a classroom, a noisy workplace, or must listen at some distance from the speaker (Flexer, Wray, & Ireland, 1989).

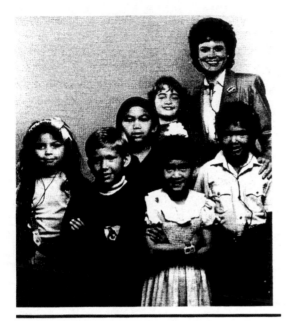

FIGURE 14.3 A mild gain, low-power output personal FM unit with Walkman headphones, can be used to make the teacher's speech clearer and more redundant. Courtesy of Phonic Ear, Inc.

Mild gain, low-power output personal FM units have been used successfully for persons who have normal or near-normal peripheral hearing but who have trouble focusing on spoken communica-tion (Blake, Field, Foster, Platt, & Wertz, 1991; Pappas, Flexer, & Shackelford, 1994; Wenzinger, Nemec, DePompei, & Flexer, 1991). The FM unit typically is fit with Walkman earphones.

The purpose of using an FM unit for persons with normal peripheral hearing sensitivity is not to make the signal louder, but to improve the S/N ra-tio, thereby enhancing the signal's saliency and re-dundancy, and focusing attention on spoken communication. An FM system can be very help-ful for persons with multiple disabilities.

Sound-field FM amplification systems are small, high fidelity public address systems that are self-contained within a single room—usually a classroom (Berg, 1993; Crandell, Smaldino, & Flexer, 1995; Flexer, 1994). The teacher wears a small, unobtrusive wireless microphone. The teacher's speech is frequency modulated onto a carrier wave that is sent from the transmitter to the receiver where it is demodulated and delivered to the students through one to five wall or ceiling mounted loudspeakers.

The purpose of the equipment is to provide a clear and consistent signal to all persons in the room no matter where they or the teacher/speaker are located. The positioning of the remote micro-phone close to the mouth of the teacher or other desired sound source creates a favorable S/N ra-tio; approximately a 10 to 15 dB improvement in

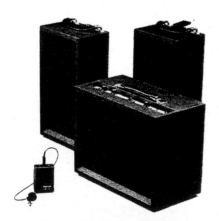
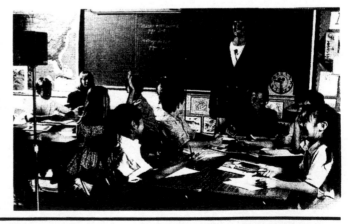

FIGURE 14.4 (L) Sound-field FM amplification systems are small, high fidelity public address systems that are self-contained in a single room. Courtesy of Audio Enhancement. (R) Sound-field FM units amplify the classroom by providing a clear and consistent signal to everybody in the room. Courtesy of Phonic Ear, Inc.

S/N ratio. It is important to note that a 10 to 15 dB improvement may not be enough for some persons with more severe hearing losses or for some persons with multiple disabilities. A well-fit personal FM system can provide a S/N ratio of +20 dB or more (Hawkins, 1984).

To summarize, it is critical to improve the S/N ratio to facilitate the listening environment for all persons with multiple disabilities. The more clearly a person can detect speech, the better opportunity that person will have to communicate and to learn. In addition to creating the quietest possible learning environment, ways to enhance the S/N ratio include moving closer to the ear of the person, or if that is not possible, using the remote microphone of either a personal or a sound-field FM system.

THE TEAM EFFORT: A DYNAMIC PROCESS

Service Provision

As of 1990, the Individuals with Disabilities Education Act required that the educational needs of all students with disabilities be addressed by a collection of professionals through the development of **Individualized Educational Programs (IEPs)** for school-age students, Individualized Family Service Plans (IFSPs) for infants and toddlers, and **Transitional Plans** for students above 16 years until age 22 or upon graduation. The professionals and persons involved in the decision-making process are those who most understand the unique needs of the student. Parents are an integral part of the team and must be invited to participate. The IEP committee is chaired by a Service Coordinator, typically the Special Education Director of the school district. Ironically, it is not unusual for this Chairperson to have never encountered or assessed the student in question. Nevertheless, the vast majority of individuals present at the IEP meeting are quite familiar with the student (Lewis & Newman, 1993). One of those professionals most knowledgeable about the student's language abilities is the speech–language pathologist.

Communication specialists are experiencing invigorating changes at this time. Insightful suggestions for the changing role of speech–language pathologists as they evolve into more classroom-based communication specialists are offered by Simon (1987). Simon has proposed that communication specialists need to expand the platforms from which they operate. Confining one's domain to the "third floor speech room" is not going to improve the efficacy of a student's IFSP/IEP/ Transition Plan, particularly for the student with multiple disabilities. The communication specialist's voice needs to be heard. Consequently, communication specialists have taken an important place in the ranks of professionals providing quality services to students with multiple disabilities (Lewis & Newman, 1993). Today, speech–language pathologists are expanding their scope of practice by acting as advocates, service coordinators, collaborators, facilitators, and increasingly, as administrators.

As with most aspects of special education, there are various options and models defining how professionals approach the educational planning process. The selection process often requires a willingness to learn about creative concepts and resourceful programs. The selection of a program should not be to defend professional territory, thereby limiting the effectiveness of a student's program, but rather to explore a variety of options that may be most appropriate and least restrictive.

The Multidisciplinary Approach

In a multidisciplinary model, numerous professionals all serve the same student. However, they do so independently of one another. The student is assessed by the professionals relevant to the case, and subsequent interventions are conducted in isolation. One drawback to this approach is the lack of communication between those delivering services to the student (English, 1994). Consequently, services and ultimately outcomes can become fragmented and uncoordinated. This method of operation continues to exist today, and is most reminiscent of the teaming that existed when Public Law 94-142 was first implemented. Lewis and Newman (1993) paint a much different picture of the current multidisciplinary team in the schools. In fact, what they describe characterizes the transdisciplinary model that will be discussed shortly.

The Interdisciplinary Approach

In this approach to collaborating, the student continues to be assessed independently; however, professionals make an effort to communicate with one another. Each professional realizes what the other is striving toward, although the interventions continue to be independent and possibly unrelated to one another. While goals may be addressed at the initial IEP meeting, there is no discussion as to how these goals will be achieved. The student continues to undergo a series of daily pullout programs that are not likely to be coordinated with other professionals, nor with the objectives established by the classroom teacher (English, 1994).

The Transdisciplinary Approach

This type of team effort epitomizes the current philosophy in special education. In the transdisciplinary model, all professionals make a concerted effort to learn enough about the other individuals' specialties to provide a cohesive, coordinated service plan. Communication is deemed a high priority, and services rendered support the student's classroom instruction within the class, as much as possible. Unfortunately, the transdisciplinary model often may not exist in practice. There continue to be "turf" issues that tend to make professionals uncomfortable and defensive (English, 1994). Much of this difficulty with *role release,* as English refers to it, may be attributed to training programs' reluctance to let go of the "expert model."

In the expert approach, the client identifies a problem and seeks out a trained professional for a diagnosis. There is no expectation on the client's part that communication will take place among others involved, nor are the professionals involved necessarily bound to the idea that sharing insights might work to create more effective programming.

On the other hand, the transdisciplinary approach strives for unity and cohesion among its members for the benefit of the student. The team's interactional style is collaborative in nature and serves to benefit both students and professionals. For students, there is less pullout, more integration of programming, and a sense by parents that the team is synchronizing its efforts. The professionals gain additional knowledge from the team-teaching and collaborating that may be taking place in and out of the classroom. Each professional is not pressured to be omnipotent regarding every field in an age of technologic and information explosions (Thousand, Villa, Paolucci-Whitcomb, & Nevin, 1992). In addition, professionals can be more efficient in planning proactive strategies to circumvent student difficulties, rather than spending inordinate amounts of time addressing major dilemmas in a reactive state (English, 1994). Thus, all team members are part of the problem-solving, which is not an event, but a process. Transdisciplinary thinking is most pervasive in training texts today, and more closely reflects the current nature of the multidisciplinary team. To promote collaborative planning, many school districts have established Intervention Assistance Teams (Neidecker & Blosser, 1993). These teams function in a capacity similar to that of the transdisciplinary model in that open communication is treated as a high priority.

The following section describes the types of professionals that a communication specialist may encounter on an IFSP/IEP/Transition team, regardless of the team's selected approach or philosophy (see Table 14.1). The key members of the service delivery team are those individuals who must be present at the student's IFSP/IEP meeting, as required by federal law. They include the parents (unless they waive their right to attend the IFSP/IEP meeting), the school principal, the regular classroom teacher and/or special education teacher(s), and the special education director. The remaining team members are referred to as itinerant due to the fact that they usually provide services to numerous schools and travel from building to building. They may or may not be part of the service delivery team.

TABLE 14.1 Service Providers

KEY MEMBERS	ITINERANT MEMBERS
Parents	Speech–Language
Principal	Pathologist
Regular Classroom	Educational Audiologist
Teacher	Resource Teacher
Special Education	Teacher of Children who
Teacher	are Hearing Impaired
Special Education	Early Intervention Specialist
Director	School Nurse
	School Psychologist
	School Counselor
	Bureau of Vocational
	Rehabilitation Counselor
	Occupational Therapist
	Physical Therapist
	Adaptive Physical
	Education Teacher
	Interpreter

Key Team Members

Parents. The student's parents may be the most knowledgeable of all the team members in terms of knowing best those factors that motivate the student, their preferences, dislikes, health history, temperament, familial background, personal goals, and so on. Parents have a legal right to participate in the programming for the student, as well as a lifetime of time and effort invested in their child. Thus, parents may often be passionate advocates and participants during the student's educational programming.

Principal. A key person on the team is the principal. The principal not only sets the tone for the program meetings, but is often the individual who is assigned the responsibility of overseeing the implementation of the IEP and Transition Plan.

Classroom Teacher. The classroom teacher is the professional who works in the "trenches." The teacher must know how to implement the program that is so painstakingly created by the team. However, given the information explosion that has oc-

curred over the last 10 years, the classroom teacher may not be adequately prepared to be all things to all students, therefore, support from other personnel is critical.

Special Education Director. These professionals may or may not have a background in special education. They typically serve as the service manager for the student's IEP or Transition Plan, and they direct the meeting. The director may have never met the student for assessment or intervention purposes.

Special Education Teacher. These teachers' certification may be in specific areas such as learning disabilities, multiple disabilities, developmental disabilities, or severe behavior disorders, or they may have a noncategorical certificate that enables them to work with students having different disabilities. In most instances, they teach in a segregated classroom, instructing students in small groups. Various degrees of mainstreaming occur contingent on the abilities of the students. Tutors known as learning disability tutors or resource professionals also may fall within this category.

Itinerant Members

Speech–Language Pathologist. The speech–language pathologist is specifically trained to assess communication skills and design speech and language intervention programs if necessary. In addition, the speech–language pathologist may (1) provide inservices to faculty in the areas of normal speech and language development and the impact of communicative disorders on social and cognitive development; (2) make referrals to the appropriate sources that may be beyond the domain of the speech–language pathologist's expertise; (3) act as an advocate for the student's communicative needs; (4) provide counseling to students and families with members having communicative disorders; and (5) function as key members of school district committees that make decisions regarding curricula, early intervention, community education, liaisons, and so on. There are numerous delivery models that the speech–language pathologist may employ. For instance, they may pull out the student from class, work within the classroom with students individually or in small groups, or the speech–language pathologist may operate on a consultative basis only. They generally travel to several schools.

Educational Audiologist. The educational audiologist may travel between numerous school districts. The educational audiologist's role is multifaceted and includes (1) identification audiometry which includes pure tone audiometric and immittance measures; (2) threshold audiometric evaluations; (3) selection and evaluation of hearing aids, FM systems, **cochlear implants,** vibrotactile devices, and other hearing assistance technology; (4) assessing classroom acoustics and implications for the learning environment; (5) written and verbal interpretation of auditory assessments; (6) IFSP/IEP planning and team management; (7) consultation and collaboration with classroom teachers and others regarding hearing loss and its impact on academic and psychosocial skills; (8) counseling for families and individuals who have hearing loss; (9) selection and maintenance of audiological equipment; and (10) implementation of inservice training for staff and support personnel (DeConde Johnson, 1995). Unfortunately, there are only about 700 audiologists to serve the country's 16,000 school districts (Neidecker & Blosser, 1993).

Resource Teachers. Resource teachers provide additional or concentrated assistance to students in a particular content area, usually reading or math. They provide the necessary small group or individual instruction to augment classroom instruction. In addition to using a pullout model, the resource teacher, like the speech–language pathologist, may also work within the regular classroom. The resource teacher has much to offer in the way of expertise to the communication specialist, and plans by both professionals should be closely coordinated.

Teachers of Children who are Hearing Impaired. Typically the teacher of children who are hearing impaired has received general education teacher's training with a specialty in hearing impairment. Many of these teachers conduct special, segregated day classes in which small groups of students are instructed in the academic areas. Many are working consultatively with regular education teachers (English, 1994).

Early Intervention Specialists. These professionals work primarily with infants and toddlers from birth to age three. They are frequently in attendance at an IEP meeting for a school-age student to assist with the transition that must take place between the student's preschool and home school. The early intervention specialist generally assumes a more active role in the planning of the IFSP for infants and toddlers.

School Nurses. Today's school nurse is assuming a much more diverse role involving a wide range of health issues, including screenings for vision, hearing, scoliosis, and so on; the provision of medical services, from simple first aid to the dispensing of medications to the treatment of acute and chronic conditions; and the control of infectious conditions such as head lice, influenza, ringworm, and so forth. They can serve as crucial liaisons between the school, home, and health community through their knowledge of medical services that may be available.

School Psychologist. This professional is responsible for the administration and interpretation of a battery of psychometric assessments, primarily standardized intelligence, psychosocial, and aptitude evaluations. They are expert in the area of behavior, and devote most of their time to referral, test, and placement activities. Currently, the emphasis is starting to shift to include psychological intervention on an assistive basis in collaboration with the classroom teacher.

School Counselor. The school counselor's domain is also becoming more diverse. Traditionally, school counselors function as academic advisors, providing information regarding college admissions, course selection, vocational training, and job placement. They also address issues pertaining to interpersonal problems with teachers, peers, or family as a crisis interventionist. Due to social changes, they are becoming more involved in social issues and physical and health development.

Vocational Rehabilitation Counselor. These counselors serve on the Transition Team with a primary emphasis on bridging the gap between the school and real world settings. They address questions pertaining to job counseling and training, funding in higher education for people who are disabled, and assessment of employment potential. In short, they assist greatly in the creation of transitional goals and begin focusing the team's thinking toward lifespan issues and objectives.

Occupational Therapist. Occupational therapists (O/T) use a student's activity and adapted surroundings to facilitate the student's independent living skills. They assess and provide services to students with disabilities that affect large and small motor functioning with the focus being on daily living skills such as self-care and adaptation of the environment (English, 1994).

Physical Therapist. The physical therapist (P/T) provides services to students having disabilities that affect large muscle groups, such as cerebral palsy, scoliosis, spina bifida, and pulmonary disorders. The emphasis is generally on mobility, as compared to the O/Ts emphasis, which mainly addresses adaptability. While P/Ts and O/Ts may have similar treatment goals, their treatment modalities may differ.

Adaptive Physical Education Teacher. This teacher (APE) is responsible for a child's physical fitness, growth, development of spatial awareness, and eye-hand coordination (Cratty, 1989). The APE adapts equipment so that students with disabilities can be actively involved in exercises,

games, and developmental activities related to growth and fitness.

Interpreter. A sign language interpreter may be present at the meetings to interpret for parents who may have hearing loss or to interpret for a student with hearing loss who elects to be present. In addition, an oral interpreter who repeats messages to provide adequate speech reading for a student having a hearing loss may be available for a student who does not sign, but rather, needs to lipread the speaker's information.

Obviously, no professional will be designing a student's educational program alone. The key is to enter the process with a collaborative mindset believing that the decision-making will be a type of shared ownership, with all members contributing a valuable piece to the educational puzzle. The important point to keep in mind is that all parts can fit. By pooling the expertise of many individuals and breaking the traditional rigidity of discipline boundaries, an educational program that is comprehensive, appropriate, and effective for the student can become a reality.

SUMMARY

The audiologist and the speech–language pathologist need to recognize how their professional contributions relate to other disciplines, and how all disciplines together combine to value the whole person. That is, the contributions of various disciplines need to be blended to achieve the goal of enhancing individuals' functions throughout the day, and across the lifespan. Never before have audiologists and speech–language pathologists assumed such critical roles.

Major Points of Chapter

- Multiple disabilities can include combinations of neuromotor disorders, sensory impairments such as blindness and/or deafness, orthopedic problems, and other health-related deficits.
- Early intervention using a team approach is an effective way of increasing functional

communication skills for people with multiple disabilities.

- Manipulation of the environment to compensate for the disabilities is critical for optimal listening, speaking, and academic progress.
- Clinical intervention may include augmentative communication systems, assistive listening technologies, as well as speech, language, and hearing services.

Discussion Guidelines

1. Use the acoustic filter phenomenon to discuss how a mild hearing loss can have negative developmental consequences.
2. Describe what is meant by the concept of "normalization," and how it affects the treatment of multiply handicapped individuals across the lifespan.
3. Describe the impact of sensory impairment on the language learning process. Contrast visual and auditory deficits and their specific effects on learning.

REFERENCES

Batshaw, M. L., & Perret, Y. M. (1993). *Children with disabilities: A medical primer.* Baltimore, MD: Paul Brookes.

Berg, F. S. (1987). *Facilitating classroom listening: A handbook for teachers of normal and hard of hearing students.* Boston: College-Hill Press/Little Brown.

Berg, F. S. (1993). *Acoustics and sound systems in schools.* San Diego: Singular Publishing Group.

Blake, R., Field, B., Foster, C., Platt, F., & Wertz, P. (1991). Effect of FM auditory trainers on attending behaviors of learning disabled children. *Language, Speech, and Hearing Services in Schools, 22,* 111–114.

Capute, A. J., & Accardo, P. J. (1991). *Developmental disabilities in infancy and childhood.* Baltimore, MD: Paul Brookes.

Compton, C. L. (1993). Assistive technology for deaf and hard-of-hearing people. In J. Alpiner & P. McCarthy (Eds.). *Rehabilitative audiology: Children*

and adults (2nd ed., pp. 441–468). Baltimore, MD: Williams & Wilkins.

Crandall, C., Smaldino, J., & Flexer, C. (1995). *Sound-field FM amplification: Theoretical foundations and practical application.* San Diego: Singular Publishing Group.

Cratty, B. (1989). *Adapted physical education in the mainstream.* (2nd ed.). Denver, CO: Love Publishing Co.

Davis, J. (Ed.). (1990). *Our forgotten children: Hard-of-hearing pupils in the schools.* Bethesda, MD: Self Help for Hard of Hearing People.

DeConde Johnson, C. (1995). Competencies for educational audiologists. *Audiology Today, 7* (3), 24–25.

Education of the Handicapped Children Act Amendments of 1990. (1990, October 30) P.L. 101–476. United States Statues at Large, 104, 1103–1151.

Eiben, R. M., & Crocker, A. C. (1983). Cerebral palsy within the spectrum of developmental disabilities. In G. H. Thompson, I. L. Rubin, & R. M. Bilenker (Eds.), *Comprehensive management of cerebral palsy* (pp. 19–23). New York: Grune & Stratton.

English, K. (1994). *Educational audiology across the lifespan: Serving all learners with hearing impairment.* Baltimore, MD: Brooks Publishers.

Erber, N. (1982). *Auditory training.* Washington, D.C.: The Alexander Graham Bell Association for the Deaf.

Flexer, C. (1994). *Facilitating hearing and listening in young children.* San Diego: Singular Publishing Group.

Flexer, C., Wray, D., & Ireland, J. (1989). Preferential seating is NOT enough: Issues in classroom management of hearing-impaired students. *Language, Speech and Hearing Services in Schools, 20,* 11–21.

Fredricks & Baldwin (1987). Individuals with sensory impairments: Who are they? How are they educated?. In L. Goetz, D. Guess, & K. Stremel-Campbell (Eds.), *Innovative program design for individuals with dual sensory impairment* (pp. 3–12). Baltimore, MD: Paul Brookes.

Gillette, Y. (1989). *Ecological programs for communicating partnerships: Models and cases.* Chicago: Riverside.

Gillette, Y. DePompei, R., & Blosser, J. (1994). *ECO: Schools Project: Ecological communication training for school speech–language pathologists.* A Proposal to the U.S. Dept. of Special Education, Personnel Preparation.

Goetz, L., Guess, D., & Stremel-Campbell, K. (1987). *Innovative program design for individuals with dual sensory impairment*. Baltimore, MD: Paul Brookes.

Hagberg, B., & Hagberg, G. (1984). Prenatal and perinatal risk factors in a survey of 681 Swedish cases. In F. Stanley & E. Alberman (Eds.), *The epidemiology of the cerebral palsied* (pp. 116–134). Philadelphia: J. B. Lippincott.

Harris, L. G., & Shelton, I. S. (1993). *Desk reference of assessments in speech–language pathology*. Tucson AZ: Communication Skill Builders.

Hawkins, D. B. (1984). Comparisons of speech recognition in noise by mildly-to-moderately hearing-impaired children using hearing aids and FM systems. *Journal of Speech and Hearing Disorders, 49,* 409–418.

Kirk, S. A., Gallagher, J. J., & Anastasiow, N. J. (1993). *Educating Exceptional Children* (7th ed.). Boston: Houghton Mifflin Company.

Light, J. (1989). Toward a definition of communication competence for individuals using augmentative and alternative communication systems. *Augmentative and Alternative Communication, 5,* 137–144.

Light, Dattilo, J., English, J., Gutierrez, L., & Hartz, J. (1992). Instructing facilitators to support the communication of people who use augmentative communication systems. *Journal of Speech and Hearing Research* (35) 4, 865–875.

Ling, D. (1989). *Foundations of spoken language for hearing impaired children*. Washington, D.C.: The Alexander Graham Bell Association for the Deaf.

Love, R. J., & Webb, G. W. (1992). *Neurology for the speech-language pathologist*. Boston: Butterworth-Heinemann.

MacDonald, J. (1989) *Becoming partners with children*. Chicago: Riverside.

MacDonald, J. D., Gillette, Y., & Hutchinson, T. A. (1989). *ECO scales manual: Assessment scales for planning and conducting communication programs*. San Antonio: Special Press.

Neidecker, E. A., & Blosser, J. L. (1993). *School programs in speech language: Organization and management*. (3rd ed.). Englewood Cliffs, NJ: Prentice-Hall.

Pappas, D. G., Flexer, C., & Shackelford, L. (1994). Otological and habilitative management of children with Down syndrome. *Laryngoscope, 104,* 1065–1070.

Ramsdell, D. A. (1978). The psychology of the hard-of-hearing and deafened adult. In H. Davis & S. R. Silverman (Eds.), *Hearing and Deafness* (4th ed). New York: Holt, Rinehart and Winston.

Ross, M., Brackett, D., & Maxon, A. (1991). *Assessment and management of mainstreamed hearing impaired children*. Austin, TX: Pro-Ed.

Ross, M., & Calvert, D. R. (1984). Semantics of deafness revisited: Total communication and the use and misuse of residual hearing. *Audiology, 9,* 127–145.

Siegel-Causey, & Downing (1987). Nonsymbolic communication development: Theoretical concepts and educational strategies. In L. Goetz, D. Guess, & K. Stremel-Campbell (Eds.), *Innovative program design for individuals with dual sensory impairment* (pp. 3–12). Baltimore, MD: Paul Brookes.

Simon, C. (1987). Out of the broom closet and into the classroom: The emerging SLP. *Journal of Childhood Communication Disorders, 2,* 41–46.

Simon, C. S. (1985). *Communication skills and classroom success*. San Diego: College-Hill Press.

Simonds, R. J., & Rogers, M. F. (1992). Epidemiology of HIV Infection in children. In A. Crocker, H. Cohen, & T. Kastner (Eds.), *HIV and developmental disabilities: A resource guide for service providers*. Baltimore, MD: Paul Brookes.

Thousand, J., Villa, R., Paolucci-Whitcomb, P., & Nevin, A. (1992). A rationale for collaborative consultation. In W. Stainback & S. Stainback (Eds.), *Controversial issues confronting special education: Divergent perspectives.* (pp. 223–232). Boston: Allyn and Bacon.

Wenzinger, K. S., Nemec, S. A., DePompei, R., & Flexer, C. (1991). The audiologist: An essential member of the rehabilitation team for traumatic brain injury. *NeuroRehabilitation, 1*(3), 41–51.

Wolfensberger, W. (1995). Of "normalization", lifestyles, the Special Olympics, deinstitutionalization, mainstreaming, integration, and cabbage and kings. *Mental Retardation, 33,* 128–131.

APPENDIX A

MODEL PROGRAMS

This appendix provides examples of some model communication intervention programs commonly used with individuals who have multiple disabilities. They include the Ecological Communication (ECO) Program (MacDonald, 1989; Gillette, 1989; MacDonald & Gillette, 1989; MacDonald, Gillette, & Hutchinson, 1989), Light's (1989) program addressing communicative competence for individuals using augmentative and alternative communication (AAC) systems, and Siegel-Causey and Downing's (1987) program for developing nonsymbolic communication.

The Ecological Communication (ECO) Program

The ECO Program was designed to address the communication development needs of persons who fit one of the following profiles:

1. An individual who does not interact meaningfully with others
2. An individual who interacts with others in play or daily life, but who does not successfully send messages to others in any form (i.e., gesture, sign, speech, or assistive device)
3. An individual who communicates, but does so with gestures or sounds, rather than linguistic forms such as words, signs, or symbols (used on some communication devices)
4. An individual who does use linguistic forms to communicate, but who does not have the skills needed to initiate, participate in, or terminate a conversation
5. An individual who has some limited conversation skill, but does not generalize it across a range of persons or activities

Such profiles are commonly found in persons with multiple disabilities. Children in wheelchairs, who are often placed alone in front of a television, will not have experience interacting with others, whatever their linguistic skills may be. Adults with visual and hearing impairments who have always had family members conduct their conversations with the outside world will have little experience communicating independently.

ECO is built around five competency areas: play, turntaking, communication, language, and conversation. The ECOScales, the program's assessment tool, specifies client goals, communication problems, and partner strategies for each competency area. ECO provides answers to the question, "How can partners interact and communicate so clients can communicate more effectively with them?" The answers are provided in the form of five principles:

1. **Be a Balanced Partner:** Engage the individual in interactions in which each person shares the lead.
2. **Be a Matched Partner:** Act and communicate at the individual's level of current communicative competence and relate these actions and communications to the person's interests.
3. **Be Responsive to Emerging Interactions:** Learn to read the individual's primitive bids for social and communicative interactions.
4. **Be Nondirective:** Allow individuals to express their communicative needs in a nondemanding, give-and-take style.
5. **Be Emotionally Attached:** Experience and express enjoyment and appreciation of individuals in interactions, so the individual seeks out and enjoys the partner.

ECO changes the interactive and communicative behavior of individuals with multiple disabilities only when their partners make significant changes in their behavior with the individual. Consequently, all interventions are conducted with the individual and the individual's significant others. ECO prescribes the following systematic approach to conducting intervention sessions with clients and partners:

> **Update:** A review of recent progress and concerns.
>
> **Plan/Educate:** Plans are based upon information obtained within the update and in-

volve making selections of client goals and partner strategies from the ECOScales. During plan/educate, professionals may provide partners with information to assist them in understanding the plan and its components.

Practice: Selecting routines and the messages to facilitate the routines. The professional and partner practice the routine together to determine how practical it is. In this way, the partner has a successful model developed with a professional that can be practiced in the natural setting.

Integrate: Partners incorporate the routines into their natural environment with the client and monitor progress and concerns. This information is shared at the next update.

The ECO program is not disability-specific but can be used with a wide range of persons with multiple disabilities. The ECOScales include skills that range from random movements to conversational participation. The methods it recommends focus the programs in the natural environment with speech–language pathologists providing support.

Communicative Competence for Augmentative Alternative Communication (AAC) Users Program

Light's program addresses the concerns of individuals who use AAC devices. It is much more difficult to communicate with technology than verbally. For example, maximum speeds that can be achieved with AAC devices are approximately 15 words a minute, while human conversation takes place at 120 to 250 words a minute. This program provides guidance to speech–language pathologists and their clients faced with concerns about message sending through technology. The program addresses four competencies required for successful AAC use: operational, linguistic, social, and strategic.

Operational competence addresses the skills the client and the facilitator will need to make maximal use of the device. Typically, this involves at least six operations: (1) keeping vocabulary up-to-date; (2) constructing overlays or other displays as needed; (3) protecting the device from damage; (4) securing needed repairs; (5) modifying the system as the clients' needs change and skills grow; and (6) making sure the device is available and operational.

Linguistic competence involves the use of the native language as well as the symbol system or linguistic code used for the AAC device display to access messages. When the need for AAC occurs as a result of a disability acquired after language is learned, the use of language itself is not an issue. However, when the individual has a developmental disability such as cerebral palsy, the individual may not have the advantage of linguistic competence. For these individuals, learning to use language and learning to use AAC occur together. For some individuals, language learning is a difficult task since the symbols used to access the messages programmed in the device are not the same as the verbal symbols partners use to communicate with them. AAC devices typically use letters, icons, or pictures to access messages.

Social competence involves skills in sociolinguistics. This includes skills in (1) initiating, maintaining, and terminating conversations; (2) communicating a variety of functions such as comments, questions, replies, requests; and (3) engaging in coherent and cohesive interactions. Social skills can be particularly problematic for individuals who have been passive communicators most of their lives. Suddenly, they have a voice but may be too timid to use it or lack the experience to initiate a conversation of their own choosing. These skills require the support of professionals and of the facilitator to provide practice opportunities in natural contexts.

Strategic competence involves the ability to use coping strategies that facilitate the use of an electronic device in natural conversation. For example, since AAC is slow, some partners will rush ahead at any pause and take the conversation down a wrong turn. The AAC user needs to have a message or nonverbal strategy that signals the listener to wait. Some users appreciate it when partners complete messages for them, while others prefer to send the message on their own without assistance. These strategic competencies need to be worked out individually so that users can communicative more effectively. Light's program addresses the unique communicative concerns of individuals who use AAC. The program recognizes the need for intervention in any competency area that may inhibit the communicative success of an AAC user.

Nonsymbolic Communication Programs

Siegel-Causey and Downing developed a program for dual sensory impaired individuals who are not verbal. The goal of the program is to promote behaviors that lead from unintentional to intentional communication at a nonsymbolic level. Examples of nonsymbolic messages might be positioning a hand outward to signal "stop," or smiling to show pleasure. This program specifies environmental factors to facilitate learning, such as (1) teaching the behaviors within the routines in which they would naturally occur; (2) teaching in a setting that includes peers who are not disabled; and (3) providing activities that promote communication throughout the day.

Once the environmental factors are in place, the program recommends these specific intervention strategies:

1. Sensitivity to individual preferences and dislikes
2. Compensation for the lack of distance senses
3. Responsivity to the individual's attempts to communicate

4. Consistency in instructional structure and format
5. Providing contingencies
6. Creating a need to communicate
7. Incorporating time-delay into adult responses
8. Establishing a cooperative social environment
9. Increasing expectations for communicative behavior (1987, p. 30–31).

Each strategy is complemented with further explanations and examples, for example, emphasizing the importance of touch and physical experience to the learner with dual sensory impairments. This program recognizes the need to provide learning experiences that are functional right from the start. Such a program is ideally suited to the needs of persons with dual sensory impairments because they frequently have difficulty learning from abstract experiences.

Summary of Model Programs

Persons with multiple disabilities often benefit from speech–language pathologist services when intervention addresses the individual in natural contexts. The contexts include naturally occurring routines as well as daily communication partners. All three of the programs outlined here address communication intervention from this perspective. Speech–language pathologists must be effective communicators in order to enlist the cooperation of the individual's often already overburdened partners. A successful communication intervention program will provide its own reward in improved relationships between individuals with multiple disabilities and their daily communication partners.

15

DEAF, DEAFENED, AND HARD-OF-HEARING INDIVIDUALS: COMMUNICATION, EDUCATION, AND REHABILITATION

NEITA K. ISRAELITE AND MARY BETH JENNINGS

This chapter introduces the reader to the lives of **deaf, deafened,** and **hard-of-hearing** individuals as they make their way across the lifespan through a world based on sound.

The chapter begins with the theory of social construction as it applies to individuals with **hearing loss.** It then turns to a more traditional study of deaf, deafened, and hard-of-hearing individuals with reviews of audiological dimensions of hearing loss; **speech, verbal language,** and **literacy** development; working with children; and working with adults. The chapter closes with a return to the notion of hearing loss as social construction and its implications for education, habilitation, and rehabilitation.

THE SOCIAL CONSTRUCTION OF HEARING LOSS

Is sound a physical reality or a social construction? Most hearing individuals would answer that sound is indeed a physical reality, and that their language and communication are based on sound. But for those whose hearing is limited, sound takes on different meanings. For those who have never heard, sound may have no meaning at all.

According to the theory of symbolic interaction (Blumer, 1969), reality is socially constructed through the process of human interaction. Thus, people create sound through the way they respond to it, the meanings they attach to it, and the value they place on it. From this perspective, much of what professionals traditionally have accepted as immutable truths about sound, hearing, and hearing status are, in fact, social constructions. Thus, hearing loss can be thought about in at least two ways: as a category of disability (traditional) or as a social difference (social construction).

Hearing Loss as a Disability

The perspective of hearing loss as a disability holds that because sound is such an important part of everyone's lives, hearing loss is a deficit that must be fixed or cured through medical procedures, hearing aids, and/or intensive speech, language, or hearing therapy. This construction of hearing loss is based on a medical model, which has "the assumption that differences in physical, sensory, or mental capabilities necessarily produce a defective member of society" (Kyle & Pullen, 1988, p. 50).

345

A critical dimension of the medical model is the notion of power. Labeling hearing loss as a disability gives permission to those who are not disabled to take charge. The medical approach to hearing has long been a dominant force in the education and rehabilitation of individuals with hearing loss.

Hearing Loss as a Difference

The difference construction perspective views hearing loss not as a category of disability, but as a social identity. According to this view, deaf persons are individuals with hearing loss who identify with the attitudes, values, traditions, mores, and ideologies of deaf culture, and who use a native sign language as their primary language (Padden & Humphries, 1988). Individuals who construct their identity in this way are referred to as **culturally deaf.**

Native sign languages are visual–spatial languages "structured to accommodate the visual capabilities of the eye and the motor capabilities of the body" (Paul & Jackson, 1993, p. 45). Native sign languages are rule-governed, with similarities to each other and to spoken languages. Signs are produced by movements of the hands, arm, face, and body. One sign can correspond to a single English word, a phrase, a sentence, or a complete idea. **American Sign Language (ASL)** is the native sign language of culturally deaf individuals in English-speaking North America.

Culturally deaf individuals base their interpretations of the world on what they see. Most do not choose to wear hearing aids or to use speech as their primary mode of communication. Instead, they use ASL, reading, and writing to communicate. These individuals expect to be viewed as a cultural and linguistic minority rather than as a category of disability. In their view, to describe a person based on hearing status is unnatural.

Being Hard of Hearing as a Difference. From a social constructionist perspective, hard of hearing people are individuals with a hearing loss who use speech as their primary means of communication,

regardless of their hearing abilities (Laszlo, 1994). Hard-of-hearing individuals use both sight and sound to communicate. They stress the importance of face-to-face interactions and clear lines of vision as well as consistent use of hearing aids and other assistive listening devices.

Hard-of-hearing individuals tend to be associated with the construction of hearing loss as a disability (Lane, 1995). Indeed, a prevailing view is that these individuals must be labeled as disabled in order to receive services and supports that facilitate spoken communication. Personal choice, however, is an important dimension of social construction (Bogdan & Biklen, 1992). Hard-of-hearing people can choose to construct their hearing status as a category of social difference while maintaining supports they view as essential.

AUDIOLOGICAL DIMENSIONS OF HEARING LOSS

This section describes **audiological** dimensions of hearing loss, including demographic information, a description of the process of hearing, types and causes of hearing loss, audiological assessment, and assistive technology.

Demographics of Hearing Loss

Hearing loss is considered to be the most common of all physical disabilities. It is estimated that 24 million Americans have some degree of hearing loss. About two million of these individuals have a loss of hearing so significant that they can hear little or no sound (audiologically deaf); the remaining 22 million have a more limited loss of hearing (audiologically hard of hearing). About three million individuals with hearing loss are children of school-age. Of this group, 50,000 are audiologically deaf and the remaining 2.5 million are audiologically hard of hearing (National Center for Health Statistics, 1994; Schein & Delk, 1974).

Hearing loss affects individuals across the lifespan. By the age of two, about 75 percent of all children have experienced a temporary hearing loss due to middle ear infection (otitis media), the most common disease in early childhood (Northern & Downs, 1984). Between kindergarten and high school graduation, about one child in five experiences a hearing loss in one or both ears stemming from otitis media or one of the many other etiologies that result in hearing loss, such as viral or bacterial infections.

The incidence of hearing loss increases with age, and many elderly individuals develop a hearing loss as part of the aging process. According to a 1990–1991 survey by the National Center for Health Statistics, approximately 25 percent of individuals age 65 to 74, and 40 percent of individuals over the age of 75 have a hearing loss (National Center for Health Statistics, 1994).

Several sets of terms are used to describe the time when a hearing loss occurs. A **congenital loss** is one that is present at birth or occurs during the birth process; an **acquired loss** is one that occurs following birth (i.e., during childhood or adulthood). Some, but not all, congenital losses are due to hereditary (inherited) factors.

A **prelingual loss** is one that is present at birth or occurs prior to the development of spoken language (before about the age of two). A **postlingual loss** is one that occurs after the development of spoken language (after about the age of two). The period between birth and the age of two is considered to be an important early developmental period for spoken language (Paul & Jackson, 1993).

Each year, about 15,000 adults experience sudden, irreversible significant hearing loss due to disease or trauma (Vernon & Andrews, 1990). They are referred to as (postlingually) deafened. Many more adults gradually develop a hearing loss through the normal processes of aging. They are said to have acquired adult-onset hearing loss.

The Process of Hearing

In their book *The Speech Chain,* Denes and Pinson (1993) trace a spoken message from its inception in the mind of a speaker to its reception and comprehension in the mind of a listener. When a person speaks, nerve impulses set vocal muscles in motion, producing pressure changes—called sound waves—in the surrounding air. The speaker's sound waves travel to the ear of the listener where they activate the hearing mechanism. The waves are converted into nerve impulses that travel to the listener's brain, where they are decoded.

The following sections review concepts related to the physics of sound, the basics of speech production, and the role of the hearing mechanism in the speech chain.

The Physics of Sound

When vibrations occur in air, they impinge on the air molecules around them, pushing or compressing the molecules more closely together. This action leaves behind spaces with fewer molecules than would normally be the case, resulting in a partial vacuum or rarefaction. The alternation of compressions and rarefactions make up sound waves. **Intensity** is the amount of energy per unit volume of air. **Frequency** refers to the number of compressions and rarefactions in a given time period.

Intensity is expressed in terms of **decibels** (dB) that describe a ratio referenced to sound pressure level. When the intensity of a sound increases, sound wave pressure increases as well. This is perceived as an increase in loudness, the perceptual correlate of intensity.

Frequency is described in terms of the number of complete cycles of compressions and rarefactions per second (cps). Cycles per second are usually expressed as **hertz** (Hz). The perceptual correlate of frequency is pitch. Increases in frequency cause a listener to hear increases in pitch. The human ear can detect frequencies between 20 and 20,000 Hz. The frequencies most useful for understanding speech are between 125 and 8000 Hz.

Pure tones are sounds that consist of only one frequency. Speech and other natural sounds are **complex tones** consisting of a fundamental frequency, (the lowest frequency in the complex wave); harmonics, (multiples of the fundamental frequency); and formants, (peaks of energy at different harmonics). Vowels and consonants are complex tones produced by vibrating air passing through the oral cavity.

The Hearing Mechanism

The ear is made up of three main parts: the **outer ear,** the **middle ear,** and the **inner ear** (see Figure 15.1).

The Outer Ear. The outer ear is made up of the pinna, the external appendage seen on the side of the head, and the ear canal (external auditory meatus). The pinna gathers sound waves from the environment and directs them into the ear. The sound waves travel down the ear canal to the eardrum (tympanic membrane), the point of division between the outer and middle ears. The ear canal is lined with skin and hair and contains several glands that produce earwax (cerumen). The eardrum is made of strong thin tissue that stretches across the ear canal to close it off at the internal

end. Sound waves that make their way down the ear canal set the eardrum into vibration.

The Middle Ear. The middle ear includes the eardrum and the air-filled space behind it. Three small bones (ossicles) and attached muscles and ligaments are housed in this space and connect the eardrum to the oval window of the inner ear. These bones, the smallest in the human body, are called the hammer (malleus), anvil (incus), and stirrup (stapes). When the eardrum vibrates, the ossicles are set into motion and carry sound waves, in the form of mechanical energy, to the inner ear.

The Eustachian tube runs between the middle ear space and the back of the throat. It is normally closed, which may cause a build up of pressure differences between the middle ear and the outside atmosphere. At these times, yawning, swallowing, or sneezing opens the Eustachian tube and permits air pressure in the middle ear space to equalize with atmospheric pressure. If the Eustachian tube becomes blocked, a vacuum is created in the mid-

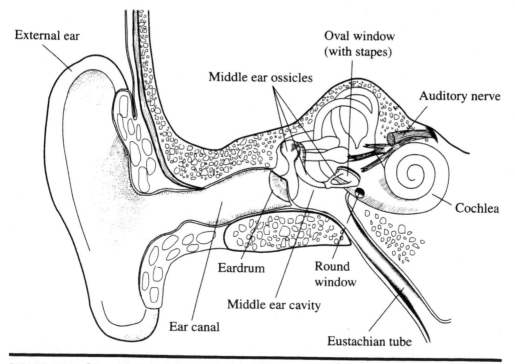

FIGURE 15.1 Cutaway view of the external, middle and inner ear.

dle ear space that may result in an accumulation of fluid drawn from the surrounding tissue.

The Inner Ear.   The inner ear is a small complex system of fluid-filled canals and chambers in the bones of the skull. It consists of the vestibular system, the sensory organs for balance and equilibrium, and the **cochlea,** the sensory organ for hearing. The focus here is on the snail-shaped cochlea, which is responsible for transforming mechanical vibrations from the middle ear into electrical signals and sending them to the brain.

The entrance to the inner ear is the oval window of the cochlea. A membraneous labyrinth divides the cochlea into three fluid-filled ducts: the scala vestibuli (the area above the membraneous labyrinth), the scala media (the area within the membraneous labyrinth), and the scala tympani (the area below the membraneous labyrinth). The scala media houses the receptor organ for the sense of hearing, called the organ of Corti. The organ of Corti contains rows of finely tuned hair cells that respond to specific frequencies of sound.

The sound waves transmitted by mechanical energy from the middle ear set the fluid in the inner ear into motion. Stimulated by this motion, the hair cells in the organ of Corti convert the mechanical energy into electrochemical pulses that are carried by neurons along the auditory nerve to the brainstem and auditory cortex, where they are interpreted as sound.

Types and Causes of Hearing Loss

The following section describes the four general types of hearing loss by location of the damage (site of lesion), major causes (etiologies), and time of onset. Most losses involve both ears (bilateral losses). Losses involving one ear (unilateral losses) may cause problems such as sound localization and difficulty in speech reception in noisy environments.

Conductive Loss.   **Conductive loss** is a disruption in the ability of the ear to conduct sound that occurs as a result of damage to the outer or middle ear. The volume of the sound is affected, but the clarity is retained. Conductive loss can generally be reversed through medical or surgical treatment.

One of the largest single causes of hearing loss is otitis media. This disorder is common in young children as a result of upper respiratory infection or poor eustachian tube function. It is typically treated with antibiotics or, in chronic cases, with surgery. During bouts of otitis media, young children experience a mild fluctuating hearing loss that may interfere with oral language input. As a result, they may be susceptible to delays in spoken language acquisition and difficulties with school learning.

Otosclerosis is a hereditary bone disease that occurs in adulthood. New bone growth in the region in front of and below the oval window causes a fixation of the footplate of the stapes in the oval window. Because the stapes cannot move freely, vibrations are not effectively transmitted to the fluid in the inner ear. Hearing loss caused by otosclerosis may be improved through surgical treatment.

Other causes of conductive hearing loss include etiologies such as congenital malformations of the outer or middle ear and occlusion of the ear canal due to excessive cerumen.

Sensorineural Loss.   **Sensorineural hearing loss** is usually permanent, resulting from damage to the hair cells and/or nerve fibers in the cochlea. The number and location of damaged elements typically determine the severity of the loss and the frequencies affected. Sensorineural loss typically causes problems not only with volume, but also with clarity. Sound is distorted and individuals may have difficulty understanding speech even when it is amplified at a comfortable listening level. A lack of tolerance for loud sounds, a condition known as loudness recruitment, may cause additional problems. Sensorineural losses are usually irreversible, but may be aided through amplification and therapeutic and/or educational intervention.

Hereditary factors are the most common cause of sensorineural hearing losses, including congenital losses that are evident at birth and progressive losses that may not show up until later in life. There are more than 150 types of genetic deafness (Vernon & Andrews, 1990). The nature of genetic transmission determines whether deafness is passed on from generation to generation. The rarity of this occurrence is shown in current estimations that fewer than 10 percent of deaf children are born to deaf parents.

Other congenital causes are prematurity, maternal viral infections that are acquired by the fetus, such as German measles (rubella), blood incompatibilities between mother and fetus, and lack of oxygen (anoxia) or trauma during the birth process. Acquired sensorineural losses may be due to factors such as noise exposure, ototoxic medications, tumors, and trauma.

Some of the factors that cause hearing loss may also cause other disabling conditions. For instance, rubella acquired in utero may cause visual problems and mental retardation in addition to hearing loss. Meningitis may cause neurological damage as well as acquired deafness. For many sensorineural hearing losses, the etiology is unknown. (See Chapter 14 for more detailed information.)

Presbycusis, the most common hearing loss in adults, is caused by the natural process of aging. It may include progressive deterioration of the cochlea due to chemical and mechanical changes in the ear, breakdown of inner ear structures, and/or degenerative changes in the auditory nerve, brainstem, and auditory cortex. These changes cause both a sensorineural hearing loss that affects the perception of spoken language and a central auditory deficit that affects comprehension.

Mixed Hearing Loss.   **Mixed hearing loss** refers to the combination of a sensorineural and a conductive component. For example, an individual may have a sensorineural loss due to hereditary factors as well as a conductive loss due to otitis media. Although the conductive component could be resolved, the sensorineural loss would not be medically treatable.

Central Auditory Processing Deficit.   This disorder is caused by damage to the auditory network that includes the path along the auditory nerve through the brainstem and auditory cortex. It may occur independent of peripheral hearing loss. **Central auditory processing deficit** typically affects comprehension and the use of auditory information and thus may have a negative affect on a child's development of language and academic achievement. As mentioned previously, this disorder also may be a component of presbycusis.

Audiologic Assessment

The **audiologist** is responsible for evaluating hearing. The audiologist also may recommend and fit hearing aids and **assistive listening devices.** (For further discussion on the role and responsibilities of audiologists, refer to Chapter 14.)

Pure-tone Audiometry.   Pure-tone audiometric tests are behavioral measures that assess how well an individual hears pure tones generated by an *audiometer.* Pure-tone testing compares the auditory thresholds of individuals with suspected hearing loss to the thresholds of individuals with normal hearing. A threshold is generally defined as the level of sound so soft that it can only be detected approximately 50 percent of the time. The range of frequencies tested is typically from 125 to 8000 Hz.

Pure-tone assessment includes testing by bone conduction and air conduction. In air conduction testing, headphones are placed over the pinnae. Sounds waves are carried through the outer ear and middle ear and into the inner ear where they are converted to electrochemical pulses and transmitted along the auditory nerve to the brain. In bone conduction testing, a vibrator is placed on the bone behind the pinna (mastoid process) or on the forehead. The sound bypasses the outer and middle ear and is primarily conducted to the inner ear.

Results of pure-tone testing for each ear are recorded on a graph called an audiogram. In Figure 15.2, sound frequency levels, expressed in Hz, are shown across the top of the graph. Hearing threshold levels, expressed in dB, are shown

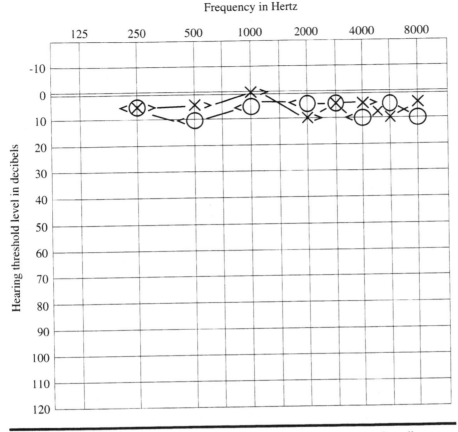

FIGURE 15.2   Audiogram illustrating normal hearing in both ears. Note that all thresholds are 10 dB HL or lower (better) for all frequencies in both ears by both air conduction and bone conduction.

along the side. The intensity range used for audiograms is from -10 (very soft) to 110 dB (very loud). The horizontal line at 0 dB hearing level (HL) represents the level of sound at the hearing threshold for average young adults. Some individuals, however, can hear sounds below this level.

Speech Audiometry.   Speech audiometry provides information about the individual's ability to receive and understand speech presented in a quiet, acoustically treated environment. Speech reception threshold (SRT) and speech discrimination tests are included in routine audiological as-

sessments and recorded on the audiogram. The SRT identifies the intensity at which listeners can hear and identify simple speech materials about 50 percent of the time. It is used to verify the results of pure-tone testing. Speech discrimination tests measure how well listeners can repeat monosyllabic words presented at comfortable listening levels. Katz and White (1992) cautioned that because these tests are typically based on single-word stimuli presented in ideal conditions, they do not represent recognition and/or discrimination of connected speech; nor do they take into account the situational, linguistic and visual cues that aid in comprehension.

Objective Measures.   **Objective measures** assess various aspects of hearing through electroacoustic and electrophyisiologic procedures that do not require a voluntary response. Acoustic immittance (impedance) tests provide information on middle ear function by measuring how resistant the middle ear system is to sound. These tests are useful in confirming the presence of conductive hearing loss in conjunction with pure-tone testing.

Auditory-evoked potentials measure activity along the auditory pathways. The auditory brainstem response (ABR) technique assesses hearing by monitoring the neural activity of the auditory nerve and the central auditory system. The ABR and other auditory-evoked potential procedures are also used for site-of-lesion testing.

A recent approach to behavioral assessment of hearing involves the use of evoked otoacoustic emissions (OAEs). OAEs are low level signals that are generated in the cochlea and detected as sound in the ear canal. In ears with normal hearing, evoked OAEs occur involuntarily in response to acoustic stimulation. They are not typically present in ears with sensorineural or mild conductive losses. This discrepancy forms the basis of diagnostic testing with evoked OAEs.

Degree of Hearing Loss.   Degree of hearing loss is generally reported as the average of the pure-tone thresholds for the frequencies most important for the perception of speech: 500, 1000, and 2000 Hz. The seven categories of hearing loss based on this average are shown in Table 15.1.

TABLE 15.1   Categories of Hearing Loss

DEGREE OF LOSS	DESCRIPTION
–10 to 15 dB	Normal
16 to 25 dB	Slight
26 to 40 dB	Mild
41 to 55 dB	Moderate
56 to 70 dB	Moderately-Severe
71 to 90 dB	Severe
91 dB and above	Profound

Source: Yantis, 1994.

Functional Categories of Hearing Loss

The effects of hearing loss are very complex, and there are wide variations in how people make functional use of audition. Individuals who have developed language and communication primarily through audition and who rely on the auditory channel for their primary mode of communication, are referred to as **functionally hard of hearing,** regardless of the degree of hearing loss. Individuals who have developed language and communication primarily through vision and who rely on the visual channel for their primary mode of communication, are referred to as **functionally deaf,** regardless of the degree of hearing loss (Ross, Brackett, & Maxon, 1991).

Individuals with any degree of hearing loss in either functional category are sometimes referred to as *hearing impaired.* Many people prefer, however, to refer to these individuals as *deaf and hard of hearing,* as this description is less deficit-based.

Factors Influencing the Impact of Hearing Loss

Major factors influencing the impact of a hearing loss are the degree of loss, the age of onset, and the rapidity of onset.

Degree of Loss.   In general, the more severe the hearing loss, the more severe the communicative consequences. Thus, the speech, language and literacy development of deaf children, and in turn, their academic progress, may be seriously affected. Hard-of-hearing children tend to experience similar difficulties, but to a lesser degree (Ross et al., 1991).

Age at Onset.   Children born with severe to profound hearing losses often miss out on auditory stimulation during the optimal period for language learning that occurs in the first few years of life. Restricted spoken language experiences during this important time may have a significant impact on oral communication and English language development.

Acquired hearing loss may have a number of psychosocial implications for adults. Deterioration in the ability to understand conversations may lead to a decrease in social interactions and difficulty with activities of daily living. Elderly adults, in particular, tend to be vulnerable to discontinuities in their lives and face the risk of lowered life satisfaction and reduced well being because of a hearing loss.

Rapidity of Onset. Individuals with a gradual loss may not realize they are developing one because of the slow progression. In fact, it is often family or friends who first become aware of the problem. Trychin and Busacco (1991) indicated that the average delay between onset of acquired hearing loss and identification is between five and seven years.

In contrast, life may become chaotic for deafened adults whose hearing loss is sudden or whose loss occurs within a short period of time. They are faced with the prospect of making significant adjustments to a well-established life pattern.

Other Factors. Other factors affecting deaf and hard-of-hearing children include age at identification, age at amplification, parental involvement, type of educational program, primary mode of communication, ethnic background, and the presence of other handicapping conditions (Moeller & Carney, 1993; Moores & Moores, 1989; Wolk & Schildroth, 1986). Children with chronic or fluctuating losses due to otitis media, permanent mild losses, and unilateral losses may be at risk for communication and educational problems. Some children with slight losses may also experience similar problems (Ross et al., 1991).

With adults, other factors influencing the impact of hearing loss are degree of acceptance, personality, motivation, occupation, and environmental conditions (Katz & White, 1992).

Assistive Technology

Following the audiometric assessment, the next consideration is the use of assistive technology,

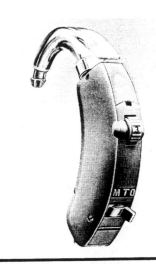

FIGURE 15.3 Ikon—Mini BYE aid. Courtesy of Unitron Industries, Limited.

including personal hearing aids, implants, vibrotactile aids, assistive listening devices (ALDs), and other technological devices and services (see Ross, 1994a, for an extensive review of assistive technology).

Personal Hearing Aids. Hearing aids are available in various types and styles (see Figure 15.3). It is the responsibility of the audiologist or licensed hearing aid dispenser to fit individuals with the aid best suited to their needs. Most audiologists favor binaural (two-ear) amplification over monaural (one-ear) amplification, when appropriate, chiefly because of the enhanced potential for sound localization and speech discrimination.

Conventional hearing aids have common components: (1) a microphone that converts acoustic energy into an electrical signal; (2) an amplifier that increases the magnitude of the electrical signal; and (3) a receiver that converts the amplified signal back into acoustic energy. These components are powered by a battery. User-controlled switches allow for adjustment by the user; internal controls must be adjusted by the audiologist or hearing aid dispenser.

Some hearing aids have a t-switch, which disables the microphone and activates a telecoil within the aid that is sensitive to the electromagnetic waves generated by telephone receivers.

Direct audio input (DAI) is a special option that is available on some hearing aids, cochlear implants, and tactile aids. DAI technology reduces distortion and poor intelligibility caused by background noise, reverberation, and distance from the speaker by connecting the hearing aid directly to assistive listening devices.

Behind-the-Ear Aid (BTE). The BTE aid is used by children and adults. Its components are housed in a unit that fits behind the ear. Amplified sound leaves the aid through an earhook and travels to the custom-fitted earmold through a short plastic tube. The BTE aid typically has a t-switch and DAI.

The BTE is the hearing aid of choice for children for several important reasons. It is durable and easy to handle. The controls are easy to manipulate. Infants and young children in rapid growth stages require new earmolds as often as every three to six months. With the BTE aid, earmolds can be replaced without having to replace the entire device. The BTE also has the advantage of DAI, which enables coupling to assistive listening devices.

In-the-Ear Aid (ITE). The ITE aid is another type of aid worn by children and adults. Its components are housed in a small custom-made unit that fits directly into the ear like an earmold. A t-switch is optional on some models.

Canal Aids. In-the-canal (ITC) and completely-in-the-canal (CIC) aids are the smallest devices currently available. They are custom designed to fit entirely into the ear canal and are fairly unobtrusive. They typically do not have a t-switch.

Body and Eyeglass Aids. The body aid is made up of a body-worn unit housing most of the aid's components, including a t-switch, and is attached to a receiver and custom earmold. It may be appropriate for individuals with poor manual dexterity. The eyeglass aid has its components built into the temple of the individual's prescription glasses. Both styles are currently used less than they were in the past.

Bone Conduction Hearing Aids. The air conduction aids described above account for nearly all the hearing aids used by deaf and hard-of-hearing individuals. Bone conduction aids, however, may be prescribed for individuals who cannot tolerate an earmold due to an ear infection or a congenital malformation of the outer or middle ear. A bone conduction vibrator is placed on the mastoid process and powered by a BTE or body style aid. Mechanical vibrations are then transmitted directly to the inner ear through the skull.

Digitally Programmable Hearing Aids. The response characteristics of digitally programmable aids are set by an external computer or programming unit. From one to eight memories can be programmed independently into the aid to provide a wide range of characteristics appropriate to different listening situations (e.g., listening in quiet environments, listening in background noise, listening to music). The user is able to change memories by pushing a button on the hearing aid or by using a remote control.

Implants

Cochlear Implants. **Cochlear implants** are devices that bypass damaged cochlear structures to provide auditory sensation through low-level electrical stimulation of the auditory nerve fibers. Several implant systems have been approved by the Food and Drug Administration (FDA) for use with adults and/or children. Although they may work in different ways, all have similar basic components. Common external components include a speech processor, a microphone, and a transmitter; internal components include a receiver/stimulator surgically implanted under the skin in the mastoid bone (behind the ear) and attached electrode(s) implanted in the inner ear. Cochlear implants use one electrode or an array of electrodes. They incorporate a single channel or multiple channels of information. Most multi-channel electrode arrays are inserted directly into the cochlea.

One of the most commonly used devices is the Nucleus 22 Channel Cochlear Implant System (see Figure 15.4), which has been implanted in more than 10,000 adults and children worldwide (Staller, Beiter, & Brimacombe, 1994). It works in the following way. Sounds in the environment are picked up by the microphone and sent to the speech processor. The speech processor selects, amplifies, and digitally codes the elements of the acoustic signals most useful for speech. These signals are sent to the transmitter, which then sends the codes across the skin to the implanted receiver/stimulator. The receiver/stimulator converts the codes into electrical signals and delivers them to specific electrodes along the array, programmed for various frequencies and intensities. The electrodes stimulate different auditory nerve fibers in the cochlea, resulting in the sensation of sound (Staller et al., 1994).

Cochlear implants are used with young prelingually deaf children and deafened adults and children. Candidates for implantation must have profound bilateral sensorineural hearing loss and must be unable to benefit from hearing aids. At this time, there is no way of predicting in advance who will benefit from implantation.

The goal of implantation in young, prelingually deaf children is to improve speech perception and facilitate the acquisition of spoken language. Geers and Moog (1994a) edited a monograph reporting on a three-year research project on sensory aids, conducted at the Central Institute for Deaf (CID). Subjects were 39 profoundly deaf children divided into three groups: 13 using Nucleus 22 Channel cochlear implants, 13 using vibrotactile aids (described below), and 13 using conventional hearing aids.

Results of studies conducted by several researchers indicated significant improvement for implanted children in speech perception (Geers & Brenner, 1994), speech production (Tobey, Geers, & Brenner, 1994), acquisition of English vocabulary and syntax (Geers & Moog, 1994b), and

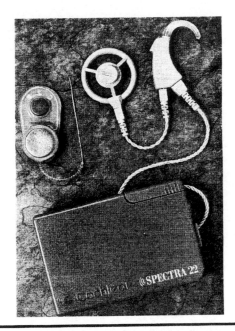

FIGURE 15.4   Courtesy of Cochlear Corporation.

speech intelligibility (Osberger, Robbins, Todd, & Riley, 1994). Children who received instruction in speech and oral language and had good family support appeared to make the most gains.

Research with deafened adults typically shows postimplantation improvement in speech-reading and speech perception, but with considerable variation among users. Research by Cohen, Waltzman, and Fisher (1993) suggested that multichannel implants are superior to single channel implants for understanding speech.

Most people support cochlear implants for postlingually deafened adults and for children who actively choose this option. A major source of contention, however, is the implantation of young prelingually deaf children. Culturally deaf people, represented by consumer groups such as the National Association of the Deaf (NAD), have expressed serious concern about this practice, citing factors such as the role of cochlear implants in delaying parental acceptance of their child and the child's own acceptance of deafness (Vernon & Alles, 1994).

Auditory Brainstem Implants. The auditory brainstem implant (ABI) is a recent advancement in implant technology. It was designed for adults diagnosed with a particular nervous system disease (Neurofibromatosis-2) with an acoustic tumor. The procedure to remove the tumor eliminates residual hearing. Therefore, the ABI is implanted in an attempt to provide auditory sensation. It includes an electrode array placed within the lateral recess of the brainstem, over the surface of the cochlear nucleus, and connected to an external receiver/stimulator. The major reported benefits of the ABI are detection of environmental sounds and enhancement of lipreading ability. It has not received FDA approval to date (Staller, Otto, & Menapace, 1995).

Vibrotactile Aids

Vibrotactile aids code speech as vibratory sensations on the skin by frequency, intensity, and time pattern. They are used by individuals who are unable to access speech through audition alone due to the severity of the hearing loss. Data from studies summarized by Weisenberger and Percy (1994) indicated that these devices may provide useful information to supplement speechreading for speech perception and speech production tasks. Eilers, Fishman, Oller, and Steffens (1993), for example, reported significant differences in the phonological productions of young profoundly deaf children using vibrotactile aids in addition to amplification, as compared to children using amplification alone. In the CID sensory aid study (Geers & Moog, 1994a), however, children with cochlear implants made more gains in speech production and spoken language development than children with tactile aids. Moreover, children with tactile aids, all of whom also wore hearing aids, did not improve significantly in spoken language, as compared to children wearing hearing aids alone.

Assistive Listening Devices (ALDs)

Hearing aids work best in quiet environments, where the acoustics are good and where the listener is close to the sound source. For large noisy settings such as schools, theaters, meeting halls, courtrooms, and houses of worship, personal and group ALDs are required. ALDs "pick up sound at or close to its source, amplify it, and deliver it to the listener's ear without extraneous sound, reverberation, and distortion" (Stone & Hurwitz, 1994, p. 245). Listeners connect to ALDs through listening attachments such as headphones, DAI, silhouette inducers, neckloop induction, and button receivers.

Radio Frequency Modulated Systems (FM). The FM is the ALD most widely used in educational settings. It operates like a miniature FM radio station. "The teacher broadcasts to a child or a group of children on a specific FM radio frequency; the children tune into the teacher's 'station' on their wearable radio receivers" (Sanders, 1993, p. 185). The system is portable, and more than one channel can be used in the same area. A new development in this technology is a device that combines a BTE aid with an FM system (Ross, 1995).

Major disadvantages of the FM system include its susceptibility to interference by external radio transmissions, the need to have the same channel for both the transmitter and receiver, and the potential for interference from other systems used in the same building within the transmission range.

Infrared Light Systems. These systems are frequently found in theaters and other public places. They convert sound into light waves that are transmitted throughout the room. The signal is picked up by an infrared receiver that converts the light waves back into sound, amplifies them, and sends them to the listener's ears. Infrared systems have excellent sound quality. However, they cannot be used outdoors or in rooms with significant amounts of natural light due to interference from the infrared rays of the sun.

Electromagnetic Loop Induction Systems. These systems rely on a loop of wire placed around a selected area. The wire has a magnetic core that creates an electromagnetic field. The sound from the microphone is transmitted by the magnetic field into the area inside the loop. Listeners access the sound through devices sensitive to magnetic field changes such as hearing aids with a t-switch or portable induction receivers.

Major disadvantages include variation in signal strength depending on the location of the listener within the loop, and interference from systems located in close proximity within the same building.

Hardwire Systems.   With these systems, listeners and speakers are directly wired to an amplifier, hence the term "hardwire." Hardwire systems are used for one-to-one listening, individual television viewing, and as a substitute for hearing aids for elderly individuals with reduced manual dexterity and mobility. The major disadvantage of these systems is that the mobility of both listeners and speakers is restricted.

Other Technological Devices and Services

Telephone Amplifiers.   Telephones that are hearing aid compatible (i.e., emit strong electromagnetic field signals) can be used with hearing aids that have a t-switch. Some telephones can be purchased with built-in amplifiers and controls to adjust the frequency of the signal and the ring. Special amplifiers can be added to the telephone, including portable amplifiers that strap onto the earpiece.

TTYs.   The **TTY** is an acoustic coupler that allows individuals to transmit and receive typed messages through regular telephone lines. TTY relay systems enable individuals who use their voices on the telephone to communicate with individuals who use the TTY via a relay operator.

Voice carry over (VCO) enables a hard-of-hearing individual to speak directly to a hearing caller instead of typing on the TTY. The relay operator types the reply so that the hard-of-hearing individual can read it.

Computers.   Advances in personal computer technology such as electronic mail systems, na-tional telecommunication systems, and the Internet greatly enhance the individual's access to information and interpersonal communication.

Closed Captioned Decoders.   **Captioning** is a process by which the audio portion of a television show is coded in written form (i.e., subtitles) and transmitted over line 21 of the television signal. Closed caption decoders are required to receive captioning. Since July 1993, all television sets with screens larger than 13 inches sold in the United States have been equipped with these devices.

Alarms and Alerting Devices.   Alarms and alerting devices use vibratory devices or visual signals such as flashing lights for smoke and fire alarms, doorbells, and telephones.

THE DEVELOPMENT OF SPEECH, VERBAL LANGUAGE, AND LITERACY

In the following section, **speech** refers to the individual's ability to produce spoken or oral English. **Verbal language** refers to the internalized knowledge of spoken English or ASL. Deaf individuals may have good verbal language (oral or signed), but speech that is difficult to understand.

Speech Perception

Hearing individuals rely on audition as the primary source of input for oral language. To make sense of a spoken message, they detect speech signals, discriminate among the acoustic/phonetic elements of speech, identify familiar patterns, and use their knowledge of linguistic, paralinguistic, and situational cues to comprehend the intended meaning. This process is known as *auditory speech perception.*

Deaf and hard-of-hearing individuals may have difficulty at any of these levels. They may not detect a speech signal at all, or the signal may be distorted, making discrimination and identification difficult. They also may not have extensive linguistic knowledge to bring to the comprehension process.

Auditory speech perception is related to degree of hearing loss. Hard-of-hearing individuals generally have better speech perception skills than deaf individuals, but their error patterns are quite similar. Most deaf and hard-of-hearing speakers have little difficulty in vowel perception. Consonants have higher frequency components than vowels and are more difficult to discriminate. The most common errors are consonants that differ by place of articulation (such as /b, d, g/; /p, t, k/). These errors occur more frequently with consonants in the word-final position because sounds in that position are acoustically weaker. Deaf and hard-of-hearing individuals have less difficulty perceiving voicing, nasality, and manner of articulation (See reviews in Nerbonne & Schow, 1989; Ross et al., 1991).

The auditory speech perception of many deaf and hard-of-hearing children and adults may be improved through auditory learning, which teaches individuals to make maximum use of amplified residual hearing for the comprehension of spoken language (Ling, 1986). Auditory learning is encouraged for individuals wearing hearing aids for the first time. It is especially important for children and adults with cochlear implants, who must learn to make sense of the auditory sensations the implant provides.

The Role of Visual Speech Perception

Although auditory information is usually sufficient for comprehension of speech by hearing listeners, visual information provides additional support useful to deaf and hard-of-hearing people who receive diminished and/or distorted information through hearing alone. Visual speech perception is dependent upon personal and environmental factors that affect visual acuity, such as eyesight, lighting conditions, distance from the speaker, and viewing angle. Another set of factors relating to the visual characteristics of speech include influences of rate of speech, variation among speakers, and visibility and visual similarities of speech sounds (Sanders, 1993).

Visemes (Fisher, 1968) are speech sounds that have been classified by their visually distinguishable characteristics, namely place of articulation and shape of the mouth. There are four generally agreed upon consonant viseme groups: *labiodentals* (/f, v/), *bilabials* (/p, b, m/), *rounded labials* (/w, r/), and *nonlabials* (/t, d, n/, and so on). Consonants within each group look the same and are called *homophemes.*

There are no comparable viseme groupings for vowels, as each has a unique mouth shape (Jackson, 1986). However, research reviewed by Hipskind (1989) suggested that errors in visual perception of vowels are common, especially with vowels that have similar lip positions and movement.

Because of the homophenous nature of speech, accurate perception through visual information alone is usually not possible. The individual must be able to make extensive use of linguistic knowledge to fill in the gaps (Boothroyd, 1988).

Auditory and Visual Speech Perception Combined

Research reviewed by French-St.George and Stoker (1988) indicated that audition is a major factor in speech perception for prelingually deaf children and deafened adults. These individuals may still benefit, however, from using visual cues to enhance comprehension.

Speechreading is defined as "the ability to understand a speaker's thoughts by watching the movements of the face and body and by using information provided by the situation and the language" (Kaplan, Bally, & Garretson, 1988, p. 1). The components of speechreading include gestures and body language, facial expression, situational cues, and linguistic factors related to the redundancy of language. *Lipreading,* the ability to identify what is being said by viewing lip movements alone, is only one of the necessary components of the speechreading process. Speechreading is a common focus of instruction for individuals with adult-onset hearing loss. With prelingually deaf children, speechreading is used as a supplement to auditory learning in many programs.

There is debate in the field as to the benefits of instruction in speechreading. Results for adults are mixed (Gagné, 1994), and it is not clear how effectively they transfer skills acquired in training to their everyday lives. Some researchers question whether young deaf and hard-of-hearing children can learn to make maximum use of auditory cues if both audition and speechreading are consistently used in combination (Ling, 1986).

Speech Production

Intelligible speech requires the development of an internal auditory-articulatory feedback loop so that individuals can monitor their own speech and voice patterns. Deaf and hard-of-hearing individuals have difficulty with self-monitoring due to problems with this feedback loop. As a result, most deaf and hard-of-hearing individuals, except those with slight losses, typically have problems with speech production.

Deaf Speakers. Deaf individuals present characteristic errors in production of both the segmental and suprasegmental elements of speech. Many of these errors were initially identified by Hudgins and Numbers (1942) and confirmed and further described by later researchers.

The segmental elements of speech are the phonemes, including vowels and consonants. The most common errors in vowel production are neutralization, in which different vowels are produced in a manner that makes them sound similar to the schwa vowel (/ə/), and prolongation, in which vowels are unnaturally elongated. Deaf speakers also typically neutralize or prolong *diphthongs,* vowel-like speech sounds produced when two vowels are blended within the same syllable (such as /au/).

Consonants are more difficult than vowels for deaf speakers to produce. Common consonant errors include voicing problems, in which voiced consonants are substituted for their voiceless cognates; omissions of consonants in word-initial and word-final positions and blends; and consonant distortions and nasalization.

Even when vowel and consonant production is satisfactory, problems with suprasegmentals may make the speech of deaf people difficult to understand. *Suprasegmentals* are the prosodic aspects of speech, including elements such as pitch, intonation, loudness, duration, and rhythm. The temporal aspects of speech, including elements such as rate of speech, duration of phonemes, and pausing within and between phrases, may also be affected.

Many deaf and hard-of-hearing individuals present abnormal breath patterns for speech (McGarr & Whitehead, 1992). This makes for problems with *duration,* the length of audible sound for syllables in a breath group, and **intensity,** the volume of a sound produced by a speaker. Other problems include reduced vocal intensity resulting in a breathy voice or excessive vocal intensity resulting in an abnormally loud voice.

Pitch is the perception of a sound relative to its frequency. Control of pitch is necessary for production of intonation patterns. Deaf speakers have difficulty establishing appropriate pitch levels and varying pitch to communicate meaning.

Deaf speakers demonstrate problems with nasality. *Hypernasality,* when the voice sounds too nasal, occurs when too much air is emitted through the nose during speech. *Hyponasality,* a lack of nasal resonance, occurs when insufficient air is emitted through the nose during the production of nasalized sounds.

For a more extensive survey of this literature, the reader is referred to Seyfried, Hutchinson, and Smith (1989) and Stoker and Ling (1992).

Hard-of-Hearing Speakers. Hard-of-hearing individuals are usually able to use audition to monitor their productions of vowels, suprasegmentals, and voice quality. For these elements, their speech tends to be comparable to hearing peers. The most common errors of hard-of-hearing speakers are the omission of consonants, especially in the word-final position. The final consonant error illustrates the relationship between speech perception and speech production (i.e., final consonants are difficult to perceive because they are often unstressed or acoustically weak). Other common errors are substitutions of one consonant sound for another and distortions, especially with affricates and fricatives (See reviews in Ross et al., 1991; Seyfried, Hutchinson, & Smith, 1989).

Deafened Speakers.   Deafened speakers tend to experience gradual deterioration of speech due to a breakdown in the auditory feedback loop necessary for self-monitoring of speech production. Factors affecting the quality of speech production include degree of hearing loss, age at onset, history of amplification, and other influences (Cowie, Douglas-Cowie, & Kerr, 1982; Jackson, 1992). Typical errors include problems with sibilants (/s, z/), final consonants, voice quality, loudness control, and rhythm.

Assessing Speech

Comprehensive assessment of the speech of deaf and hard-of-hearing individuals should describe strengths and weaknesses in speech production as well as intelligibility. The most comprehensive procedures for assessing the speech of deaf and hard-of-hearing children is the Phonetic-Phonologic Speech Evaluation Record (Ling, 1991). This inventory determines the child's repertoire of sound production (phonetic level) and then assesses how these sounds are used in meaningful communication (phonologic level).

The phonetic level evaluation (PLE) specifies an order to the evaluation of speech skills based on Ling's (1976) developmental model. It relies on teacher or clinician categorization and rating of children's imitative or prompted productions. The PLE is the tool most widely used to assess the speech of deaf and hard-of-hearing children (Abraham, Stoker, & Allen, 1988) although several recent studies have questioned the adequacy of the PLE as an accurate assessment tool.

Tests developed for hearing speakers, such as the Goldman Fristoe Test of Articulation (Goldman & Fristoe, 1969), Fisher-Logemann Test of Articulation Competence (Fisher & Logemann, 1971), and the Assessment of Phonological Processes (Hodson, 1986) may be useful evaluations for hard-of-hearing individuals, whose speech tends to resemble the speech of hearing peers.

When assessing deaf and hard-of-hearing individuals, it is always important to compare results to the audiogram and to the individual's auditory perception capabilities. Patterns of production as compared to perceptual strengths and difficulties should inform intervention goals and strategies.

Teaching Speech

The most widely used model for teaching speech to children with hearing disorders was developed by Ling (1976; 1989). The Ling approach works at both the phonologic and the phonetic levels. It acknowledges the importance of the auditory channel for spoken language learning and emphasizes early consistent amplification. Sounds are taught through audition first, with the addition of visual and tactile cues as necessary. Activities based on this approach can be incorporated into both informal and formal teaching situations, used in conjunction with other speech programs (See, for example, Waling & Harrison, 1987), and modified for work with adults. Research findings have shown the success of the Ling approach in promoting spoken language development (Ling & Milne, 1981; Novelli-Olmstead & Ling, 1984; Perigoe & Ling, 1986). (See Stoker & Ling, 1992, for an extensive review of theory and practice in speech production.)

Verbal Language

Hearing children all over the world acquire the spoken language of their society in a consistent, predictable, and relaxed manner, and in a relatively short period of time. Language acquisition begins at birth and continues throughout childhood, adolescence, and adulthood. Young hearing children use complex sentences by the time they are three and are sophisticated language users by the time they enter school.

The same principles hold true for young deaf children of deaf parents acquiring the native sign language of their community. Their process of language learning corresponds to the way that hearing children learn spoken languages with regard to progression through developmental stages and rate of acquisition (See reviews in Hoffmeister, 1990; Israelite, Ewoldt, & Hoffmeister, 1992).

This is not the case, however, for the majority of deaf and hard-of-hearing children learning spoken language. Although many eventually acquire sufficient skill to communicate effectively with hearing people, they typically have serious difficulty in this area.

The Role of Early Interactions

Young children acquire language through interacting with caregivers in their environment as well as listening and/or watching as other people interact. Hearing caregivers communicate with hearing children in a natural and relaxed manner, using grammatical phrases and sentences that are short, syntactically simple, repetitive, and related to the child's world. They encourage their child to initiate communication and participate in conversations by using interrogatives and long pauses between utterances (Bloom & Lahey, 1978; deVilliers & deVilliers, 1979).

When hearing parents discover their child's deafness, the nature of the communicative interaction changes. Parents typically become more directive and controlling. They speak less, do not engage in verbal play, and seem less comfortable when communicating with their deaf child. These kinds of interactions appear to negatively influence language development. In contrast, interactions between deaf parents and deaf children are very similar to the interactions of hearing parents and hearing children. There is more evidence of child-initiated communication and apparent enjoyment of communication by all participants (see review in Meadow-Orlans, 1990).

Research consistently shows that deaf children of deaf parents outperform deaf children of hearing parents in language, literacy, and social development as well as in academic achievement (Moores, 1987). It is hypothesized that a major reason for this difference is the natural and smooth early communication that can occur in a climate of parental acceptance when parents provide their children with a complete visual language such as ASL, from birth.

The Acquisition of English

When learning English, deaf children follow normal patterns of development, but at a delayed rate. This trend is seen in the development of syntax (the grammatical system of language), semantics (the meaning system), and pragmatics (the use of language in context). Although deaf children typically can use simple syntactic, semantic, and pragmatic functions effectively in English, difficulties become more apparent with linguistic tasks requiring more complex coding strategies. (See McAnally, Rose, & Quigley, 1994, for a review of this literature.)

Hard-of-hearing children typically acquire language at a rate more comparable to hearing peers, although some delays may still be evident. They appear to have particular difficulty with vocabulary acquisition and complex syntactic structures (Ross et al., 1991).

Assessing Language

A variety of specialized tests are used to assess the English language skills of deaf and hard-of-hearing students, including many originally designed and normed on hearing populations. Three widely used tests developed specifically for deaf and hard-of-hearing students are the Grammatical Analysis of Elicited Language (GAEL)—Simple Sentence Level (Moog & Geers, 1985) and Complex Sentence Level (Moog & Geers, 1980) and the Teacher Assessment of Grammatical Structures (TAGS) (Moog & Kozak, 1983). Several tests of ASL acquisition are in development or nearing completion.

Many speech–language pathologists favor detailed analysis of spoken, signed, or written language samples as the assessment of choice. Schirmer (1994) provides a comprehensive description of procedures for language sampling and formats for analysis.

Facilitating Language Development

Speech–language pathologists and teachers formulate language goals and activities based on the results of their assessments and observations. Many educators recommend natural, conversational approaches to language instruction based on principles of normal language development. Language is acquired through authentic communication that is meaningful for the child, and not through drill and practice.

Deaf and hard-of-hearing children often may need coaching and practice in using language appropriately in context. Language-rich environments with opportunities to communicate and good language models provide a natural setting for learning about holding successful conversations and repairing communication breakdowns. The ultimate goal of all language instruction should be communicative competence.

Literacy Development

For purposes of this discussion, **literacy** refers to reading and writing in English. **Deaf cultural literacy,** which includes story-telling, drama and poetry in ASL, is not addressed.

English language proficiency is an important factor in the **literacy** development of deaf and hard-of-hearing students. When and how this proficiency is established in relation to reading and writing instruction is a matter for debate in the literacy field.

The traditional reading readiness position assumes that proficiency with verbal language, be it spoken or signed, is a prerequisite to the development of reading and writing. In contrast, the emergent literacy position holds that proficiency in verbal language and written language develop simultaneously, and that children learn a great deal about these processes long before they begin for-

mal literacy instruction (Harste, Woodward, & Burke, 1984). Recent research with young deaf children supports the emergent literacy perspective. For example, in studies by Ewoldt (1990) and Williams (1994), young deaf children made gains comparable to hearing children of similar ages in their knowledge and use of written language. Sign and/or oral language improved concomitantly.

Despite such positive beginnings, many deaf and hard-of-hearing school-age children have difficulty with literacy and may achieve at levels well below their hearing peers. Literacy levels remain a concern in postsecondary programs and in adult continuing education.

The Reading Readiness Explanation

The reading readiness position suggests that the poor literacy attainments of deaf and hard-of-hearing students are a result of their being taught to read and write before they have developed an internalized language system and sufficient knowledge of English syntax and phonology. This view informs an approach to readiness that focuses to a great extent on developing verbal language proficiency, especially in spoken English, and literacy instruction that often focuses on teaching isolated skills.

The Emergent Literacy Explanation

The emergent literacy position offers an alternate perspective. It suggests that the problem lies in a mismatch between instructional practices based on reading readiness and deaf students' abilities to bypass syntax and phonology and construct meaning semantically, directly from print. Several studies have demonstrated the facilitative effect of sufficient contextual support and background knowledge on deaf children's reading comprehension (Israelite & Helfrich, 1988; Yurkowski & Ewoldt, 1986). Research has shown that deaf children can and do learn language through literacy.

Early access to written language and meaningful literacy events is important for deaf and hard-of-hearing children, many of whom receive incomplete messages in English or linguistically different messages in ASL. Holistic approaches such as whole language (see Goodman, 1986) and process writing (see Graves, 1983) support the development of both verbal and written language for any child. They are strongly recommended for deaf and hard-of-hearing students. For further discussion of methods to facilitate literacy development, the reader is referred to Schirmer (1994).

WORKING WITH DEAF AND HARD-OF-HEARING CHILDREN

This section explores some of the major issues related to working with deaf and hard-of-hearing children, including factors related to identification of hearing loss and early education, communication philosophies and educational approaches, and options in educational placements.

Identification

When parents initially approach the family doctor or pediatrician with worries about their child's unresponsiveness to sound or delay in speaking, it is not uncommon for the doctor to ascribe the parents' concern to overreaction, and to recommend that they ignore the situation. As a result, identification of hearing loss is sometimes delayed until the child is between one and three years old (Vernon & Andrews, 1990).

The Interdisciplinary Team

Once the loss has been identified, hearing parents require the understanding and support of professionals with different areas of expertise as they adjust to the situation and begin to consider options. Because audiologists are often the first professional with whom hearing parents come in contact, they often take on counseling and educational roles in addition to their diagnostic responsibilities. Speech–language pathologists and teachers of the deaf and hard-of-hearing may be involved in helping parents explore communication philosophies and educational options. Social

workers, counselors, and psychologists may provide ancillary support as necessary.

Parents of recently identified deaf and hard-of-hearing children should be encouraged to meet other parents who have raised deaf children. Deaf, deafened, and hard-of-hearing adults, including members of the deaf community, can provide support, information, and a wealth of firsthand experiences (Vernon & Andrews, 1990).

Early Education

It is important that infants and young deaf and hard-of-hearing children be enrolled in early education programs to maximize opportunities for language and communication during these critical years. Current models of early education are based on the view that young children learn language best at home, through meaningful interactions with their families. Federal legislation mandates that early intervention programs take a family-centered approach and that parents have an active role in decision-making.

Communication Philosophies and Educational Approaches

A major decision for parents is what language/communication option and educational approach to choose for their young deaf child. The language/communication options include American Sign Language (ASL), spoken English, and sign systems that were developed to represent English visually. The educational approaches are bilingual, oral, and total communication. The language/communication issue is highly contentious and has been the focus of much discussion and debate for many years. The major options, educational approaches, and some of the controversies are presented in this section.

Oral Approaches. Oral approaches advocate the use of English in its spoken form to support acquisition of speech, oral language, and literacy. They focus on understanding language through the visual information provided through speechreading and/or the auditory information provided through amplified residual hearing.

There are two major approaches that emphasize vision and hearing to varying degrees. Auditory–oral communication is the traditional approach to oral education. It combines the use of visual information (i.e., speechreading) and auditory information with intensive instruction in speech production (Ling, 1989). Auditory–verbal communication focuses on the acquisition of speech and language primarily through amplified residual hearing (Estabrooks, 1994; Goldberg, 1993). A third approach, cued speech (Cornett, 1967), uses hand cues to make English sounds or phonemes visible as a supplement to auditory–oral communication.

Research over the years has shown oral methods to be highly successful for select children. In a study by Geers and Moog (1989), 100 orally educated deaf students were superior to nonorally educated deaf students in reading, writing, and academic achievement. Some children taught through oral methods, including those with moderate, severe, and profound hearing losses, have developed highly intelligible speech (Ling, 1989).

From the late 1800s until the 1960s, most deaf children were educated in oral programs. The majority of oral programs were abandoned, however, because of continuing concerns about the poor **oral communication,** academic achievement, and social adjustment of many of their graduates.

Total Communication. **Total Communication** (TC) is both a philosophy and a methodology that may incorporate all modes of communication including speech, fingerspelling, invented sign forms of English (described below), ASL, gestures, and written English. In common practice, however, TC typically is a combination of spoken English and an invented sign form.

In the 1960s and 1970s, with increasing concerns about the effectiveness of oral programs, the decision was made to supplement spoken language with signs, assuming that this added support would result in increased levels of academic achievement. Invented sign systems that attempted to represent English morpheme units in a visual form were created for classroom use. The creators of these systems combined ASL signs with invented signs and chose to follow English word order rules. The most common of these **manually coded English (MCE)** systems include Signed English (Bornstein, Hamilton, Saulnier & Roy, 1975), Seeing Essential English (SEE I) (Anthony, 1971), and Signing Exact English (SEE II)(Gustason, Pfetzing, & Zawolkow, 1972).

MCE systems, as well as ASL, are augmented by *fingerspelling,* a system of handshapes that represent individual letters. Fingerspelling is used to spell proper nouns borrowed from English. Some TC programs also incorporate the use of **pidgin sign English** (PSE), which consists of ASL signs in English word order.

Concerns have begun to surface about the total communication approach. It is argued that (1) attempts to combine a temporal system (speech) with a visual–spatial system (sign) violate the integrity of both systems; (2) difficulty in producing invented signs and speech simultaneously may cause teachers and students to use fragmented, incomplete versions of both systems; and (3) total communication has not brought about the hoped for increases in academic achievement (Johnson, Liddell, & Erting, 1989). These concerns, however, have been challenged (Hyde & Power, 1991; Luetke-Stahlman, 1988; Martin, 1994), and presently, the majority of educational programs for deaf students are still based on the total communication approach.

Bilingual/Bicultural Approaches. Since the early 1980s, there has been increasing interest in **bilingual/bicultural education** for deaf students. This approach promotes knowledge and use of two languages (e.g., ASL and English) and two cultures (deaf culture and hearing culture). In most bilingual/bicultural programs, ASL is recognized as the native language and is used as the basis for classroom communication and instruction in read and written English. The study of deaf culture is an integral part of the curriculum, with deaf adults serving as role and language models. Deaf teachers and administrators are important members of the educational team. Parent education is viewed as an essential component of the program (Israelite et al., 1992). Instruction in spoken English (speech, speechreading, auditory learning) may be presented as an individual option. Bilingual/bicultural programs also use PSE to facilitate communication between individuals who are fluent in ASL and individuals who are fluent in English.

Advocates of bilingual/bicultural education assert that sign language should be considered the native language of most deaf children because of the poor match between the characteristics of oral language and deaf children's processing capabilities. ASL, they argue, presents sign language users with an intact visual–motor feedback loop similar to the auditory-articulatory feedback loop of spoken language users (Cicourcel & Boese, 1972).

There is a movement toward bilingual/bicultural education for deaf students in the United States and Canada among the deaf community and some deaf educators. Bilingual/bicultural education is mandated by law in Sweden and is widely accepted, although not mandated, in Denmark. Theoretical papers and position papers in favor of this approach frequently appear in the literature, as do reports of successful programs. (See Mahshie, 1995, for a review of bilingual/bicultural education for deaf children.)

Much of the theoretical basis supporting bilingual/bicultural education for deaf students is premised on the work of researchers such as Cummins (1984; 1989), who has studied the relationships between the acquisition of first and second languages with both spoken and written forms, and their educational implications. The Cummins model has been widely applied to the situation of deaf students learning English (Cummins & Danesi, 1990; Israelite et al., 1992; Schirmer, 1994). Recent papers by Akamatsu (1995) and Mayer and Wells (1996), however, question the appropriateness of this application. Because sign languages have no written form, deaf learners cannot develop literacy skills in their first language (ASL) that can be used as a basis for acquiring literacy skills in their second language (English). These authors suggest that a naturally occurring signed form of spoken English (as opposed to invented sign systems, e.g. Fischer, 1995) may provide the bridge between ASL and English literacy.

The Oral–Manual Controversy. For more than a century, educators have been embroiled in an ongoing debate about what communication approach is best for deaf students. This debate, called the **oral–manual controversy,** started out in the early days of deaf education as an argument between *oralists,* who believed that deaf children should learn to speak, and *manualists,* who believed that deaf children should learn sign language. The advent of total communication approaches added an additional layer to the debate. As one might expect, each position has its own proponents and its own strong arguments. The debate is fueled by the fact that no one method is superior for all children and some children taught through each method excel in language, literacy, and academic achievement.

Although the current trend is toward bilingual/bicultural education, auditory–oral approaches appear to be recapturing interest because of recent advances in technologies such as sensory aids (e.g., cochlear implants) and computer-based speech perception and speech production training aids. These technologies have the potential to strengthen the auditory-articulatory feedback loop and improve perception and production of speech for children and adults (Berg, 1992; Stoker & Ling, 1992).

Options in Educational Placements

Historical Perspectives. The first schools for the deaf in North America were mostly segregated residential institutions. Children lived at the school from age four or five until high school graduation, going home only for major holidays and summer vacation. Until the 1960s and 1970s, the only other option in most locales was for children with hearing loss to attend regular school with no support services. Thus, because of a lack of viable alternatives, many deafened or severely hard-of-hearing children attended residential schools.

Until World War II, residential schools were the major learning institutions for deaf people in North America, Britain, and Europe. Since then, several significant developments have profoundly affected the pattern of educational placements for deaf children. Highly mechanized warfare in World War II resulted in a large proportion of soldiers returning home with noise-induced hearing losses. Their rehabilitation needs sparked interest in the development and refinement of hearing aids. This trend led to the development of increasingly sophisticated aids that have benefitted many individuals who previously could not benefit from these devices.

During the postwar period, people began to recognize the wide variety and degree of hearing loss, as well as the effects of hearing loss and the individualized needs of deaf and hard-of-hearing children. Increases in the number of school-age children, growing population centers, improved transportation, and changes in the role of the parent and parental expectations necessitated a much wider range of educational options and greater demand for services at the local level.

Another major factor was the Education of the Handicapped Act (PL 94-142), passed by Congress in 1975. **The Individuals With Disabilities Education Act** (IDEA) (PL 101-476), was passed by Congress in 1990 and mandated a free appropriate education for all students with disabilities in the least restrictive environment and as close to the mainstream as possible. The enactment of this legislation and the other factors cited above resulted in a sharp increase in programs for deaf and hard-of-hearing children in local school districts and a concomitant decrease in the number of children attending residential schools. By 1992, about 80 percent of deaf and hard of hearing students in the United States were educated in local schools and only 20 percent in residential schools. Of the students attending local schools, about 33 percent attended special classes, while 47 percent attended regular classes with hearing students (U.S. Department of Education, 1993).

Placement Options.   Moores (1987) identified five basic classifications that represent the typical range of school placements for deaf and hard of hearing students. *Residential schools* provide living arrangements as well as educational and social programs. Children who attend residential schools have the opportunity to be immersed in the language and culture of deaf people. *Day schools* are typically found in metropolitan areas. Here, children live at home and commute to school daily. Some deaf children may attend residential schools as day students.

Day classes are often located in public schools where the majority of the children are hearing. Many deaf and hard-of-hearing children frequently spend part or most of their day in regular classes; others may have most or all of their instruction in self-contained classes.

In the past, only children with the most residual hearing and best oral communication were placed in the mainstream. Today, however, many signing deaf children attend regular classes accompanied by sign language interpreters.

Many deaf and hard-of-hearing children who are mainstreamed receive support through *itinerant programs*. Itinerant teachers may work directly with deaf and hard-of-hearing students, or on a consultative basis with the students' classroom teachers. Other mainstreamed deaf and hard-of-hearing children may go to *resource rooms* where they receive academic support on an as needed basis.

Hearing and Speech Services.   The listening needs of deaf and hard-of-hearing students should be supported by educational audiologists. Their role includes functions such as monitoring personal hearing aids and ALDs, monitoring classroom acoustics, working with classroom teachers, and providing direct instruction to deaf and hard-of-hearing students. Some educational audiologists also assess hearing, and fit and monitor hearing aid use.

Some deaf and hard-of-hearing students may also use the services of speech–language pathologists. These professionals assess language and speech, develop intervention programs, consult with teachers, and provide direct instruction to deaf and hard-of-hearing students.

Academic Achievement

Although research on the cognitive development of deaf individuals shows they have the same achievement potential as hearing individuals (Martin, 1994), academic performance is an area of continuing concern. Deaf students tend to perform more poorly than hearing peers on standardized tests of achievement such as the Stanford Achievement Test (SAT) (Gardner, Rudman, Karlsen, & Merwin, 1982). Performance is better in mathematics than in reading-related areas. Hard-of-hearing students tend to perform at higher levels than deaf peers; however, they typically do not achieve as well as hearing students (Ross, 1990).

The mismatch between the cognitive abilities of deaf and hard-of-hearing students and their academic achievements has called into question the appropriateness and effectiveness of specialized educational methodologies for teaching deaf and hard-of-hearing students in segregated settings (Johnson et al., 1989) as well as the type and quality of support services available in the mainstream (Ross et al., 1991).

Research shows that deaf and hard-of-hearing children who are mainstreamed tend to achieve at higher levels than those who attend residential schools (Allen, 1986; Holt, 1994; Holt & Allen, 1989). A study by Holt (1994), for example, examined achievement in reading comprehension and mathematical computation for deaf and hard-of-hearing students in a range of school settings. The results showed a significant effect for degree of integration.

Studies comparing academic achievement in different settings, however, typically do not take into account student performance prior to class placement. Deaf and hard-of-hearing students may have been selected for regular classes because of their already high levels of academic achievement. Thus, the actual influence of mainstreaming is difficult to ascertain (Holt, 1994).

What Is Least Restrictive for a Deaf Child?

There is a major controversy regarding whether the least restrictive environment for a deaf student is a residential school or a mainstream setting. At the residential school, deaf children are exposed to deaf role models and deaf peers. They have full access to the academic program and can readily take an active role in student clubs and organizations, sports, and cultural events. In the mainstream, on the other hand, deaf students often have limited access to the academic program and extracurricular activities. They report feeling socially isolated and alone (Foster, 1989). Indeed it is a common observation that the deaf student's primary communicative and social partner in a mainstream class is often the sign language interpreter. These factors have caused some researchers, educators, deaf and hard-of-hearing students, and parents to view the residential school as the least restrictive environment. To many other members of these stakeholder groups, however, the least restrictive environment remains the regular classroom.

Full Inclusion.   More recently, there has been a move toward full or total inclusion of deaf students in regular education programs. Few people would disagree that inclusion in regular education with appropriate support services should be an option for deaf students. Many, however, are concerned that the terms *full* and *total* imply, and will lead to, all deaf children being enrolled in regular education classes despite the appropriateness of the placement (Corson & Stuckless, 1994). Stinson and Lang (1994) argued that full inclusion may only serve to increase the social isolation that deaf students in mainstream programs so commonly report.

Choosing Among the Options

When considering educational options, the primary concern should be ensuring that children are placed in programs consistent with their individual needs, abilities, and aspirations. Central to such decisions are in-depth understanding of the hearing loss; the linguistic, academic, and social potentials; the family and cultural considerations; and the availability of appropriate support services. Parents and their children should make these decisions together, in partnership with members of the interdisciplinary team. The firsthand experiences of deaf, deafened, and hard-of-hearing adults may be of invaluable assistance.

Postsecondary Education

There are numerous options available for deaf and hard-of-hearing students at the postsecondary level. Gallaudet University, in Washington, D.C., was established more than a century ago as the first liberal arts institution for deaf students in the world. Since the mid-1960s, the National Technical Institute for the Deaf (NTID) at the Rochester Institute of Technology in Rochester, New York, has provided technical and academic programs in both integrated and segregated settings. Many other colleges and universities offer educational support services for deaf and hard-of-hearing students. In addition, select community colleges and vocational schools provide a range of programs and services for these individuals.

Of particular concern to adults with hearing loss is the effect on employment. The job picture for deaf individuals has traditionally been characterized by underemployment rather than unemployment (Moores, 1987). In difficult economic times, however, employers may be reluctant to hire and/or retain workers they perceive to be disabled. Thus, access to high quality postsecondary education and training is imperative.

Educational Support Services

Support services enable the participation of deaf, deafened, and hard-of-hearing individuals in educational, vocational, social, and cultural activities. Such services were mandated with passage of the **Americans with Disabilities Act** of 1990 (ADA), which requires, among other provisions, communication access for individuals with hearing loss (Strauss, 1994). Prior to this legislation, other federal and state laws mandated similar accommodations, but not to as great an extent as ADA has done.

This section reviews services that provide visual and text-based representations of spoken language, including manual notetaking, electronic notetaking, and interpreting. Other educational services include supports such as tutoring, peer-support groups, and ALDs (described previously). These services are provided individually or in combination depending on the needs of the student.

Interpreting. Interpreters facilitate communication between individuals who are deaf, deafened, or hard-of-hearing and individuals who are hearing. They have become an important part of the interdisciplinary team, working with students in elementary, secondary, and postsecondary settings. Interpreters are responsible for conveying information; they do not participate in the dialogue as contributing members of the communication. Sign language interpreters (1) translate spoken information into sign language (ASL) or a sign system, depending on the preferences of the deaf, deafened or hard-of-hearing individual; and (2) translate sign language into spoken information for individuals not familiar with manual communication.

Oral interpreters use nonvocalized lip movements, gestures and body language to convey spoken communication. This process facilitates communication for individuals who rely on *speechreading* in settings in which speechreading the speaker is difficult.

Manual Notetaking. Manual notetaking involves summarizing and transcribing spoken information into written form. In educational settings, hearing students enrolled in the same classes as deaf, deafened, and hard-of-hearing students frequently serve as notetakers on a volunteer or paid basis.

Electronic Notetaking. Vivran (1991) described the two types of electronic notetaking: computerized notetaking and real-time captioning. In computerized notetaking, a typist summarizes spoken information on a personal/portable computer. The notes appear on a monitor, a television, or an overhead screen and can later be accessed as hard copy. Depending on the skills of the typist and the speaker's rate of speech, the notes can vary from summary information to near-verbatim captions.

In real-time captioning, a court reporter creates and transmits verbatim captions of spoken information using a stenotype system of shorthand notation. Specialized equipment instantly converts the notations into text form, which is then displayed in real time.

WORKING WITH ADULTS

This section focuses on hard-of-hearing adults who seek out aural rehabilitation programs and services. The majority of these individuals have adult-onset, acquired hearing loss. Their ages range from young adult to elderly. The severity of their losses vary from mild to profound; the progression of their losses, from gradual to sudden. Adults who are hard-of-hearing since birth also participate in aural rehabilitation; culturally deaf adults typically do not.

The first step in aural rehabilitation is the recognition of the possibility of a hearing loss, followed by an audiological assessment. Next is the audiological prescription and fitting of hearing aids, as appropriate, and orientation to ALDs and other assistive technology.

Hearing tests and the provision of hearing aids, however, are usually not enough to solve the problems that the loss creates. Individuals require information about aids and other technical devices, strategies for maximizing auditory–visual speech reception, suggestions for reducing barriers to communication, and support in adjusting to any psychosocial, educational, and/or occupational effects. These supports and services are the purview of aural rehabilitation. The goal of aural rehabilitation is to increase the likelihood and effectiveness of communication for hard-of-hearing individuals within the limits that their hearing loss creates.

Aural rehabilitation professionals include audiologists, speech–language pathologists, and occasionally, teachers of the deaf and hard-of-hearing. They provide services such as (1) identifying and evaluating sensory capabilities (auditory, visual and tactile-kinesthetic); (2) interpreting results of assessments; (3) counseling individuals and/or families; (4) helping individuals maintain and/or improve expressive and receptive communication; and (5) serving as the liaison between hard-of-hearing individuals, their families, agencies, and other members of the interdisciplinary team (ASHA, 1984).

Aural rehabilitation takes an ecological focus (Noble & Hétu, 1994). This means it achieves its goal by working not only with hard-of-hearing individuals, but also with significant others (e.g., spouses, family members, employers, caretakers) and physical environments (e.g., private homes, places of business, residential care facilities).

Aural Rehabilitation Programs

Aural rehabilitation programs are offered to hard-of-hearing individuals and significant others in several formats: therapy sessions for individuals; modules for large groups, consisting of single sessions focusing on one topic (e.g., assistive devices, speechreading, communication strategies); and group aural rehabilitation courses for small groups, consisting of weekly sessions with a set curriculum. Format selection depends on the needs and preferences of the individual. One individual may participate in more than one format simultaneously.

Group Aural Rehabilitation. Group aural rehabilitation courses typically cover topics such as (1) hearing loss and communication; (2) hearing aids and technical devices; (3) communication and coping strategies; (4) speechreading principles and practice; and (5) advocacy and assertiveness. Methods of instruction are lecture, discussion, group problem-solving, and role playing. The group format is highly recommended because of the benefits of the group experience to the individual (Montgomery, 1993).

Speechreading is often a focus of interest for many hard-of-hearing individuals who mistakenly believe that it can replace audition as a primary means of comprehending spoken language. A major goal of group aural rehabilitation is to help individuals recognize that auditory–visual speech reception is improved when other communication strategies and assistive devices are used in addition to, or in combination with, speechreading.

Aural rehabilitation curricula and methods may be adapted to meet the needs of various groupings of hard-of-hearing individuals such as students in postsecondary programs, adults in the workforce, active seniors, and seniors in residential care facilities. Spouses, family members, friends, and associates may also be accommodated.

Working with Older Adults

Aural rehabilitation programs designed for seniors include topics specific to their life circumstances and the communication problems caused by presbycusis. Active seniors benefit from the peer interaction and social support of group aural rehabilitation classes. Many attend Elderhostel programs for hard-of-hearing seniors, which combine group aural rehabilitation with social and cultural activities.

Older seniors in residential care facilities typically require a different sort of programming. Because of their generally frail condition and the presence of other health problems, services based on an ecological model are best delivered on-site. Participation of caretakers is essential as modifications to the residential environment and caregiving practices are often necessary and may significantly improve seniors' communication and quality of life. Service delivery is also facilitated when caregivers are aware of the communication requirements of this population (Jennings & Head, 1994).

Consumer Groups

It is important that individuals advocate for their own needs at home, at school, at work, and in the community. In the past few years there has been increased interest in **consumer groups** for deafened and hard-of-hearing individuals, such as the Association for Late-Deafened Adults (ALDA)

and Self Help for the Hard of Hearing, Inc. (SHHH). Consumer groups such as these provide leadership and support to individuals in their self-advocacy efforts. Ross (1994b) recommended that consumer groups be viewed as "adjuncts and extensions" that put "the primary AR [aural rehabilitation] responsibility where it belongs: with the involved individuals themselves" (p. 593). In the deaf community, consumer groups such as the NAD have long been involved in advocacy and political action. Social and fraternal organizations also are common.

Issues in Assessment

In addition to audiometric testing, assessment in aural rehabilitation typically relies on speechreading tests and self-report communication scales. The goals of speechreading tests, such as the Utley Test (Utley, 1946) and the Denver Quick Test of Lipreading Ability (described in Alpiner & Schow, 1993), are to assess basic speechreading ability and the effects of training. Giolas (1994) argues against the use of these tests because they place too much emphasis on discrete skills and not enough on the role of speechreading in the communication process.

The goal of self-report communication scales such as the Communication Profile for the Hearing Impaired (CPHI) (Demorest & Erdman, 1987) and the Hearing Handicap Interview for the Elderly (HHIE) (Ventry & Weinstein, 1982) is to determine how hearing loss affects the individual's everyday life. They are often used as pre- and posttests to measure the individual's progress in aural rehabilitation and the success of the program. Little, if any, change is typically shown on these quantitative tests, however, despite qualitative evidence of substantial progress in adjusting to hearing loss and using productive communication strategies.

A major difficulty is that communication scales and speechreading tests may not be sensitive to the elements of everyday communication faced by hard-of-hearing individuals. There is a mismatch between scores on tests/rating scales and how people function in their day-to-day lives. Qualitative research and evaluation are needed to more thoroughly understand the personal meanings that individuals in aural rehabilitation construct from their experiences. Results of qualiative research indicate that hard-of-hearing individuals and significant others are profoundly affected by hearing loss (Hallberg & Carlsson, 1991; Jones, Kyle, & Wood, 1987). Several qualitative studies show that group aural rehabilitation supports hard-of-hearing individuals and significant others in the adjustment process. In two recent studies, hard-of-hearing individuals in group aural rehabilitation classes progressed in their use of productive communication strategies and assertive behaviors (Israelite & Jennings, 1995; Jennings & Israelite, 1994). Spouses in other qualitative studies developed greater understanding of the impact of hearing loss on their hard-of-hearing partners and the marital relationship through group aural rehabilitation (Getty & Hétu, 1991).

The progress that individuals make in aural rehabilitation appears to be the product of a complex set of interacting factors related to the nature of the curriculum, the unique aspects of each individual, the experiences they bring to the aural rehabilitation course, and the meanings they construct. Hearing loss and the aural rehabilitation process thus are highly personalized experiences that are continually constructed through real life social interactions. This helps to explain why quantitative tests and measures are not effective ways of showing improvement and/or deciding if aural rehabilitation "works."

THE SOCIAL CONSTRUCTION OF EDUCATION AND REHABILITATION

Throughout this chapter, hearing loss is seen as socially constructed in two ways: as a category of disability or as a social difference. Proponents of the construction of hearing loss as a disability argue that hearing loss must be labeled as deficit so that it can be cured through sound-based assistive devices, such as personal hearing aids and ALDs, and education that emphasizes oral communication.

Culturally deaf individuals are typically proponents of the construction of hearing loss as a social difference perspective. Most reject hearing aids and ALDs because, in their view, there is no deficit to cure. They are interested in assistive devices such as TTYs and support services such as sign language interpreting that provide visual access to communication.

Culturally deaf individuals object to what they call the "hearing agenda" in deaf education, i.e., education based on the disability construction. Many value an educational approach that teaches deaf children to communicate with each other through ASL and with hearing individuals primarily through written English. They want to ensure that children learn about deaf culture and take pride in being deaf. They strive for more deaf community involvement in education and for the increased preparation and hiring of deaf administrators and teachers (Lane, 1992).

The preferences of deafened and hard-of-hearing individuals complicate the distinctions between the two perspectives. Many of these individuals use sound-based assistive devices such as hearing aids and ALDs, vision-based assistive devices such as TTYs, and support services such as computerized notetaking and sign language and/or oral interpreting. As well, some choose to obtain cochlear implants or use tactile aids.

Deafened and hard-of-hearing individuals identify with the language, culture, and values of the hearing majority. They may choose to attend programs to improve their speech, speechreading, use of residual hearing, and coping strategies. Choosing these programs, however, should not be equated with choosing the disability construction of hearing loss. The value and appropriateness of programs and services depend on the individuals involved, their needs and potentials, and the choices they make.

The individual's sociocultural affiliation is another important factor to consider. Deaf, deafened, and hard-of-hearing individuals may identify not only with cultures and communities based on hearing status, but with their home cultures as well. The beliefs, values, and attitudes of the family's cultural group may strongly influence communication practices and educational choices.

A culturally deaf individual may view speech or hearing therapy as disempowering. A deafened or hard-of-hearing individual may find the same therapy empowering. Participation in education and rehabilitation programs that support oral communication should be viewed as choices that individuals make to enable their participation in the hearing world. The increased interest in consumer groups such as the NAD, SHHH, and ALDA demonstrates how individuals with hearing loss are becoming empowered to take control of their lives. From this perspective, it is possible to construct not only being deaf, but also being deafened or hard-of-hearing, as categories of social difference.

Major Points of Chapter

- Hearing loss can be described as either a category of disability or as a social difference.
- The major types of hearing loss are categorized by location of damage, cause, and age of onset.
- Factors influencing the impact of a hearing loss include the degree of loss, age of onset, rapidity of loss, and age at the time of amplification.
- Current rehabilitative methods include assistive listening devices, digitally programmable hearing aids, cochlear implants, and vibrotactile aids.
- Oral approaches to rehabilitation are contrasted with manual and/or total communication perspectives.
- Important issues include cultural aspects of deafness, language and literacy, academic achievement, and workplace integration of people with hearing impairment.

Discussion Guidelines

1. Contrast the medical approach to deafness with the social constructionist point of view. State both sides of the argument, and justify why you agree or disagree with the arguments.
2. Describe the factors that impede the acquisition of language and literacy in children with hearing loss.
3. Describe rehabilitation goals for children who are prelingually deafened, and compare them with the goals for adults who are postlingually deafened. Outline approaches used for both populations.

REFERENCES

Abraham, S., Stoker, S., & Allen, W. (1988). Speech assessment of hearing-impaired children and youth: Patterns of test use. *Language, Speech, and Hearing Services in Schools, 19,* 17–27.

Akamatsu, C. T. (1995, July). *Thinking with and without language: What is necessary and sufficient for school-based learning.* Paper presented at the International Congress on Education of the Deaf, Tel Aviv, Israel.

Allen, T. E. (1986). Patterns of academic achievement among hearing impaired students: 1974 and 1983. In A. N. Schildroth & M. A. Karchmer (Eds.), *Deaf children in America* (pp. 161–206). San Diego, CA: College-Hill.

Alpiner, J. G., & Schow, R. L. (1993). Rehabilitative evaluation of hearing-impaired adults. In J. G. Alpiner & P. A. McCarthy (Eds.), *Rehabilitative audiology: Children and adults* (pp. 237–283). Baltimore, MD: Williams & Wilkins.

American Speech-Language-Hearing Association (1984). *Definition of and competencies for aural rehabilitation.* Position Statement. *ASHA 26*(5), 37–41.

Anthony, D. A. (1971). *Seeing essential English (1 & 2).* Anaheim, CA: Education Services Division, Anaheim Union School District.

Berg, F. S. (1992). Educational management of children who are hearing impaired. In R. H. Hull (Ed.), *Aural rehabilitation* (pp. 120–132). San Diego, CA: Singular Publishing Group.

Bloom, L., & Lahey, M. (1978). *Language development and language disorders.* New York: Wiley.

Blumer, H. (1969). *Symbolic interactionism: Perspective and method.* Eaglewood Cliffs, NJ: Prentice-Hall.

Bogdan, R., & Biklen, S. (1992). *Qualitative research for education* (2nd ed.). Boston: Allyn & Bacon.

Boothroyd, A. (1988). Linguistic factors in speechreading. In C. L. De Filippo & D. G. Sims (Eds.) *New reflections on speechreading* [Monograph]. *The Volta Review, 90,* 77–98.

Bornstein, H., Hamilton, L., Saulnier, K., & Roy, H. (1975). *The signed English dictionary for preschool and elementary levels.* Washington, D.C.: Gallaudet College Press.

Cicourcel, A., & Boese, R. (1972). Sign language acquisition by Spanish-speaking parents of hearing-impaired children. In C. Cazden, V. John & D. Hymes (Eds.), *Functions of language in the classroom* (pp. 32–62). New York: Teachers College, Columbia University.

Cohen, N. L., Waltzman, S. B., & Fisher, S. G. (1993). A prospective randomized study of cochlear implants. *New England Journal of Medicine, 328,* 233–237.

Cornett, R. O. (1967). Cued speech. *American Annals of the Deaf, 112,* 3–13.

Corson, H. J., & Stuckless, E. R. (1994). Special programs, full inclusion, and choices for students who are deaf: Introduction. *American Annals of the Deaf, 139,* 148–149.

Cowie, R., Douglas-Cowie, E., & Kerr, A. G. (1982). A study of speech deterioration in post-lingually deafened adults. *Journal of Laryngology and Otology, 96,* 101–112.

Cummins, J. (1984). *Bilingual and special education: Issues in assessment and pedagogy.* Clevedon, UK: Multilingual Matters.

Cummins, J. (1989). A theoretical framework of bilingual special education. *Exceptional Children, 56,* 111–119.

Cummins, J., & Danesi, M. (1990). *Heritage languages: The development and denial of Canada's linguistic resources.* Toronto: Our Schools/Our Selves Education Foundation.

Demorest, M. E., & Erdman, S. A. (1987). Development of the communication profile for the hearing impaired. *Journal of Speech and Hearing Disorders, 52,* 129–143.

deVilliers, P. A., & deVilliers, J. G. (1979). *Early language.* Cambridge, MA: Harvard University Press.

Denes, P. B., & Pinson, E. N. (1993). *The speech chain* (2nd ed.). New York: W. H. Freeman.

Eilers, R. E., Fishman, L. M., Oller, D. K., & Steffens, M. L. (1993). Tactile vocoders as aids in speech production in young hearing impaired children. *The Volta Review, 95,* 265–293.

Estabrooks, W. (1994). *Auditory-verbal therapy for parents and professionals.* Washington, D.C.: A. G. Bell Association for the Deaf.

Ewoldt, C. (1990). The early literacy development of deaf children. In D. F. Moores & K. P. Meadow-Orlans (Eds.), *Educational and developmental aspects of deafness* (pp. 85–114). Washington, D.C.: Gallaudet University.

Fischer, S. (1995, July). *Critical periods for language acquisition: Consequences for deaf education.* Paper presented at the International Congress on Education of the Deaf, Tel Aviv, Israel.

Fisher, C. G. (1968). Confusions among visually perceived consonants. *Journal of Speech and Hearing research, 11,* 796–804.

Fisher, H. B., & Logemann, J. A. (1971). *The Fisher-Logemann Test of Articulation Competence.* Boston: Houghton Mifflin.

Foster, S. (1989). Reflections of a group of deaf adults on their experiences in mainstream and residential school programs in the United States. *Disability, Handicap and Society, 4,* 37–56.

French-St.George, M., & Stoker, R. (1988). Speechreading: An historical perspective. In C. L. De Filippo & D. G. Sims (Eds.), *New reflections on speechreading* [Monograph]. *The Volta Review, 90,* 17–31.

Gagné, J-P.(1994). Visual and audiovisual speech perception training: basic and applied research needs. In J-P. Gagné & N. Tye-Murray (Eds.), *Research in audiological rehabilitation: Current trends and future directions* [Monograph]. *Journal of Academy of Rehabilitative Audiology, 27,* 133–159.

Gardner, E. F., Rudman, H. C., Karlsen, B., & Merwin, J. (1982). *Stanford Achievement Test* (7th ed.). New York: Harcourt Brace Jovanovich.

Geers, A., & Brenner, C. (1994). Speech perception results: audition and lipreading enhancement. Effectiveness of cochlear implants and tactile aids for deaf children: The sensory aids study at Central Institute for the Deaf [Monograph]. *The Volta Review, 96,* 97–108.

Geers, A., & Moog, J. (1989). Factors predictive of the development of literacy in profoundly hearing-impaired adolescents. *The Volta Review 91,* 69–86.

Geers, A. E., & Moog, J. S. (Eds.) (1994a). Effectiveness of cochlear implants and tactile aids for deaf children: The sensory aids study at Central Institute for the Deaf [Monograph]. *The Volta Review, 96.*

Geers, A. E., & Moog, J. S. (1994b). Spoken language results: Vocabulary, syntax and communication. In A. E. Geers & J. A. Moog (Eds). Effectiveness of cochlear implants and tactile aids for deaf children: The sensory aids study at Central Institute for the Deaf [Monograph]. *The Volta Review, 96,* 131–148.

Getty, L., & Hétu, R. (1991). Development of a rehabilitation program for people affected with occupational hearing loss: 2. Results from group intervention with 48 workers and their spouses. *Audiology, 30,* 317–329.

Giolas, T. (1994). Aural rehabilitation of adults with hearing impairment. In J. Katz (Ed.) *Handbook of clinical audiology* (4th ed.) (pp. 776–790). Baltimore, MD: Williams & Wilkins.

Goldberg, D. M. (1993). Auditory-verbal philosophy: A tutorial. *The Volta Review, 95,* 181–186.

Goldman, R., & Fristoe, M. (1969). *The Goldman-Fristoe test of articulation.* Circle Pines, MN: American Guidance Service.

Goodman, K. (1986). *What's whole in whole language.* Portsmouth, NH: Heinemann.

Graves, D. (1983). *Writing: Teachers and children at work.* Portsmouth, NH: Heinemann.

Gustason, G., Pfetzing, D., & Zawolkow, E. (1972). *Signing Exact English.* Rossmoor, CA: Modern Signs Press.

Hallberg, L., & Carlsson, S. (1991). A qualitative study of strategies for managing a hearing impairment. *British Journal of Audiology, 25,* 201–211.

Harste, J., Woodward, V., & Burke, C. (1984). *Language stories and literacy lessons.* Portsmouth, NH: Heinemann.

Hipskind, N. M. (1989). Visual stimuli in communication. In R. L. Schow & M. A. Nerbonne (Eds.). *Introduction to aural rehabilitation* (2nd. ed.) (pp. 125–180). Boston: Allyn & Bacon.

Hodson, B. (1986). *Assessment of phonological processes: Revised.* Danville, IL: Interstate Press.

Hoffmeister, R. (1990). ASL and its implications for education. In H. Bornstein (Ed.) *Manual communication: implications for education.* (pp. 81–107). Washington, D.C.: Gallaudet University Press.

Holt, J. (1994). Classroom attributes and achievement test scores for deaf and hard of hearing students. *American Annals of the Deaf, 139,* 430–437.

Holt, J. A., & Allen, T. A. (1989). The effects of schools and their curricula on the reading and mathematics achievement of hearing impaired students. *International Journal of Educational Research, 13,* 547–562.

Hudgins, C. V., & Numbers, F. C. (1942). An investigation of the intelligibility of speech of the deaf. *Genetic Psychology Monographs, 25,* 289–392.

Hyde, M. B., & Power, D. J. (1991). Teachers' use of simultaneous communication. *American Annals of the Deaf (136),* 381–387.

Israelite, N. K., Ewoldt, C., & Hoffmeister, R. (1992). *Bilingual/bicultural education for deaf and hard-of-hearing students.* Toronto: MGS Publication Services.

Israelite, N. K., & Helfrich, M. A. (1988). Improving text coherence in basal readers: Effects of revisions on the comprehension of hearing impaired and hearing readers. *The Volta Review, 90,* 261–276.

Israelite, N. K., & Jennings, M. B. (1995). Participant perspectives on group aural rehabilitation: A qualitative inquiry. *Journal of the Academy of Rehabilitative Audiology, 28,* 26–36.

Jackson, P. L. (1986). The theoretical minimal unit for visual speech perception: Visemes and coarticulation. *The Volta Review, 90,* 99–115.

Jackson, P. L. (1992). A psychosocial and economic profile of the hearing impaired and deaf. In R. H. Hull (Ed.), *Aural rehabilitation,* 42–49. San Diego, CA: Singular Publishing Group.

Jennings, M. B., & Head, B. G. (1994). Development of an ecological audiologic rehabilitation program in a home-for-the-aged. *Journal of the Academy of Rehabilitative Audiology, 27,* 73–88.

Jennings, M. B., & Israelite, N. K. (1994, November). *Studying the efficacy of group aural rehabilitation: A qualitative inquiry.* Paper presented at the American Speech-Language-Hearing Association annual convention, New Orleans, LA.

Johnson, R., Liddell, S., & Erting, C. (1989). *Unlocking the curriculum: Principles for achieving access in deaf education.* Gallaudet Research Institute Working Paper 89–3. Washington, D.C.: Gallaudet University.

Jones, L., Kyle, J., & Wood, P. (1987). *Words apart.* London: Tavistock Publications.

Kaplan, H., Bally, S. J., & Garretson, C. (1988). *Speechreading, a way to improve understanding.* Washington, D.C.: Gallaudet University Press.

Katz, J. & White, M. A. (1992). Introduction to the handicap of hearing impairment. In R. H. Hull (Ed.), *Aural rehabilitation* (2nd ed.) (pp. 15–27). San Diego, CA: Singular Publishing Group.

Kyle, J. & Pullen, G. (1988). Culture in contact: Deaf and hearing people. *Disability, Handicap and Society, 3,* 49–61.

Lane, H. (1992). *The mask of benevolence: Disabling the deaf community.* New York: Alfred Knopf.

Lane, H. (1995). Constructions of deafness. *Disability & Society, 10,* 171–189.

Laszlo, C. (1994). Is there a hard-of-hearing identity? *Journal of Speech-Language Pathology and Audiology, 18,* 248–252.

Ling, D. (1976). *Speech and the hearing-impaired child: Theory and Practices.* Washington, D.C.: A. G. Bell Association for the Deaf.

Ling, D. (1986). Devices and procedures for auditory learning. In E. Cole & H. Gregory (Eds.), Learning auditory training [Monograph]. *The Volta Review, 88,* 19–28.

Ling, D. (1989). *Foundations of spoken language for hearing-impaired children.* Washington, D.C.: A. G. Bell Association for the Deaf.

Ling, D. (1991). *The phonetic-phonologic speech evaluation record.* Washington, D.C.: A. G. Bell Association for the Deaf.

Ling, D., & Milne, M. (1981). The development of speech in hearing-impaired children. In F. Bess, B. A. Freeman, & J. S. Sinclair (Eds.), *Amplification in education* (pp. 98–108). Washington, D.C.: A. G. Bell Association for the Deaf.

Luetke-Stahlman, B. (1988). Documenting syntactically and semantically incomplete bimodal input to hearing-impaired subjects. *American Annals of the Deaf (133),* 230–234.

Mahshie, S. N. (1995). *Educating deaf children bilingually.* Washington, D.C.: Pre-College Programs, Gallaudet University.

Martin, D. S. (1994). Cognitive development and deafness. In R. C. Nowell & L. E. Marshak (Eds.), *Understanding deafness and the rehabilitation process,* (pp. 35–49). Boston: Allyn & Bacon.

Mayer, C., & Wells, G. (1996). Can the linguistic interdependence theory support a bilingual-bicultural model of literacy education for deaf students? *Journal of Deaf Studies and Deaf Education, 1,* 93–107.

McAnally, P., Rose, S., & Quigley, S. P. (1994). *Language learning practices with deaf children* (2nd ed.). Austin, TX: Pro-Ed.

McGarr, N. S., & Whitehead, R. (1992). Contemporary issues in phoneme production by hearing-impaired persons: Physiological and acoustic aspects. In R. G. Stoker & D. Ling (Eds.), Speech production

in hearing-impaired children and youth [Monograph]. *The Volta Review, 94,* 33–45.

Meadow-Orlans, K. P. (1990). The impact of childhood hearing loss on the family. In D. F. Moores & K. P. Meadow-Orlans (Eds.), *Educational and developmental aspects of deafness,* (pp. 321–33). Washington, D.C.: Gallaudet University Press.

Miskiel, L. W., Carney, A. E., Johnson, C. J., & Carney, E. (1994). An analysis of the Phonetic Level Evaluation: Age and task factors. *Language, Speech, and Hearing in Schools. 25,* 165–173.

Moeller, M. P., & Carney, A. E. (1993). Assessment and intervention with preschool hearing-impaired children. In J. G. Alpiner & P. A. McCarthy (Eds.), *Rehabilitative audiology: Children and adults* (pp. 106–135). Baltimore, MD: Williams & Wilkins.

Montgomery, A. A. (1993). Management of the hearing-impaired adult. In J. G. Alpiner & P. A. McCarthy (Eds.) *Rehabilitative audiology: Children and adults* (2nd ed.) (pp. 311–330) Baltimore, MD: Williams & Wilkins.

Moog, J. S., & Geers, A. E. (1980). *Grammatical analysis of elicited language: Complex sentence level.* St. Louis, MO: Central Institute for the Deaf.

Moog, J. S., & Geers, A. E. (1985). *Grammatical analysis of elicited language: Simple sentence level.* St. Louis, MO: Central Institute for the Deaf.

Moog, J. S., & Kozak, J. (1983). *Teacher assessment of grammatical structures.* St. Louis, MO: Central Institute for the Deaf.

Moores, D. (1987). *Educating the deaf: Psychology, principles, and practices* (3rd ed.). Boston: Houghton Mifflin.

Moores, J. M. Y., & Moores, D. F. (1989). Educational alternatives for the hearing impaired. In R. L. Schow & M. A. Nerbonne (Eds.). *Introduction to aural rehabilitation* (pp. 271–291). Boston: Allyn & Bacon.

National Center for Health Statistics (1994). Prevalence and characteristics of persons with hearing trouble, United States, 1990–91. *Vital and health statistics.* Hyattsville, MD: U.S. Department of Health and Human Services.

Nerbonne, M. A., & Schow, R. L. (1989). Auditory stimuli in communication. In R. L. Schow & M. A. Nerbonne (Eds.). *Introduction to aural rehabilitation* (pp. 81–123). Boston: Allyn & Bacon.

Noble, W., & Hétu, R. (1994). An ecological approach to disability and handicap in relation to impaired hearing. *Audiology, 33,* 117–126.

Northern, J. L., & Downs, M. P. (1984) Medical aspects of hearing loss, In J. L. Northern & M. P. Downs (Eds.). *Hearing in children* (3rd ed.) (pp. 51–91). Baltimore, MD: Williams & Wilkins.

Novelli-Olmstead, T., & Ling, D. (1984). Speech production and speech discrimination by hearing-impaired children. *The Volta Review, 86,* 72–80.

Osberger, M. J., Robbins, A. M., Todd, S. L., & Riley, A. I. (1994). Speech intelligibility of children with cochlear implants. In A. E. Geers & J. A. Moog (Eds). *Effectiveness of cochlear implants and tactile aids for deaf children: The sensory aids study at Central Institute for the Deaf* [Monograph]. *The Volta Review, 96* (5), 169–180.

Padden, C., & Humphries, T. (1988). *Deaf in America: Voices from a culture.* Cambridge, MA: Harvard University Press.

Paul, P. V., & Jackson, D. W. (1993). *Toward a psychology of deafness.* Boston: Allyn & Bacon.

Perigoe, C., & Ling, D. (1986). Generalization of speech skills in hearing-impaired children. *The Volta Review, 88,* 351–366.

Ross, M. (1990). Definitions and descriptions. In J. Davis (Ed.). *Our forgotten children: Hard-of-hearing children in the schools* (2nd Ed.) (pp. 3–17). Washington, D.C.: Self Help for Hard of Hearing People.

Ross, M. (Ed.)(1994a). *Communication access for persons with hearing loss: Compliance with the Americans with disabilities act.* Baltimore, MD: York Press.

Ross, M. (1994b). Overview of aural rehabilitation. In J. Katz (Ed.) *Handbook of clinical audiology* (4th ed.) (pp. 587–595). Baltimore, MD: Williams & Wilkins.

Ross, M. (1995). Developments in research and technology. *SHHH, 16,* 2–32.

Ross, M., Brackett, D., & Maxon, A. B. (1991). *Assessment and management of mainstreamed hearing-impaired children.* Austin, TX: Pro-Ed.

Sanders, D. A. (1993). *Management of hearing handicap. Infants to elderly* (3rd. ed.). Englewood Cliffs, NJ: Prentice-Hall.

Schein, J. D., & Delk, M. T. (1974). *The deaf population in the United States.* Silver Spring, MD: National Association of the Deaf.

Schirmer, B. R. (1994). *Language and literacy development in children who are deaf.* New York: Macmillan.

Schow, R. G., & Nerbonne, M. A. (1982). Communication screening profile: Use with elderly clients. *Ear & Hearing, 3,* 135–147.

Seyfried, D. N., Hutchinson, J. M., & Smith, L. L. (1989). Language and speech of the hearing impaired. In R. L. Schow & M. A. Nerbonne (Eds.), *Introduction to aural rehabilitation* (pp. 181–239). Boston: Allyn & Bacon.

Shaw, S., & Coggins, T. E. (1991). Interobserver reliability using the Phonetic Level Evaluation with severely and profoundly hearing-impaired children. *Journal of Speech and Hearing Research, 34,* 989–999.

Staller, S. J., Beiter, A. L., & Brimacombe, J. A. (1994). Use of the Nucleus 22 Channel Cochlear Implant system with children. In A. E. Geers & J. A. Moog (Eds). *Effectiveness of cochlear implants and tactile aids for deaf children: The sensory aids study at Central Institute for the Deaf* [Monograph]. *The Volta Review, 96,* 15–39.

Staller, S., Otto, S., & Menapace, C. (1995). Clinical trials of the auditory brainstem implant. *Audiology Today, 7*(4), 9–12.

Stinson, M. S., & Lang, H. G. (1994). Full inclusion: A path for integration or isolation. *American Annals of the Deaf, 139,* 156–159.

Stoker, R., & Ling, D. (Eds.). (1992). *Speech production in hearing-impaired children and youth* (Monograph). *The Volta Review, 94.*

Stone, H. E., & Hurwitz, T. A. (1994). Accessibility to the hearing world: Assistive devices and specialized support. In R. C. Nowell & L. E. Marshak (Eds.), *Understanding deafness and the rehabilitation process* (pp. 239–267). Boston: Allyn & Bacon.

Strauss, K. P. (1994). The ADA: The law, communication access, and the role of audiologists. In M. Ross (Ed.), *Communication access for persons with hearing loss: Compliance with the Americans with disabilities act* (pp. 1–16). Baltimore, MD: York Press.

Tobey, E., Geers, A., & Brenner, C. (1994). Speech production results: Speech feature acquisition. In A. E. Geers & J. A. Moog (Eds). *Effectiveness of cochlear implants and tactile aids for deaf children: The sensory aids study at Central Institute for the Deaf* [Monograph]. *The Volta Review, 96,* 109–129.

Trychin, S., & Busacco, D. (1991). *Manual for mental health professionals, part 1.* Washington, D.C.: Gallaudet University.

U.S. Department of Education (1993). *To assure the free appropriate education of all children with disabilities: Fifteenth annual report to Congress on the implementation of the individuals with disabilities act.* Washington, D.C..

Utley, J. (1946). A test of lipreading ability. *Journal of Speech and Hearing Disorders, 11,* 109–116.

Ventry, I. J., & Weinstein, B. (1982). The hearing handicap tool for the elderly: A new tool. *Ear and Hearing, 3,* 128–134.

Vernon, M., & Alles, C. D. (1994). Issues in the use of cochlear implants with prelingually deaf children. *American Annals of the Deaf, 139,* 485–492.

Vernon, M., & Andrews, J. F. (1990). *The psychology of deafness.* New York: Longman.

Vivran, B. (1991). You don't have to hate meetings— Try computer-assisted notetaking. *SHHH Journal,* Jan.–Feb., 1991.

Waling, S., & Harrison, W. (1987). *A speech guide for teachers and clinicians of hearing impaired children.* Tuscon, AZ: Communication Skill Builders.

Weisenberger, J. M., & Percy, M. E. (1994). Use of the Tactaid II and Tactaid VII with children. In A. E. Geers & J. A. Moog (Eds). *Effectiveness of cochlear implants and tactile aids for deaf children: The sensory aids study at Central Institute for the Deaf* [Monograph]. *The Volta Review, 96,* 41–57.

Williams, C. L. (1994). The language and literacy worlds of three profoundly deaf preschool children. *Reading Research Quarterly, 29,* 125–155.

Wolk, S. & Schildroth, A. N. (1986). Deaf children and speech intelligibility: A national study. In A. N. Schildroth & M. A. Karchmer (Eds.), *Deaf children in America,* (pp. 139–159). San Diego, CA: College-Hill.

Yantis, P. A. (1994). Pure tone air conduction threshold testing. In J. Katz (Ed.). *Handbook of clinical audiology* (pp. 97–108) (4th ed.). Baltimore, MD: Williams & Wilkins.

Yurkowski, P., & Ewoldt, C. (1986). A case for the semantic processing of the deaf reader. *American Annals of the Deaf, 131,* 243–247.

GLOSSARY

Abduct   To move away from the midline.

Abduction   The act of moving away from the midline; movement away from the middle of the body; opening of the vocal folds.

Abductor   A muscle that moves a bone or cartilage away from the midline.

Abductor Spasmodic Dysphonia   One of three manifestations of a rare neurological voice disorder characterized by breathy or whispered voice produced when the vocal folds move away from the midline during phonation so that the phonation is interrupted.

Abscess   Swollen, inflamed area of body tissue.

Abstract language   The ability to use and understand vocabulary and utterances in a nonliteral sense.

Accommodation   Children's ability to adapt existing mental structures (or schemata) to changing real life experiences.

Acetylcholine   An excitatory neurotransmitter that is important for any excitatory function (e.g., muscle movement).

Acoustic filter effect of hearing impairment   Hearing impairment acts like an invisible acoustic filter that distorts, smears, or eliminates incoming sounds; the negative impact of this filter on spoken communication, reading, academics, and independent function causes the problems associated with hearing impairment.

Acquired hearing loss   Hearing loss that occurs following birth (i.e., during childhood or adulthood).

Adduct   To move toward the midline.

Adduction   The act of moving toward the midline; movement toward the middle of the body; closing of the vocal folds.

Adductor   A muscle that moves a bone or cartilage toward the midline.

Adductor Spasmodic Dysphonia   One of three manifestations of a rare neurological voice disorder characterized by voice arrests, rough, effortful voice and a strained-strangled voice quality produced with increased vocal folds stiffness and medial compression.

Aditus laryngis   Entrance to the larynx.

Affect   The outward expression of emotion that can be observed by others.

Agrammatism   Loss of the ability to produce function words.

Aided augmentative communication systems   Nonspeech communication system that involves something other than the nonspeaking communicator, such as some signaling device or letter board that contains pictures, letters, or symbols.

Air reservoir   Volume of air temporarily stored in the upper third of the esophagus for the purpose of voicing.

Alaryngeal speech   Any form of oral communication produced without a larynx.

American Sign Language (ASL)   Native sign language of culturally deaf individuals in English-speaking North America.

Americans with Disabilities Act (ADA)   Federal legislation requiring, among other provisions, communication access for individuals with hearing loss.

Amino acid   A small molecule building block of protein. There are 20 different amino acids which make up proteins; however, there are many other amino acids.

Amygdala nucleus   A nucleus located in the medial temporal lobe region, anterior to the hippocampus. The hippocampus connects to the amygdala, making the amygdala functionally a part of the memory system.

Amyloid precursor protein   A protein that undergoes some alteration (becomes separated) prior to becoming an amyloid protein.

Amyotrophic lateral sclerosis (ALS)   A degenerative motor neuron disease causing muscular atrophy and weakness.

Aneurysm Sac formed by an enlargement of an arterial wall.

Ankylosis Fixation of a joint.

Anomaly Abnormality.

Anoxia Lack of oxygen.

Anterior commissure Point of attachment for the vocal folds on the inner surface of the thyroid cartilage just below the thyroid notch.

Aorta Main artery of the body, carries blood from the left ventricle of the heart to all parts of the body except the lungs.

Apgar score A score given to a newborn infant by a nurse or physician, usually at one and five minutes following delivery. It is a useful means of communicating the newborn's general status and adaptation to extrauterine life. The maximum Apgar score is 10.

Aphasia An acquired impairment of language processes underlying receptive and expressive modalities caused by damage to areas of the brain primarily responsible for language function.

Aphonia An abnormal involuntary whisper or complete loss of voice; voice that is produced without an observable definable quasiperiodical laryngeal sound.

Apnea A prolonged pause in respiration, often accompanied by a slowing of the heart rate (bradycardia) or a blue color to the skin (cyanosis).

Apolipoprotein E A protein whose allele is inherited from each parent.

Appropriate for gestational age Birth weight that is appropriate for a child's gestational age.

Apraxia An inability to make voluntary skilled movements, in the absence of weakness or paralysis in the musculature.

Apraxia of speech Neurologically based disorder that affects the ability to program and plan speech movements.

Arcuate fasciculus White matter pathway connecting Wernicke's area to Broca's area.

Arteries Branching tubes that carry blood from the heart to all parts of the body.

Aryepiglottic folds Bundles of connective tissue and muscle running from the sides of the epiglottis to the apex of each arytenoid cartilage.

Arytenoid cartilages Pair of pyramidal shaped cartilages located on the posterior superior surface of the cricoid cartilage.

Aspiration Entry of food, liquid, or saliva into the airway below the true vocal folds.

Assimilation Children's ability to adapt their growing perception of the world to their existing system (or schemata).

Assistive Listening Device (ALD) Any of a number of pieces of equipment used to augment hearing or to assist the hearing aid in difficult listening situations; through the use of a remote microphone, assistive listening devices provide a superior signal-to-noise ratio that enhances the clarity (intelligibility) of the speech signal.

Associated somatic symptom Muscular or skeletal tension which can be observed.

Astrocytes A type of neuroglia that supports the membrane of the neuron and may be involved in transporting substances between blood vessels and neurons.

At risk Possessing a grouping or constellation of risk factors that may be accompanied by developmental delay.

Ataxia Defect of posture or gait, caused by a disorder of the cerebellum.

Atherosclerosis Disease of the arteries in which fatty plaques develop on the inner walls eventually leading to blood flow obstruction.

Atrium Space below the vocal folds.

Attention

Focused Ability to respond discretely to specific visual, auditory, or tactile stimuli

Sustained Ability to maintain consistent behavioral response during continuous repetitive activities

Selective Ability to maintain a behavioral set in the presence of distracting extraneous stimuli

Alternating Ability to shift the focus of attention and move between tasks with different behavioral requirements

Divided Ability to respond simultaneously to multiple task demands

Audibility Being able to hear but not necessarily distinguish among speech sounds.

Audiogram A graph of a person's peripheral hearing sensitivity with frequency (pitch) on one axis and intensity (loudness) on the other.

Audiology Science of hearing.

Audiometer An instrument that delivers calibrated pure tone or speech stimuli for the measurement of sound detection and speech detection, recognition, and identification.

Auditory processing skills The capacity of processing language through the auditory channel.

Basal nuclei   Gray matter structures embedded deep within the white matter of the cerebrum, rich in neural connections to the cortex and thalamus, and involved with control of motor behavior.

Basilar artery   Artery at the base of the brain formed by a union of the two vertebral arteries.

Behavior disorders   Also known as externalizing disorders, these cause pain, distress, or discomfort to others.

Bernoulli principle   Aerodynamic principle stating that air increases in velocity and decreases in pressure when going through a narrow constriction.

Bilingual/bicultural deaf education   An approach that promotes knowledge and use of two languages (e.g., ASL and English) and two cultures (deaf culture and hearing culture).

Blepharospasm   Involuntary tight contraction of the eyelid.

Body   Innermost portion of the vocal folds, consisting of the thyroarytenoid muscle.

Botulinum Toxin Injection   (BTX injection therapy) A treatment for the symptoms of spasmodic dysphonia with a nerve toxin produced by the bacterium Clostridium botulinum found in improperly smoked, canned, or refrigerated foods. From the bacterium Clostridium botulinum toxin is extracted, processed, and injected into the vocal folds resulting in weakened movements of the vocal folds.

Brainstem   Enlarged upward extension of the spinal cord, consisting of the medulla, pons, and midbrain.

Breathiness   Voice quality in which there is an audible escape of air during phonation.

Broca's area   Portion of the motor cortex in the left frontal lobe responsible for the initiation of speech movements.

Bronchopulmonary Dysplasia (BPD)   Disease characterized by chronic lung changes including decreased lung capacity.

CPAP (Continuous positive air pressure)   A term used to describe the process of assisted ventilation in which a continuous positive air pressure is applied to the infant's lungs.

Candidiasis   An infection caused by candida, a yeast-like fungus.

Capillaries   Tiny blood vessels that connect arteries with veins.

Captioning   Process by which the audio portion of a television program is coded in written form (i.e., subtitles) and transmitted over line 21 of the television signal.

Carcinoma in-situ   Replacement of normal cells by malignant cells only on epithelial surfaces.

Cardiovascular   Biological system that includes the heart, lungs, and blood vessels.

Career education   Ongoing implementation of training and education throughout the lifespan of persons with developmental disabilities in all experiential phases (e.g., academics, activities of daily living, independent living skills, menu planning, recreational skills, vocational training, and so on).

Carotid artery   Major blood vessel from the heart that supplies the brain with blood.

Cell-mediated immunity   One type of immunity that protects against viruses, fungi, and cancer.

Central Nervous System (CNS)   Part of the nervous system that includes the brain and spinal cord.

Central auditory disorder   An auditory disorder that causes difficulty with perception or deriving meaning from incoming sounds. The source of the problem is in the brainstem or in the brain, not in the peripheral hearing mechanism (outer, middle, or inner ear) and not related to auditory reception.

Cerebellum   Large part of the brain bulging back behind the pons, essential for maintaining muscle tone, balance, and coordination of voluntary muscle activity.

Cerebral cortex   Sheets of gray matter that cover the entire surface of cerebral hemispheres.

Cerebral palsy   A movement and posture disorder due to an immature brain defect.

Cerebrovascular accident (CVA)   Sudden and severe disruption of blood to the brain. Popular term is *stroke.*

Cerebrum   White matter of the brain, consisting of two hemispheres.

Childhood disintegrative disorder   A disorder of childhood characterized by a clinically significant loss of previously acquired skills in a number of areas which may include two of the following: expressive or receptive language, social skills or adaptive behavior, bladder control, play, or motor skills. Qualitative impairment in social interaction, qualitative impairment in communication, and/or restricted or stereotyped patterns of behavior may also be present.

Cholinergic   Describing nerve fibers that release acetylcholine as a neurotransmitter.

Choreoathetosis A form of cerebral palsy characterized by variable muscle tone and involuntary movements.

Circle of Willis Circle of vessels at the base of the brain formed by linked branches of arteries that supply the brain.

Cleft Space or opening.

Clinical retardation Levels of function ranging from moderate to severe to profound; often occurs in conjunction with structural abnormality or dysmorphism, with some identifiable central nervous system (CNS) pathology.

Clostridia botulinum Bacterium found in contaminated food.

Cochlea Portion of inner ear responsible for converting sound waves from the middle ear into electrochemical impulses that are sent to the brain.

Cochlear implant A device that delivers electrical stimulation to the VIIIth cranial nerve (auditory nerve) via an electrode array surgically implanted in the cochlea.

Cognition Related to the mind, information processing, information in memory, and the processes involved in acquiring, retaining, and using the information.

Cognitive rehabilitation Treatment regimen aimed at increasing functional abilities in everyday life by improving an individual's capacity to process and interpret incoming information.

Cognitive-developmental theory Theory of learning that stresses the individual as an active participant who obtains knowledge via a dynamic process of interacting with people and/or objects within the environment, using assimilation and accommodation.

Coma Prolonged period of unconsciousness in which individual displays minimal, if any, purposeful response to the external environment, resulting from a disruption of the reticular activating system.

Communicative competence Ability of an individual to integrate and use appropriate phonology/morphology/syntax (form), semantics (content), and pragmatics (use) in a language to both convey and receive information to and from other speakers.

Communicative design Ability to take into account the background knowledge and informational needs of a listener in order to construct an appropriate message.

Community integration Deinstitutionalized placement of an individual with developmental disabilities into the community. Residential placements may include foster care facilities, intermediate care facilities (group homes), nursing homes, or independent apartments. Vocational/work placements may include day treatment, day training, sheltered workshops, and/or competitive employment settings.

Comorbidity Disease state co-occurring with other disease, i.e., attention deficit hyperactivity disorder (ADHD) with obsessive-compulsive disorder (OCD).

Compensatory errors Maladaptive articulation errors (usually substitutions) associated with velopharyngeal insufficiency and usually associated with the cleft palate population, including glottal stops, pharyngeal fricatives, nasal snorting, and others; sometimes referred to as *cleft palate speech.* These errors are not directly caused by an anatomic defect and can only be corrected with speech therapy.

Complex tones Tones consisting of more than one frequency, such as speech.

Computerized Axial Tomography (CT scan) Radiological examination of the soft tissues of the body.

Conductive hearing loss Disruption in the ear's ability to conduct sound that occurs as a result of damage to the outer or middle ear.

Congenital Occurring prior to birth.

Congenital hearing impairment A hearing impairment that occurs prior to the development of speech and language; usually before or at birth.

Consolidation Theoretical stage of memory that involves the integration of new memories within an individual's existing stored information.

Consumer groups Groups that provide leadership and support to individuals with hearing loss in their self-advocacy efforts. Examples include: Association for Late-Deafened Adults (ALDA), Self Help for Hard of Hearing People, Inc. (SHHH), and the National Association of the Deaf (NAD).

Content of language What the message consists of.

Context of language Where language occurs and with whom.

Continuum of risk A principle that implies that risk for developmental delay can have very early origins or later onset during the preschool years.

Contra coup Damage in closed head injuries to the side of the brain opposite from the point of impact due to subsequent rebound effects.

Corniculate cartilages Pair of small cartilages located on top of the apex of each arytenoid cartilage.

Cornu Horn, or small projection of bone or cartilage.

Corpus callosum Mass of white fibers that connect the cerebral hemispheres.

Corpus striatum Part of basal nuclei located in the subcortical gray matter.

Cortex External layer of grey matter covering the cerebrum.

Corticobulbar tract Monosynaptic pathway descending from the motor area of the cerebral cortex to the medulla.

Corticospinal tract Monosynaptic pathway descending from the motor area of the cerebral cortex to the spinal cord.

Coup Damage in closed head injuries from the inward compression of the skull at the point of impact.

Cover Outermost portion of the vocal folds, comprised of the epithelium and superficial layer of the lamina propria.

Craniofacial anomaly Abnormality of the skull (cranium) and/or face.

Cricoarytenoid joint Joint that allows the arytenoid cartilages to move in various ways, and thus to abduct and adduct the vocal folds.

Cricoid cartilage Signet-ring shaped cartilage located directly above the trachea.

Cricopharyngeal (CP) region Valve into the esophagus. This area may be known as the *upper esophageal sphincter (UES)*, or *pharyngoesophageal segment (PE segment)*.

Cricothyroid joint Joint that allows downward movement of the thyroid cartilage, and is involved in pitch change.

Cuneiform cartilages Paired elastic wedges of cartilage found in the aryepiglottic folds.

Cyclothymic A psychopathological disturbance involving depressed and elevated mood, not severe enough to qualify as bipolar disorder and separated by periods of normal mood.

Cytomegalovirus (CMV) A congenital infection communicated from mother to infant.

Deaf cultural literacy Story-telling, drama, and poetry in ASL.

Deaf person (audiological definition) Individual with a hearing loss of at least 71 dB.

Deaf person (sociocultural definition) Individual with a hearing loss who identifies with the attitudes, values, traditions, mores, and ideologies of deaf culture, and who use a native sign language as the primary language.

Deafened persons Individuals who experience sudden, irreversible significant hearing loss due to disease or trauma.

Decibel (dB) Unit of intensity used in audiometry.

Developmental coordination disorder Marked impairment in the development of motor coordination that is substantially below that expected for age and level of intelligence, and that is not due to a generalized medical condition.

Diabetes Disease characterized by high levels of blood sugar and many other chemical abnormalities.

Diagnostic and Statistical Manual of Mental Disorders IV (DSM IV) A descriptive, multiaxial, diagnostic framework that identifies and lists essential features of different mental disorders.

Diencephalon A structure of the brain that is located between the cerebral hemispheres that serves as a relay center for sensory impulses.

Diffuse axonal injury Stretching, shearing, and tearing of blood vessels and nerve fibers caused by rapid rotation of the brain in the skull resulting in widespread brain dysfunction.

Diffuse Widespread, as when damage to the brain occurs in several anatomic regions.

Diplegia Paralysis of limbs on both sides of the body, with the legs usually being more affected.

Direct fiber tract Pathway comprised of the corticobulbar and corticospinal tracts mediating discrete voluntary movement.

Discourse Language structure beyond the sentence level.

Discrimination The ability to differentiate among sounds of different frequencies, durations, or intensities.

Distance hearing The ability to monitor environmental events and to "overhear" conversations; an ability that is severely reduced by hearing impairment.

Dopamine An inhibitory neurotransmitter that is produced in the substantia nigra (a nucleus in the midbrain).

Dopaminergic System that utilizes the inhibatory neurotransmitter dopamine.

Dysarthria Collection of speech disorders characterized by weakness in the muscles that control respiration, phonation, resonance and articulation.

Dysmetria Inability to control the range of movement.

Dysphagia Condition in which the action of swallowing is difficult to perform.

Dysphonia   A disorder of the voice that includes deviation in pitch, loudness, or quality.

Dyspnea   Shortness of breath, breathing difficulty.

Dyssynergia   Lack of coordination characterized by clumsy, uncoordinated movements.

Dysthymia   Chronically depressed mood, not severe enough to qualify as full blown depression.

Dystonia   A neurological disorder that affects motor control; involuntary contractions of the muscles result in fast or slow twisting and turning movements.

Efficacy   The study of the effectiveness of the services provided to children and their families.

Electrolarynx   Extrinsic electronic device containing a vibratory mechanism which, when applied to the neck or oral cavity, generates voicing for speech.

Embolism   Obstruction of a blood vessel by foreign material.

Emotional disorders   Also known as internalizing disorders, these cause pain or distress to the individual with the disorder.

Encephalopathy   A disturbance of brain function.

Encoding   Analysis performed by an individual on material to be remembered to facilitate its later recall.

Encopresis   Repeated passage of feces into inappropriate places, after the age of 4 years.

Endoscopy   Insertion of a small viewing instrument called an endoscope into an orifice; the procedure in which an endoscope is inserted through the nose to view the vocal tract or larynx is referred to as nasal endoscopy or nasopharyngoscopy.

Entorhinal cortex   A portion of the parahippocampal gyrus. The entorhinal cortex is a region that transitions into the head of the hippocampus.

Enuresis   Repeated voiding of urine into the bed or into cloth, during the day or night, in a child of at least 5 years of chronological or mental age.

Epidemiology   The study of the distributions and determinants of health-related states and events in populations, and the application of the study to control health problems.

Epiglottis   Unpaired cartilage of the larynx that closes over the entrance to the larynx during swallowing.

Epithelium   Thin layer of cells which is almost fluid-like in its composition; outermost tissue of the vocal folds.

Eructated   Belched.

Esophageal voice   Phonation produced when air trapped in the upper third of the esophagus passes through the P–E sphincter causing it to vibrate.

Established risk   A grouping or constellation of risk factors that are generally accompanied by developmental delay.

Etiology   Cause.

Executive function   Composite of activities related to achievement/completion of a goal, including anticipation, goal formulation, planning, implementation of plan, self-monitoring, and use of feedback.

Expiratory Effort   An impression of involuntary increased resistance to the flow of air during speech; an involuntary increase in perceived labor in the production of phonation.

Extension   A straightening movement.

Extirpation   Removal.

Extrapyramidal   Involved in subconscious, automatic motor coordination.

Extrinsic muscles   Muscles with one attachment to the larynx or hyoid bone, and one attachment to some other structure such as the sternum or clavicle.

Failure to thrive   A condition describing children who gain weight at a slower than normal rate in infancy and early childhood in comparison to their peers.

Feeding disorder of infancy and childhood   Persistent failure to eat adequately as reflected by a significant failure to gain weight.

Fetal alcohol syndrome   A condition describing children exposed to maternal ingestion of alcohol during pregnancy in sufficient amounts to cause craniofacial dysmorphism, growth retardation, and central nervous system dysfunction.

Fetal death   Death taking place at 20 weeks gestation or later and before birth.

Fingerspelling   System of handshapes that represent individual letters of the alphabet.

Fistula   Abnormal congenital or acquired opening between two surfaces or between a hollow structure and the outside.

Flexion   A bending movement.

Flight of ideas   The flow of rapid, continuous verbalizations or play on words which produce a constant shifting from one idea to another.

Floppy infant   An infant who assumes atypical postures, has excessive range of motion of the joints, and offers little resistance to passive movement.

Focal   Discrete, as when damage to the brain is localized to one area or one anatomic structure of the brain.

Fragile X syndrome   A genetic syndrome that includes mental retardation, flaring ears, elongated faces, a slightly reduced cranial perimeter, normal stature, and enlarged testes.

Frequency Modulation (FM) The frequency of transmitted waves is alternated in accordance with the sounds being sent; radio waves.

Frequency response The way that each hearing aid or ALD shapes the incoming (speech) sounds; the amount of amplification provided by the hearing aid at any frequency.

Frequency Number of complete cycles of compressions and rarefactions of a sound wave, per second. The perceptual correlate of frequency is pitch.

Frontal lobe Anterior part of each cerebral hemisphere.

Functional communication skills Skills that are useful to the person in meeting environmental and communicative demands.

Fundamental frequency Rate at which the vocal folds vibrate during phonation.

Gastroesophageal reflux Condition in which contents of the stomach flow upward through the esophagus and pharynx.

Ghost tangles Bundled neurofibrillary tangles.

Globus pallidus A nucleus that is part of the extrapyramidal system.

Glossoptosis Collapse of the back of the tongue into the airway related to small mandible, usually associated with Robin sequence.

Glottal stop Maladaptive compensatory articulation error produced by abrupt adduction of the vocal folds, usually used as a substitution for stop consonants.

Glottal Pertaining to the space between the vocal folds.

Glottis Space between the vocal folds, divided into membraneous and cartilaginous portions.

Glucose Important source of energy in the body and the brain.

Granulation tissue Rough grainy tissue that may develop around an ulcer.

Gravida Refers to a pregnant woman; she is called gravida 1 during the first pregnancy, gravida 2 during the second, and so on.

Gray matter Darker colored tissue of the central nervous system, primarily composed of cell bodies and dendrites.

Gyrus Prominent rounded elevations that form the cerebral hemisphere.

Hard-of-hearing person (audiological definition) Individuals with a hearing loss between 26 dB and 70 dB.

Hard-of-hearing person (sociocultural definition) Individual with a hearing loss who uses speech as the primary means of communication, regardless of hearing abilities.

Harshness Voice quality characterized by strain and tension.

Hearing aids Miniature public address systems that amplify and shape incoming sounds to make them audible to an ear that would not otherwise detect them.

Hearing impairment Lessened or loss of hearing sensitivity caused by disease or damage to one or more parts of one or both ears.

Hearing loss Loss of sound sensitivity due to an abnormality in the auditory system.

Hemiplegia Spasticity on one side of the body.

Hemorrhage Escape of blood from a ruptured vessel.

Hertz (Hz) Unit of frequency used in audiometry.

Hippocampus A gyrus located in the medial and inferior portion of the temporal lobe. It is shaped like a seahorse and is important in memory functioning.

HIV-1 infection A human retrovirus that suppresses the immune system resulting in opportunistic infections and tumors.

Hoarseness Voice quality characterized by roughness and raspiness.

Hyoid bone U-shaped bone from which the larynx is suspended.

Hyperactivity (hyperkinesis) Restless, aggressive, destructive activity, often associated with some underlying organic pathology.

Hyperadduction Condition in which the vocal folds close with excessive force.

Hypernasality Excessive nasal resonance during production of vowels; often associated with but not the same as nasal escape of air; usually caused by velopharyngeal insufficiency.

Hypertension High blood pressure.

Hypertonia Extreme tension of muscles.

Hypoadduction Condition in which the vocal folds close with insufficient force.

Hypomanic An abnormally and persistently elevated, expansive, or irritable mood, but not to the degree of mania.

Hyponasality Denasality; insufficient nasalization of nasal phonemes; usually associated with nasal obstruction or congestion.

Hypotonia Decreased muscle tone and decreased resistance to passive movement.

Idioms Expressions which have meaning based on abstract language that goes beyond the literal translation of words.

Inadequate prenatal care Fewer than five prenatal visits for pregnancies less than 37 weeks, fewer than eight visits for pregnancies 37 weeks or longer, or care beginning after the first four months of pregnancy.

Incidence The number of new events in a given period of time.

Inclusion/effective schooling Theoretical educational model that stresses the full integration of all children within the same classroom, regardless of etiological background or functional level.

Indirect fiber tract Pathways linking the motor strip of the cortex with subcortical structures including the basal nuclei and cerebellum.

Individualized Education Program (IEP) The written plan designed and implemented by the school district and the IEP team describing the educational needs and services that are unique to a student with a disability.

Individuals with Disabilities Education Act (IDEA) Federal law mandating a free appropriate education for all students with disabilities in the least restrictive environment and as close to the mainstream as possible (formerly PL. 94–142).

Indwelling semipermanent prothesis Prosthesis used in voice restoration that can remain in the fistula tract for long periods before replacement is necessary.

Infant mortality statistics The study of death rates, and incidence and prevalence of death for children under one year of age.

Infant A child during the first year of life.

Infarct (Infarction) Death of tissue that occurs when the artery carrying its blood supply is obstructed.

Inferior division Space below the vocal folds.

Inflammation Body's response to injury involving pain, heat, redness, swelling, and loss of function of the affected part.

Inner ear Portion of the ear buried deep in the bones of the skull. Includes the cochlea (sensory organ for hearing) and the vestibular system (sensory organs for balance).

Inspiration The act of moving air into the lungs.

Insufflate Fill with air.

Insula Region of the brain buried within the lateral fissure.

Intelligibility The ability to detect differences among speech sounds (e.g., to hear words such as "vacation" and "invitation" as separate and distinct words).

Intensity Sound vibration energy per unit volume of air. The perceptual correlate of intensity is loudness.

Interdisciplinary A clinical model in which a number of disciplines participate in making a clinical diagnosis and provide treatment options in cooperation with each other.

Intrauterine Within the uterus.

Intraventricular hemorrhage (IVH) Bleeding into the fluid-filled spaces of the brain.

Intrinsic muscles Muscles with both their attachments within the larynx; there are five intrinsic muscles of the larynx.

Ischemia (Ischemic) Inadequate flow of blood caused by a constriction or blockage of the blood vessels.

Jaundice A yellowish color of the skin and whites of the eyes caused by an accumulation of bilirubin, a byproduct of the breakdown of red blood cells.

Jitter Cycle-to-cycle variability in frequency of vocal fold vibration.

L-dopa Precursor to dopamine, used in the treatment of Parkinson's disease.

Lamina propria Mucous membrane surrounding the thyroarytenoid muscle, composed of superficial, intermediate, and deep layers.

Laryngeal Dystonia A movement disorder characterized by action-induced involuntary spasms of the laryngeal muscles. There are three types: adductor spasmodic dysphonia, abductor spasmodic dysphonia, and mixed spasmodic dysphonia.

Laryngeal ventricle Space between the ventricular folds and vocal folds.

Laryngectomee Individual who has had the larynx surgically removed.

Laryngectomy Surgical removal of the laryngeal mechanism.

Laryngopharynx Area between the glottis and pharynx.

Laterality Notion that a particular function can be represented on the left or right side of the brain.

Lead pipe rigidity Increased muscular tone that persists through flexion and extension.

Learning disorders Disorders in which performance in reading, mathematics, or written expression is substantially below that expected for age, schooling, and level of intelligence.

Lewy body An outer region of loosely packed neurofilaments and an inner region of tightly packed neurofilaments found in the cells of the substantia nigra.

Lexigrams   Symbols used on an aided augmentative communication device. May include pictures, photographs, letters, numbers, Blissymbolics, Rebus symbols, and so on.

Linguistics   Study of language.

Literacy   Reading and writing.

Localization   Notion that control of a particular function is represented in a certain area of the brain.

Loop FM system   A frequency modulated (FM) system that features magnetic (loop) induction and telecoil reception of the transmitted signal.

Low birth weight   Birth weight below 2,500 grams (5.5 lbs.).

Lower motor neuron   Spinal and cranial nerves transmitting impulses to and from the periphery.

Magnetic Resonance Imaging (MRI)   Technique for visualizing brain structure.

Mainstreaming   Educational practice of integrating children with disabilities into nonhandicapped classrooms in certain subject areas.

Maneuvers   Voluntary controls exerted over selected neuromuscular aspects of the pharyngeal stage of swallow.

Manually coded English (MCE)   Sign systems invented to represent English morpheme units in a visual form.

Mapping   Initial forming of some mental representation of a person or event or life experience in the memory of a child.

Meconium   A thick, sticky, brown substance that normally is passed in a bowel movement during the first few days of life. Passage of this material before delivery is one sign of fetal distress.

Medial compression   Force exerted by the adductor muscles of the larynx that brings the vocal folds together at the middle.

Medulla oblongata   Upper end of the spinal cord, forming the lowest part of the brainstem.

Mental status examination   Part of the clinical assessment that describes the sum total of the examiner's observations and impressions of a psychiatric patient at the time of the interview.

Metabolic disorder   A disturbance or impairment in any part of the body's metabolism.

Metaphor   Figurative use of language in which an attribute is used to describe an entity not literally associated with the attribute.

Metastasis   Spread of cancer cells from a primary site to a distant one through blood vessels or the lymphatic system.

Microglia   A type of neuroglial cell that is small in size. They proliferate in response to injury within the central nervous system and are scavengers for foreign bodies and injured tissue.

Microphone/Transmitter   An electroacoustic transducer that changes a sound (acoustic) stimulus to electrical energy.

Microtubule   Long tubelike filament structures inside a neuron, extending through the neuronal processes (axon and dendrites) that assist transportation of synthesized proteins.

Midbrain   Small portion of the brainstem excluding the pons and medulla.

Middle ear   Middle section of the ear housing the ossicles (malleus, incus, stapes). Carries sound vibrations to the inner ear.

Midline   The center.

Milieu training   "Incidental" language teaching that occurs between an adult and a child in a naturalistic setting.

Mixed hearing loss   Combination of a sensorineural and a conductive hearing loss.

Modelling/Expansion/Re-direction   Key elements of *motherese,* language teaching strategies used by adult caregivers in the home environment that either model a particular sound, word, or syntactic/morphologic form for a child; provide additional phrase or sentence elements in an expansion of the child's original utterance; or bring the child's attention back to a previous utterance or topic.

Motherese   Code employed by adult caregivers, characterized by the use of age-appropriate vocabulary, simpler sentence patterns, more pronounced intonational patterns, and repetitions of previously produced utterances, as needed to aid in the child's language comprehension and expression.

Motor unit   Nerve pathway that carries impulses outward from the brain to bring about activity in a muscle.

Mucosal wave   Rolling, wave-like motion of the cover of the vocal folds during vibration.

Muscular process   Small projection on the base of the arytenoids forming the attachment for various intrinsic muscles.

Myelomeningocele   A developmental defect in which the spinal cord projects through a cleft in the vertebral column

Myoelastic-aerodynamic theory Theory that explains vocal fold vibration in terms of the relationship between muscular and elastic tissue forces and aerodynamic forces.

Nasal emission Passive nasal escape of air during production of nonnasal speech sounds; usually an obligatory error noted during production of pressure consonants but may be a maladaptive compensatory error in some cases.

Nasal regurgitation Food coming out of the nose during feeding.

Nasal snort Maladaptive compensatory articulation error produced by forcing air out the nose; it is often associated with phone-specific velopharyngeal insufficiency and is usually substituted for sibilant and fricative sounds.

Native sign languages Visual–spatial languages used by deaf communities throughout the world.

Necrotizing Enterocolitis (NEC) Serious intestinal disorder due to injury to the intestinal wall, bacteria, or early formula feeding when the infant's gut is immature.

Neocortex The outermost 5mm of the brain, which is composed of 6 layers of cells. The neocortex is divided into lobes.

Neolung See *Air reservoir.*

Neonatal Of the first 27 days of life.

Neonatology A medical subspecialty dealing with diseases of the newborn, particularly related to infants of low birth weight and prematurity.

Neoplasm (Neoplastic) Spontaneous and abnormal growth of tissue; a tumor that may be malignant or benign.

Neural tube An embryological structure which develops into the brain and spinal cord.

Neurofibrillary tangles A neurofibril is a filament-like structure found in a neuron that extends into a dendrite and axon, that becomes twisted and tangled in Alzheimer's disease.

Neuroglia A cell in the nervous system that supports the function of neurons by regulating the environment outside the neuron. There are several types of neuroglia including microglia, astrocytes, and oligodendroglia.

Neurolinguistics Study of how language functions are organized in the brain.

Neuron A cell in the nervous system that contains basically four regions: a cell body, dendrites, an axon, and a presynaptic terminal.

Neuroscience Interdisciplinary science that examines the brain and behavior.

Noise Any unwanted or unintended sound or electrical signal that interferes with communication or transmission of energy; may be disturbing, and/or hazardous to hearing health.

Noise reduction A process of acoustical treatments and structural modifications whereby the intensity in dB of unwanted sound is reduced in a room.

Normalization Practices such as including children with special needs in standard classrooms.

Nuclei Collection of nerve cell bodies within the central nervous system.

Nucleus Part of a cell found inside the neuron, contains chromatin deposits consisting largely of deoxyribonucleic acid or DNA, the genetic material.

Nystagmus Rapid involuntary movements of the eyes that may be from side to side, up and down, or rotary.

Obesity Condition in which excess fat has accumulated in the body.

Objective measures Tests that assess various aspects of hearing and the hearing mechanism through the use of electroacoustic and electrophysiologic procedures that do not require a voluntary response.

Obligatory errors Articulation distortions directly resulting from an anatomic deviation that are not responsive to speech therapy.

Obsessive compulsive disorder Pervasive pattern of preoccupation with orderliness, perfectionism, and mental and interpersonal control.

Obturators Artificial devices (prostheses) like acrylic plates that are used to close an opening without surgery (see *speech bulb* and *palatal lift*).

Occipital lobe Region of the cortex involved in visual processing.

Occlusion Closing or obstruction of a vessel.

Occult submucous cleft palate (OSMCP) Flattening or grooving of the nasal surface of the soft palate reflecting deficiency or absence of the musculus uvulae (m.u.) without any oral signs of submucous cleft palate.

Oncologist Physician who specializes in the treatment of cancer.

Operant behaviorism Learning model of choice when the concern is for teaching a concrete task that can be readily sequenced, such as the buttoning of a shirt or the putting together of two or more hardware pieces in a vocational training task.

Oral communication   Philosophy that advocates the use of English in its spoken form to support acquisition of speech, oral language, and literacy.

Oral–manual controversy   Ongoing debate about what communication approach is best for deaf students.

Orientation   Individual's awareness of four spheres: person, place, time, and circumstance.

Orthopedic   Pertaining to the bones or joints.

Otolaryngologist   Physician who specializes in the treatment of diseases in the head and neck.

Outer ear   Outermost section of the ear, including the pinna and the external auditory meatus (ear canal). Carries sound to the middle ear.

Overall severity   An estimate of the global severity of a disorder.

Overextension   Use of the same term to refer to a variety of referents that share certain salient features.

Palatal lift   Prosthetic device for management of velopharyngeal insufficiency that contains a palatal retainer and finger-like extension that does not extend beyond the palate and elevates the palate.

Para   Refers to a woman who has borne a live child. A para 2 is a woman who has borne two live children, and so on.

Parahippocampus   A gyrus located in the inferior, medial temporal lobe. It sends axons out that communicate with the hippocampus.

Parietal lobe   Region of each cerebral hemisphere lying behind the frontal lobe, above the temporal lobe, and in front of the occipital lobe.

Passavant's ridge   Localized area of motion of the posterior pharyngeal wall that contributes to velopharyngeal closure in about 20 percent of individuals, and may constrict the vocal tract in others.

Pedunculated   (Growths) that are perched on a thin stalk.

Penetration   Entry of food, liquid or saliva into the entrance to the airway (larynx) no lower than the top surface of the true vocal folds.

Peptide   A series of amino acids.

Perception   Understanding the meaning of incoming sounds; occurs in the central auditory system (brainstem and cortex).

Perinatal   Of events occurring during the process of birth.

Perinatal death   Both fetal and neonatal deaths.

Peripheral   Located away from the center.

Peripheral auditory mechanism   The part of the ear that includes the outer, middle, and inner ear and functions to receive incoming sounds.

Peripheral Nervous System (PNS)   All parts of the nervous system lying outside the brain and spinal cord, including the cranial and spinal nerves.

Personal FM system   A radio system that delivers frequency modulated signals and has individual wearable receiver units.

Personal hearing aids   External devices, worn on or in the ear, that are used to amplify sound.

Pervasive developmental disorders   Disorders characterized by impairment in the development of reciprocal social interaction and verbal and nonverbal communication skills. Associated features may include abnormal sensory and motor behaviors, abnormalities in eating, drinking, or sleeping, and self-injurious behaviors.

Pharyngeal flap   Surgical procedure in which a flap of tissue from the posterior pharyngeal wall is inserted into the soft palate to correct velopharyngeal insufficiency.

Pharyngeal fricative   Maladaptive compensatory articulation error produced by constriction of the vocal tract or constriction between the retracted tongue and pharynx to create frication; usually substituted for fricatives.

Pharynoesophageal sphincter   Muscular valve separating the pharynx from the esophagus.

Phonation   The act of sound production in the larynx; the act of transforming energy from moving air into acoustic energy by the vibration of the vocal folds.

Phonation-Neutral   A position and stiffness of the vocal folds coordinated with appropriate expiratory drive that results in gentle initiation of phonation.

Phonatory   Relating to the production of voiced sound resulting from vibration of the vocal folds.

Phone-specific velopharyngeal closure   Articulation disorder in which velopharyngeal closure is achieved on only one sound or one class of sounds during speech; during production of other oral sounds, velopharyngeal insufficiency is present.

Phone-specific velopharyngeal insufficiency   Articulation disorder in which velopharyngeal insufficiency is present during production on one sound or one class of sounds (usually sibilants), but closure is achieved during production of all other oral phonemes.

Phonosurgery Term for a group of surgical procedures aimed at preserving or restoring optimal voice function.

Photophobia Abnormal sensitivity of the eyes to light.

Pica Persistent eating of nonnutritive substances.

Pick bodies Dense structures found in diseased conditions, that displace the nucleus, pushing it toward the outside of the cell.

Pick cells Inflated or enlarged neurons.

Pidgin sign English (PSE) ASL signs in English word order.

Pons Portion of the brainstem that links the medulla and the midbrain.

Positron Emission Tomography (PET) Technique used to evaluate metabolic activity of brain tissue.

Postlingual hearing loss Hearing loss that occurs after the development of spoken language (after about the age of two).

Postnatal Of events occurring after birth.

Prelingual hearing loss Hearing loss that is present at birth or occurs prior to the development of spoken language (before about the age of two).

Premature infant Child born at or before the 36th week of gestation.

Prematurity Any pregnancy lasting fewer than 38 weeks.

Premaxilla Portion of the maxilla anterior to the incisive foreman. This area anchors four teeth—the central and lateral maxillary incisors. Although this part of the maxilla is contiguous with the palate, it is embryologically part of the lip and individuals with complete cleft lip have cleft alveolus but not necessarily cleft palate. In bilateral cleft lip, the premaxilla is unattached from the alveolar segments on both sides, and is often referred to as a "floating" premaxilla.

Premotor area Area of the cerebral cortex directly in front of the motor strip.

Prenatal Of events occurring during the gestational period.

Prenatal Substance Abuse The use of one or more illicit drugs during pregnancy that contributes to a pattern of developmental delay following the birth of the child.

Prevalence The total percentage of a given event in a given population.

Preventative education Theory underlying many specialized preschool early intervention programs that provide educational and therapeutic services to children with developmental disabilities. Children are provided with language training, as well as cognitive, social skill, and perceptual-motor developmental training.

Primary motor cortex Term used synonymously with motor strip.

Problem-solving Process involving recognition of problem, strategy selection, application of strategy for resolution of the problem, and evaluation of the outcome.

Prosthodontist Dentist or orthodontist with additional special training in the construction of artificial teeth and devices.

Protein A working molecule of a cell. Proteins provide structural rigidity, control membrane permeability, regulate the amounts of metabolites, recognize and bind with other molecules, and control gene function. Proteins are made up of amino acids.

Psycholinguistics Study of the psychological processes that underlie language functioning.

Psychosocial stressor A psychosocial or environmental problem which may contribute to a mental health problem.

Ptosis Drooping of the upper eyelid.

Pure tone Tone consisting of only one frequency.

Pyramidal (direct) tract The pathway of nerve fibers originating in the cortex and terminating at the medulla or spinal cord.

Pyriform sinuses Spaces created by the way in which the inferior pharyngeal constrictors attach to the outside of the larynx.

Quadrate lamina Back portion of the cricoid cartilage.

Quadriplegia Movement difficulties affecting all four limbs.

Reasoning

  Deductive Drawing conclusions based on the premises of general principles

  Inductive Formulation of solutions given information that leads to but does not necessarily support a general conclusion

Reception The detection of sound that occurs in the inner ear.

Recurrent laryngeal nerve A branch of the vagus nerve responsible for activating the muscles in the vocal folds.

Recurrent laryngeal nerve section A surgical procedure performed to improve the voice quality of patients with spasmodic dysphonia; the recurrent laryngeal nerve is cut on one side of the larynx causing the vocal fold to be paralyzed on that side.

Redundancy   The part of a message that can be eliminated without loss of information.

Reinke's space   Another name for the superficial layer of the lamina propria.

Residual hearing   The hearing that remains after damage or disease in the auditory mechanism; there is almost always some residual hearing, even with the most profound hearing impairments.

Residue   Food that is left behind in the mouth or pharynx when the swallow is completed.

Resonance   Characteristic of the speech signal that results from the way in which physical characteristics of the pharynx and movement of the velopharyngeal muscles modify the vocal signal from the larynx.

Respiration   The act of breathing.

Respiratory Distress Syndrome (RDS)   The most common disorder of prematurity resulting from immature lung development generally secondary to preterm birth.

Reticular activating system   System within the brainstem responsible for the initiation, maintenance, and degree of wakefulness on which higher nervous functions depend.

Retinitis pigmentosa   A group of diseases associated with the degeneration of the retina of the eye that leads to blindness.

Retinopathy   A degenerative disease of the retina.

Retrovirus   A virus that uses RNA to make DNA (this is the reverse process of a "normal" virus). The viral DNA is replicated, killing the host cell.

Rett's disorder   A pervasive developmental disorder in which multiple specific deficits develop after a period of normal functioning following birth.

Robin sequence (formerly "Pierre Robin Syndrome")   Common sequence associated with cleft palate in which failure of the mandible to grow properly in utero prevents the tongue from lowering into its normal position which interferes with palatal closure resulting in an incomplete cleft palate. Diagnosis is based on the presence of a small mandible, cleft palate, and neonatal breathing difficulties due to glossoptosis.

Rough voice quality   An abnormal voice quality that sounds harsh, hoarse, raspy, coarse, or uneven.

Rubella   German measles.

Rumination disorder   Repeated regurgitation and rechewing of food.

Scaffolding   Providing a structure (e.g. simple terminology, redundancy) to the verbal interaction with a person who has difficulty maintaining an adequate level of communicative proficiency.

Seizure   A transient, paroxysmal, pathophysiological disturbance of cerebral function caused by a spontaneous, excessive discharge of cortical neurons.

Senile plaques   A deposit found outside the neuron. It has a center core composed of an amyloid peptide and it is surrounded by abnormal dendrites and axons.

Sensorineural hearing loss   Permanent hearing loss resulting from damage to the inner ear, auditory nerve, or both.

Sequence   Two or more anomalies occurring together in which the primary etiology caused the first anomaly and in which the first anomaly caused the second one.

Sessile   (Growths) having a broad base.

Shimmer   Cycle-to-cycle variability in amplitude of vocal fold vibration.

Sickle-cell disease   Hereditary blood disease that primarily affects people of African descent. Characterized by the production of an abnormal type of hemoglobin.

Signal-to-Noise Ratio or Speech-to-Noise Ratio (S/N Ratio)   The relationship between the intensity of the speech signal and any sound that the person does not want to hear.

Silastic   Synthetic material used as an implant to move a paralyzed vocal fold toward the midline.

Small for Gestational Age (SGA)   An infant whose birth weight falls below the 10th percentile for gestational age.

Social communication spectrum disorders   Group of psychiatric disorders including autism, pervasive developmental disorders, schizotypal personality disorder, schizophrenia, and psychosis.

Somatic   Relating to the body.

Sound-field (classroom) amplification systems   Electronic equipment that amplifies an entire (class)room through the careful positioning of two to four loudspeakers; the teacher wears an FM microphone/transmitter.

Spasmodic Dysphonia   A rare voice disorder that has three manifestations: abductor, characterized by breathy or whispered voice, adductor, characterized by voice arrests and a rough, effortful, strained-strangled voice quality, and mixed characterized by a combination of adductor and abductor symptoms.

Speech Spoken or oral English.

Speech bulb Prosthetic device for management of velopharyngeal insufficiency that contains a palatal retainer and pharyngeal extension terminating in a bulb usually made of acrylic; it functions in the same way as a pharyngeal flap.

Speech intelligibility The degree of overall clarity with which an utterance is capable of being understood by the average listener.

Speech rate The speed of producing utterances; reduced speed is related to lengthened consonants and vowels or to unexpected pauses between sounds, syllables, or words; increased speed is related to shortened consonants and vowels or to shortened pauses between sounds, syllables, or words.

Speechreading Making sense of a spoken message by watching facial and body movements and by using situational and linguistic cues.

Spinal cord Portion of the central nervous system enclosed in the vertebral column containing nerves that connect all parts of the body to the brain.

Splinter skills Unusual or preconscious cognitive or visual motor abilities or islets of precocity, sometimes seen in autism and mental retardation.

Stenosis Narrowing of a tube or opening.

Stoma blast Noise produced when pulmonary air is forcefully exhaled through the opening in the neck.

Strabismus Inward or outward deviations of the eye.

Strained-strangled An abnormal voice quality that is squeezed and effortful.

Stridor Noisy breathing due to some kind of airway obstruction.

Stroke Sudden attack of weakness on one side of the body caused by an interruption to the flow of blood to the brain.

Subglottal cavity Space below the vocal folds.

Subglottal pressure Pressure of the air below the vocal folds, which increases when the vocal folds are closed.

Submucous cleft palate (SMCP) Form of cleft palate in which the overlying oral tissues are intact but there is a cleft of the palatal bones and/or muscles.

Substantia nigra Collection of nerve cells in the midbrain, anatomically and functionally related to the basal nuclei, involved in the creation of dopamine.

Sulcus Groove.

Supplementary motor area Area of the cerebral cortex involved in integration of motor and sensory information.

Support network Collection of people providing assistance and support to a person with developmental disabilities. This group may include the person's family, friends, teachers, therapists, clergy, and so on.

Surfactant Chemical substance needed in the lungs of infants to prevent air sacs in the lungs from closing.

Synapse Minute gap at the end of a nerve fiber across which nerve impulses pass from one neuron to the next.

Syndrome A constellation or grouping of factors that define a known medical condition.

Tardive dyskinesia Disorder characterized by involuntary abnormal movements that is caused by the prolonged use of antipsychotic drugs.

Tau A protein that is associated with microtubules.

T-cells A common name for the immune cell, CD4+ T lymphocytes, that are critical to defending a cell against a variety of microbes.

Telecoil A series of interconnected wire loops in a hearing aid that respond electrically to a magnetic signal.

Telecoil switch An external control (switch) on a hearing aid that turns off the microphone and activates a telecoil in the hearing aid that picks up magnetic leakage from a telephone or the loop of an ALD.

Telephone Device For the Deaf (TTY/TDD) Acoustic coupler that allows individuals to transmit and receive typed messages through regular phone lines.

Temporal lobe Region of the cerebral cortex involved in audition and memory.

Teratogen Agent that passes from mother to the developing embryo or fetus through the placenta and that has the potential to interfere with normal prenatal development.

Thalamus Ovular masses of gray matter that lie deep within the cerebral hemispheres.

Thought disorder Abnormal or deviant thinking expressed through expressive and receptive language and indicative of certain types of psychiatriatric diagnoses, such as schizophrenia or psychosis.

Thrombosis Clotting within a blood vessel that may cause an infarction of brain tissue supplied by that vessel.

Thyroepiglottic ligament Ligament attaching the epiglottis to the thyroid cartilage.

Thyroplasty Surgical technique of changing the position of the vocal folds through an opening made in the thyroid cartilage.

Tonic bite A sustained contraction of the muscles that are responsible for the biting movement, resulting in a sustained bite.

Topographic A description of any part of the body.

Torticollis Involuntary turning movement of the head to one side of the body caused by muscle spasm.

Total communication Philosophy that may incorporate multiple modes of communication including speech, fingerspelling, invented sign forms of English, American Sign Language, gestures, and written English.

Toxemia A condition of pregnancy characterized by high blood pressure, protein in the urine, and fluid retention.

Toxoplasmosis An infectious disease that can lead to severe fetal malformations.

Tracheoesophageal voice Phonation produced when pulmonary air, diverted from the trachea into the esophagus, passes through the P–E sphincter, causing it to vibrate.

Tracheostoma (stoma) Surgically created opening in the neck through which an individual may breathe.

Transdisciplinary approach Intervention approach in which professionals from a variety of backgrounds (e.g., educational, medical, therapeutic) function not only within their own disciplines but also contribute input across disciplines, to provide integrated treatment.

Transient Ischemic Attack (TIA) Acute neurologic deficit of vascular origin, lasting less than 24 hours.

Transition Portion of the vocal folds between the outermost cover and the innermost body, made up of the intermediate and deep layers of the lamina propria. Also known as the vocal ligament.

Transitional plans Services included in the IEP that will assist in moving the student from school to postschool work or continued education, independent living, and community participation.

Transmitter An apparatus that sends out electromagnetic rays; the M system component that modulates the frequency of the radio signal in an audio frequency signal and sends the radio waves through the air to the antenna of the amplifier/receiver.

Transneoglottic air flow Flow of air passing through the P–E sphincter (neoglottis).

Traumatic brain injury Classified as open or closed head injuries depending on whether or not the meninges remain intact.

Open head injury Results when scalp and skull are penetrated

Closed head injury Results from acceleration and deceleration injuries leading to coup, contra coup, and diffuse axonal injuries; meniges remain intact

Primary damage Caused by impact to head, may range from large brain lesions to microscopic damage

Secondary damage Results from such factors as infection, lack of oxygen to the brain, brain swelling, excessive intracranial pressure, and so on

Tremor Rhythmic alterations in frequency and/or amplitude of vocal fold vibration, perceived as a quavery quality in the voice.

Troubleshooting (hearing aids or ALDs) Performing various visual and listening inspections to determine whether an amplification unit is malfunctioning and, if so, evaluating the nature and severity of the malfunction.

Tuberous sclerosis A genetic disorder generally and chiefly characterized by mental retardation, epilepsy, and skin lesion.

Unaided augmentative communication systems Nonspeech communication system that involves only the nonspeaker, without additional static supports (e.g. American Sign Language, Amer-Ind, Signing Exact English, Cued Speech, and so on).

Upper aerodigestive tract Area of the body consisting of the oral cavity, nasal cavity, pharynx, larynx, cervical esophagus, and trachea.

Upper motor neuron Collective term for the direct and indirect motor systems.

Vagus nerve Cranial nerve that innervates the larynx, having three branches: the pharyngeal nerve, the superior laryngeal nerve, and the recurrent laryngeal nerve.

Valleculae Space between the base of tongue and epiglottis.

Vascular occlusion See *occlusion.*

Veins Blood vessel carrying blood toward the heart.

Velopharyngeal closure Process by which the nasal branch of the vocal tract is separated from or coupled with the rest of the vocal tract.

Velopharyngeal insufficiency (VPI) Lack of closure of the space between the palate and throat that must occur during normal swallowing and production of oral speech sounds.

Ventricles A series of interconnecting cavities in the brain that contain cerebrospinal fluid that is produced by specialized cells (choroid plexus). The lateral ventricle is located inside the hemisphere, the third ventricle is located at the level of the thalamus, the cerebral aqueduct is located at the level of the midbrain, and the forth ventricle separates the pons and medulla from the cerebellum.

Ventricular folds Also known as the false vocal folds, located parallel but superior to the true vocal folds.

Verbal language Internalized knowledge of spoken English or American Sign Language.

Vermis Central portion of the cerebellum, lying between its two lateral hemispheres.

Vertebral arteries Major blood vessels that pass through the upper cerebral vertebra en route to the brain.

Vestibule Uppermost cavity of the larynx, extending from the aditus laryngis to the ventricular folds.

Vocal fold A paired structure that projects into the airway just below the level of the thyroid notch. The vocal fold is inferior to and thinner than the ventricular vocal fold and consists of a vocal ligament, the thyroarytenoid muscle, and squamous cell epithelium. The vocal fold vibrates and produces a buzzing sound that is shaped into speech by the articulators.

Vocal ligament The mid-portion of the vocal folds, also known as the transition, formed by the intermediate and deep layers of the lamina propria.

Vocal process Small projection on the base of each arytenoid cartilage, to which the vocal folds attach posteriorly.

Voice Signal that results from respiratory and laryngeal activity.

Voice arrest An abnormal unexpected interruption in voice production during a voiced sound suggesting either the impedance of airflow by closing the vocal folds too tightly, or decreased resistance to airflow by suddenly opening the vocal folds.

Voice tremor An abnormal involuntary voice quality due to rapidly occurring fluctuations in pitch and/or loudness resulting in a quavering sound similar to a vibrato.

Wernicke's area Auditory association cortex located in the temporal lobe.

White matter Nerve tissue of the central nervous system that is paler in color than gray matter because it contains more nerve fibers.

Wireless system An FM transmitter and FM receiver; radio waves, not wires, connect the speaker and listener.

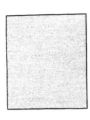

NAME INDEX

Abbeduto, L., 42, 45
Abbs, J., 176
Abraham, S., 360
Abrahamsen, A., 40
Accardo, P. J., 11, 321
Ackmajian, A., 148
Adamovich, B. L. B., 110, 114, 118, 125, 127, 128, 154
Adams, R., 182
Adamson, L., 40
Affolder, F., 51
Agramaso, R. V., 212, 217
Akamatsu, C. T., 365
Albert, M. L., 85, 101, 157
Albert, M. S., 94
Alessi, N. E., 51
Alexander, M. P., 111, 112, 116, 125, 144
Allen, D., 31
Allen, E. L., 314
Allen, T. A., 367
Allen, T. E., 367
Allen, W., 360
Alles, C. D., 355
Alpiner, J. G., 370
Alzheimer, A., 84–86
Amaro, H., 18
Amato, J., 206
Ambinder, A., 103
Aminoff, M. J., 305
Anastasiow, N. J., 323
Anderson, J. C., 54, 60, 61, 68
Anderson, M., 215
Anderson-Levitt, K., 30, 43
Andersson, L., 60
Andreason, N. C., 65, 68
Andrews, J. F., 347, 350, 363
Ang, L. C., 99
Angel, M., 216
Ansell, B. J., 123, 124
Anthony, D. A., 364

April, M. M., 260
Aram, D. M., 22, 55, 60
Arbodela, C., 68
Arlazoroff, A., 99
Arnold, G. E., 305, 308, 309
Aronson, A. E., 144, 166, 168, 173, 181, 182, 188, 301–313
Aten, J. L., 151, 159
Audet, L., 52
Audet, T., 154
Auerbach, S., 114, 118, 125, 128, 145
Avery, M., 11
Azen, C., 18
Azorin, J. M., 99

Bacellar, H., 95
Bacon, M., 308
Baer, D., 36
Bailey, B. J., 273, 275
Bailey, L., 35
Baker, L., 51–56, 58, 60–62, 69, 70
Baldwin, 324
Ball, M. J., 86
Bally, S. J., 358
Balsara, G., 261
Baltaxe, C. A. M., 6, 51–83, 53, 54, 56–65, 67–70
Bambara, L., 36
Bandur, D. L., 160
Bankier, A., 203
Banks, G., 96
Barcz, D., 291
Bardach, J., 213
Baribeau, L. J., 257
Barnes, M., 199
Baron-Cohen, S., 65
Barresi, B., 160
Bartolucci, G., 64
Bartus, R. T., 87
Basili, A. G., 154, 295
Bastian, R. W., 239

Batshaw, M. L., 11, 17, 320–325
Baum, G., 241
Baumeister, J. J., 59
Bayles, K., 102
Beard, A. W., 59
Beckenham, E. J., 216
Becker, J. T., 96
Becker, M. R., 124, 125
Becker, R. E., 90
Beckman, P., 38
Bedrosian, J., 43
Begelman, A., 238
Beitchman, J. H., 51, 54, 58, 60, 61, 68–70
Beiter, A. L., 355
Bell, K., 182, 188
Bell, K. R., 117
Bell-Dolan, D., 66
Bellman, A., 21
Bellussi, G., 302
Benedict, R. H. B., 130, 133
Bennett, S., 288
Benninger, M. S., 247
Benowitz, L., 154
Benson, D. E., 84, 92
Benson, D. F., 116, 125
Benson, E., 96
Benson, F., 116
Benton, A. L., 111, 127
Benton, H. L., 113
Ben-Yishay, Y., 130, 133
Berg, F. S., 332–334, 365
Bergner, L. H., 290
Bergsma, D., 11
Berkman, M. D., 205
Berko-Gleason, J. B., 148, 152, 158
Berry, G. A., 205
Berry, W., 182
Berstein, B. A., 132
Bertha, G., 100
Beukelman, D. R., 117, 182, 188

SUBJECT INDEX